HANDBOOK OF
Adult
Rehabilitative
Audiology

Second Edition

HANDBOOK OF
Adult Rehabilitative Audiology

SECOND EDITION

Jerome G. Alpiner, Ph.D.
Editor

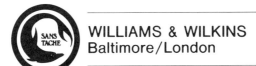

WILLIAMS & WILKINS
Baltimore/London

Copyright ©, 1982
Williams & Wilkins
428 East Preston Street
Baltimore, MD 21202, U.S.A.

First edition, 1978

Library of Congress Cataloging in Publication Data

Main entry under title:

Handbook of adult rehabilitative audiology.

    Includes bibliographies and indexes.
    1. Deaf—Rehabilitation. 2. Audiology.
I. Alpiner, Jerome G., 1932–   . [DNLM: 1. Audiology—Handbooks. 2. Commu-
nication—Handbooks. 3. Deafness—Rehabilitation—Handbooks. WV 270 H235]
RF297.H36 1982   362.4′283   81-15980
ISBN 0-683-00076-4   AACR2

Composed and printed at the
Waverly Press, Inc.
Mt. Royal and Guilford Aves.
Baltimore, MD 21202, U.S.A.

Dedication

Writing the second edition of this book represented a real challenge for me, first because of covering the continuing neglected area of rehabilitative audiology for adults. Secondly, my wife passed away during the writing of this edition; she was a major inspiration to me in writing a text on adult rehabilitation as well as on my life. I dedicate this book to my beloved wife, Judy. I also dedicate it to my wonderful children, Steven, Susan, Sharon, David, and Carol who kept me inspired by their support and love.

Preface

The second edition of this book continues its attempt to fill the literature void for those persons who have contact with hearing-impaired adults. There has been no other text devoted to adults to emerge since the first edition. Primary use is intended for students in audiology, speech-language pathology, and for practicing audiologists. An effort has been made to deal comprehensively with the rehabilitation process for adults with hearing loss. This handbook can be used most efficiently when the basic material is complemented with current literature and research.

Chapter 1 considers the present status of rehabilitative audiology for adults, emphasizing the rationale for remediation procedures. The strengths and weaknesses of present philosophies are reviewed.

Assessment procedures for evaluating how clients function in communication situations is the basis for Chapter 2. Measuring techniques and speechreading methodologies are discussed to assist the audiologist in planning a remediation program. Primary emphasis is on case management, and information presented should enable the audiologist to obtain baseline information on how clients progress relative to pre- and post-therapy.

The hearing aid is a major component in rehabilitation. Drs. Kasten and Mc-Croskey consider this aspect in Chapter 3. Quite often, after audiologic assessment, there is significant need to work with clients to obtain the maximum benefits from amplification. This chapter emphasizes pre- and post-hearing aid orientation as well as the rehabilitative aspects involved in the hearing aid evaluation process.

Chapters 4 and 5 are concerned with the remediation process as well as psychologic and counselling aspects. Various techniques will be presented including the methodologies available to the clinician involved in therapy. Hearing loss and subsequent communication difficulties are only a part of rehabilitation. Communication deficits caused by hearing loss may manifest themselves in psychologic problems such as withdrawal from society or attempts to deny the problems that may exist. Audiologists need to know the kinds of situations which may arise and how to counsel clients effectively through problem areas. This aspect of rehabilitation permits the clinician to treat the client as a total person rather than dealing only with hearing loss *per se*. Dr. McCarthy shares the chapter on the therapy process with this author. Dr. Wylde deals with the psychologic and counselling aspects of the hearing-impaired individual.

The need to provide rehabilitation for senior citizens with hearing loss has increased in importance. It is discussed in Chapter 6. Reasons for greater awareness of this population include the increasing number of senior citizens in this country as well as our desire to help them lead more productive lives. Remediation methodologies suggested for this age group often differ from the usual procedures for younger adults and are presented in this chapter.

Drs. Johnson and Crandall present a broad overview of the deaf client in Chapter 7. The congenitally deaf adult is now receiving services from audiologists on a more frequent basis. Such persons generally have serious speech problems and greatly reduced hearing acuity which preclude "normal" communication ability. Many rely on manual communication or total communication. The clinician needs to understand the communication potential of these persons and the manner in which they may be helped. Techniques for therapy differ significantly from routine procedures and must be understood by the audiologist if any degree of success can be anticipated. The chapter focuses on the ways in which the audiologist may deal with this group.

Ms. Linda Hirsch has added a new dimension to the book with her insightful Chapter 8 on the adult deaf-blind. This area is one in which many of us know little but should know more when encountering this type of client.

Rehabilitation of many hearing-impaired clients may involve more than the services rendered by the audiologist. The roles of ancillary professions and individuals is considered in Chapter 9 by Dr. Garstecki. To treat the client as a total person, it may be necessary to involve vocational rehabilitation counselors, physicians, social workers, and others. This chapter presents some ways in which they may assist the audiologist in a total approach to rehabilitation.

Chapter 10 discusses community adult aural rehabilitation programs. Any successful rehabilitation program should attempt to identify adults with hearing loss. Of the few such programs in the United States at the present time, most are public school oriented. This chapter shows the audiologist how he may learn what community needs exist, approaches by which adults can be reached for identification of hearing loss, and types of rehabilitation programs which may be established.

One of the weakest areas in adult hearing rehabilitation has been research activity. Criticism has long been directed at adult rehabilitation because of its lack of sophisticated methodologies. Intensive research to assist audiologists in developing more meaningful approaches to rehabilitation is needed. In Chapter 11, Dr. Tobias identifies and explores research approaches.

Many individuals have contributed both directly and indirectly to the writing of this book. I am indebted to the numerous students who have been members of my adult rehabilitative audiology classes. As we searched together for philosophies of adult hearing rehabilitation, these students helped me to achieve differing insights regarding the need for substance in therapy. Without them, there would have been no motivating force for writing the book. In addition, I must thank the countless hearing-impaired adults with whom I have worked whose input indicated a significant role for audiologists in rehabilitation. I also acknowledge with appreciation the efforts of Emily Boswell, who edited the manuscript, and my marvelous secretary, Michelle Guerdan, who typed the manuscript. Finally, I extend a sincere thanks to two of my graduate assistants, Florence Davenport and Susan Holmes, who read the manuscript and provided me with significant input.

Jerome G. Alpiner, Ph.D.

Acknowledgments

Donald D. Johnson and Kathleen E. Crandall express their gratitude to Frank C. Caccamise, R. Greg Emerton, Charles Layne, Gerard Walter, Joanne D. Subtelny, Jaclyn Gauger, E. Ross Stuckless, Deborah Veatch, Kathleen Martin, Carolyn S. Dunn, Lynne Williams, Charles A. Parker, and William A. Welsh for their advice, guidance, and support throughout the preparation of Chapter 7. The many other NTID faculty and staff who provided them directly and indirectly with data and information have their papers cited in the references. Thanks are also extended to the many persons who provided typing, especially Dorris Fox, and other processing support services.

Linda M. Hirsch acknowledges gratitude to the administration of the Helen Keller National Center for Deaf-Blind Youths and Adults for their cooperation in the preparation of Chapter 8. In addition, thanks are extended to Dr. Deena Bernstein and to Dr. Robert J. Smithdas for allowing access to their unpublished materials; to Ms. Gertrude Queen for her library assistance; and to the National Eye Institute, American Foundation for the Blind, Dr. Jerome Schein, Linda Kates, Grune & Stratton, Inc., and the Helen Keller National Center for allowing her to cite generously from their publications. Appreciation is also extended to Deanna Morton, Melissa Malis Shapiro, Sharon Grossman, and Dr. Harry Levitt for their review and suggestions concerning various sections of the chapter, as well as to the Ph.D. Program in Speech and Hearing Sciences at the City University of New York for allowing time to prepare this chapter during her enrollment there.

Contributors

Jerome G. Alpiner, Ph.D., Director, Speech and Hearing Department, Porter Memorial Hospital, Denver, Colorado 80210. (*Chapters 1, 2, 4, 6, 10*)

Kathleen E. Crandall, Ph.D., Associate Dean and Director, Communication Program, National Technical Institute for the Deaf, Rochester Institute of Technology, P.O. Box 9887, Rochester, New York 14623. (*Chapter 7*)

Dean C. Garstecki, Ph.D., Associate Professor of Audiology and Hearing Impairment, Department of Communicative Disorders, Northwestern University, Evanston, Illinois 60201. (*Chapter 9*)

Linda M. Hirsch, M.S., Doctoral Student, Audiology and Hearing Impairment, Northwestern University, Evanston, Illinois, 60201; formerly Audiologist, Helen Keller National Center for Deaf-Blind Youths and Adults, Sands Point, New York 11050. (*Chapter 8*)

Donald D. Johnson, Ph.D., Professor, Communication Program, National Technical Institute for the Deaf, Rochester Institute of Technology, P.O. Box 9887, Rochester, New York 14623. (*Chapter 7*)

Roger N. Kasten, Ph.D., Professor of Communicative Disorders and Sciences, Wichita State University, Wichita, Kansas 57206. (*Chapter 3*)

Patricia A. McCarthy, Ph.D., Assistant Professor, Speech Pathology and Audiology, the University of Georgia, Athens, Georgia 30602. (*Chapter 4*)

Robert L. McCroskey, Ph.D., Professor of Communication Disorders and Sciences, Wichita State University, Wichita, Kansas 67206. (*Chapter 3*)

Jerry V. Tobias, Ph.D., Director, Industrial Audiology, Norman, Oklahoma 73070. (*Chapter 11*)

Margaret A. Wylde, Ph.D., Associate Professor, Department of Communicative Disorders, The University of Mississippi, University, Mississippi 38677. (*Chapter 5*)

Contents

1

Adult Rehabilitative Audiology: An Overview

Jerome G. Alpiner, Ph.D.

Regardless of the whys and hows of audiologic site-of-lesion assessment, we are confronted with a communicative breakdown, the causative factors of which encompass the entire communicative event, not merely the hearing sensitivity curve of the patient. In fact, the patients' reported symptoms primarily describe manifestations responsible for . . . inefficient communication (Regan, 1977). The role of the audiologist engaged in rehabilitation, therefore, is to help the hearing-impaired adult overcome his inefficient communication.

Who are these adult clients who come to us for help and how do they feel about therapy? In the first edition of this book, Alpiner (1978) presented the results of a questionnaire administered to clients 1 year after they had received lipreading (aural rehabilitation) instruction at a university speech and hearing center. Three general open-ended questions were asked.

1. Will you describe as completely as possible how our lipreading groups have helped you?
2. What do you think we could do to improve our lipreading sessions?
3. What aspects of the lipreading sessions did you like most? Which did you like least?

To minimize the effects of bias, clients were asked not to identify themselves on the ques-

tionnaires. Several prevailing attitudes surfaced.

It was frequently revealed that clients initially considered lipreading an exact science, to be learned as one learns a foreign language. As instruction progressed, they felt that there were general guidelines for improving communication but the degree of success achieved was an individual matter.

Another frequent opinion was that learning how to lipread through vision alone was one of the most difficult tasks ever undertaken. At first, these clients had assumed it would be possible to achieve success in "visual hearing." They recommended that lipreading instruction be retained but used in conjunction with audition to utilize residual hearing more effectively.

Third, clients felt that it was important to be part of a therapy group. Group participation reduced their personal feelings of being the only ones affected by hearing loss. They particularly liked sharing common problems of communication breakdown and learning of similarities of problems. The difficulty of trying to understand speech in noisy situations, for example, was one which many clients had experienced. Many clients stressed that it was easier to adjust to wearing an aid because they were not the only ones with that "electronic gadget" in the group setting. After the experience of wearing the hearing aid in a group in which others were utilizing similar devices, they found it was less "emotionally" difficult to wear the hearing aid around people with normal hearing.

A fourth opinion was that therapy dealing with improvement in listening ability, increased awareness of facial expressions and gestures, and increased attention to environmental cues taught clients to be aware of these "common sense" factors in communication.

Fifth, clients stated that it was a relief when they could finally admit they had a hearing loss. They indicated that previously it had been difficult to admit to others, "I have a hearing loss." Prior to this admission, communication difficulty was attributed to the "softly spoken speaker," "the mumbler," or noisy situations. Therapy sessions helped the clients accept the fact that hearing loss can interfere with some of their everyday family, social, and vocational roles. Although it generally took the entire therapy term for most adults to reach this stage, they felt that behavior modification techniques should be stressed for all hearing-impaired clients even if initial resistance was encountered.

TERMINOLOGY CONSIDERATIONS

Audiologists engaged in remediation often disagree about what to call their classes, their services, and themselves. Titles such as rehabilitative audiologist, clinical audiologist, hearing clinicians, or simply audiologist are currently in use. The variety may confuse those seeking therapy as well as students of rehabilitative audiology (or audiologic remediation, or aural rehabilitation, or remediation audiology). The relative youth of audiology accounts for this abundance of synonyms. The American Speech-Language-Hearing Association uses only the term audiologist for the professional person engaging in audiologic practice. The area of emphasis for the audiologist then follows. For example, an individual is an audiologist who emphasizes rehabilitation, diagnostics, pediatrics, and so forth.

Historically, adult therapy has consisted of lipreading and auditory training. This traditional approach represents a limited view of remediation. As one reads this text, it will become apparent that rehabilitation is much broader and concerns itself with a number of other aspects that represent our efforts to assist the adult who is hearing-impaired.

Terminology considerations are stressed in this text for the benefit of readers who may be confused by the variety of nomenclature currently used. As the student gains experience, he will better understand the definition problems inherent in the profession. For the present, we need to define what is meant by the words used in audiology.

The remediation process will be referred to as rehabilitative audiology, except when the word habilitative is used for specific situations. The audiologist's role will be remediation-oriented. Keeping in mind that audiologists also engage in diagnosis and research, we will designate these roles specifically.

Speechreading, lipreading, visual listening, and visual hearing will be used synonymously. Aural rehabilitation will be used synonymously with rehabilitative audiology. This procedure will facilitate understanding of various literature references cited throughout the text. Any deviations from these definitions will be indicated.

GUIDELINES FOR REHABILITATIVE AUDIOLOGY

The Committee on Rehabilitative Audiology of the American Speech and Hearing Association (ASHA) (1974) has adopted guidelines for the audiologist in the habilitation of the auditorily handicapped. Some of the designated responsibilities are pertinent to the remediation process for adults.

ASHA uses the term "auditorily handicapped" in reference to individuals with auditory disabilities of varying degrees. In this text, "hearing impairment" is used synonymously with "auditory handicap." An individual may have a hearing loss which does not result in a communication handicap.

The ASHA Committee (1974) states that audiologic habilitation is designed to help individuals with auditory disabilities realize their optimal potential in communication regardless of age. This same committee replaces the term "aural rehabilitation" with "audiologic habilitation" on the rationale that aural rehabilitation was restricted to programs of lipreading and auditory training.

The term habilitation has not been universally accepted as a replacement for rehabilitation either medically or legally. We will use rehabilitation as a restoration process of the communication function. It is our belief that habilitation should be defined as the process of developing communication function, a skill not previously possessed by an individual. Habilitation is frequently used, for example, with congenitally deaf children. For the adult with acquired loss of hearing, remediation procedures are aimed at restoring, as nearly as possible, that function the client had previous to the loss of hearing. With limited modifications of the ASHA Committee guidelines, the plan for comprehensive audiologic rehabilitation may include any or all of the following components.

1. Selection of an amplification system to make available as much undistorted sensory information as possible.
2. Development, remediation, or conservation of receptive and expressive language abilities.
3. Counselling for client and family.
4. Continuing re-evaluation of auditory function.
5. Assessment of the effectiveness of rehabilitative procedures.

PRESENT STATUS OF REHABILITATIVE AUDIOLOGY

Oyer and Frankmann (1975) have stressed the need to approach the various aspects of rehabilitative audiology from a conceptual framework. They believe that it is necessary to proceed from a number of assumptions in order to more effectively understand and develop a meaningful remediation process. Their assumptions appear reasonable since we are interested in rehabilitating the "total" person who may have been handicapped by hearing loss. Their assumptions follow.

1. Aural rehabilitation is one facet of the multidisciplinary problem area referred to as audiology, just as clinical hearing measurement or the experimental approach to the study of the normal processes of audition are facets.
2. Aural rehabilitation is a psychosocial education process, and therefore lends itself to analysis within a conceptual framework.
3. Aural rehabilitation, as a process, must be examined as a dynamic interrelated flow of events, and therefore cannot be studied meaningfully as events occurring in isolation.
4. Communication handicaps stemming from auditory deficit can be alleviated in varying degrees through the process of aural rehabilitation.

5. Self-adjustment that has been distorted by the effects of hearing loss can be modified through the process of aural rehabilitation.
6. Social adjustment that has been adversely affected by a hearing loss can be modified through the process of aural rehabilitation.
7. Every aspect of the process of aural rehabilitation can be further clarified through rigorous empirical and experimental investigation.
8. There is at present no available well-organized conceptual framework by which to study the process of aural rehabilitation.
9. Given the proper attention through thoughtful conceptualization, pooled clinical impressions, and rigorous scientific research, the success of the aural rehabilitation process can be predicted for individuals within a specific range.

The above assumptions prompt the question, "If we know so little about the rehabilitative audiology process, how do we know our methodologies are appropriate?" After all, we have been providing rehabilitation services for adults in this country since about 1900. The majority of therapy has focused on speechreading and auditory training, yet little information is available on the results of therapy using these techniques (O'Neill and Oyer, 1973). We find ourselves, therefore, utilizing techniques which have no supportive documentation for their success. We have relied heavily on subjective clinical impressions. As reported by Alpiner (1978), 89 of 100 hearing-impaired clients reported that they were better communicators. This was verified by the use of the Denver Scale of Communication Function. However, pre- and post-therapy lipreading test results indicated no significant improvement. It would appear that Oyer and Frankmann (1975) are quite correct in their recommendation for rigorous scientific research.

In view of the above situation, it may very well be that the hearing aid is the major aspect of rehabilitative audiology. Schow and Nerbonne (1980) have emphasized that a common factor in aural rehabilitation is a recognition that hearing aid adjustment, orientation, and general communication help are the central issues. Aural rehabilitation, then, in most cases will center on amplification aspects whereas extensive speechreading and auditory training are occasional ancillary procedures. This philosophy, if correct, could extensively change our approach to rehabilitative audiology.

PRE-REHABILITATION CONSIDERATIONS

Ideally, the adult client is referred to the speech and hearing center by an otologist or personal physician who has ruled out medical or surgical treatment. It is this writer's opinion that the audiologist should also see the self-referred client. By taking the opportunity to counsel him regarding the importance of otologic examination, we reduce the risk that he remain untreated and establish our concern for the overall welfare of the client.

Following a medical referral, audiologic procedures can be implemented with the understanding that either the hearing impairment is non-reversible or it has been medically minimized to the fullest extent possible.

The first step in the audiologic process is evaluation, which includes pure tone and speech audiometry and any special tests indicated. If the hearing impairment appears significant in terms of communication ability, the client will receive a hearing aid evaluation to determine if amplification will be beneficial. This test assumes that the reader has a working knowledge of audiologic assessment and hearing aid evaluation procedures, topics covered in other sources (Davis and Silverman, 1978; Newby, 1979; Pollack, 1980; Rose, 1978). The results of these evaluations are important to the rehabilitation techniques covered in this handbook.

During the audiologic process, the audiologist will be making judgments regarding necessary remediation methodologies. Techniques include evaluation of the hearing impairment (whether or not amplification is indicated), assessment of communication function, hearing aid orientation when amplification has been recommended, and remediation including therapy and counseling. It may be necessary to obtain assistance from other resources such as the psychologist, social worker, or rehabilitation counsellor. Special considerations for the deaf, deaf-blind, or geriatric client must also be taken into account.

EVALUATION OF COMMUNICATION FUNCTION

Stephens (1980) has emphasized that it is important to thoroughly evaluate a hearing-impaired client before beginning a program of auditory rehabilitation for the client. Further, the determination of the individual's psychosocial function and the concomitant difficulties encountered is a necessary requisite if the rehabilitation program is to be structured to meet individual needs. Such an evaluation will permit the audiologist to have baseline information so that communication improvement can be evaluated.

Since most individuals take hearing for granted, it is difficult for the hearing-impaired to accept their fate; humans are reticent about their shortcomings and usually attempt to camouflage their deficiencies (Hipskind, 1978). He also states that, regardless of the emphasis of the therapy rendered, the audiologist must be aware of several preliminary procedures that should precede or accompany any aural rehabilitation approach.

1. The procurement of a complete otologic and audiologic evaluation.
2. A thorough explanation of the auditory mechanism to the client.
3. A detailed description of the auditory disorder to the client.
4. An assessment of how, when, and where the client is experiencing difficulty because of the hearing loss.
5. A determination of the client's needs, as he perceives them.
6. An explanation to the patient of the general techniques that will be utilized to accomplish the desired results.
7. An explanation to the client's family of the nature of his hearing loss and the importance of cooperation and involvement of the family in assisting in the alleviation of the deleterious effects of the auditory impairment.

Clearly, assessment of communication difficulty is an integral aspect of the rehabilitation process. As Hipskind (1978) states, these procedures should prove conducive to establishing a positive clinician-client relationship. This relationship will evolve from the clinicians's knowledge of the client's needs, understanding of his hearing loss, and the reasons for the ensuing therapy, as well as the family's understanding of its role in the rehabilitative process.

Stephens (1980) suggests that many clients will respond more openly to a computer-based presentation and also to a relatively anonymous questionnaire which they may be sent and asked to return when they come for their first appointment. The difficulty with the latter is that it is often associated with a poor response rate. However, it is an approach which provides the client with an opportunity to consider unhurriedly what his real problems are in the security of his home environment rather than in an audiology clinic. Stephens sent questionnaires to all persons seen in the Department of Auditory Rehabilitation of the Royal National Throat, Nose, and Ear Hospital. The questionnaires were sent to clients seeking a hearing aid for the first time. The results indicated were based on the first 500 responses received. Almost one-half of the respondents complained of difficulty hearing television and/or the radio. The next most common problem was difficulty in conversation. Another major problem was that of employment difficulties at work because of hearing loss. It also appears that personality changes occur in many adults as a result of hearing impairment. It is suggested that hearing handicap scales be utilized to more intensively evaluate these problems. On the basis of available information, the audiologic evaluation battery should include assessment procedures for determining specific communication breakdowns and resultant attitudinal difficulties.

HEARING AIDS AND REHABILITATION

For some time, audiologists have been concerned about the client's purchase of a hearing aid and his subsequent rehabilitation. The ASHA Committee on Rehabilitative Audiology (1974) states that the hearing aid evaluation process is an integral part of rehabilitative audiology. For successful hearing aid use, it is imperative that the client receive follow-up service after purchase of the instrument. It is interesting to note the referral sources for hearing aids in terms of post-purchase remediation opportunities. Following is a list of hearing aid sales to clients from certain referral sources (Cranmer, 1981).

Source	Percentage
Medical referrals	32.36
Audiologist referrals	12.82
Customer referrals	19.85
Repeat customers	21.10
Advertising	13.87

Cranmer also reports on whether or not referring agents request the client to return after the hearing aid is issued. The response from both dispensing audiologists and hearing aid specialists follows.

	Dispensing Audiologist	Hearing Aid Specialist
Yes	56.2%	52.73%
No	34.78%	34.55%
N/A	8.70%	12.73%

From the above information, it appears that a sizeable number of individuals may not be receiving any aural rehabilitation service. This could be due to the nature of some of the referral sources as well as the fact that some referring agents do not wish to see clients after the aid is purchased. In addition, it is reported that 17.39% of dispensing audiologists and 23.64% of hearing aid specialists do not send follow-up letters to the referring sources.

The important considerations here are pre- and post-test procedures for the client purchasing an instrument. All persons who provide aids should be aware that there may be a need for rehabilitation, including both pre- and post-hearing aid orientation. In addition, physicians, audiologists, and others should be cognizant of the potential value of rehabilitative audiology for their clients. Anyone with a handicapping hearing loss should be referred to the audiologist for remediation. Obviously, there is a need to improve the client's communication function to a level as near normal as possible, whether or not a hearing aid has been recommended. Hearing aids and other rehabilitative procedures are not perfect substitutes for normal ears but the combination can significantly help the client improve his communication ability.

REMEDIATION ASPECTS FOR THE HEARING-IMPAIRED ADULT

The specific speechreading techniques of Mueller-Walle (Bruhn, 1949), Jena (Bunger, 1961), Kinzie and Kinzie (1931), and Nitchie (1950) are still evident to some degree in rehabilitation programs. Publications describing these techniques may be purchased today but little information can be found on their effectiveness.

The Mueller-Walle Method is based primarily on rapid identification of syllables through rhythmic drills. In this method, the observer is trained to pay close visual attention to lip movements, associating them with sounds in syllables. The lipreader is encouraged to become familiar with charts which classify the sounds according to the ways they are formed.

The Jena approach employs kinesthetic and visual cues. It emphasizes the patterns and rhythms of speech production while encouraging the client to become kinesthetically aware of the different sounds by producing them himself. In the first two lessons, the client studying the Jena Method learns vowel and consonant charts illustrating the visual characteristics of sounds. Subsequent lessons emphasize the three basic principles of kinesthesis, imitation, and rhythm.

Nitchie's approach includes awareness of lip movements for producing consonants, vowels, and diphthongs, but stresses training with key words, sentences, and short stories. Ordman and Ralli (1957) reported that, with the Nitchie approach, "The pupil is led, by the use of clue words, to lipread a series of simple associated sentences and without conscious effort, to analyze the distinctive characteristics of the various movements."

The Kinzies developed a method combining the Mueller-Walle and Nitchie Methods. They developed a series of graded lessons in lipreading which were designed to provide lipreading instruction for both children and adults at different levels of ability.

The above methods of lipreading may be classified as predominantly analytic or synthetic in their approach. Generally, the analytic approach stresses close attention to the speaker's lip movements in order to recognize individual sounds. The synthetic approach stresses comprehension of the message by recognizing key words and employing associational and contextual cues. Historically, the Jena and Mueller-Walle methods are considered primarily analytic with emphasis on sentence drills and recognition of individual sound units. The Kinzie and Nitchie approaches are predominantly synthetic and emphasize the thought or general idea of the message.

As indicated previously, no published research has proved or disproved the effectiveness of any of these methods. Perhaps the lack of a research base for evaluating lipreading instruction accounts for the scarcity of new formal methods being introduced in the United States.

Williams (1979) investigated the relationship between reading and lipreading, examining specific reading strategies which might be used by both readers and lipreaders as they attempted to comprehend written and/or spoken material. In order to facilitate the achievement of this purpose and to ensure maximum clarification of the nature and extent of the relationship between reading and lipreading, this study was also concerned with the relationship between the efficiency with which the readers used these strategies and reading ability.

The major conclusions drawn from the data were as follows. (1) There are similarities in the strategies used by readers and lipreaders in their approach to comprehension of spoken and written material. (2) There is a significant relationship between reading ability and lipreading ability. (3) While good readers may be either good or poor lipreaders, poor readers are more likely to be poor lipreaders than good lipreaders. (4) Word-by-word reading appears to be a salient characteristic of both poor reading and poor lipreading ability. (5) Good readers and lipreaders do not engage in word-by-word reading but rather employ a combination of visual and linguistic cues to interpret messages.

Viewed historically, a transition seems to have occurred during this century in the rehabilitative audiology process. During this period of time, services were being provided for hearing-impaired adults, but there were philosophical changes in the methods of therapy. In the first 30 years, therapy emphasized the formal lipreading methods mentioned previously. The lack of sophisticated amplification systems may have resulted in heavy reliance on the visual modality for communication.

In the late 1940s, the emphasis shifted to assessment of lipreading ability using words and sentences. Lipreading materials such as the Utley test (1946), the Mason Film Series (1942), the Morkovin Life Situation Film (1948), and a variety of others appeared. Unsuccessful efforts were made to validate these lipreading tests. During the 1940s and the 1950s, attempts were made to correlate lipreading ability with such attributes as intelligence, severity of hearing loss, duration of hearing loss, and so forth. The intent, in part, was to lend research sophistication to the rehabilitative process. Since the lipreading tests employed were not valid, the results of the studies were questionable.

In the 1960s and the 1970s, research was directed toward studying the visual aspects of speech. Other research emphasized bisensory approaches to therapy, that is, the utilization of both visual and auditory modalities. Binnie (1976) has been instrumental in advocating the bisensory approach and its application in the therapy process.

We enter the present era with a continued emphasis on lipreading training for our clients. The practical applied aspects of bisensory instruction, however, have increased in therapy. There seems to be a trend toward a more Progressive approach to adult rehabilitative audiology, in comparison to earlier Traditional techniques which relied so heavily on lipreading.

Fleming's Communication Therapy Program (1972) is an example of what this writer refers to as a Progressive approach. She illustrates the contrast between this and the Traditional approach. According to Fleming, the Traditional approach includes the following.

1. The hard-of-hearing individual is recognized through the clinical program. Medical and surgical problems are dealt with and prostheses are provided as indicated.

2. If the audiologist or the client still report some difficulty in the communication process, the client agrees to attend an aural rehabilitation program.

3. The client describes for the audiologist his hearing disability and the situations where he has the most difficulty understanding.

4. This self-evaluation, along with clinical reports, is used to develop a visual and auditory training schedule to incorporate the individual into a group program. The training would include visual awareness with and without distractions, auditory training with and without distractions, visual and auditory memory training, understanding of the physical loss, suggestions on how to control situations to make communication easier to understand, and a session with family members to help them better understand the ramifications of the individual's hearing loss and how they might help him.

5. The goal of this program is to provide supportive therapy with reinforcement.

In Fleming's Communication Therapy Program philosophy, the structure of the program changes after Point 3, the point at which the client indicates what his problem is as related to his hearing loss and outlines the situations where difficulties most often occur. The client is counselled about the accessibility of a program in which the aim is to make him a more effective communicator. Emphasis in this approach is not on lipreading or auditory training but rather on learning where the communication breakdown occurs.

The client will then join one of two groups. In Group One, a family member or friend with whom the client has difficulty communicating attends all sessions. Group Two is for the hard-of-hearing only, because the people with whom they have difficulty communicating cannot or will not take the time to attend.

A group consists of 10–12 clients plus the audiologists and a psychologist. The clients are informed that they will be expected to function as a group with each person equally responsible for the program's accomplishment. The professional staff is considered a part of the group. The clients are asked to make a contract with themselves and with the group defining what they want to accomplish during a given session. Examples of such contracts, as indicated by Fleming, are as follows.

1. To be able to hear in noise better.
2. To get my teenage children not to say "skip it" when I do not hear them.
3. To be able to function better in group meetings.

The goal of the Communication Therapy Program is to provide supportive therapy. There is also an emphasis on removing the hearing loss as a crutch, giving clients an opportunity to recognize honestly where their communication problems exist. It needs to be reiterated that speechreading and auditory training are not a part of this approach, representing a significant difference from the traditional methods.

Pengilley (1980) perceives three approaches in Aural Rehabilitation.

1. The well-known Traditional Approach: Auditory Training, Lipreading, and Speech Conservation.
2. The Progressive Approach (Alpiner, 1978), which is primarily a counselling-oriented methodology. Pengilley agrees with Alpiner but does not feel his definition is broad enough. She sees it

also as a problem-solving-information-giving method. It implies client self-responsibility.

3. The Community Method, which implies that the community—which includes family, friends, work-structure associates and members of support organizations—takes responsibility for the hearing impaired population by providing adequate "hearing services." Imagine an ideal society. A person receives appropriate hearing assessment, and a free aid. Theatres, public buildings, and community centers provide hearing devices. Aids are available in places of work and in church groups. Television sets provide teletext services and captioning. Amplified phones are installed in public buildings. Clear speech is a community concern to assist migrants, aging adults and hearing-impaired people. Oral and written literacy are equally important! Visually oriented information is also freely available. In this case, the main approach to rehabilitation is through information-giving: people need to be aware of resources and How To Use Them. The community needs to be aware of How To Assist people with hearing impairments. The community adopts tactics for "sound" communication. Finally, the community accepts aging as a natural process, and people are not afraid of aging with dignity. They are able to wear an aid—with dignity. The ideal method is, of course, a combination of all three approaches. It is easier for individuals to change when family relationships are supportive, when friends, community systems, and political governmental organizations are informed and caring.

PSYCHOLOGIC AND COUNSELLING ASPECTS

When one considers that hearing loss results in sensory deprivation, it should be understood that there may be concomitant problems for the adult. Hearing loss has often been referred to as the invisible handicap, since the person with impairment looks like an individual with normal hearing. This differs from other handicapped individuals such as those with cerebral palsy, cleft palate, loss of physical structure, and so forth. The person with a hearing impairment, however, may have feelings that interfere with his personality adjustment. Men may feel less masculine and women less feminine because of the loss of normal auditory function. Since the hearing-impaired adult looks like anyone else in his environment, others may not realize that psychologic problems may exist because of auditory deprivation.

Psychologic problems resulting in the need for counselling may necessitate a period of readjustment. Adults need to accept their loss,

realize their potential, and engage in a therapy process in order to assume positive roles in all aspects of their everyday living activities.

Unfortunately, most of the literature focuses on the deaf adult. Little is written about the problems encountered by the adult with acquired hearing impairment. Early approaches to rehabilitation emphasized lipreading and auditory training with only secondary emphasis on the counselling aspects, the assumption being that persons learning to lipread would have no related problems. This assumption is refuted on the basis that it is not possible to compensate totally through the visual modality for a deficient auditory system. Clinicians in any rehabilitation program should be aware of the possible need to counsel hearing-impaired adults. Our approach to rehabilitation, therefore, attempts to deal realistically with the total human being.

REHABILITATION FOR SENIOR CITIZENS

In today's society, there is a greater awareness of the need to provide remediation for senior citizens because our lifespan has been increased and the aging process is the most common cause of hearing loss. Methodologies in remediation for this age group may differ from the usual procedures for younger adults, but little information is available regarding successful programs for this population.

In university training programs, students seem to prefer working with children rather than "old people." Obviously, we do not dispute the need to habilitate youngsters, but wish to stress that senior citizens constitute an increasingly large segment of society's human resources. Classroom discussions invariably lead to such moral issues as the practicality of therapy for the non-productive senior citizen. This insensitivity fails to consider whether there are other roles for the senior citizen who is no longer employed. For the older adult, still physically and mentally able, confined to a home for the aged (nursing home, retirement center, extended care facility, or care center), the basic question is whether such a home is able to provide more than the basic needs of food, clothing, and shelter. It is this writer's opinion, based on experience, that most nursing homes and care centers in the United States provide only enough for survival.

From a practical point of view, it would seem reasonable to keep the senior citizen productive as long as possible. As a moral issue, there should be little question as to what we should do for those who are physically and mentally capable of communication activity. We need to do away with arbitrary levels of old age and concern ourselves with capabilities rather than limitations.

THE DEAF ADULT

In recent years, audiologists have become increasingly concerned with deaf adults and deaf-blind adults. It was previously believed that little could be done to improve intelligibility of their verbal output and receptive input. The general attitude was to leave these clients to their own environments. Since the attitudes of many audiologists have changed during the past several years, two sections on these individuals are included in this text.

For a general understanding of hearing loss, a classification of hearing impairment is presented in Table 1.1. Classification is based on numerical audiologic data. It is also important to consider discrimination difficulty,

benefits derived from amplification, and specific communication difficulties encountered by individual clients.

In general, we categorize a deaf client with a congenital hearing loss under either a Class E or Class F handicap. Although some of these individuals possess a Class E handicap, congenital handicaps will have prevented the client from learning linguistic and syntactic concepts necessary for normal speech and language development. A deviant auditory input system will result in defective verbal output for most deaf people. To assess an individual's hearing handicap it is necessary to consider the evaluation factors previously mentioned. A tentative decision can then be made concerning whether the client functions as a deaf person (an inability to utilize oral-aural communication as a primary communication mode) or a hearing-impaired individual (oral-aural communication as a primary communication mode). Special considerations are necessary for deaf-blind clients.

ROLE OF ANCILLARY PROFESSIONS

Experience has shown that there is often a need to convince both physicians and disseminators of hearing aids of the importance of

Table 1.1
Classes of Hearing Handicap[a]

Hearing Threshold Level	Class	Degree of Handicap	Average Hearing Threshold Level for 500, 1000, and 2000 Hz in the Better Ear*		Ability to Understand Speech
			More Than	Not More Than	
dB			dB	dB	
ISO					
25	A	Not significant		25	No significant difficulty with faint speech
40	B	Slight handicap	25	40	Difficulty only with faint speech
55	C	Mild handicap	40	55	Frequent difficulty with normal speech
70	D	Marked handicap	55	70	Frequent difficulty with loud speech
90	E	Severe handicap	70	90	Can understand only shouted or amplified speech
	F	Extreme handicap	90		Usually cannot understand even amplified speech

* Whenever the average for the poorer ear is 25 dB or more greater than that of the better ear in this frequency range, 5 dB are added to the average for the better ear. This adjusted average determines the degree and class of handicap. For example, if a person's average hearing threshold level for 500, 1000, and 2000 Hz is 37 dB in one ear and 62 dB or more in the other his adjusted average hearing threshold level is 42 dB and his handicap is Class C instead of Class B.

[a] Reprinted by permission from DAVIS, H., and SILVERMAN, S. R., *Hearing and Deafness*. 4th Ed. New York: Holt, Rinehart and Winston (1978).

rehabilitative audiology. McCarthy (1976) devised a series of questions and answers indicating why rehabilitation is important for many clients. This approach focuses on a situation in which many audiologists have found themselves attempting to justify rehabilitative services.

McCarthy's defense of audiology emphasizes the following points.

1. While the hearing aid dealer's experience in fitting aids is undoubtedly vast, the audiologist has more intensive knowledge of the entire hearing process. Audiologists are trained to rehabilitate the hearing-impaired person by educating him to his hearing aid, demonstrating to him how to adjust to his hearing aid, and demonstrating to him how to adapt to environmental, facial, gestural, and listening clues. We cannot justify fitting a client with a hearing aid and allowing him to struggle with it and the adjustment process on his own. It is our training in dealing with the client after the hearing aid evaluation that, in large part, differentiates us from the hearing aid dealer.

2. The main benefit of lipreading groups is to give hearing-impaired individuals an opportunity to interact with their peers, exchanging feelings and attitudes in an atmosphere of mutual understanding. With the guidance of the audiologist, they can learn about their hearing loss, its ramifications, and available remediation procedures. While dealers or physicians can answer certain questions for them, it may be more meaningful to hear responses from others experiencing similar problems. Lipreading groups do not create good lipreaders. The main purpose of teaching lipreading is to develop better communicators through therapy processes which may include counseling.

3. Modification of attitudes toward hearing losses, families, and jobs is of great importance for improving communication ability. Improvement may be demonstrated by various scales of communication function (Alpiner, 1975; Sanders, 1975). McCarthy (1976) summarizes by saying that audiologists have the technical skill and education to do hearing aid evaluations and the training to help the client become a better communicator.

The audiologist, whatever his specialty, cannot be all things to all hearing-impaired adults. Hearing loss may result in other problems for the hearing-impaired person. Psychologic, vocational, medical, and social difficulties, for example, may result from the breakdown in the communication process. The audiologist should know when to make the appropriate referrals. Our interactions with other disciplines can be more effective if we know when, how, and to whom a referral should be made. Conversely, persons in other professional disciplines may encounter the same problem with regard to our services. The diversity of our audiologic activities and the variety of audiology titles further complicate our interactions with others.

A questionnaire study (Reese and Alpiner, 1976) was devised to determine how vocational rehabilitation counselors regard audiology, specifically rehabilitative audiology. The purpose of the study was to assess the working relationship between the audiologist and the vocational rehabilitation counsellor. The vocational counsellor's function, in part, is to help hearing-impaired and deaf clients find appropriate employment.

Questionnaires were sent to state divisions of vocational rehabilitation in each state and the District of Columbia. Each questionnaire included instructions and defined a hearing-impaired person as an individual with a hearing loss. It also listed the services provided by rehabilitative audiologists as follows: lipreading instruction, auditory training, counseling, manual communication training, and speech therapy. Each counsellor was asked to answer the following questions.

1. What percentage of your total caseload per year is hearing-impaired?
2. Of this group of hearing-impaired clients, what percentage of your cases communicates either predominantly by manual communication or predominantly by oral communication?
3. What percentage of your predominantly manual hearing-impaired caseload are you able to place in jobs per year? What percentage of your predominantly oral hearing-impaired clients are you able to place in jobs per year?

The vocational counsellors were also asked what percentage of their clients they referred to the audiologist for rehabilitation.

Thirty of the 51 questionnaires were returned. Table 1.2 summarizes these results and shows a wide range in the percentage of predominantly oral-aural or manual caseloads, communication means, and job placement. Of the 30 vocational rehabilitation counselors responding, 5 use the service of the rehabilitative audiologist for manual communication training, 12 for lipreading instruction, 16 for speech therapy, and 4 for

Table 1.2
Vocational Rehabilitation Caseload and Placement Data Study Results

Responses	Hearing-Impaired Caseload Per Year Compared to Total Caseload	Cases Communicating Primarily by Manual Communication	Cases Communicating Primarily by Oral-Aural Communication	Vocational Placement Per Year of Primarily Manual Hearing-Impaired	Vocational Placement Per Year of Primarily Oral-Aural Hearing-Impaired
	%	%	%	%	%
1	40 public school students; 20 others	40	60	50	50
2	40	70	30	50	70
3	5	5	95	25	30
4	7	50	50	60	20
5	80	50	50	50	50
6	2	100	0	25	50
7	5–7	2.5	4	33	45
8	100	75	25	11	3
9	4	25	75	18–20	15
10	no response	no response	no response	no response	no response
11	8	no data	no data	no data	no data
12	2.2	no data	no data	no data	no data
13	4.5	90	10	no response	no response
14	4.5	66	34	17	13
15	20	60	40	60	80
16	31	66	34	25	50
17	no response	25	75	90	95
18	100	95	5	25	10
19	6.2	15	85	1.5	4.7
20	·40	no response	no response	no response	no response
21	2	70	30	80	50
22	5–7	30	70	no response	no response
23	3–9	no data	no data	no data	no data
24	50	60	40	90	90
25	1	25	75	30	30
26	100	30	70	no data	no data
27	99	90	10	50	?
28	100	70	30	75	75
29	2.3	40	60	20	33
30	100	60	40	50	70

other services. Referral percentages were low for all respondents, with the highest being 50%. Referrals averaged about 10%. The vocational rehabilitation counsellors made almost no referrals for any of the services listed in the questionnaire.

Many rehabilitation counsellors did not know what services were provided by the audiologist. The general opinion reported was that audiologists are involved only with diagnostic services. Several of the counsellors indicated that it was the speech pathologist who taught lipreading and thought manual communication training was done by teachers of the deaf, other deaf persons, and interpreters. It appears that the audiology profession has failed to make the range of its services known to vocational rehabilitation agencies.

Our relationship with the medical profession is equally limited. Binnie (1976) has aptly stated that the medical profession must be made aware of the full scale of aural rehabilitative services within a speech and hearing center. He indicated further that we need to establish more effective referral services between audiologists and physicians. Medical personnel need to know the full extent of our services and that their patients are receiving appropriate therapy from audiologists. He believes that effective and relevant aural rehabilitation should result in spontaneous comments from clients which would instill confidence in the minds of any referring physicians. Cooperation between audiologists and other allied professionals is of the utmost importance for providing optimal service to the hearing-impaired client.

COMMUNITY AURAL REHABILITATION PROGRAMS

Approximately 20 million children and adults in the United States have hearing loss (Chalfant and Sheffelin, 1969). The incidence of hearing loss increases with age (U. S. Department of Health, Education, and Welfare, 1962). In those persons 25–55 years of age, the incidence of hearing loss is 2.2 per thousand persons. The incidence rises to 277.4 per thousand for persons age 75 years and above.

In terms of hearing conservation, school age children are generally in an enviable situation because their hearing is tested on a periodic basis in most schools. The typical adult American, however, is not automatically tested unless he assumes the initiative for periodic examination. Most adults seem to be either unaware of the need for hearing tests or not interested in receiving them. Even those adults who receive annual medical examinations may or may not have hearing testing as part of the examination procedure. Fortunately, many employees are required by various industries and governmental agencies to receive periodic hearing tests.

Since hearing loss is often a gradual process due to such factors as noise exposure and the aging process (presbycusis), most adults may not be aware of an impairment during its early stages. This occurs primarily because the higher frequencies, which may not affect the understanding of speech, are generally the first frequencies which begin to diminish. An individual with an emerging hearing impairment may accuse those speaking to him of not speaking loudly enough or of mumbling. The tendency is to blame the breakdown in communication on the speaker rather than the recipient of the message.

There are millions of adults in the mainstream of society who are not being tested, including thousands of senior citizens living in care facilities. Their difficulties in communication commonly are attributed to mental deterioration. Obviously, there is a need to seek development of community hearing rehabilitation programs to reach all adults.

For the purpose of obtaining some basic information on public knowledge and attitudes about hearing, a pilot study (Holanov, 1976) was devised to determine if any trends could be observed. A survey was administered to 30 adults in the waiting room of a metropolitan airport. Ten adults, 5 men and 5 women, were interviewed in each of the following age groups: 20–30 years, 35–45 years, and 55–65 years. Of the 30 persons interviewed, 16% had 12 or less years of education, 70% had 13–16 years of education, and approximately 13% had more than 16 years of education. Each person responded that his last physical examination had been within the past 4 years. Of the total group, 40% had their hearing tested at that time.

Fifty-three percent of the total group responded that their hearing had been tested by some person in the last 10 years. Of these individuals, 62.5% were men and 37.5% were women.

It is important to note that while the total group had received routine physical examinations in the past 4 years, 66% of the men and only 13% of the women had received hearing tests during these examinations. This may be due to the fact that the majority of women were examined by gynecologists.

Regarding their knowledge about audiologists, no one reported any rehabilitative responses in their answers. Approximately 36% indicated some awareness that the audiologist engaged in hearing testing. Of this group, 55% stated that they responded as they did by determining what the word must mean; that is "audio has to do with hearing." Two persons said they had read something about the field. No one had learned about the profession by having his hearing tested by an audiologist. Half of the total group interviewed responded that they did not know what an audiologist was (and did not care to guess). Approximately 20% of the group stated that a rehabilitative audiologist must be involved in some aspect of rehabilitation. It is assumed that these responses were due to the adjective "rehabilitative" preceding audiologist rather than to actual knowledge of the audiologist's role.

The total group was asked if they had any

idea how much training would be necessary for the audiologist. Zero to 4 years of college was the guess of 23% of the respondents, with the lowest figure given by a woman who believed that only a few special courses would qualify a person to test someone's hearing. Thirty percent felt that 5–7 years of college would be necessary, and another 23% indicated that, like medicine, 8 or more years were needed. Twenty-three percent would not guess.

Twenty-three percent of the respondents had no idea what a hearing aid dealer does. Forty-eight percent said they were acquainted with hearing aids through some form of advertising in the media. When asked about the training necessary to become a hearing aid dealer, most responses were guesses. Twenty-six percent of the group stated that there probably would be no educational or training requirements. Twenty percent thought 2–4 years of college was necessary. One person believed that more than 4 years of college was required. Two subjects mentioned either a technical school or a special training program requirement. Seven subjects were unwilling to make a guess.

Another survey item dealt with the question, "What is lipreading?" Two women responded that it was speechreading. Their answers were consistent with the definitions appearing in audiology textbooks. Eighty-three percent responded that it was being able to understand what people said by reading lips. Three persons had no idea what the process involved. Forty percent said they would go to a speech and hearing center for training in lipreading. Sixty percent had no idea where to go for instruction.

After the survey was completed and the subjects had some increased awareness of the profession, they were asked how audiologists could more effectively inform the general public about audiologic services. Responses stressed more publicity for speech and hearing centers, the use of the media for public service announcements, and increased contact between the audiologist and the public.

In general, this public sample knew little about hearing disorders and available services. Specifically, they had little knowledge of audiology. There was some awareness of hearing aids but this was not related to audiology. It is expected that results similar to those obtained in this survey would be obtained nationally.

Brown (1980) attempted to determine how the hearing-impaired perceive the problems which exist between them and the societal structure. Are these problems perceived as resulting from their own deficiency, or are they perceived as resulting from outside themselves? If these problems are perceived as resulting from something outside their individual deficiency, then what are they, and what are the indicators?

The population sampled was the non-institutionalized hearing-impaired of the Greater Rochester, New York area. A questionnaire was mailed to the target population to gather economic and demographic data. From the respondents, a stratified random sample of 50 subjects was selected to be interviewed. The focus of each interview was on the following four major areas of interaction between the hearing-impaired adult and the social structure: dissemination of information, attitudes toward hearing peers, community identification, and delivery of services.

The resultant recommendations for community education programming were based upon the way the different groups appeared to view the individual deficiency paradigm operating within the four areas of this study. The recommendations emphasized the importance of heterogeneous grouping, educational development, broadening the currently planned community education program, and preliminary planning for community education programs. The hearing impaired of Rochester are developing community education programs which they view as a viable means for solving their problems within the existing societal structure.

It has been reported (Alpiner *et al.*, 1973) that the issues related to community programs in rehabilitation are fairly complex. Guidelines need to be established for such programs. The audiologist must assume the responsibility for educating the public about the value of community hearing conservation programs and be prepared to deal with the following.

1. Location of community program.
2. Population to be served.
3. Actual types of programs to be established.
4. Personnel to engage in community programs.

5. Financing of community programs.

6. Selling of community programs to physicians.

7. Identification of mechanisms for locating the hearing-impaired.

8. Short term and long term goals of community rehabilitative audiology programs.

RESEARCH ASPECTS OF REHABILITATIVE AUDIOLOGY

Binnie and Alpiner (1969) attempted to determine whether any significant differences in lipreading methods could be found. They wanted to assess the value of different approaches in lipreading instruction. Further, they desired information on the usefulness of the Utley film, a lipreading test known as "How Well Can You Read Lips?" (1946). An underlying purpose of the project was to evaluate what happens when non-valid methods are used in lipreading instruction and then to compare the effectiveness of these methods with the non-valid Utley test. The Utley was used because other lipreading tests developed since 1946 were validated on the basis of this particular instrument. It was hypothesized that this pilot study would reveal the present status of lipreading instruction and therapy evaluation.

Fifteen adult subjects, aged 35–65 years, with sensorineural hearing loss, were selected for this study. All subjects had received an audiologic examination at the University of Denver Speech and Hearing Center. None had participated in any previous lipreading instruction.

The 15 subjects were randomly divided into three groups of 5 each. Group One received instruction in the Jena Method during a 9-week course for 1 hour each week. Group Two was assigned to the Nitchie program and those individuals also received a 9-week course in lipreading instruction for 1 hour each week. Group Three, the control group, received no formal training in lipreading and provided the basis for comparison with Groups One and Two. Group Three also was used to rule out the possible effects of learning on test performance.

Before and after therapy, the subjects' lipreading abilities were assessed in their respective groups of 5. They received the Utley silent film word and sentence test. In addition to this test, individual phonemes (vowels and consonants) were selected from the International Phonetic Alphabet and were recorded on video tape (Ampex VR-7000) by a male speaker. Subjects were seated in a semi-circular arrangement approximately 10 feet from the screen or television monitor. The test materials were presented inaudibly. Subjects were instructed to watch the speaker's lip movements and write the responses on prepared answer sheets. One point was allowed for each item correctly identified. The homophoneity of responses was considered on the consonant and vowel test. For example, if the stimulus item was /p/ and the response was /b/ or /m/, the response was counted as correct.

A test for significance of difference between means of small samples (Spence et al., 1968) demonstrated no significant differences between the pre- and post-test treatment conditions. This suggests that the Control Group's scores in lipreading did not show improvement and rules out the effect of practice (that is, viewing the same test on two occasions) as a basis for possible improved scores. Neither the Jena nor the Nitchie Groups demonstrated significantly better scores on the lipreading tests administered in this study after 9 weeks of training. The lipreading methodology employed did not seem to make a difference in terms of demonstrating better performance in lipreading ability.

To demonstrate the difference between treatment (Jena and Nitchie Groups) and no treatment (Control Group), the difference scores of the pre- and post-tests were pooled for the treatment groups and compared to those of the control group. Statistical analysis failed to demonstrate any significant difference. The treatment groups could not identify test materials any better than the group with no formal lipreading experience.

This study contained a number of limitations which could have influenced the difference scores. They are discussed for the value they may have in future studies of this nature. First, research of this type should be carried out with large samples of the hearing-impaired population. Second, more intensive lipreading sessions, over a longer time period, should be completed before assessing the value of lipreading instruction. The appropriate number of sessions a client should receive in lipreading instruction has never been determined.

The most important limitation of this study may be the tests which were used. The Utley continues to be utilized for validation criteria and to assess lipreading ability because it contains reliability standardization data and is commercially available. It appears to be a very difficult film test, however, and not necessarily a good measure of lipreading ability. Characteristics necessary for successful lipreading have never been determined. The Word section of the Utley test contains 36 items but standardization data demonstrate a mean score of only 6.8 and a standard deviation of 3.7. The Sentence section contains 125 items with a mean score of only 33.6 and a standard deviation of 16.3 (Utley, 1946). These data would indicate that lipreading performance, as measured by this test, is quite restricted and extremely variable.

DiCarlo and Kataja (1951) reported that the Utley test was so difficult that only 19% of the items could be answered correctly. One of the reasons for this difficulty could be the manner of presentation. The test items are administered inaudibly. Considering that only about one-third of our English sounds are visible, it may not be surprising that the Utley scores are low.

The Utley test stimulated further investigative endeavors in measuring lipreading ability. The Barley Speechreading Test (Barley, 1964) was developed using Central Institute for the Deaf (CID) Everyday Sentences (Davis and Silverman, 1978). Jeffers and Barley (1971) reported that the Barley Test, Form A, was indicated to be a valid test of speechreading using the Utley Test, Form B, as the criterion test. Results obtained with these two tests were very similar. A second study indicated high correlations between both forms of the Barley Test and the Utley Sentence Test, Form A. When comparing the Barley Test, Form A, with the Utley Test, Form A, correlations were 0.79. When the Barley Test, Form B, was compared to the Utley Test, Form A, correlations were 0.83.

The subjects' low scores on both the Barley and Utley tests might be explained by the medium used. Jeffers and Barley (1967) report that one of the limitations of the Utley Sentence Test may be due to inherent difficulties in film presentation rather than in the content of the film *per se*. They administered the Utley Test to college students and to hearing-impaired adults, using both a film and "live" presentation without voice. The college students did twice as well as the hearing-impaired groups with the film version and three times as well with the "live" presentation. While the "live" version tested the same skill as the filmed version, it needs to be emphasized that it still is not known what skills are being measured and how the lipreading test relates to clients' communication function either pre- or post-therapy. Other lipreading tests continue to use the non-valid Utley test for validation.

Pelson and Prather (1974) studied three groups of adult subjects, differing primarily in age and auditory status, performing two speechreading tasks. One task consisted of speechreading sentences in which the only cues provided were those from the speaker's face and lips. In the other task, a related picture was presented just prior to speechreading a given sentence. Results indicated that while message-related pictures markedly enhanced speechreading performance for all groups, the older hearing-impaired subjects improved more than the two groups of normal-hearing subjects, regardless of age. In terms of absolute speechreading performance, however, the younger normal-hearing subjects speechread better than either of the two older groups while the older adults with hearing impairment tended to speechread better than the older subjects with normal hearing.

Clouster (1976) studied the factors of vowel consonant ratio and sentence length in order to determine their relationship to the lipreading ability of normal and hearing-impaired subjects. It was determined that there is no relationship between vowel consonant ratio and lipreading ability for either normal or hearing-impaired subjects. It was determined that there is a relationship between sentence length and lipreading ability for both normal and hearing-impaired subjects. Three-word sentences were found to be easier to lipread than six- or nine-word sentences, and six- and nine-word sentences were of equal difficulty. The normal and the hearing-impaired group of subjects did not differ in their ability to lipread the sentences of different lengths.

It should be determined whether future efforts should be directed toward measuring lipreading ability or measuring communication function. Practically, audiologists should be able to predict communication ability with a valid lipreading test. To date, there is no such lipreading instrument. Development of such tests should be a high priority in audiology.

The remediation value of visual cues as a supplement to audition, under adverse listening conditions, was examined by Neely (1956), O'Neill (1954), and Sumby and Pollack (1954). These studies demonstrated that the listener can increase his receptive communication ability by giving visual attention to the speaker. Dodds and Harford (1968) found that a bisensory auditory and visual listening condition provided the best scores for Utley sentences. Preliminary investigation by Binnie and Barrager (1969) demonstrated that scores for monosyllabic words presented visually only were approximately 25%. Bisensory articulation function curves, however, demonstrated the following pattern.

0	dB	SL—55%
8	dB	SL—85%
16	dB	SL—95%

Consequently, Binnie and Barrager (1969) recommended that lipreading tests be devised employing some auditory cues to complement the restricted visual channel.

Future research should demonstrate the amount of sound required to complement lipreading for optimum identification of speech. Since most hearing-impaired adults have some degree of residual hearing, this approach may be more realistic than traditional lipreading.

References

ALPINER, J. G., *Handbook of Adult Rehabilitative Audiology*. Baltimore: Williams and Wilkins (1978).

ALPINER, J. G., Hearing aid selection for adults. In M. Pollack (Ed.), *Amplification for the Hearing Impaired.* New York: Grune & Stratton (1975).

ALPINER, J. G., MUSSEN, E., NORTHERN, J., REED, D., and SODERBERG, M., Community aural rehabilitation programs. *J. Acad. Rehab. Audiol.,* **6,** 31–34 (1973).

ASHA COMMITTEE ON REHABILITATIVE AUDIOLOGY, AMERICAN SPEECH AND HEARING ASSOCIATION, The audiologist: responsibilities in the habilitation of the auditorily handicapped. *ASHA,* **16,** 68–70 (1974).

BARLEY, M., CID everyday sentences test of speechreading ability. In J. Jeffers, and M. Barley, *Speechreading (Lipreading).* Springfield, Ill: Charles C Thomas (1971).

BINNIE, C. A., Relevant aural rehabilitation. In J. L. Northern (Ed.), *Hearing Disorders.* Boston: Little, Brown and Co. (1976).

BINNIE, C. A., and ALPINER, J. G., A comparative investigation of analytic versus synthetic methodologies in lipreading training. Paper presented at the annual convention of the American Speech and Hearing Association, Chicago (1969).

BINNIE, C. A., and BARRAGER, D. C., Bi-sensory established articulation functions for normal hearing and sensorineural hearing loss patients. Paper presented at the annual convention of the American Speech and Hearing Association, Chicago (1969).

BROWN, A. T., JR., An analysis of the perceptions of the hearing-impaired regarding their relationship with their community. Unpublished dissertation, Syracuse University (1980).

BRUHN, M. D., *The Mueller-Walle Method of Lipreading.* Washington, D. C.: The Volta Bureau (1949).

BUNGER, A. M., *Speech Reading—Jena Method.* Danville, IL: The Interstate Printers and Publishers, Inc. (1961).

CHALFANT, J. C., AND SHEFFELIN, M. A., *Central Processing Dysfunctions in Children.* Bethesda, MD.: U. S. Department of Health, Education, and Welfare (1969).

CLOUSTER, R. A., The effect of vowel consonant ratio and sentence length on lipreading ability. *Am. Ann. Deaf,* **121,** 513–518 (1976).

CRANMER, K., Hearing aid dispensing—1981. *Hearing Instruments,* **32,** 11–13 (1981).

DAVIS, H., and SILVERMAN, S. R., *Hearing and Deafness.* New York: Holt, Rinehart and Winston (1978).

DICARLO, L. M., and KATAJA, R., An analysis of the Utley Lipreading Test. *J. Speech Hear. Disord.,* **16,** 226–240 (1951).

DODDS, E., and HARFORD, E., Application of a lipreading test in a hearing aid evaluation. *J. Speech Hear. Disord.,* **33,** 167–173 (1968).

FLEMING, M., A total approach to communication therapy. *J. Acad. Rehab. Audiol.,* **5,** 28–31 (1972). (Copyright 1972, *Journal of the Academy of Rehabilitative Audiology.*)

HIPSKIND, N. M., Aural rehabilitation for adults. *Otolaryngol. Clin. N. Am.,* **11,** 823–834 (1978).

HOLANOV, S., Public attitudes of adults regarding hearing. Paper presented at University of Denver Seminar on Rehabilitative Audiology (1976).

JEFFERS, J., and BARLEY, M., *Speechreading (Lipreading).* Springfield, Ill.: Charles C Thomas (1971).

JEFFERS, J., and BARLEY, M., A re-evaluation of the Utley Lipreading Sentence Test. Paper presented at the annual convention of the American Speech and Hearing Association, Chicago (1967).

KINZIE, C. E., and KINZIE, R., *Lip-reading for the Deafened Adult.* Philadelphia: John C. Winston Co. (1931).

MASON, M. K., Teaching and testing visual hearing by the cinematographic method. *Volta Rev.,* **44,** 703–705 (1942).

MCCARTHY, P., Questions to rehabilitative audiologists. Paper presented at University of Denver Seminar on Rehabilitative Audiology (1976). (Copyright, 1976, Patricia McCarthy.)

MORKOVIN, B. V., *Life-situation speechreading through the cooperation of senses.* Los Angeles: University of Southern California (1948).

NEELEY, K. K., Effect of visual factors on the intelligibility of speech. *J. Acoust. Soc. Am.,* **28,** 1275–1277 (1956).

NEWBY, H. A., *Audiology*, Englewood Cliffs, New Jersey: Prentice-Hall, Inc. (1979).

NITCHIE, E. H., *New Lessons in Lipreading*. Philadelphia: J. B. Lippincott Co. (1950).

O'NEILL, J. J., Contributions of the visual components of oral symbols to speech comprehension. *J. Speech Hear. Disord.*, **19**, 429–439 (1954).

O'NEILL, J. J., and OYER, H. J., Aural rehabilitation. In J. Jerger (Ed.), *Modern Developments in Audiology*. New York: Academic Press (1973).

ORDMAN, K. A., and RALLI, M. P., *What People Say: the Nitchie School Basic Course in Lipreading*. Washington, D. C.: The Volta Bureau (1957).

OYER, H. J., and FRANKMANN, J. P., *The Aural Rehabilitation Process*. New York: Holt, Rinehart and Winston (1975).

PELSON, R. O., and PRATHER, W. F., Effects of visual message-related cues, age, and hearing impairment on speechreading performance. *J. Speech Hear. Res.*, **17**, 518–525 (1974).

PENGILLEY, P., Hearing tactics: the strategy of coping with a hearing problem. Paper presented at the 4th National Conference, Audiological Society of Australia, 1980.

POLLACK, M. C., *Amplification for the Hearing Impaired*. New York: Grune & Stratton (1980).

REESE, N., and ALPINER, J. G., The rehabilitative audiologist's role in vocational placement of the hearing impaired. *J. Rehab. Deaf* **10(2)**, 1–8, (1976).

REGAN, D. E., Problem reduction approach to aural rehabilitation. *Audiol. Hear. Educ.*, **3(6)**, 6–7, 48 (1977).

ROSE, D. E., *Audiological Assessment*. Englewood Cliffs, New Jersey: Prentice-Hall, Inc. (1978).

SANDERS, D. A., Hearing aid orientation and counseling. In M. Pollack (Ed.), *Amplification for the Hearing Impaired*. New York: Grune & Stratton (1975).

SCHOW, R. L., and NERBONNE, M. A., *Introduction to Aural Rehabilitation*. Baltimore: University Park Press (1980).

SPENCE, J., UNDERWOOD, B., DUNCAN, C., and CANTON, J., *Elementary Statistics*. New York: Appleton-Century-Crofts, Inc. (1968).

STEPHENS, S. D. G., Evaluating the problems of the hearing impaired. *Audiology*, **19**, 205–220 (1980).

SUMBY, W. H., and POLLACK, I., Visual contributions to speech intelligibility in noise. *J. Acoust. Soc. Am.*, **26**, 212–215 (1954).

U. S. DEPARTMENT OF HEALTH, EDUCATION, AND WELFARE, NATIONAL CENTER OF HEALTH STATISTICS, *Hearing level of adults by age and sex, United States*. Series 11, No. 11. Washington, D. C. (1960–62).

UTLEY, J., Factors involved in the teaching and testing of lipreading ability through the use of motion pictures. *Volta Rev.*, **38**, 657–659 (1946).

WILLIAMS, A. M., The relationship between two visual communication systems: reading and lipreading. Unpublished dissertation, Hofstra University (1969).

2

Evaluation of Communication Function

Jerome G. Alpiner, Ph.D.

The complex mechanism by which we acquire knowledge and communicate with others can be likened to a computer. Hearing and other senses provide the input; the brain is programmed to store and interpret the information; behavior, including speech, is the output. The audiologist is deeply involved with human communication, and restoration of communication function to as normal a status as possible is his fundamental concern. Obtaining numerical audiologic data is only one part of the process. For effective remediation, assessment should focus on the communication breakdown caused by the auditory deficit.

Adults exist in a variety of environments: social, vocational, avocational, and familial. Evaluation of how hearing impairment affects communication in diverse situations allows us to plan an effective rehabilitation program. This chapter suggests some ways to evaluate communication function. Modifying the experience and learning of the organism (as the teacher does when he attempts to have the patient learn a new language with a new set of sensory receptors) is one way to improve the client's communication ability (Hirsh, 1951).

AUDIOLOGIC TEST BATTERY

In attempting to modify experiences and learning through rehabilitation, audiologists should obtain as much information about clients as possible. Although we are not specifically concerned with clinical audiologic assessment here, we need to be aware of its relationship to rehabilitation. A routine test battery usually begins with pure tone air and bone conduction audiometry. Pure-tone audiometry provides the initial picture of auditory system function. It shows the severity of hearing loss, whether it is low frequency, high frequency, or flat in nature, and whether the type of hearing loss is conductive, sensorineural, or mixed.

Speech audiometry supplies information which substantiates pure-tone speech frequency averages with speech reception thresholds. Discrimination testing at suprathreshold levels measures the ability to understand speech stimuli which are presented at comfortable hearing levels. Monosyllabic words are generally used in discrimination testing although various sentence lists may be used. The general trend in speech and hearing centers is to recommend lipreading and auditory training following audiologic evaluation. Except for speculation from case history information (onset of hearing loss, etiology, medical data, general communication problems) and subjective interpretation of numerical test results, little consideration is given to communication difficulties encountered in the client's environment. We are beginning to realize, however, that numerical data are not a precise indicator of communication success and initial client input is too limited for effective therapy planning.

COMMUNICATION SCALES

There has been continuing interest in the expansion of the routine audiologic test battery to evaluate a client's handicap (Alpiner, 1975; Giolas, 1970; High *et al.*, 1964; Koniditsiotis, 1971; Noble, 1972; Sanders, 1975; Kaplan *et al.*, 1978; Giolas *et al.*, 1979; McCarthy and Alpiner, 1980; Schow and Nerbonne, 1980). Although communication evaluation efforts have not been perfected, they have generated interest in more comprehensive evaluation methods. The measures which have been developed are subjectively interpreted and therefore should be used with caution. Schow and Nerbonne (1980) suggest that a hearing handicap measurement tool can be a valuable part of the audiologist's armamentarium by telling how an individual feels about his hearing loss.

The Social Adequacy Index was an early attempt by Davis (1948) to develop a scale based on the relationship between speech reception thresholds and discrimination scores. Davis (1948) indicated that the scale was not effective because the phonetically balanced (PB) recording used had not been sufficiently standardized to measure discrimination as accurately as hearing threshold levels may be measured. He stated that we need more knowledge about the relationship between hearing and understanding connected speech. Although the concept of the index was worthwhile, its reliance on numerical data lacked sufficient emphasis on differences in individual behavioral characteristics.

The Hearing Handicap Scale (HHS) Forms A and B (High *et al.*, 1964) is a self-report scale designed to assess the effects of hearing loss on an individual's performance in everyday living activities. It consists of formalized questions and standardized client responses. The scale lends itself to quantification of subject responses, allowing for self and group comparisons on a periodic basis.

Two limitations of the HHS are cited by its authors. First, responses may be easily falsified since there is no internal method to determine the validity of answers given. Second, the questions are similar and designed to focus on only one aspect of hearing handicap. Psychologic, vocational, and other problems caused by hearing loss are not considered (Giolas, 1970; Sanders, 1975). Despite its limitations, the HHS can still be considered a tool in the rehabilitative program and a motivational factor in encouraging additional research.

Form A of the scale is presented in Appendix 2A. Options for each item are as follows.

      ____ 1. Almost always
      ____ 2. Usually
      ____ 3. Sometimes
      ____ 4. Rarely
      ____ 5. Almost never

In a limited study by Koniditsiotis (1971), the relationship between audiometric data and actual performance was investigated. Three therapists used a performance test (Appendix 2B) to rate the hearing of 9 subjects. Hearing sensitivity, as measured by pure tone audiometry and speech reception thresholds, was the better index of actual performance. An important consideration in this type of evaluation is that the client's feelings about the communication situation are ignored. Further, it would be helpful to know how individual clients functioned in pre- and post-therapy.

Another test procedure, the Hearing Measurement Scale (HMS) (Noble, 1972; Noble and Atherley, 1970), was devised for the assessment of handicap due to industrial noise. Although the scale was planned for use with an industrial population, the authors suggest that it can probably be used for any group of hearing-impaired persons with sensorineural disorders. The scale (Appendix 2C) was modified from its original form to include seven sub-categories.

    1. Speech-hearing
    2. Acuity for non-speech sound
    3. Localization
    4. Reaction to handicap
    5. Speech distortion
    6. Tinnitus
    7. Personal opinion of hearing loss

There is an attempt to include all possible areas of difficulty for the individual with hearing loss. The authors stress that client reactions to hearing loss should have a definite place in an overall evaluation of each "individual" problem.

The Denver Scale of Communication Function (Appendix 2D) (Alpiner *et al.*, 1974) is a tool designed to help the clinician make a subjective assessment of communication attitudes of adults with acquired hearing loss. Based on the assumption that lipreading tests fail to assess communication difficulties, the purpose of this scale is to focus attention on improving the client's communication function, regardless of his lipreading ability. The present form is not designed to be used for senior citizens in extended care facilities (see Chapter 7 for evaluation scales for this population).

The scale should be administered before initiating therapy to avoid influencing client responses. After reviewing the samples, the client uses a semantic differential type continuum for each of 25 statements to judge his own communication function in four categories: family, self, social-vocational, and general communication experience. To encourage "first impression" responses, a time limit of 15 minutes to administer the scale is suggested.

Client responses are recorded on a Profile Form (Fig. 2.1) with the desired responses at the top end of the ordinate axis, much like an audiogram. The abscissa points represent each statement on the questionnaire. To plot the curve, the points on the abscissa between agree and disagree are marked according to each response and connected with a straight line.

Pre- and post-service testing compares the client with himself, not his therapy counterparts or any other norms.

To determine the initial reliability of the Denver Scale, it was administered to 10 hearing-impaired adults at the termination of a rehabilitative audiology group (McNeil and Alpiner, 1975) and repeated 1 week later. When all items of both tests were correlated for all subjects, an overall correlation of 0.729 was obtained. Each of the four categories of the two test administrations was correlated, with the following results.

Category	Correlation Coefficient
Family	$r = 0.962$
Self	$r = 0.767$
Social-vocational	$r = 0.917$
Communication	$r = 0.930$

The initially obtained r of 0.729 represented an acceptable level of test reliability. By tradition, and by virtue of the nature and purpose of the test, an r of 0.700 or above is considered satisfactory test-retest reliability.

Schow and Nerbonne (1980) investigated both the Hearing Handicap Scale (HHS) and a modification of the Denver Scale of Communication Function (the Quantified Denver Scale, QDS) in terms of audiologic scores obtained in hearing evaluations. The mean pure tone averages were in the slight-to-mild hearing loss category and were about 8 dB poorer than the mean speech reception thresholds. The authors attribute this discrepancy to a strict use of the three-frequency average (500, 1000, and 2000 Hz). The results show approximately a 10-point difference between pure tone average and HHS score. These scores appear to be consistent with categories suggested by Schow and Tannahill (1977) for interpretation of HHS scores. They found that most candidates for hearing aid eligibility or aural rehabilitation will have scores of 41% or higher (Table 2.1).

The same procedure was used by Schow and Nerbonne (1980) for the Quantified Denver Scale (Appendix 2E). There were 50 subjects with a mean age of 55.8 years. The subjects were divided into three groups based on the pure tone average in the best ear. One group of 14 subjects had a pure tone average of 0 to 15 dB HL; a second group of 20 had a pure tone average of 16 to 26 dB HL; the third group of 16 subjects had a pure tone average of 27 to 40 dB HL. The Quantified Denver Scale was administered to all subjects. A raw score was calculated for each QDS and then converted to percent by subtracting 25 points from the raw score. In this study, all scores obtained were in an unaided condition. Table 2.2 indicates the results for each of the three groups. It appears that the degree of handicapping condition increased as a function of greater pure tone averages. The subjects with better hearing had a mean score of 6.5%, those with intermediate hearing sensitivity had a mean score of 21.3%, and those with poorer hearing had a mean score of 37.7%. Of interest is the fact that the scores on the Quantified Denver Scale were in close agreement with the obtained pure tone averages.

Hutton (1980) analyzed responses to a Hearing Problem Inventory (HPI-A) (At-

THE McCARTHY-ALPINER SCALE OF HEARING HANDICAP

by

Patricia McCarthy, Ph.D., V.A. Medical Center, No. Chicago, Ill.

and

Jerome Alpiner, Ph.D., University of Mississippi, University, MS

NAME ______________________ SS# ______________________ AGE ________

DATE ______________________ SEX ________ AUDIOLOGIST ______________________

PROFILE FORM

	PSYCHOLOGICAL										SOCIAL														VOCATIONAL									
	N 1	N 2	N 3	N 4	P 5	N 6	N 7	P 8	N 9	N 10	N 11	N 12	P 13	N 14	P 15	N 16	N 17	N 18	P 19	N 20	N 21	P 22	N 23	P 24	N 25	N 26	N 27	N 28	N 29	P 30	N 31	P 32	N 33	P 34
1																																		
2																																		
3																																		
4																																		
5																																		

DIRECTIONS: Items are worded negatively & positively and scored from 1 point to 5 points with 5 points indicating maximum handicap. Negative items are coded as "N" and positive items are coded as "P". For "N" items, calculate always=5 pts. usually=4 pts. sometimes=3 pts. rarely=2 pts. and never=1 pt. For "P" items, calculate always=1 pt. usually=2 pts. sometimes=3 pts. rarely=4 pts. and never=5 pts.

LEGEND: Responses of hearing impaired individual = X
Responses of family member = 0

Figure 2.1. Profile scoring form, the McCarthy-Alpiner Scale of Hearing Handicap. (Reprinted by permission from McCarthy, P. A., and Alpiner, J. G., The McCarthy-Alpiner Scale of Hearing Handicap, 1980, unpublished study.)

lanta). The data for this report were made available from HPI-As filled out by patients who received hearing aids in 1977 and 1978. (The HPI-A form is found in Appendix 2F). Responses by 329 patients to a 51-item self-administered HPI-A were examined in order to identify some of the influences on patients' perceptions of their problems and on the amount of time aids were worn. The data were pooled into 4 groups: (1) the pre-data from patients receiving initial fittings, (2) the post-data from patients receiving initial fittings, (3) the pre-data for those receiving replacement fittings, and (4) the post-data for those receiving replacement aids.

Experience wearing a hearing aid was shown to have substantial influence on both problem perception and hearing aid use. The effects of hearing loss were large for the inexperienced users and small for the experienced users. Older persons reported increases in problems and decreases in wearing

time. Employment was also examined. Employed persons had slightly higher problem scores and longer hours of hearing aid use. Employment was higher for experienced hearing aid users than for those receiving their initial fittings.

The comparisons of pre- and post-data showed reductions in self-assessed problems by persons who were receiving their initial fittings, counseling, and orientation training. Experienced hearing aid users showed smaller pre-post reductions in HPI-A scores. Hearing aid wear time increased progressively from the post-wear times of the initial users to the wear times reported on the pre-HPI-As of the experienced users to the post-wear times of the latter. For patients receiving replacement aids, both the pre- and post-results showed a decrease in wear time above age 54. There is also a decrease in aid wear of roughly an hour per day per decade above age 55 which may have implications for hearing aid design and for the rehabilitative process. For instance, wear time is also influenced by "psycho-social" factors.

The relationship between severity ratings of hearing problems and hours of use of hearing aids was very complex. For all groups of persons, hours of wear increased as hearing loss increased. Problem scores went up only for inexperienced users. Age and employment increased problem scores, age decreased wear time, and employment increased wear time.

Table 2.1
Categories and Associated Percentage Scores for Use in Classifying HHS Performance (Schow and Tannahill, 1977)

Category	Percentage Scores
No handicap	0–20
Slight hearing handicap	21–40
Mild-moderate hearing handicap	41–70
Severe hearing handicap	71–100

Table 2.2
Summary of Means, Standard Deviations (S.D.), and Ranges for Various Groups of the Study with Respect to Age, Pure-Tone Average (PTA), and Quantified Denver Scores

Groups	N	Age			PTA[a]				Quan. Denver		
		Mean	S.D.	Range	Mean	S.D.	Mean	S.D.	Mean	S.D.	Range
		yr			dB				%		
Subgroup 1 (extremely sensitive hearing (0–15 dB HL))	14	43.5	20.3	19–74	10.8	4.3	14.1	5.8	6.5	8.4	0–25
Subgroup 2 (intermediate hearing sensitivity (16–26 dB HL))	20	59.9	13.6	32–78	22.3	4.4	23.0	4.5	21.3	24.2	0–77
Subgroup 3 (hearing-impaired (27–40 dB HL))	16	61.6	12.2	28–73	41.3	19.9	34.6	5.2	37.7	20.3	5–69
Total group	50	55.8	16.9	19–78	25.1	16.8	24.2	9.5	22.4	22.8	0–77

[a] Re ANSI, 1969.

The effect on problem perception and hearing aid use was shown to be greater for non-hearing loss factors, a finding consistent with other recent reports. For this reason, the primary goal of the hearing aid fitting, counselling, and adaptation process should be changed from that of maximizing the acoustical match of the aid to the patient to that of maximizing the number of hours the aid is worn by the person.

The Hearing Performance Inventory (HPI) was developed to assess hearing performance in problem communication areas experienced in everyday listening (Giolas *et al.*, 1979). The inventory items were divided into six categories: (1) understanding speech, (2) intensity, (3) response to auditory failure, (4) social, (5) personal, and (6) occupational. The authors indicated that the HPI is intended to provide the following.

1. An indication whether the hearing impairment has manifested itself as a communication problem.
2. A detailed analysis of the communication breakdown allowing a more tailor-made management program to emerge sooner than is now possible.
3. A quantitative measure of performance both for initial assessment and for evidence of progress.

The basic format of the HPI consists of presenting listeners with everyday situations and asking them to judge their listening performance according to the following categories: practically always, frequently, about half the time, occasionally, and almost never. Numbers from 1 to 5 are assigned to the descriptive categories for scoring and statistical summaries. Examples of items from the HIP are as follows.

1. You are with a male friend or family member in a fairly quiet room. Can you understand him when his voice is loud enough for you and you can see his face?
2. Can you understand what a woman is saying on the telephone when her voice is loud enough for you?
3. You are at home reading in a quiet room. Do you hear the telephone ring when it is in another room?
4. At the beginning of a conversation, do you let a stranger know that you have a hearing problem?
5. Does your hearing problem interfere with helping or instructing others on the job?

The present form of the inventory (Experimental Form II) consists of 158 items. Administration time is said to be about 30 to 45 minutes.

An example of the profile answer sheet for the HPI is shown in Fig. 2.2. The authors presently are obtaining additional normative data before making any revisions of the HPI. They indicate that the inventory can be useful as a tool at this time.

It appears that there are a number of ramifications in both the utilization and development of scales to assess hearing-impaired adults. There is a need to focus on the specific client problems and attitudes which may have developed from the sensory deficit of the auditory system.

We should consider the question of scale validity. Giolas (1970) put this problem in proper perspective when he stated:

The question of validity for any measure attempting to assess handicap can always be raised. The complexity of human behavior is such that cause and effect information of the type that is necessary when measuring the effect of a hearing loss on human behavior is almost impossible to demonstrate. On the other hand, such validity is not central in this situation. The goal is to obtain information about the kinds of problems a particular person is experiencing and not a measure of group or typical behaviors. All that is necessary are items representative of typical problems experienced by hard of hearing persons and good test—re-test reliability. In this way, reliable information about a particular person's hearing handicap can be ascertained in order to evolve a personalized rehabilitative program. When measuring progress, the individual can be used as his own control.

It should be stressed in this context that the above scales are subjective tools for the audiologist to use. Their successful use depends on the audiologists' judgment, not on tests of validity.

ATTITUDES AND PROBLEM ASSESSMENT

Two scales are recommended as part of a complete audiologic assessment: the McCarthy-Alpiner Scale of Hearing Handicap (the M-A Scale, 1980) and a measurement scale developed by Sanders (1975). The M-A Scale was designed to develop a measuring tool which would validly and reliably assess the psychologic, social and vocational effects of adult hearing loss.

HEARING PERFORMANCE INVENTORY (EXPERIMENTAL FORM II)

NAME ____________________ AGE ________ DATE ________

ADDRESS ____________________ PHONE ________

TEST LOCATION ____________________ SEX ________ MARITAL STATUS ________

EMPLOYED ____________ EDUCATION ____________ HEARING AID WEARER: Yes ☐ No ☐

PRIOR AURAL REHABILITATION COURSE EXPERIENCE? ____________ IF YES, WHEN? ________

Answer Sheet

	1 Practically Always	2 Frequently	3 About Half The Time	4 Occasionally	5 Almost Never		6 Does Not Apply		1 Practically Always	2 Frequently	3 About Half The Time	4 Occasionally	5 Almost Never		6 Does Not Apply
1.	☐	☐	☐	☐	☐	—	☐	33.	☐	☐	☐	☐	☐	—	☐
2.	☐	☐	☐	☐	☐	—	☐	34.	☐	☐	☐	☐	☐	—	☐
3.	☐	☐	☐	☐	☐	—	☐	35.	☐	☐	☐	☐	☐	—	☐
4.	☐	☐	☐	☐	☐	—	☐	36.	☐	☐	☐	☐	☐	—	☐
5.	☐	☐	☐	☐	☐	—	☐	37.	☐	☐	☐	☐	☐	—	☐
6.	☐	☐	☐	☐	☐	—	☐	38.	☐	☐	☐	☐	☐	—	☐
7.	☐	☐	☐	☐	☐	—	☐	39.	☐	☐	☐	☐	☐	—	☐
8.	☐	☐	☐	☐	☐	—	☐	40.	☐	☐	☐	☐	☐	—	☐
9.	☐	☐	☐	☐	☐	—	☐	41.	☐	☐	☐	☐	☐	—	☐
10.	☐	☐	☐	☐	☐	—	☐	42.	☐	☐	☐	☐	☐	—	☐
11.	☐	☐	☐	☐	☐	—	☐	43.	☐	☐	☐	☐	☐	—	☐
12.	☐	☐	☐	☐	☐	—	☐	44.	☐	☐	☐	☐	☐	—	☐
13.	☐	☐	☐	☐	☐	—	☐	45.	☐	☐	☐	☐	☐	—	☐
14.	☐	☐	☐	☐	☐	—	☐	46.	☐	☐	☐	☐	☐	—	☐
15.	☐	☐	☐	☐	☐	—	☐	47.	☐	☐	☐	☐	☐	—	☐
16.	☐	☐	☐	☐	☐	—	☐	48.	☐	☐	☐	☐	☐	—	☐
17.	☐	☐	☐	☐	☐	—	☐	49.	☐	☐	☐	☐	☐	—	☐
18.	☐	☐	☐	☐	☐	—	☐	50.	☐	☐	☐	☐	☐	—	☐
19.	☐	☐	☐	☐	☐	—	☐	51.	☐	☐	☐	☐	☐	—	☐
20.	☐	☐	☐	☐	☐	—	☐	52.	☐	☐	☐	☐	☐	—	☐
21.	☐	☐	☐	☐	☐	—	☐	53.	☐	☐	☐	☐	☐	—	☐
22.	☐	☐	☐	☐	☐	—	☐	54.	☐	☐	☐	☐	☐	—	☐
23.	☐	☐	☐	☐	☐	—	☐	55.	☐	☐	☐	☐	☐	—	☐
24.	☐	☐	☐	☐	☐	—	☐	56.	☐	☐	☐	☐	☐	—	☐
25.	☐	☐	☐	☐	☐	—	☐	57.	☐	☐	☐	☐	☐	—	☐
26.	☐	☐	☐	☐	☐	—	☐	58.	☐	☐	☐	☐	☐	—	☐
27.	☐	☐	☐	☐	☐	—	☐	59.	☐	☐	☐	☐	☐	—	☐
28.	☐	☐	☐	☐	☐	—	☐	60.	☐	☐	☐	☐	☐	—	☐
29.	☐	☐	☐	☐	☐	—	☐	61.	☐	☐	☐	☐	☐	—	☐
30.	☐	☐	☐	☐	☐	—	☐	62.	☐	☐	☐	☐	☐	—	☐
31.	☐	☐	☐	☐	☐	—	☐	63.	☐	☐	☐	☐	☐	—	☐
32.	☐	☐	☐	☐	☐	—	☐	64.	☐	☐	☐	☐	☐	—	☐

Figure 2.2. Answer Sheet for Hearing Performance Inventory (Experimental Form II). (Reprinted by permission from Giolas, T. G., Owens, E., Lamb, S. H., and Schubert, E. D., Hearing performance inventory. *J. Speech Hear. Disord.*, **44,** 169–195, 1979.)

In order to test the validity of the scale, it was proposed that a family member also complete a parallel form of the scale. By correlating the responses of the hearing-impaired individual with a family member, it was hypothesized that the validity of the items could be assessed. This method was based on the Campbell and Fiske (1959) multitrait-multimethod matrix analysis which requires independent methods of measurement. In this study, the responses of the family member and the hearing-impaired individual were used to measure convergent validity. In addition to measuring the validity of the scale, it was felt that use of a family member would be the initial, formal attempt to quantify the feelings of the family members of hearing-impaired individuals.

PILOT STUDY

Initially, 100 items representing psychologic, social, and vocational effects of hearing loss were generated and organized into a self-assessment scale format. Items were presented in statement form to which the subject responded always, usually, sometimes, rarely, or never. Wording of the items included positive and negative directions with the response representing the greatest handicap equal to 5 points.

The first procedure in the pilot study involved determining optimal "recall time" in order to measure test-retest reliability for the 100 items. The scale was administered and a randomized version of the scale was readministered to normal hearing subjects at varying time intervals. Subjects were required to indicate how many of the items were remembered by them during the second administration of the scale. A criterion of 5% was set for the total number of allowable remembered items. Optimal "recall time" was defined as that time period which came closest to achieving the 5% criterion and yet, did not introduce internal validity problems (history, maturation, etc). Two weeks was determined to be the optimal "recall time" for this scale.

The scale was then administered to 100 adults (21–50 years) with acquired sensorineural hearing loss ($\geq$30 dB at 2 or more octave interval frequencies 250–4000 Hz in the better ear according to ANSI, 1969). A randomized form of the scale was readministered after 2 weeks. From the responses, Pearson product-moment correlation coefficients were computed for each of the items in order to determine test-retest reliability of the 100 original items. Thirty-four items fit the proposed criteria with $\geq$0.80 correlation. Internal consistency reliability using Cronbach's alpha method was shown to fit the criteria ($\geq$0.80) for the psychologic, social, and vocational traits. Items which did not fit the criteria were eliminated from the scale with the remaining 34 items incorporated into a scale which was used in the formal study (Appendix 2G).

FORMAL STUDY

The purpose of the formal study was to determine the validity of each of the items. Validity was measured by using the multitrait-multimethod matrix analysis (Campbell and Fiske, 1959). This statistical method is based on 4 aspects of the validation process. First, validation is typically convergent, a confirmation by independent methods of measurement. Second, discriminant validity is needed so tests will not be invalidated by too high correlations with other tests from which they are supposed to differ. Third, each trait measured is influenced by the method of measurement resulting in a "trait-method" unit. And fourth, in order to examine discriminant validity and to estimate the relative contributions of trait and method variance, it is necessary to use more than one trait and more than one measurement method. In order to implement these four aspects of validation, a matrix incorporating the intercorrelations of each of the traits and each of the methods is devised.

In this study, the traits being measured were the psychologic, social, and vocational effects of acquired sensorineural hearing loss. The two methods used were the administration of the scale to both the hearing impaired subject and to a family member. These family members had to be adults who resided in the same household as the subject. The family members were given an identical form of the scale, but written in the third person (Appendix 2H). No collaboration was allowed.

The three traits were then measured by the two methods, generating six variables. The correlations were set up into a matrix table for analysis. In addition, partial correlation coefficients were generated partialling on the variables of age, hearing aid use, and degree of hearing impairment. Matrices were produced for each of these analyses.

Reliability results using Cronbach's alpha method for internal consistency showed high correlations for each of the traits measured for the self-assessment and family member assessment. However, results of the multi-trait-multimethod analysis showed a general lack of convergent or discriminant validity for the psychologic, social, or vocational traits. That is, the general level of agreement in responses between subjects and family members was consistently low. Negatively worded items appeared to show higher correlations, but did not meet the requirements for convergent or discriminant validity. In addition, the variables of age, degree of hearing loss, and hearing aid usage did not have an influence on the validity of the items.

While several factors may have contributed to the lack of validity, it appears that perhaps the most dominant factor is the difference in perception between the subject and his family. This study required that the subject introspectively respond about his own feelings and behaviors while the family member was asked to objectively respond about the hearing-impaired individual's feelings and behaviors. Their perspectives, of course, were from totally different viewpoints. Each individual's perceptions of the situation were shaped by his own life experience. It cannot be stated, therefore, that one's perception of a situation was correct while the other individual's was inaccurate.

The rehabilitative purpose of the scale was to validly define areas of difficulty caused by hearing impairment. However, even though validity was not shown through a level of agreement between subjects and family members, it cannot be conclusively stated that these items do not represent problem areas or that these problem areas do not exist. Rather, the results obtained may have uncovered other problem areas associated with hearing loss and may present a more important use for the scale.

Several limitations in the interpretation of the hearing scale appear to emerge: (1) the hearing-impaired individual's failure to accept, understand, or deal with his hearing problems while the member of his family is keenly aware of the handicapping effects, (2) the family member's inability to recognize, understand, or deal with the individual's hearing impairment, (3) the failure of the two persons to agree on what are the problem areas, and (4) any combination of the above three.

Because the individuals in this study were closely involved in the problems being examined, it may be erroneous to assume that one's response can either validate or invalidate the other's responses. Therefore, the low correlations obtained may not have been due to the invalidity of the scale items themselves, but rather to the method used to measure validity.

Despite the negative findings relative to validity, several positive findings arose from this study. These findings not only offer immediate clinical applicability for aural rehabilitation, but also offer directions for additional research.

Perhaps the most significant information obtained in this study related to the counseling needs for both hearing-impaired individuals and family members. Pollack (1978) has stated that any counseling of the hearing-impaired individual should involve the family. This study represents the initial effort to systematically determine the attitudes and relationships of family members with hearing-impaired individuals. The low level of agreement of responses in this study supports the need to include family members in the rehabilitation process. Family involvement can contribute to a more complete rehabilitation program for hearing-impaired persons.

It appears that this scale fulfills at least 3 objectives. It provides an index of whether the organic hearing loss has manifested itself as a handicap, it provides diagnostic data with rehabilitative implications, and the information provided by the scale provides for a detailed analysis of psychologic, social, and vocational problem areas. Future research should focus on quantifying a client's progress as the result of aural rehabilitation and/or hearing aid usage. Further, research is needed to assess the impact of each of the individual items.

This study demonstrates the present clinical application of the scale. It is suggested that the scale routinely be administered to both hearing-impaired adults and family members. A comparison of the responses can outline problem areas of difficulty which can be addressed in the therapy process.

The second measurement scale recommended was developed by Sanders (1975). The three profile questionnaires (Appendices 2I to 2K) to be used with adults rate communicative performance in the home, occupational, and social environments. Using both scales should enable the audiologist to subjectively assess attitudes caused by hearing impairment and the specific communication difficulties encountered. When these scales are given pre- and post-remediation, we may plan therapy and evaluate its success in terms of the client's individual needs. Regarding the use of scales, Sanders (1975) stated:

The Audiologist must decide for himself how to generate needed information. He should, however, seek information about both performance and attitudes. Compare, for example, the outline I have suggested with the information obtained by the Denver Scale. Notice that although these two approaches seek to achieve the same goal, the Denver Scale approaches the task in a different manner. The information it generates is heavily weighted in terms of how the client feels about the effect of his hearing loss on his performance in communication and how he feels others react to him. It provides valuable information for adjustment counseling that my outlines do not generate. On the other hand, the Denver Scale does not provide specific information about specific types of situations peculiar to a particular person's environment. For this reason, I feel these two approaches are complementary, with only a small area of overlap.

We believe that the M-A Scale fulfills, in similar manner, the original concept of the Denver Scale. Use of the recommended instruments (McCarthy and Alpiner, 1980; Sanders, 1975) constitutes part of a diagnostic rehabilitative battery allowing audiologists to assess attitudes as well as specific difficulties confronting the hearing-impaired adult.

ASSESSMENT OF LIPREADING ABILITY

Lipreading or speech reading can be defined as the skill enabling a person, regardless of his hearing ability, to understand language by attentively observing the speaker (Hardy, 1970). Ideally, lipreading implies visual comprehension for an auditory deficit, either partially or completely. Historically, Trask (1917) proposed levels of lipreading ability.

1. Good lipreading ability. The lipreader can understand most people with whom he comes in contact. He can sometimes follow sermons or lectures.
2. Fair lipreading ability. The lipreader has little difficulty in understanding his family or friends.
3. Poor lipreading ability. The lipreader can understand a few people readily and a few more a little.

In more contemporary terminology, Jeffers and Barley (1971) relate lipreading to a total process which involves three steps: (1) sensory reception of the motor or movement pattern, (2) perception of the pattern, and (3) association of the pattern with meaningful concepts.

They emphasize that the reader of speech movements is receiving limited visual information. The lipreader must mentally "fill in" information not received in order to complete the process indicated. The hearing-impaired adult is told that it is important to understand the thought or idea of the communication conveyed to him; it is not necessary to identify every spoken word. This concept is theoretically sound but, unfortunately, data are lacking to validate this process.

O'Neill and Oyer (1981) provide several reasons for the use of lipreading tests.

1. They are useful in the measurement of basic lipreading ability.
2. They can be used as instruments to measure the effects of lipreading training. Although one cannot always be certain of all the factors that bring about improvement, many persons will increase their skills as a result of practice.
3. They can be used in the proper placement of individuals within a training program. For diagnostic purposes, it is necessary to categorize the acoustically handicapped who are excellent, average, and poor lipreaders.
4. They can be used to help decide which teaching methods, or combinations of methods, are most appropriate.

The difficulties of relying solely on the visual modality for understanding speech are borne out in a study on perceptual features of lipreading (Farran and Danhauer, 1978). Ninety young, adult, normal-hearing college-age students served as subjects. The stimuli consisted of 24 inter-vocalic English sounds presented in the context /a C (consonant) a/. The consonants were /p, b, t, d, k, g, f, v,

θ, ð, s, z, ʃ, ʒ, tʃ, dʒ, m, n, y, r, l, w, j, h/. Four randomized lists, each containing the 24 phonemes, were constructed. The stimuli were presented on videotape using a 24-inch video monitor. Four subjects were tested at one presentation and seated about 5 feet from the monitor. The results of this study indicated subject use of distinctive features in perceptual judgments. Features relating to the visual modality were heavily weighted such as closed-bilabial, velar, dental, labial, and easy-to-see/hard-to-see, relating more to place of articulation than to manner and voicing characteristics. Phonemes produced toward the front of the mouth were categorized as easy to see: /r, w, p, b, m, dʒ, tʃ, ʃ, θ, ð, f, v/. Those described as hard to see included /s, z, t, d, ʒ, m, g, h, l, k, j/. Further, the results show that all but about 30% of these stimuli can be correctly identified and suggest that other sensory modalities such as audition can be helpful to the hearing-impaired in understanding speech. These results are generally similar to those found by Woodward and Barber (1960), Erber (1975), Walden et al. (1974b), and Danhauer and Appel (1976) regarding the place of articulation feature in lipreading.

With knowledge of these concepts of lipreading, it is necessary to examine different ways it can be measured. Reference may be made to studies in which lipreading tests, without voice, were administered to adults (Jeffers and Barley, 1971; DiCarlo and Kataja, 1951; Jeffers and Barley, 1967; Lowell, 1958; Taaffe, 1957). These studies evaluated the Barley Speechreading Test, the John Tracy Clinic Test, and the Utley Lipreading Test. In these studies, scoring was not based on correct identification of the thought or idea of each sentence but only on the number of words identified correctly in each sentence. This evaluation approach is contrary to the definition of lipreading (the emphasis is how well individuals understand communication, not individual words).

Erber (1977) has proposed a conceptual model for the evaluation of lipreading. Although this model is designed for children, it may have clinical application for use with adults. This system previously has been used for auditory tasks. A simple matrix (Fig. 2.3) summarizes the variety of the different types of speech stimuli which can be used: speech

	SPEECH ELEMENTS	SYLLABLES	WORDS	PHRASES	SENTENCES	CONNECTED DISCOURSE
DETECTION						
DISCRIMINATION						
RECOGNITION						
COMPREHENSION						

Figure 2.3. A lipreading skills matrix for hearing-impaired children. The child's visual speech-perception abilities are evaluated at each level of stimulus/response complexity. These measures are used to specify goals for instruction in visual communication.

elements, syllables, words, phrases, sentences, and connected discourse. There are four response tasks used in this matrix: detection, discrimination, recognition, and comprehension. Each box in Fig. 2.3 describes the interaction between a particular type of visual speech stimulus and a specific manner of response. Detection is the ability to respond differently to the presence and absence of speech articulation. Visual detection of articulatory movements should result in the individual orienting to the speaker's mouth for gaining more information from him visually as well as indicating the presence of post-dental consonants in certain vowel contexts. Discrimination requires a same-different response or the ability to perceive similarities and differences between two or more speech samples. Recognition is the ability to reproduce a visual speech stimulus by naming or identifying it in some way. Comprehension is the ability to understand the meaning of speech stimuli within an individual's language ability. The information obtained from the use of this procedure may be helpful in planning aural rehabilitative therapy.

Another application was suggested by Dodds and Harford (1968) in a study using the Utley test as part of a hearing aid evaluation. This test was used to evaluate how well clients understand sentences under visual and auditory-visual conditions. In this study, Form A of the Utley sentence test was presented unaided, and Form B was presented with auditory and visual cues. The latter condition resulted in greater understanding of the stimuli materials.

To assist in homogeneous therapy placement, Donnelly and Marshall (1971) used the John Tracy Film Test of Lipreading as a multiple-choice test for a college age deaf population. The emphasis in this study was how well individuals understood sentences as opposed to isolated words, the important consideration in lipreading evaluation.

A variety of reliable lipreading tests is available and the choice of which measuring instrument to use will probably be made according to the personal preference of the audiologist. Whether the test will be presented live, or by film, and whether or not sound will be used will also be at the discretion of the audiologist.

Although film or videotape administrations are more standardized, there are some questions regarding their use. Production qualities of film tests can leave much to be desired. Criticisms include the following.

1. The distractions caused by the tester on the film holding up a card with the number of the item.
2. The stolid appearance of the presenter.
3. The usual presentation mode of showing the speaker from the shoulders upward.
4. The erratic rate of presentation of stimulus materials.
5. The dated clothing and hair styles which may prove distracting to the client.

These factors create an artificial test environment. In addition, as indicated by Jeffers and Barley (1967, 1971), it appears that a live presentation yields significantly better scores than a film presentation.

Obviously, there are limitations to any manner of presentation. The personal preference of this writer is to present lipreading tests through a live modality. This approach requires considerable practice on the part of the audiologist. Items should be presented in as true-to-life a manner as possible since in the environment this is the way in which clients ultimately receive communication.

A lipreading test for adults was devised at the University of Denver Speech and Hearing Center. The Denver Quick Test of Lipreading Ability (Table 2.3) is comprised of 20 com-

Table 2.3
The Denver Quick Test of Lipreading Ability

University of Denver Speech and Hearing Center The Denver Scale Quick Test Answer Key
Rehabilitative Audiology (adults)

1. Good morning.
2. How old are you?
3. I live in (state of residence).
4. I only have one dollar.
5. There is somebody at the door.
6. Is that all?
7. Where are you going?
8. Let's have a coffee break.
9. Park your car in the lot.
10. What is your address?
11. May I help you?
12. I feel fine.
13. It is time for dinner.
14. Turn right at the corner.
15. Are you ready to order?
16. Is this charge or cash?
17. What time is it?
18. I have a headache.
19. How about going out tonight?
20. Please lend me 50 cents.

mon, everyday expressions and scored on the basis of correct identification of the thought or idea of the sentence. Each sentence has a value of 5%. The Quick Test was administered live, without voice, to 40 hearing-impaired adults. Results were compared to scores for the Utley Sentence Test, presented live, without voice. Correlation between the two tests was 0.90, indicating good reliability.

Our own experience in utilizing lipreading tests, under a visual-only condition, continues to show no outstanding improvement in lipreading ability when comparing pre-service scores to post-service scores. Further, there does not appear to be any relationship between scores on lipreading tests and success in communication ability as determined by assessment scales of communication function.

This pattern, i.e. lack of significant improvement with the use of the visual modality, has been observed regardless of the lipreading test used. This was consistent with clients' subjective opinions that they had made substantial improvement as communicators. Although the clients were not good lipreaders, they reported they were better communicators.

Why should we administer lipreading tests in the visual only condition? They have been used as a diagnostic tool. Low scores suggest that lipreading instruction should be continued to improve the visual perception of speech. It is assumed that clients who score well in the visual only modality have less difficulty understanding communication and should have fewer concomitant difficulties often associated with hearing loss. Continuing research is suggested so that clients may be evaluated on a longitudinal basis.

BISENSORY EVALUATION

This writer feels that testing in a visual-only condition is not adequate. Assessment should utilize a bisensory evaluation, allowing the client to utilize both his visual and auditory modalities. Binnie (1973) indicates that auditory-visual scores might suggest how individuals receive person-to-person speech in general conversation situations. Since this is the general mode of communication for most people, the information would be useful to the clinician in planning a realistic remediation program. In addition, further diagnostic information becomes available to the clinician regarding the contribution of audition to the visual modality.

In this approach to lipreading evaluation, test materials can be presented not only in a quiet condition, but in the presence of different background noises which often create major difficulties for the hearing-impaired adult. Numerous clients state that they seem to do well in one-to-one quiet environmental situations, but simply cannot understand what is being said when there is background noise. Binnie (1973) demonstrates the benefits of the bisensory approach. He states that the level at which the best auditory-visual score is obtained may serve as the starting point for rehabilitative audiology. The data in Tables 2.4 and 2.5 show the effects of auditory and auditory-visual presentations at various sensation levels.

With a combined sensory modality presentation, the contribution of visual speech cues to auditory-visual speech perception was found to increase as the speech-to-noise (s/n) ratio was decreased (O'Neill, 1954). In other words, as noise increased, the visual modality played a greater role in the individual's understanding of speech. In a study by Sanders

Table 2.4
Effect of Auditory Presentations at Various Sensation Levels[a]

Sensation Level of Presentation*	AUDITORY Sensorineural Loss Cases					Mean Scores for Normals
	1	2	3	4	5	
	%					%
0	30	22	20	46	42	21
8	64	40	46	86	38	59
16	74	62	60	90	54	80
24	84	84	78	94	36	94

* Re: Sound field SRT.
[a] Reprinted by permission from Binnie, C. A., *J. Acad. Rehab. Audiol.*, **6**, 43–53, copyright 1973, *Journal of the Academy of Rehabilitative Audiology.*

Table 2.5
Effect of Audio-Visual Presentations at Various Sensations Levels[a]

Sensation Level of Presentation*	AUDIO-VISUAL Sensorineural Loss Cases					Mean Scores for Normals
	1	2	3	4	5	
	%					%
−20	22	14	12	8	18	23
0	66	58	46	76	72	57
8	70	76	68	84	84	85
16	88	82	86	98	74	94

* Re: Sound field SRT.
[a] Reprinted by permission from Binnie, C. A., *J. Acad. Rehab. Audiol.*, **6**, 45–53, copyright 1973, *Journal of the Academy of Rehabilitative Audiology.*

and Goodrich (1971), speech was presented through a 400-Hz low-pass filter. Recognition of words increased from 24 to 78% with the addition of vision to the perception process. Neely (1956) found that addition of visual cues to auditory cues increased the intelligibility of received speech by approximately 20%.

Sumby and Pollack (1954) found an increase in intelligibility scores when audition was supplemented with vision. They indicated that, as the S/N ratio decreases, the importance of visual cues to listener intelligibility increases. Prall (1957) found significant differences in intelligibility of speech through combined audio-visual channels when compared to audition or vision only. Hutton (1959) and Hutton *et al.* (1959) found that more information was received by auditory stimuli than by visual stimuli, but both separately fell short of the scores obtained by using combined methods. Siegenthaler and Gruber (1969) indicate that the use of audition and vision combined resulted in higher scores by 19% than when either vision or lipreading was used alone.

Walden *et al.* (1974a) found that hearing-impaired adults were able to distinguish visually within the Woodward and Barber consonant categories (1960). These consonant categories are as follows.

1. Bi-labial: /p, b, m/
2. Rounded labial: /ʍ, w, r/
3. Labio-dental: /f, v/
4. Non-labial: /t, d, n, θ, ð, ʃ, h, dʒ, s, z, k, n, ʒ, g/

Brannon (1961) indicates that words of less visibility are harder to lipread than words of greater visibility. His study suggests that a synthetic approach to lipreading, in which additional clues are provided, is more effective for developing lipreading ability.

The research cited emphasizes the need to evaluate lipreading through a bisensory approach. Since most persons perceive speech in this way, it would appear to be a realistic consideration. Erber (1975) states that most clinical evaluations have been dominated by auditory measures, often to the exclusion of testing visual and auditory-visual capabilities.

The work of Binnie *et al.* (1974) provides substantive data for bisensory assessment. They studied 16 consonants in which 5 distinct homophonous categories were apparent.

1. Bi-labials: /p, b, m/
2. Labio-dentals: /f, v/
3. Interdentals: /θ, ð/
4. Rounded labials: /ʃ, ʒ/
5. Linguals: /s, z, t, d, n, k, g/

Stimuli were presented in auditory, auditory-visual, auditory in quiet, and visual-only conditions. S/N ratios used for auditory and auditory-visual conditions were −18 dB, −12 dB, and −6 dB, employing a broad-band masking noise. The results of their study demonstrate that identification of consonants under noise conditions improves significantly with vision. The auditory-visual condition approaches the results of materials presented in quiet. The visual-only condition indicates

the difficulties posed when relying only on this modality. Table 2.6 summarizes their results.

As indicated by the research of Woodward and Barber (1960), Walden *et al.* (1974a), and Binnie *et al.* (1974); subjects were able to distinguish consonants within group categories. That is, they could identify whether a consonant fell into a certain homophonous category. For this reason, Binnie *et al.* (1974) suggested that the primary emphasis in hearing rehabilitation should be on auditory training. Most normal and hearing-impaired persons obtain near perfect lipreading results in identifying place of articulation.

Erber's research (1975) suggests that evaluation of each client's auditory-visual perception of speech can be helpful in the following areas.

1. Most hearing-impaired patients typically receive speech through both auditory and visual modalities during everyday communication. This means they usually watch the speaker's mouth and face to maximize perception of speech information. Auditory-visual evaluation in the clinic can give the audiologist a valid estimate of the patient's ability to communicate socially in this manner.

2. Auditory-visual testing may provide a more realistic indication of how much more a hearing aid helps a patient than would auditory testing alone, especially for profoundly deaf persons who typically score low on auditory word identification tests. Research is required to determine whether it

Table 2.6
Results of Stimuli Presentations under Auditory, Auditory-Visual, Auditory in Quiet, and Visual-Only Conditions[a]

Condition	Correct Responses
	%
Auditory	
S/N ratio: −18	6
S/N ratio: −12	34
S/N ratio: −6	54
Auditory-visual	
S/N ratio: −18	47.7
S/N ratio: −12	83.5
S/N ratio: −6	88.7
Auditory in quiet	95
Visual only (overall)	43.2

[a] Reprinted by permission from Binnie, C. A., Montgomery, A. A., and Jackson, P. L., *J. Speech Hear. Res.*, **17**, 619–630, copyright 1974, *Journal of Speech and Hearing Research.*

is possible to select aids for profoundly deaf individuals by comparing their aided auditory-visual results with their lipreading scores for the same speech material.

3. If single speech elements are used as test stimuli, an analytic evaluation of the auditory and visual errors in recognition can help the audiologist determine how well the patient uses two types of sensory information to complement one another. The test results may suggest to the clinician whether the patient should receive rehabilitative emphasis in the auditory or visual modality.

4. Often, a moderately hearing-impaired patient needs to be convinced of the value of using lipreading in combination with listening through his hearing aid. A comparison of his auditory-visual score with his auditory only performance usually will demonstrate to him that he has some lipreading ability and can benefit from its use.

5. Conversely, a profoundly deaf person may reject the use of a hearing aid because of his inability to understand speech through it alone. The patient may be motivated to attend to acoustic cues, if it can be demonstrated that his speech comprehension improves when he uses the aid in combination with lipreading. It would appear that vision plays a significant role in the communication process, when utilized with audition, even though the interaction between these two modalities is not fully understood.

The data indicate that we can teach hearing-impaired adults to recognize the difference between homophonous sound categories. This information suggests the value of lipreading in therapy. The assumption is that in difficult communication situations, chances for understanding everyday communication will be improved. Fewer alternatives will be available to the client in determining what is being said. An example is "Please turn on the fan. It is very hot." If the hearing-impaired adult is able to understand everything with the expection of "fan," recognition may be made on the basis of knowing the /f/ and /v/ homophonous category with regard to articulatory placement. When the options are "fan" or "van," through available alternatives, it becomes obvious that the "fan needs to be turned on for it to be cooler."

To assess basic lipreading ability in the rehabilitative diagnosis of clients, it is recommended that the lipreading screening test devised by Binnie et al. (1976) be employed for consonant categories. The test consists of nine homophonous categories.

1. /f, v/
2. /p, b, m/
3. /w/
4. /l, n/
5. /ʃ, ʒ/
6. /r/
7. /θ, ð/
8. /t, d, s, z/
9. /k, g/

The consonants are used with the carrier /a/ so that syllables are presented to each client in an attempt to evaluate his recognition ability. The authors of this research utilized videotape for presentation of the screening test. In this study, traditional orthography was used since most of the clients would not be familiar with the International Phonetic Symbols. Information provided allows the audiologist to plan therapy according to the client's deficits in phoneme recognition. The remediation process should result in improvement of overall lipreading ability.

We have data regarding the ability to lipread phonemes according to homophonous categories. There are inadequate data about the relationship between phoneme recognition and the ability to comprehend everyday communication. Real-life situations demand that hearing-impaired individuals understand continuous speech discourse. Clinical experience has shown that clients can perceive differences in sounds according to homophonous categories. More difficulty is encountered in understanding what is said on a day-to-day basis at work, home, or in a variety of social situations.

Clients often indicate that they experience little difficulty recognizing sounds in isolated categories in therapy. Their attempts to follow general conversation in the outside environment, however, are frustated because the rate of the typical speaker may be either too fast or too slow, or his enunciation poor. In addition, it is sometimes difficult to understand what is being said because after every word in a sentence there is a shift of articulators when no sound is being conveyed. The client attempts to identify a sound when none is being produced. For example, view the sentence, "It is cold outside." Client frustration occurs when trying to identify sounds between the words "it," "is," "cold," and "outside." This example is not used to negate the value of lipreading, but to illustrate the difficulties faced by clients.

It is recommended that client evaluation should include assessment of understanding general speech discourse through both auditory and auditory-visual tests of lipreading. The Denver Lipreading Quick Test has proved useful for this. Although other lipreading tests might also provide significant information on overall lipreading performance, lipreading tests should be complemented by communication assessment scales to provide more comprehensive diagnostic and prognostic information.

ASSESSMENT OF AUDITORY DISCRIMINATION

Auditory discrimination may be defined as the ability to hear and understand clearly the sounds which make up our speech and language. Many of us have encountered the classic statement, "I hear you but I just don't understand clearly everything you say." Lack of good discrimination ability results in perceptual confusions and distortions which may inhibit or reduce the understanding of the language. This may occur whether amplification is being utilized or not. A hearing aid is an electronic device that can make speech sufficiently loud but not necessarily clear. The speech signal is still being transmitted for interpretation to the brain by way of a damaged or degenerated auditory mechanism. Persons with discrimination problems caused by hearing loss are often frustrated by this inability to hear speech clearly.

Nerbonne and Schow (1980) emphasize that an integral part of any auditory training program is the assessment of the client's performance. They cite several reasons for assessing auditory discrimination ability.

1. To determine whether or not auditory training appears warranted.
2. To provide a basis for comparing, following a period of therapy, the amount of improvement in speech perception, that has occurred.
3. To identify specific areas of speech perception difficulties that can be concentrated on in future auditory training work.

Oyer and Frankmann (1975) indicated that the primary areas of concern regarding the need for auditory training are.

1. Confusions among various sounds due to the condition of the sensorineural hearing mechanism.
2. Adjustment problems in the utilization of amplification systems due to recruitment problems.
3. Adjustment problems due to amplification

because of speech sounding unnatural (hearing aids are not precise replacements for abnormally functioning ears).

Poor discrimination results from sensorineural impairment. The individual with a conductive loss of hearing is not usually confronted with this difficulty since the etiology of the impairment is in the outer or middle ear. Once speech has been made sufficiently loud, it can be understood.

Discrimination testing may be the most useful procedure utilized in routine audiologic assessment for evaluating the communication capability of an individual. Ideally, as stated by Goetzinger (1972), ". . . the purpose of word discrimination testing is to determine how well an individual functions in a society in which the basic mode of communication is through speech." Owens (1978) analyzed consonant errors of hearing-impaired subjects and showed that 14 consonants caused most of the difficulty in consonant recognition. This study constitutes (1) a summary of auditory consonant recognition errors in a multiple choice word format for persons with sensorineural hearing loss and (2) a consideration of implications for remediation.

Items for this study consisted of a battery of consonant-vowel-consonant words. The initial position consonants show lower error-probabilities than their counterparts in the final position. Place errors were the most frequent but manner errors also were noted frequently. Substitutions tended to be the same over a wide range of pure tone configurations. Therefore, only in a few instances would the type of configuration of a given subject be of any special help in predicting those consonants particularly difficult to recognize.

This study demonstrated that auditory recognition of consonants can be improved by training. This program consists of two specially adapted cassette recorders used in combination. The control tape, recorded in the playback mode, presented each successive item through a speaker system. If the response was incorrect, the client depressed the pause button on the control recorder, automatically stopping it. The other recorder then played it back once every 10 seconds until the subject disengaged the pause button.

Visual recognition errors of normal hearers were consistent among consonants within visual groups. An approach directed to enhancement or sharpening of the recognition of consonants, *per se*, may contribute substantially to speech perception ability.

Another aspect of consonants as they relate to speech perception is the frequency of their occurrence in everyday speech. The consonants /j, n, w, r, h, l, m/ are the most easily recognized auditorily by hearing-impaired persons. The consonants /t, d, s, k, z/, on the other hand, provide auditory as well as visual difficulty. The /s/ emerges as the most troublesome in speech perception. Along with /s/ is the cognate /z/ with /k/ close behind. Owens (1978) proposes that it might be helpful to devote part of aural rehabilitation to direct auditory training work with consonants.

A variety of stimulus materials exists to ascertain an individual's discrimination ability. There is not agreement on which is best. The stimuli are presented at a level above speech reception threshold at which the client indicates speech sounds comfortable to him. Words and sentences from several sources are used for discrimination testing (Egan, 1948; Hirsh et al., 1952; Jerger et al., 1968; Tillman and Carhart, 1966; Owens and Schubert, 1977; Kalikow et al., 1977; House et al., 1965; Schultz and Schubert, 1969). We will discuss auditory discrimination assessment for purposes of therapy.

DISCRMINATION MEASUREMENT

We recommend that the audiologist evaluate the client's confusion with individual sounds and general speech discourse for the purpose of planning auditory training. Sound confusions may be assessed on the monosyllabic words used in discrimination testing. We can opt to indicate sound errors as well as whether or not a word was correctly identified. From List 1 of the Northwestern University Word Test Number 6 (Tillman and Carhart, 1966), for example, the following four words were used: bean, burn, knock, and moon. Hypothetical responses might be: bead, bird, dock, and mood. While scoring, we note that /d/ is confused with /n/. Therapy would be planned to emphasize the auditory differences between the two sounds. Discrimination word tests, already a part of the audiologic assessment battery, may be utilized. The same purpose can be accomplished with any discrimination test used in an audiologic battery. For more intensive discrimination testing between consonants, the Larson Sound Discrimination Test (Fig. 2.4) is recommended (Larson, 1950).

The California Consonant Test (CCT) also allows for the identification of discrimination errors. List 1 of the CCT is found in Appendix 2L. Schwartz and Surr (1979) conducted three experiments using the CCT. The studies were designed to (1) determine the performance intensity function for the CCT, (2) compare performance scores on the CCT with those on the Northwestern University (NU) Number 6 lists, and (3) examine internal consistency and split-half reliability of forms one and two of the CCT. The stimuli materials consisted of CCT forms one and two and recordings of the NU Number 6.

In experiment one, 12 normal hearers, 6 males and 6 females, and 12 males with sensorineural hearing loss comprised the subjects. Word/consonant discrimination was assessed with forms one and two of the CCT which were divided into four lists of 50 words. Each subject recorded written responses on a standard answer form that was presented at increasingly higher sensation levels from 0 dB to 50 dB. Preliminary data suggested that the CCT is particularly sensitive to the phoneme recognition difficulties of persons with high frequency hearing loss and would be capable of differentiating between normal hearing and those with high frequency hearing loss.

In experiment two, a comparison was made of performance scores achieved on the CCT to those obtained with the NU Auditory Test Number 6, to explore further the assumption that the CCT is a more sensitive index of minor deficits in phoneme discrimination than the NU Number 6 list for listeners with high frequency sensorineural hearing loss. The subjects were 60 males ranging in age from 20 to 78 years of age. The recorded speech materials consisted of Lists 1–4, Form B of the NU 6 lists. The subjects were subcategorized into four groups of 15 subjects such that each was assigned to receive one of four 50 word lists in a counterbalanced fashion.

The data were first analyzed for the four groups independently. The group means did not differ significantly and, therefore, the data were pooled for further examination. These data suggest that the CCT was more

Score: (Errors)

Name_____ With Aid _____

Date_____ Without Aid _____

Directions to be Given the Listener: Draw a line through the words that are pronounced to you from each box.

Box 1 f and ch		Box 2 l and z		Box 3 l and n		Box 4 d and n		Box 5 m and l	
few	chew	lip	zip	lame	name	dot	not	mine	line
fin	chin	loan	zone	light	night	die	nigh	mast	last
filed	child	dale	daze	loan	known	deed	need	moan	loan
calf	catch	mail	maze	pail	pain	ode	own	name	nail
four	chore	hail	haze	rail	rain	did	din	home	hole

Box 6 b and m		Box 7 l and v		Box 8 k and g		Box 9 p and b		Box 10 m and v	
bill	mill	lane	vane	coal	goal	pin	bin	mice	vice
boast	most	lie	vie	came	game	pie	by	ham	have
bake	make	lace	vase	coat	goat	pole	bowl	glum	glove
robe	roam	lull	love	luck	lug	cap	cap	mine	vine
tab	tam	rail	rave	rack	rag	rope	robe	mile	vile

Box 11 n and v		Box 12 sh and f		Box 13 f and k		Box 14 f and b		Box 15 s and sh	
nice	vice	show	foe	fit	kit	fun	bun	lease	leash
nurse	verse	shore	fore	four	core	fig	big	sew	show
nine	vine	shade	fade	find	kind	cuff	cub	sigh	shy
loans	loaves	cash	calf	cliff	click	call	cab	sap	ship
lean	leave	leash	leaf	laugh	lack	graph	grab	save	shave

Box 16 p and f		Box 17 s and z		Box 18 v and f		Box 19 ch and sh		Box 20 b and d	
pour	four	ice	eyes	five	fife	chop	shop	bid	did
pile	file	seal	zeal	vase	face	chair	share	big	dig
par	far	bus	buzz	leave	leaf	watch	wash	buy	die
cap	call	lice	lies	view	few	catch	cash	rob	rod
cup	cuff	juice	Jews	loaves	loafs	cheap	sheep	robe	rode

Box 21 d and g		Box 22 t and p		Box 23 l and s		Box 24 b and v		Box 25 v and z	
doe	go	tail	pail	fine	sign	bet	vet	live	lies
date	gate	cat	cap	flat	slat	dub	dove	have	has
drove	grove	cut	cup	cuff	cuss	base	vase	rave	raise
bud	bug	tar	par	knife	nice	bigger	vigor	view	zoo
dad	gag	toll	pole	lift	list	robe	rove	wives	wise

Box 26 th and f		Box 27 t and th		Box 28 k and t		Box 29 k and p		Box 30 m and n	
thin	fin	tie	thigh	kick	tick	pike	pipe	mine	nine
thirst	first	tin	thin	kite	tight	cat	pat	new	knew
three	free	trill	thrill	code	toad	crock	crop	time	tine
thought	fought	mit	myth	shirk	shirt	cry	pry	dime	dine
thrill	frill	pat	path	park	part	coal	pole	dumb	done

Box 31 Word Endings			Box 32 th and s		Box 33 th and v	
store	stores	stored	thumb	sum	than	van
will	wills	willed	truth	truce	thy	vie
start	starts	started	path	pass	that	vat
cough	coughs	coughed	thing	sing	thine	vine
cap	caps	capped	thank	sank	loathes	loaves

Figure 2.4. The Larson Sound Discrimination Test. pp. 236–237. Reprinted by permission from Sanders, D. A., *Aural Rehabilitation*. Prentice-Hall, Inc., Englewood Cliffs, NJ (1971) pp. 236–237.

sensitive in differentiating among individuals with a wide range of high frequency hearing loss than were the NU Number 6 Lists. The majority of subjects were able to recognize the words from the NU Number 6 List whereas the CCT list scores were more widely distributed.

The third experiment measured split-half reliability. The one obvious problem with the CCT is the time involved in administration of the 100 words. Two scramblings of the CCT were administered to 10 male subjects, aged 25–45 years, with high frequency hearing loss. There was a high correlation between the half-tests when analyzed for the entire groups. However, due to considerable individual variances, the study did not support the use of half-lists.

Another option available to the clinician in assessing discrimination difficulties was developed by Kelly (1973) and reprinted by the Alexander Graham Bell Association for the Deaf in 1973. Although Kelly addresses himself to tests for children, his methodology seems appropriate for adult diagnostic procedures as well. For clinical purposes, Kelly (1973) indicated that test lists should meet the following requirements.

1. Units should not be words or sentences.
2. Units should be multiple or in series.
3. Units should not involve context; one word should not facilitate recognition of the next.
4. Units should be easy enough for children to recognize (to this item, we add adults).
5. Units should be quickly presented and easily recorded, avoiding problems of spelling or pronunciation in response.
6. Units should be numerous to minimize effect of accidents in mis-identification.
7. Units should be representative samples of sounds of connected English speech associated with communication breakdown.

Kelly is of the opinion that by using alphabet letters, comparatively equal familiarity with examination units is achieved. Some of the alphabet letters are omitted because they are vocalic and no mis-identification with other alphabet letters is likely. The letters /i/, /o/, /u/, /q/, /r/, /w/, and /y/ are omitted. The remaining 19 alphabet letters fall into three groups determined by the carrier vowel.

1. Those with the vowel /i/.
2. Those with the vowel /ɛ/.

3. Those with the vowel /e/.

In this diagnostic approach, the clinician assumes the responsibility of categorizing the phonemic errors made by a given client. Examples of 2 of the 20 available lists are presented in Table 2.7. As Kelly (1973) indicates, a diagnosis of adequate listening must be related to a score above which serious communication trouble is unlikely. A person with no hearing loss will hear from 95 to 100% of the alphabet letters at a distance of 6 feet, if sounds are presented by a competent speaker. Since the person with impaired hearing will not be expected to hear normally, even with a hearing aid, a level of 90% may be considered a fairly respectable performance. This arbitrary level is satisfactory for determination of adequate listening ability for normal conversation. As scores decline, communication difficulty will increase.

In addition to assessment of individual phonemes through the auditory modality, it

Table 2.7
Examples of Diagnostic Discrimination Test Lists[a]

	List One	List Two
1.	ATZ	AKE
2.	BCS	TCT
3.	DNV	VDS
4.	TKE	NFB
5.	ZFM	MTN
6.	VFD	HJE
7.	SPT	DPC
8.	KAE	ZNE
9.	VMZ	VGN
10.	SDM	TKT
11.	FXC	AZP
12.	DKN	DMS
13.	DTN	FCN
14.	TKB	BTM
15.	NTN	DCE
16.	NTS	TKD
17.	EFM	ZCM
18.	SNZ	ETN
19.	NED	CNF
20.	SNT	TZN
21.	NPK	TEV
22.	ZBC	PZD
23.	DCE	NTN
24.	NCT	CKS
25.	EHM	DEM

[a] Reprinted by permission from Kelly, J. C., Clinician's Handbook for Auditory Training, copyright 1973, Alexander Graham Bell Association For the Deaf, Inc.

is also recommended that evaluation of ability to perceive continuous discourse be made. This procedure may be helpful in determining a client's auditory function when additional contextual information is available. The CID Everyday Speech Sentences (Davis and Silverman, 1970) are available for this purpose. These sentences are suggested for evaluation since they represent a sample of American speech of high face validity. The 10 sentence lists are presented in Appendix 2M. As indicated by Davis and Silverman (1970), certain important characteristics exist for these sentences.

1. The vocabulary is appropriate for adults.
2. The words appear with high frequency in one or more of the well-known word counts of the English language.
3. Proper names and proper nouns are not used.
4. Common non-slang idioms and contractions are used freely.
5. Phonetic loading and "tongue twisting" are avoided.
6. Redundancy is high.
7. The level of abstraction is low.
8. Grammatical structure varies freely.
9. Sentence length varies.
10. Different sentence forms are utilized, including declarative, rising interrogative, imperative, and falling interrogative.

In addition to evaluating discrimination ability for both individual phonemes and continuous speech discourse, the audiologist must consider any tolerance problems affecting the hearing-impaired adult. The ability to tolerate auditory stimuli at comfortable levels has significance for those clients utilizing or needing amplification. In evaluating discrimination ability, the test materials should be presented in an auditory only condition without the use of visual cues. Emphasis in this phase of the evaluation is assessment of the auditory modality only.

THERAPY JUDGMENTS

Results of these evaluation procedures enable the audiologist to make some rehabilitative judgments regarding specific auditory communication deficits of the client. Ramsdell (1970) describes three levels of hearing.

1. The primitive level. Sound serves as the auditory background of all daily living. At this level, we react to such sounds as the tick of a clock, the

distant roar of traffic, and vague echoes of people moving in other rooms in the house, without being aware that we do hear them.
2. The warning level. Sound serves as a direct sign or signal of events to which we make constant adjustments in daily living.
3. The symbolic level. Sound is used to comprehend language, since language is symbolic in nature.

The audiologist should plan therapy in terms of how the auditory modality affects individual clients. A prognosis can then be made permitting the clinician to determine where remediation should begin in auditory training. Four basic levels of training (Carhart, 1961) that may be considered for therapy are as follows.

1. Development of sound awareness.
2. Development of gross sound discrimination.
3. Development of broad speech discrimination.
4. Development of fine speech discrimination.

The adult with acquired hearing loss usually will begin therapy at levels 3 and 4 indicated above. Severe discrimination difficulties, however, may require working on sound awareness and gross sound discrimination. Oyer (1966) indicated that factors such as the amount of loss, the nature of the onset of the loss, and the motivation of the client will be additional factors in determining training needs. Evaluation of auditory discrimination test results enables the clinician to make a decision regarding utilization of a bisensory approach in the overall remediation process. Clinical results have not demonstrated great success in improving discrimination ability for the adult. Bisensory training, therefore, is recommended to improve overall communication ability.

Oyer (1968) indicated that in a majority of cases, auditory training will not stand alone as a method of rehabilitating the hard-of-hearing individual. It is part of a broad conceptual framework encompassing the entirety of aural rehabilitation.

DIAGNOSTIC TEST BATTERY: RECOMMENDATIONS

Information acquired from the assessment battery serves as a guide to planning remediation. The client's input is also important, as his estimate of the problem may provide a starting point for therapy. Although infor-

Table 2.8
Recommended Diagnostic Test Battery

Procedure	Rationale
1. Audiologic assessment (pure tone and speech audiometry)	Determination of type and severity of hearing loss, contribution of results to physician's diagnosis. Information on determining tolerance and discrimination abilities.
2. Hearing aid evaluation	Determination if amplification is necessary to minimize the auditory deficit.
3. McCarthy-Alpiner Scale of Hearing Handicap (Form A and Form B)	Client and family member assessment of attitudes toward psychologic, social, and vocational aspects.
4. Sander's Scales for performance in the home, occupational, and social environments	Assessment of specific problem areas in communication situations.
5. Lipreading Test for Phonemes (Binnie *et al.*, 1976)	Determination of client's ability to lipread the individual phonemes that comprise language. (Should be administered under visual and auditory-visual conditions to assess the relative contribution of vision to the auditory modality.)
6. Denver Quick Test of Lipreading	Assessment of client's ability to understand general communication. (Should be administered under visual and auditory-visual conditions.)
7. Auditory discrimination testing: (a) NU Auditory Word Tests (b) CID Everyday Sentences (c) California Consonant Test	Assessment of client's ability to discriminate phonemes and assessment of discrimination ability of everyday speech discourse through the auditory modality.
8. Plan for Remediation for Clients	Synthesis of all evaluative information to assist a client to achieve as near normal communication function as possible.

mation obtained from the client is subjective, therapy based on individual problems can be initiated, avoiding a generalized remediation approach, based on the experience of the audiologist, if necessary.

There is no "cookbook" approach. The following diagnostic battery (Table 2.8) is recommended, although a variety of other techniques may be available to the audiologist.

References

ALPINER, J. G., Hearing aid selection for adults. In M. C. Pollack (Ed.), *Amplification for the Hearing-Impaired*. New York: Grune & Stratton (1975).

ALPINER, J. G., CHEVRETTE, W., GLASCOE, G., METZ, M., and OLSEN, B., The Denver Scale of Communication Function. Unpublished study, University of Denver (1974).

ANSI (AMERICAN NATIONAL STANDARDS INSTITUTE), *Specifications for Audiometers, ANSI S 3.6–1969*. New York: American National Standards Institute (1969).

BINNIE, C. A., Bi-sensory articulation functions for normal hearing and sensorineural hearing loss patients. *J. Acad. Rehab. Audiol.*, **6**, 43–53 (1973).

BINNIE, C. A., JACKSON, P. L., and MONTGOMERY, A. A., Visual intelligibility of consonants: a lipreading screening test with implications for aural rehabilitation. *J. Speech Hear. Disord.*, **41**, 530–539 (1976).

BINNIE, C. A., MONTGOMERY, A. A., and JACKSON, P. L., Auditory and visual contributions to the perception of consonants. *J. Speech Hear. Res.*, **17**, 619–630 (1974).

BRANNON, C., Speechreading of various speech materials. *J. Speech Hear. Dis.*, **26**, 348–354 (1961).

CAMPBELL, D. T., and FISKE, D. W., Convergent and discriminant validation by the multitrait-multimethod matrix. *Psychol. Bulletin.*, **56**, 81–105 (1959).

CARHART, R., Auditory Training. In H. Davis and S. R. Silverman (Eds.), *Hearing and Deafness*. New York: Holt, Rinehart and Winston (1961).

CRONBACH, L. J., Coefficient alpha and internal structure of tests. *Psychometrika*, **10**, 297–334 (1951).

DANHAUER, J. L., and APPEL, M. A., INDSCAL Analysis of perceptual judgments for twenty-four consonants via visual, tactile, and visual-tactile sensory inputs. *J. Speech Hear. Res.*, **18**, 68–77 (1976).

DAVIS, H., The articulation area and the social adequacy index for hearing. *Laryngoscope*, **58**, 761–778 (1948).

DAVIS, H., and SILVERMAN, S. R., *Hearing and Deafness*. New York: Holt, Rinehart and Winston (1970).

DiCARLO, L. M., and KATAJA, R., An analysis of the Utley Lipreading Test. *J. Speech Hear. Disord.*, **16**, 226–240 (1951).

DODDS, E., and HARFORD, E. Application of a lipreading test in a hearing aid evaluation. *J. Speech Hear. Dis.*, **33**, 167–173 (1968).

DONNELLY, K. G. and MARSHALL, W. J. A., Development of a multiple choice test of lipreading. *J. Speech Hear. Res.*, **10**, 565–569 (1971).

EGAN, J. P., Articulation testing methods. *Laryngoscope*, **58**, 955–991 (1948).

ERBER, N. P., Developing materials for lipreading evaluation and instruction. *Volta Rev.*, **79**, 35–42 (1977).

ERBER, N. P., Auditory-visual perception of speech. *J. Speech Hear. Dis.*, **40**, 481–492 (1975). (Copyright 1975, *Journal of Speech and Hearing Disorders.*)

FARRAN, C. L., and DANHAUER, J. L., Perceptual features of speechreading. *Acta Symbolica*, **7**, 73–83 (1978).

GIOLAS, T. G., The measurement of hearing handicap: a point of view. *Maico Audiological Library Series*, VIII, 6 (1970). (Copyright 1970, *Maico Audiological Library Series.*)

GIOLAS, T. G., OWENS, E., LAMB, S. H., and SCHUBERT, E. D., Hearing performance inventory. *J. Speech Hear. Disord.*, **44**, 169–195 (1979).

GOETZINGER, C. P., Word discrimination testing. In J. Katz (Ed.), *Handbook of Clinical Audiology.* Baltimore: Williams & Wilkins (1972).

HARDY, M. D. Speechreading. In H. Davis, and S. R. Silverman (Ed.), *Hearing and Deafness.* New York: Holt, Rinehart and Winston (1970).

HIGH, W. S., FAIRBANKS, G., and GLORIG, A., Scale for self-assessment of hearing handicap. *J. Speech Hear. Disord.*, **29**, 215–230 (1964).

HIRSH, I. J., Audiology and the basic sciences. *Acta Otolaryng.*, **90**, 42–50 (1951).

HIRSH, I. J., DAVIS, H., SILVERMAN, S. R., REYNOLDS, E. G., ELBERT, E., and BENSEN, R. W., Development of materials for speech audiometry. *J. Speech Hear. Disord.*, **17**, 321–337 (1952).

HOUSE, A., WILLIAMS, C., HACKER, M., and KRYTER, K., Articulation-testing methods: consonant differentiation with a loud-set response. *J. Acoust. Soc. Am.*, **37**, 158–166 (1965).

HUTTON, C., Combining auditory and visual stimuli in aural rehabilitation. *Volta Rev.*, **6**, 316–319 (1959).

HUTTON, C., CURRAY, E. T., and ARMSTRONG, M. B., Semi-diagnostic test materials for aural rehabilitation. *J. Speech Hear. Dis.*, **24**, 318–329 (1959).

HUTTON, C. L., Responses to a hearing problem inventory. *J. Acad. Rehab. Audiol.*, **13**, 133–154 (1980).

JEFFERS, J., and BARLEY, M., *Speechreading (Lipreading).* Springfield, IL: Charles C Thomas (1971).

JEFFERS, J., and BARLEY, M., A re-evaluation of the Utley Lipreading Sentence Test. Paper presented at the annual convention of the American Speech and Hearing Association, Chicago (1967).

JERGER, J., SPEAKS, C., and TRAMMELL, J. L., An approach to speech audiometry. *J. Speech Hear. Disord.*, **33**, 318–328 (1968).

KALIKOW, D., STEVENS, K., and ELLIOT, L., Development of a test of speech intelligibility in noise using sentence materials with controlled word predictability. *J. Acoust. Soc. Am.*, **61**, 1337–1351 (1977).

KAPLAN, H., FEELY, J., and BROWN, J., A modified Denver Scale: test-retest reliability. *J. Acad. Rehab. Audiol.*, **11**, 15–32 (1978).

KELLY, J. C., *Clinician's Handbook for Auditory Training.* Washington, D.C.: Alexander Graham Bell Association for the Deaf, Inc. (1973). (Copyright 1973, Alexander Graham Bell Association for the Deaf, Inc.).

KONIDITSIOTIS, C. Y., The use of hearing tests to provide information about the extent to which an individual's hearing loss handicaps him. *Maico Audiological Library Series*, IX, 10 (1971).

LARSON, L. L., *Consonant Sound Discrimination.* Bloomington, IN: Indiana University Press (1950).

LOWELL, E. L., *Pilot Studies in Lipreading. John Tracy Clinic Research Papers VIII.* Los Angeles: John Tracy Clinic (February 1958).

MCCARTHY, P. A., and ALPINER, J. G., The McCarthy-Alpiner scale of hearing handicap. Unpublished study (1980).

MCNEIL, M. R., and ALPINER, J. G., A study of the reliability of the Denver Scale of Communication Function. Unpublished study, University of Denver (1975).

NEELY, K., Effects of visual factors of the intelligibility of speech. *J. Acoust. Soc. Am.*, **28**, 1275–1277 (1956).

NERBONNE, M. A., and SCHOW, R. L., Auditory stimuli in communication. In R. L. Schow and M. A. Nerbonne (Eds.), *Introduction to Aural Rehabilitation.* Baltimore: University Park Press (1980).

NOBLE, W. G., The measurement of hearing handicap: a further viewpoint. *Maico Audiological Library Series*, X, 5 (1972).

NOBLE, W. G., and ATHERLEY, G. R. C., The hearing measurement scale: a questionnaire for the assessment of auditory disability. *J. Aud. Res.*, **10**, 229–250 (1970).

O'NEILL, J. J., Contributions of the visual components of oral symbols to speech comprehension. *J. Speech Hear. Disord.*, **19**, 429–439 (1954).

O'NEILL, J. J., and OVER, H. J., *Visual Communication for the Hard of Hearing.* Englewood Cliffs, NJ: Prentice-Hall, Inc. (1981).

OWENS, E., and SCHUBERT, E., Development of the California Consonant Test. *J. Speech Hear. Res.* **20**, 463–474 (1977).

OWENS, E., Consonant errors and remediation in sensorineural hearing loss. *J. Speech Hear. Disord.*, **43**, 331–347 (1978).

OYER, H. J., Auditory training—significance and usage for children and adults. In J. G. Alpiner (Ed.), *Proceedings of the Institute on Aural Rehabilitation.* University of Denver (1968).

OYER, H. J., *Auditory Communication for the Hard of Hearing.* Englewood Cliffs, NJ: Prentice-Hall, Inc. (1966).

OYER, H. J., and FRANKMANN, J. P., *The Aural Rehabilitation Process.* New York: Holt, Rinehart and Winston (1975).

POLLACK, M. C., The remediation process: psychological and counseling aspects. In J. G. Alpiner (Ed.), *Handbook of Adult Rehabilitative Audiology.* Baltimore: Williams and Wilkins Co. (1978).

PRALL, J., Lipreading and hearing combined for better comprehension. *Volta Rev.*, **59**, 64–65 (1957).

RAMSDELL, D. A., The psychology of the hard-of-hearing and the deafened adult. In H. Davis and S. R. Silverman (Eds.), *Hearing and Deafness.* New York: Holt, Rinehart and Winston (1970).

SANDERS, D. A., Hearing aid orientation and counseling. In M. C. Pollack (Ed.), *Amplification for the Hearing-Impaired.* New York: Grune & Stratton (1975).

SANDERS, D. A., and GOODRICH, S. J., The relative

contribution of visual and auditory components of speech to speech intelligibility as a function of three conditions of frequency distortion. *J. Speech Hear. Res.*, **14**, 172–178, (1971).

SCHOW, R. L., and NERBONNE, M. A., *Introduction to Aural Rehabilitation.* Baltimore: University Park Press (1980).

SCHOW, R. L. and TANNAHILL, C., Hearing handicap scores and categories for subjects with normal and impaired hearing sensitivity. *J. Am. Audiol. Soc.*, **3**, 134–139 (1977).

SCHULTZ, M., and SCHUBERT, E., A multiple choice discrimination test (MCDT). *Laryngoscope*, **79**, 382–399 (1969).

SCHWARTZ, D. M., and SURR, R. K., Three experiments on the California Consonant Test. *J. Speech Hear. Dis.*, **44**, 61–72 (1979).

SIEGENTHALER, B. M., and GRUBER, V., Combining vision and audition for speech reception, *J. Speech Hear. Disord.*, **34**, 58–60 (1969).

SUMBY, W. H., and POLLACK, I., Visual contributions to speech intelligibility in noise. *J. Acoust. Soc. Am.*, **26**, 212–215 (1954).

TAAFFE, G., *A Film Test of Lip Reading. John Tracy Clinic Research Papers II.* Los Angeles: John Tracy Clinic (November, 1957).

TILLMAN, T. W., and CARHART, R., An expanded test for speech discrimination utilizing CNC monosyllabic words. Northwestern University Auditory Test Number 6, *Technical Report, SAM-TR-66-55,* USAF School of Aerospace Medicine, Brooks AFB, Texas (1966).

TRASK, A. N., More about lip-reading, and then some. *Volta Rev.*, **19**, 567–569 (1917).

WALDEN, B. E., PROSEK, R. A., and SCHERR, C. K., Dimensions of visual consonant perception by hearing-impaired observers. Paper presented at the annual convention of the American Speech and Hearing Association, Las Vegas (1974a).

WALDEN, B. E., PROSEK, R. A., and WORTHINGTON, D. W., Predicting audiovisual consonant recognition performance of hearing-impaired adults. *J. Speech Hear. Res.*, **17**, 270–278 (1974b).

WOODWARD, M. F., and BARBER, C. G., Phoneme perception in lipreading. *J. Speech Hear. Res.*, **3**, 212–222 (1960).

APPENDIX

2A

Hearing Handicap Scale (Form A)*

1. If you are 6 to 12 feet from the loudspeaker of a radio do you understand speech well?
2. Can you carry on a telephone conversation without difficulty?
3. If you are 6 to 12 feet away from a television set, do you understand most of what is said?
4. Can you carry on a conversation with one other person when you are on a noisy street corner?
5. Do you hear all right when you are in a street car, airplane, bus, or train?
6. If there are noises from other voices, typewriters, traffic, music, etc., can you understand when someone speaks to you?
7. Can you understand a person when you are seated beside him and cannot see his face?
8. Can you understand if someone speaks to you while you are chewing crisp foods, such as potato chips or celery?
9. Can you carry on a conversation with one other person when you are in a noisy place, such as a restaurant or at a party?
10. Can you understand if someone speaks to you in a whisper and you cannot see his face?
11. When you talk with a bus driver, waiter, ticket salesman, etc., can you understand all right?
12. Can you carry on a conversation if you are seated across the room from someone who speaks in a normal tone of voice?
13. Can you understand women when they talk?
14. Can you carry on a conversation with one other person when you are out-of-doors and it is reasonably quiet?
15. When you are in a meeting or at a large dinner table, would you know the speaker was talking if you could not see his lips moving?
16. Can you follow the conversation when you are at a large dinner table or in a meeting with a small group?
17. If you are seated under the balcony of a theater or auditorium, can you hear well enough to follow what is going on?

* Reprinted by permission from High, Fairbanks, and Glorig: Scale for self-assessment of hearing handicap. *J. Speech Hearing Dis.*, **29**, 215–230, © 1964, *Journal of Speech and Hearing Disorders*.

18. When you are in a large formal gathering (a church, lodge, lecture hall, etc.) can you hear what is said when the speaker does not use a microphone?
19. Can you hear the telephone ring when you are in the room where it is located?
20. Can you hear warning signals, such as automobile horns, railway crossing bells, or emergency vehicle sirens?

2B

Test of Actual Performance*

How well does he/she:

	Poor	Adequate	Good	Excellent
1. pay attention in the group? (day-dreams, restlessness, changes the subject)				
2. communicate ideas verbally?				
3. use speech intelligibly?				
4. respond to others? (shares similar experiences, agrees, disagrees)				
5. hear speech when noise was going on around him/her? (like at parties)				
6. understand speech when not able to see the speaker?				
7. monitor the loudness of his/her own speech?				

---

* Reprinted by permission from Koniditsiotis: The use of hearing tests to provide information about the extent to which an individual's hearing loss handicaps him. *Maico Audiological Library Series*, IX, 10 © 1971, *Maico Audiological Library*.

APPENDIX
2C

The Hearing Measurement Scale*

The form of the scale given here is for reference purposes only. It cannot be used without first reading the instruction manual. Copies of this and the scale are obtainable from Dr. W. G. Noble, Department of Psychology, University of New England, Armidale, N.S.E. 2351, Australia.

Section I Speech Hearing

1. Do you ever have difficulty hearing in the conversation when you're with one other person when you're at home?
2. Do you ever have difficulty hearing in the conversation when you're with one other person outside?
3. Do you ever have difficulty in group conversation at home?
4. Do you ever have difficulty in group conversation outside?
5. Do you ever have difficulty hearing conversation at work?
5a. Is this due to your hearing, due to the noise or a bit of both?
6. Do you ever have difficulty hearing the speaker at a public gathering?
7. Can you always hear what's being said in a TV program?
8. Can you always hear what's being said in TV news?
9. Can you always hear what's being said in a radio program?
10. Can you always hear what's being said in radio news?
11. Do you ever have difficulty hearing what's said in a film at the cinema?

Section II Acuity for Non-speech Sound

12. Do you have any pets at home? (Type____) Can you hear it when it____ (barks, mews, etc.)?
13. Can you hear it when someone rings the doorbell or knocks on the door?
14. Can you hear a motor horn in the street when you're outside?
15. The sound of footsteps outside when you're inside?
16. The sound of the door opening when you're inside that room?
17. Can you hear the clock ticking in the room?
18. The tap running when you turn it on?
19. Water boiling in a pan when you're in the kitchen?

Section III Localization

20. When you hear the sound of people talking and they're in another room

---

* Reprinted by permission from Noble and Atherley: The hearing measurement scale: a questionnaire for the assessment of auditory disability. *J. Aud. Res.,* **10,** 229–250, © 1970, *Journal of Auditory Research.*

would you be able to tell whereabouts this sound was coming from?
21. If you're with a group of people and someone you can't see starts to speak would you be able to tell where that person was sitting?
22. If you hear a motor horn or a bell can you always tell which direction it's sounding?
23. Do you ever turn your head the wrong way when someone calls to you?
24. Can you usually tell, from the sound, how far away a person is when he calls you?
25. Have you ever noticed outside that a car you thought, by its sound, was far away turned out to be much closer in fact?
26. Outside, do you always move out of the way of something coming up from behind, for instance a car, a trolley or someone walking faster?

Section IV Reaction to Handicap
27. Do you think you are more irritable than other people or less so?
28. Do you ever give the wrong answer to someone because you've misheard them?
29. When you do this, do you treat it lightly or do you get upset?
30. How does the other person react? Does he get irritated or make little of it?
31. Do you think people are tolerant in this way or do they make fun of you?
32. Do you ever get bothered or upset if you are unable to follow a conversation?
33. Do you ever get the feeling of being cut off from things because of difficulty in hearing?
33a.Does this feeling upset you at all?

Section V Speech Distortion
34. Do you find that people fail to speak clearly?
35. What about speakers on TV or radio? Do they fail to speak clearly?
36. Do you ever have difficulty, in everyday conversation, understanding what someone is saying even though you can hear what's being said?

Section VI Tinnitus
37. Do you ever get a noise in your ears or in your head?
37a.to 37e. A series of items on nature and incidence of tinnitus.
38. Does it ever stop you sleeping?
39. Does it upset you?

Section VII Personal Opinion of Hearing Loss
40. Do you think your hearing is normal?
41. Do you think any difficulty with your hearing is particularly serious?
42. Does any difficulty with your hearing restrict your social or personal life?
42a.to 42f. A series of items on Temporary Threshold Shift, specifically for those with chronic acoustic trauma, on the relative importance of eyesight over hearing and on other difficult hearing situations not mentioned in the interview.

It must be re-emphasized that the foregoing form of the scale cannot be used without prior reference to the manual of instructions obtainable from the principal author.

2D

The Denver Scale of Communication Function*

Pre-Service_____   Post-Service_____

Date _____   Case No. _____

Name _____Age ___Sex____

Address _____

        (City)   (State)   (Zip)

Lives Alone_____In Apartment _____Retired_____
                (if no, specify)

Occupation _____

Audiogram (Examination Date_____Agency_____)
  Pure Tone:

	250	500	1000	2000	4000	8000	Hz
RE	__	__	___	___	___	___	
LE	__	__	___	___	___	___	dB (re: ANSI)

  Speech:

SRT   DISCRIMINATION SCORE (%)

                    Quiet   Noise (S/N =)

RE_____dB   RE_____

LE_____dB   LE_____

_____

* Reprinted by permission from Alpiner, Chevrette, Glascoe, Metz, and Olsen: Unpublished study, the University of Denver, © 1974.

Hearing Aid Information

Aided_____For How Long_____Aid Type_____

Satisfaction _____

EXAMINER:_____

The following questionnaire was designed to evaluate your communication ability as you view it. You are asked to judge or scale each statement in the following manner.

If you judge the statement to be *very closely related* to either extreme, please place your check mark as follows:

Agree __X__ _____ _____ _____ _____ _____ _____ Disagree

or

Agree _____ _____ _____ _____ _____ _____ __X__ Disagree

If you judge the stagement to be *closely related* to either end of the scale, please mark as follows:

Agree _____ __X__ _____ _____ _____ _____ _____ Disagree

or

Agree _____ _____ _____ _____ _____ __X__ _____ Disagree

If you judge the statement to be only slightly related to either end of the scale, please mark as follows:

Agree _____ _____ __X__ _____ _____ _____ _____ Disagree

or

Agree _____ _____ _____ _____ __X__ _____ _____ Disagree

If you consider the statement to be irrelevant or unassociated to your communication situation, please mark as follows:

Agree _____ _____ _____ __X__ _____ _____ _____ Disagree

PLEASE NOTE: Check a scale for every statement.
                     Put only one checkmark on each scale.
                     Make a separate judgment for each statement.
ALSO: You may comment on each statement in the space provided.

1. The members of my family are annoyed with my loss of hearing.
   Agree _____ _____ _____ _____ _____ _____ _____ Disagree
   Comments:
2. The members of my family sometimes leave me out of conversations or discussions.

Agree _____ _____ _____ _____ _____ _____ _____ Disagree
Comments:

3. Sometimes my family makes decisions for me because I have a hard time following discussions.
Agree _____ _____ _____ _____ _____ _____ _____ Disagree
Comments:

4. My family becomes annoyed when I ask them to repeat what was said because I did not hear them.
Agree _____ _____ _____ _____ _____ _____ _____ Disagree
Comments:

5. I am not an "outgoing" person because I have a hearing loss.
Agree _____ _____ _____ _____ _____ _____ _____ Disagree
Comments:

6. I now take less of an interest in many things as compared to when I did not have a hearing problem.
Agree _____ _____ _____ _____ _____ _____ _____ Disagree
Comments:

7. Other people do not realize how frustrated I get when I cannot hear or understand.
Agree _____ _____ _____ _____ _____ _____ _____ Disagree
Comments:

8. People sometimes avoid me because of my hearing loss.
Agree _____ _____ _____ _____ _____ _____ _____ Disagree
Comments:

9. I am not a calm person because of my hearing loss.
Agree _____ _____ _____ _____ _____ _____ _____ Disagree
Comments:

10. I tend to be negative about life in general because of my hearing loss.
Agree _____ _____ _____ _____ _____ _____ _____ Disagree
Comments:

11. I do not socialize as much as I did before I began to lose my hearing.
Agree _____ _____ _____ _____ _____ _____ _____ Disagree
Comments:

12. Since I have trouble hearing, I do not like to go places with friends.
Agree _____ _____ _____ _____ _____ _____ _____ Disagree
Comments:

13. Since I have trouble hearing, I hestitate to meet new people.
Agree _____ _____ _____ _____ _____ _____ _____ Disagree
Comments:

14. I do not enjoy my job as much as I did before I began to lose my hearing.
Agree _____ _____ _____ _____ _____ _____ _____ Disagree
Comments:

15. Other people do not understand what it is like to have a hearing loss.
Agree _____ _____ _____ _____ _____ _____ _____ Disagree
Comments:

16. Because I have difficulty understanding what is said to me, I sometimes answer questions wrong.
    Agree _____ _____ _____ _____ _____ _____ _____ Disagree
    Comments:
17. I do not feel relaxed in a communicative situation.
    Agree _____ _____ _____ _____ _____ _____ _____ Disagree
    Comments:
18. I do not feel comfortable in most communication situations.
    Agree _____ _____ _____ _____ _____ _____ _____ Disagree
    Comments:
19. Conversations in a noisy room prevent me from attempting to communicate with others.
    Agree _____ _____ _____ _____ _____ _____ _____ Disagree
    Comments:
20. I am not comfortable having to speak in a group situation.
    Agree _____ _____ _____ _____ _____ _____ _____ Disagree
    Comments:
21. In general, I do not find listening relaxing.
    Agree _____ _____ _____ _____ _____ _____ _____ Disagree
    Comments:
22. I feel threatened by many communication situations due to difficulty hearing.
    Agree _____ _____ _____ _____ _____ _____ _____ Disagree
    Comments:
23. I seldom watch other people's facial expressions when talking to them.
    Agree _____ _____ _____ _____ _____ _____ _____ Disagree
    Comments:
24. I hesitate to ask people to repeat if I do not understand them the first time they speak.
    Agree _____ _____ _____ _____ _____ _____ _____ Disagree
    Comments:
25. Because I have difficulty understanding what is said to me, I sometimes make comments that do not fit into the conversation.
    Agree _____ _____ _____ _____ _____ _____ _____ Disagree
    Comments:

Quantified Denver Scale*

Name _____   Score:
                                 Raw score:

Age _____

Date _____

	Strongly disagree				Strongly agree
1. The members of my family are annoyed with my loss of hearing.	1	2	3	4	5
2. The members of my family sometimes leave me out of conversations or discussions.	1	2	3	4	5
3. Sometimes my family makes decisions for me because I have a hard time following discussions.	1	2	3	4	5
4. My family becomes annoyed when I ask them to repeat what was said because I did not hear them.	1	2	3	4	5
5. I am not an "outgoing" person because I have a hearing loss.	1	2	3	4	5
6. I now take less of an interest in many things as compared to when I did not have a hearing problem.	1	2	3	4	5
7. Other people do not realize how frustrated I get when I cannot hear or understand.	1	2	3	4	5
8. People sometimes avoid me because of my hearing loss.	1	2	3	4	5
9. I am not a calm person because of my hearing loss.	1	2	3	4	5

---

* Modified from Denver Scale of Communication Function (Alpiner *et al.*, 1974).

	Strongly disagree				Strongly agree
10. I tend to be negative about life in general because of my hearing loss.	1	2	3	4	5
11. I do not socialize as much as I did before I began to lose my hearing.	1	2	3	4	5
12. Since I have trouble hearing, I do not like to go places with friends.	1	2	3	4	5
13. Since I have trouble hearing, I hesitate to meet new people.	1	2	3	4	5
14. I do not enjoy my job as much as I did before I began to lose my hearing.	1	2	3	4	5
15. Other people do not understand what it is like to have a hearing loss.	1	2	3	4	5
16. Because I have difficulty understanding what is said to me, I sometimes answer questions wrong.	1	2	3	4	5
17. I do not feel relaxed in a communicative situation.	1	2	3	4	5
18. I don't feel comfortable in most communication situations.	1	2	3	4	5
19. Conversations in a noisy room prevent me from attempting to communicate with others.	1	2	3	4	5
20. I am not comfortable having to speak in a group situation.	1	2	3	4	5
21. In general, I do not find listening relaxing.	1	2	3	4	5
22. I feel threatened by many communication situations due to difficulty hearing.	1	2	3	4	5
23. I seldom watch other people's facial expressions when talking to them.	1	2	3	4	5
24. I hesitate to ask people to repeat if I do not understand them the first time they speak.	1	2	3	4	5
25. Because I have difficulty understanding what is said to me, I sometimes make comments that do not fit into the conversation.	1	2	3	4	5

APPENDIX

2F

Hearing Problem Inventory*

The purpose of this set of statements and questions is to give the audiologists who will be working with you as much information about your hearing problem as you can tell us.

Try to ask yourself each question separately and answer them one at a time. Sometimes there are different questions about different aspects of the same topic. For example, there are a number of questions about how your hearing problems affect your job. Try to answer each one separately as best as you can.

You may find that some of the questions do not apply to you. If so, please write in the reason why. For example, if the statement is "I understand what my boss says to me at work," and if you are not working, please write an answer that states you are not working. This will let us know that you do not have a problem in this area.

If the question is "How many hours a day do you wear your hearing aid?", and if you do not have a hearing aid at this time, please write an answer such as "I do not have a hearing aid."

We want to know about *you* and your problems. In this way we can do a better job of solving your specific problems. There is space at the end for you to write about problems you have which are not listed.

HEARING PROBLEM INVENTORY (ATLANTA)

1. I turn the radio or TV down before I try to carry on a conversation:
   - _____ Almost always
   - _____ Most of the time
   - _____ Half of the time
   - _____ Usually not
   - _____ Unnecessary to

2. The telephone pickup on my hearing aid is good:
   - _____ Understand almost all
   - _____ Understand most
   - _____ Miss half or more
   - _____ Cannot use on my aid
   - _____ No pickup on my aid
   - _____ Do not have aid

3. I don't have a problem hearing over the telephone at work or at home:
   - _____ Almost no difficulty
   - _____ Usually hear enough to understand

* Reprinted by permission from Hutton, C. L., Responses to a hearing problem inventory. *J. Acad. Rehab. Audiol.* **13,** 133–154 (1980).

_____ I get some but miss a lot
_____ I miss most of what is said
_____ I cannot use at all
I have a problem because: _____

4. I can understand the people that I talk with a lot, like family and friends:
   _____ Almost always
   _____ Most of the time
   _____ Half of the time
   _____ Not usually
   _____ Almost never
   Don't understand because: _____

5. I feel that listening to several people talk at the same time is too hard:
   _____ Almost always too hard
   _____ Most of the time too hard
   _____ Half of the time
   _____ Usually too hard
   _____ Almost never too hard

6. My hearing loss is embarrassing to my family, especially when we go out:
   _____ Almost never embarrassing
   _____ Half of the time
   _____ More than half
   _____ Almost always

7. My family steps in and makes decisions for me when I don't hear:
   _____ Almost always they step in
   _____ Most of the time
   _____ Half of the time they do
   _____ Usually they don't
   _____ Almost never

8. People have to talk slowly for me to understand them:
   _____ Almost everyone has to
   _____ Most people have to
   _____ About half need to
   _____ Some need to
   _____ Almost no one

9. I feel people avoid talking to me because of my hearing loss:
   _____ Everyone avoids talking to me
   _____ Most people avoid
   _____ Half of the people avoid
   _____ Most people don't avoid
   _____ Almost never avoid

10. I do not take part in social activities as much as I did before I began to lose my hearing:
    _____ Almost always I do not
    _____ Most of the time I do not
    _____ Half of the time I do not
    _____ Usually I do
    _____ Almost always I do

11. I have difficulty understanding what people say in a large room:
- _____ Almost never
- _____ Not usually
- _____ Half of the time
- _____ Most of the time
- _____ Almost always

12. I ask people to repeat when I cannot understand what they say:
- _____ Almost always I ask
- _____ Most of the time
- _____ Half of the time I ask
- _____ Not usually
- _____ Almost never

13. When I have difficulty understanding my family and friends, they go right on talking and leave me out. This happens to me:
- _____ Almost never
- _____ Several times a day
- _____ Half of the time
- _____ Most of the time
- _____ Almost always

14. I avoid meeting strangers because of my hearing problem:
- _____ Almost never avoid
- _____ Usually do not avoid
- _____ Avoid half of the time
- _____ Avoid most of the time
- _____ Avoid almost always

Avoid because: _____

15. Because I have difficulty understanding what is said to me, I say things that don't fit into the conversation. This happens to me:
- _____ Less than once a day
- _____ Several times a day
- _____ Half of the time
- _____ Most of the time
- _____ Almost always

16. My family gets annoyed when I don't understand what they say:
- _____ Almost never gets annoyed
- _____ Several times a day
- _____ Half of the time
- _____ Most of the time
- _____ Almost always

17. I wear my aid:
- _____ Almost all the time
- _____ Most of the time but have problems
- _____ Wear about half the time
- _____ Do not have an aid
- _____ Not able to wear it
- _____ Only a little bit because

Explain problems: _____

18. I can control the noise level where I live:
    _____ Almost always I can't
    _____ Most of the time I can't
    _____ Half of the time I can
    _____ Most of the time I can
    _____ Almost always I can
    I can't control it because: _____

19. The person I talk with most is easy to understand:
    _____ Almost never
    _____ Usually not
    _____ Half of the time
    _____ Most of the time
    _____ Almost always
    This person is my: _____

20. The people I talk with a lot get my attention before starting to talk to me:
    _____ Almost always do
    _____ Most of the time
    _____ Half of the time
    _____ Usually do not
    _____ Almost never do

21. People at work get my attention before they start to talk to me:
    _____ Almost always
    _____ Most of the time
    _____ Half of the time
    _____ Usually do not
    _____ Almost never
    _____ Not working

22. Trying to talk with my family makes me nervous:
    _____ Almost never does
    _____ Usually doesn't
    _____ Half of the time it does
    _____ Most of the time it does
    _____ Almost always

23. My hearing loss keeps me from going out and doing many things I want to do:
    _____ Almost always prevents me
    _____ Most of the time
    _____ Half of the time
    _____ Usually doesn't
    _____ Almost never interferes
    Cannot do: _____

24. When lots of people are talking in a large room I can't carry on a conversation:
    _____ Almost always can't hear
    _____ Most of the time I can't
    _____ Half of the time I can't
    _____ Usually can
    _____ Almost always can

25. When there are several conversations going on and I can't follow what is being said to me I feel left out and uncomfortable:
____ Almost always feel left out
____ Most of the time
____ Half of the time
____ Usually don't feel left out
____ Almost never feel left out

26. When someone talks behind me, I miss the first part of what they say:
____ Almost always miss
____ Most of the time
____ Miss half of the time
____ Usually don't miss
____ Miss less than once a day

27. I watch other people's facial expressions when talking to them:
____ Almost always
____ Most of the time
____ Half of the time
____ Not usually
____ Less than once a day

28. Except at home, trying to talk with people makes me feel uncomfortable:
____ Makes me uncomfortable almost always
____ Most of the time
____ Half of the time
____ Bothers me sometimes
____ Almost never

29. When I don't hear a whole statement, I try to guess at the words I missed and figure it out:
____ Almost always figure it out
____ Most of the time
____ Half of the time figure it out
____ Usually can't figure it out
____ Almost never

30. Other people do not seem to understand what it is like to have a hearing problem:
____ Almost never understand
____ Usually do not
____ Half of the time do
____ Most of the time understand
____ Almost always understand

31. My family and friends complain that I turn up the radio and TV too loud:
____ Almost always I do
____ Most of the time
____ Half of the time
____ Less than half the time
____ Almost never

32. Listening requires a lot of hard work and concentration for me:
____ Almost always
____ Most of the time

_____ Half of the time
_____ Not usually
_____ Hardly ever

33. I am not having problems with my hearing aid because it:
_____ Helps in almost all situations
_____ Helps in most situations
_____ Helps in half the places
_____ Helps in only a few places
_____ I can't wear an aid
_____ I don't have an aid
Describe problems: _____

34. I have difficulty understanding if I cannot see the speaker's face well:
_____ Have difficulty less than once a day
_____ Several times a day
_____ Half of the time
_____ Most of the time
_____ Almost always

35. My hearing loss causes problems for me at work:
_____ Less than once a day
_____ Several times a day
_____ Half of the time
_____ Most of the time
_____ Almost always
_____ Not working
What problems? _____

36. Noise is a problem at work:
_____ Less than once a day
_____ Usually is not
_____ Half of the time
_____ Most of the time
_____ Almost always is
_____ Not working
Describe: _____

37. I don't hear important sounds around me, like the phone ringing:
_____ Almost always don't hear
_____ Usually don't hear
_____ Hear about half of the sounds around me
_____ Usually hear sounds around me
_____ Almost always hear
Environmental sounds I miss: _____

38. Because of my hearing loss I do not enjoy my job like I used to:
_____ Almost never enjoy it
_____ Don't enjoy it most of the time
_____ Like it half as much
_____ Like it most of the time
_____ Still like it as much
_____ Not working

39. Not knowing which direction sound is coming from is a problem to me:
    _____ Almost always can't tell direction
    _____ Most of the time
    _____ Half of the time I don't know
    _____ Not usually a problem
    _____ Almost never a problem

40. When watching a speaker I should concentrate on:
    _____ His lips
    _____ The lower half of his face
    _____ His whole face and body
    _____ Should not concentrate
    _____ Don't know

41. How many hours a day do you wear your aid? _____

42. I don't understand when people try to talk with me from another room:
    _____ Understand nothing
    _____ Understand less than half
    _____ Understand about half
    _____ Understand most
    _____ Understand almost all

43. I have trouble with my earmold:
    _____ It is too loose
    _____ It hurts my ear
    _____ It is too tight
    _____ My hearing aid squeals
    _____ My earmold is OK
    _____ I don't have an earmold

44. I wash my earmold: _____ Do not have an earmold
    _____ Once a day
    _____ Once a week
    _____ Once a month
    _____ Once a year
    _____ Hardly ever

45. Check those items which might cause hearing loss:
    _____ Cold weather
    _____ Some medications
    _____ Loud noises
    _____ Certain foods
    _____ Circulation problems

46. The aid I am wearing now is:
    _____ The best I've ever had because:
    _____ One of the better ones, but needs:
    _____ About the same as most aids
    _____ Not as good as most aids
    _____ The worst aid I've had
    _____ I don't have any aid
    Explain: _____

47. I cannot carry on a conversation with people who talk softly:
   _____ Almost never can
   _____ Usually can't
   _____ Can half the time
   _____ Can most of the time
   _____ Almost always can

48. If eligible I will receive a spare aid:
   _____ In the mail in 6 months
   _____ Only if I apply for it
   _____ Don't know
   _____ Have working spare aid

49. All batteries and repair needs are handled by:
   _____ Atlanta VA Prosthetics
   _____ Local hearing aid dealers
   _____ The Denver VA Center
   _____ Don't know

50. I control the corrosion caused by moisture and perspiration by using a drying kit:
   _____ Dry out my aid regularly
   _____ Dry aid in summer
   _____ Dry it only when needed
   _____ My aid does not require
   _____ Don't know about this
   _____ Don't have an aid

51. I have learned how to adjust to and manage my hearing problems:
   _____ Successfully manage them almost always
   _____ Manage them most of the time
   _____ Manage them about half the time
   _____ Usually cannot
   _____ Almost never can
   Cannot manage these problems: _____
   _____

_____

NAME   SS#   DATE

_____

HOME TELEPHONE NUMBER   OFFICE TELEPHONE NUMBER

2G

The McCarthy-Alpiner Scale
of Hearing Handicap
(The M-A Scale)
Form A*

NAME: _____ DATE: _____

AGE: _____ SEX: _____ TIME: _____

OCCUPATION: _____ PHONE: _____

ADDRESS: _____

HEARING AID: YES _____ NO _____   ONSET OF

             TYPE _____   HEARING LOSS: _____

             HOW LONG _____

             SATISFACTION _____

AUDIOGRAM: DATE OF EXAMINATION

             _____

             EXAMINER _____

             CATEGORY OF HEARING

             LOSS _____

RIGHT EAR

	250 Hz	500 Hz	1000 Hz	2000 Hz	4000 Hz	8000 Hz
AIR						
BONE						

LEFT EAR

	250 Hz	500 Hz	1000 Hz	2000 Hz	4000 Hz	8000 Hz
AIR						
BONE						

SPEECH RECEPTION   SPEECH DISCRIMINATION:
THRESHOLD:

RIGHT EAR _____ dB HL   RIGHT EAR _____ % @ _____ dB HL

LEFT EAR _____ dB HL   LEFT EAR _____ % @ _____ dB HL

DIRECTIONS

The following questionnaire will be used to help audiologists understand what it is like to have a hearing loss and the effects of a hearing loss on your life. You are asked to give your reaction to each of the statements included in the questionnaire. For example, you might be given this statement:

People avoid me because of my hearing loss.

×

| ALWAYS | USUALLY | SOMETIMES | RARELY | NEVER |

You are asked to mark your reaction to the statement with an × on the appropriate space. Please mark every item with only one answer, as seen in the example.

In marking your answer, please keep in mind that ALWAYS means at all times or on all occasions. USUALLY refers to generally, commonly, or ordinarily. SOMETIMES means occasionally or on various occasions. RARELY refers to seldom or infrequently. NEVER means not ever or at no time.

If you are not presently employed, please respond "N/A" for not applicable.

All answers will be kept strictly confidential and used only to help audiologists to understand what it is like to have a hearing loss and the effect hearing loss has on your life.

1. I get annoyed when people do not speak loud enough for me to hear them.
   ALWAYS   USUALLY   SOMETIMES   RARELY   NEVER

2. I get upset if I cannot hear or understand a conversation.
   ALWAYS   USUALLY   SOMETIMES   RARELY   NEVER

3. I feel like I am isolated from things because of my hearing loss.
   ALWAYS   USUALLY   SOMETIMES   RARELY   NEVER

4. I feel negative about life in general because of my hearing loss.
   ALWAYS   USUALLY   SOMETIMES   RARELY   NEVER

5. I admit to most people that I have a hearing loss.
   ALWAYS   USUALLY   SOMETIMES   RARELY   NEVER

6. I get upset when I feel that people are "mumbling."
   ALWAYS   USUALLY   SOMETIMES   RARELY   NEVER

7. I feel very frustrated when I cannot understand a conversation.
   ALWAYS   USUALLY   SOMETIMES   RARELY   NEVER

8. I feel that people in general understand what it is like to have a hearing loss.
   ALWAYS   USUALLY   SOMETIMES   RARELY   NEVER

9. My hearing loss has affected my life in general.
   ALWAYS   USUALLY   SOMETIMES   RARELY   NEVER

10. I am afraid that people will not like me if they find out that I have a hearing loss.
    ALWAYS   USUALLY   SOMETIMES   RARELY   NEVER

11. I tend to avoid people because of my hearing loss.
    ALWAYS   USUALLY   SOMETIMES   RARELY   NEVER

12. People act annoyed when I cannot understand what is being said in a group conversation.

ALWAYS   USUALLY   SOMETIMES   RARELY   NEVER

13. My family is patient with me when I cannot hear.

ALWAYS   USUALLY   SOMETIMES   RARELY   NEVER

14. Strangers react rudely when I do not understand what they say.

ALWAYS   USUALLY   SOMETIMES   RARELY   NEVER

15. I ask a person to repeat if I do not hear or understand what he said.

ALWAYS   USUALLY   SOMETIMES   RARELY   NEVER

16. My hearing loss has affected my relationship with my spouse.

ALWAYS   USUALLY   SOMETIMES   RARELY   NEVER

17. I do not go places with my family because of my hearing loss.

ALWAYS   USUALLY   SOMETIMES   RARELY   NEVER

18. Group discussions make me nervous because of my hearing loss.

ALWAYS   USUALLY   SOMETIMES   RARELY   NEVER

19. People in general are tolerant of my hearing loss.

ALWAYS   USUALLY   SOMETIMES   RARELY   NEVER

20. I avoid going to movies or plays because of my hearing loss.

ALWAYS   USUALLY   SOMETIMES   RARELY   NEVER

21. I avoid going to restaurants because of my hearing loss.

ALWAYS   USUALLY   SOMETIMES   RARELY   NEVER

22. I enjoy social situations with considerable conversation.

ALWAYS   USUALLY   SOMETIMES   RARELY   NEVER

23. I am not interested in group activities because of my hearing loss.

ALWAYS   USUALLY   SOMETIMES   RARELY   NEVER

24. I enjoy group discussions even though I have a hearing loss.

ALWAYS   USUALLY   SOMETIMES   RARELY   NEVER

25. My hearing loss has interfered with my job performance.

ALWAYS   USUALLY   SOMETIMES   RARELY   NEVER

26. I cannot perform my job well because of my hearing loss.

ALWAYS   USUALLY   SOMETIMES   RARELY   NEVER

27. My co-workers know what it is like to have a hearing loss.

ALWAYS   USUALLY   SOMETIMES   RARELY   NEVER

28. I try to hide my hearing loss from my co-workers.

ALWAYS   USUALLY   SOMETIMES   RARELY   NEVER

29. I do not enjoy going to work because of my hearing loss.

ALWAYS   USUALLY   SOMETIMES   RARELY   NEVER

30. I am given credit for doing a good job at work even though I have a hearing loss.

ALWAYS   USUALLY   SOMETIMES   RARELY   NEVER

31. I feel more pressure at work because of my hearing loss.

   ALWAYS   USUALLY   SOMETIMES   RARELY   NEVER

32. My employer understands what it is like to have a hearing loss.

   ALWAYS   USUALLY   SOMETIMES   RARELY   NEVER

33. I try to hide my hearing loss from my employer.

   ALWAYS   USUALLY   SOMETIMES   RARELY   NEVER

34. My co-workers speak loudly and clearly.

   ALWAYS   USUALLY   SOMETIMES   RARELY   NEVER

2H

The McCarthy-Alpiner Scale of Hearing Handicap (The M-A Scale) Form B*

NAME: _____ DATE: _____

AGE: _____ SEX: _____ TIME: _____

OCCUPATION: _____ PHONE: _____

ADDRESS: _____

RELATIONSHIP TO HEARING IMPAIRED INDIVIDUAL: _____

DO YOU HAVE A HEARING LOSS? _____ YES _____ NO _____

DIRECTIONS

The following questionnaire will be used to help audiologists understand what it is like to have a hearing loss. A member of your family has a hearing loss. We are interested in finding out what effects the hearing loss has had on his job, his family and the social aspects of his life.

Your task is to give your reaction to each of the statements included in the questionnaire. The items all concern the effects of the hearing loss on your hearing-impaired family member. You are to answer how the hearing loss has affected him in these aspects of his life. For example, you might be given the statement:

People tend to avoid him because of his hearing loss.

		×		
ALWAYS	USUALLY	SOMETIMES	RARELY	NEVER

You are asked to mark your reaction to each of the statements as it applies to your hearing-impaired family member. Please put an × on the appropriate space. Please mark every item with only one answer as seen in the example.

In marking your answer, please keep in mind that ALWAYS means at all times or on all occasions. USUALLY refers to generally, commonly, or ordinarily. SOMETIMES means occasionally or on various occasions. RARELY refers to seldom or infrequently. NEVER means not ever or at no time.

If your family member is not presently employed, please respond "N/A" for not applicable.

All answers will be kept strictly confidential and used only to help audiologists to understand what it is like to have a hearing loss and the effects the hearing loss had on one's life.

1. He acts annoyed when people do not speak loud enough for him to hear them.

ALWAYS	USUALLY	SOMETIMES	RARELY	NEVER

2. He gets upset if he cannot hear or understand a conversation.

ALWAYS	USUALLY	SOMETIMES	RARELY	NEVER

3. He feels like he is isolated from things because of his hearing loss.

ALWAYS	USUALLY	SOMETIMES	RARELY	NEVER

4. He feels negative about life in general because of his hearing loss.

ALWAYS	USUALLY	SOMETIMES	RARELY	NEVER

5. He admits to most people that he has a hearing loss.

ALWAYS	USUALLY	SOMETIMES	RARELY	NEVER

6. He gets upset when he feels that people are "mumbling."

ALWAYS	USUALLY	SOMETIMES	RARELY	NEVER

7. He feels very frustrated when he cannot understand a conversation.

ALWAYS	USUALLY	SOMETIMES	RARELY	NEVER

8. He feels that people in general understand what it is like to have a hearing loss.

ALWAYS	USUALLY	SOMETIMES	RARELY	NEVER

9. His hearing loss has affected his life in general.

ALWAYS	USUALLY	SOMETIMES	RARELY	NEVER

10. He is afraid that people will not like him if they find out that he has a hearing loss.

ALWAYS	USUALLY	SOMETIMES	RARELY	NEVER

11. He tends to avoid people because of his hearing loss.

ALWAYS	USUALLY	SOMETIMES	RARELY	NEVER

12. People act annoyed when he cannot understand what is being said in a group conversation.

ALWAYS	USUALLY	SOMETIMES	RARELY	NEVER

13. The family is patient with him when he cannot hear.

ALWAYS	USUALLY	SOMETIMES	RARELY	NEVER

14. Strangers react rudely when he does not understand what they say.

ALWAYS	USUALLY	SOMETIMES	RARELY	NEVER

15. He asks a person to repeat if he does not hear or understand what is said.

ALWAYS	USUALLY	SOMETIMES	RARELY	NEVER

16. His hearing loss has affected his relationship with his spouse.

ALWAYS	USUALLY	SOMETIMES	RARELY	NEVER

17. He does not go places with the family because of his hearing loss.

ALWAYS	USUALLY	SOMETIMES	RARELY	NEVER

18. Group discussions make him nervous because of his hearing loss.

   ALWAYS   USUALLY   SOMETIMES   RARELY   NEVER

19. People in general are tolerant of his hearing loss.

   ALWAYS   USUALLY   SOMETIMES   RARELY   NEVER

20. He avoids going to movies or plays because of his hearing loss.

   ALWAYS   USUALLY   SOMETIMES   RARELY   NEVER

21. He avoids going to restaurants because of his hearing loss.

   ALWAYS   USUALLY   SOMETIMES   RARELY   NEVER

22. He enjoys social situations with considerable conversation.

   ALWAYS   USUALLY   SOMETIMES   RARELY   NEVER

23. He is not interested in group activities because of his hearing loss.

   ALWAYS   USUALLY   SOMETIMES   RARELY   NEVER

24. He enjoys group discussions even though he has a hearing loss.

   ALWAYS   USUALLY   SOMETIMES   RARELY   NEVER

25. His hearing loss has interfered with his job performance.

   ALWAYS   USUALLY   SOMETIMES   RARELY   NEVER

26. He cannot perform his job well because of his hearing loss.

   ALWAYS   USUALLY   SOMETIMES   RARELY   NEVER

27. His co-workers know what it is like to have a hearing loss.

   ALWAYS   USUALLY   SOMETIMES   RARELY   NEVER

28. He tries to hide his hearing loss from his co-workers.

   ALWAYS   USUALLY   SOMETIMES   RARELY   NEVER

29. He does not enjoy going to work because of his hearing loss.

   ALWAYS   USUALLY   SOMETIMES   RARELY   NEVER

30. He is given credit for doing a good job at work even though he has a hearing loss.

   ALWAYS   USUALLY   SOMETIMES   RARELY   NEVER

31. He feels more pressure at work because of his hearing loss.

   ALWAYS   USUALLY   SOMETIMES   RARELY   NEVER

32. His employer understands what it is like to have a hearing loss.

   ALWAYS   USUALLY   SOMETIMES   RARELY   NEVER

33. He tries to hide his hearing loss from his employer.

   ALWAYS   USUALLY   SOMETIMES   RARELY   NEVER

34. His co-workers speak loudly and clearly.

   ALWAYS   USUALLY   SOMETIMES   RARELY   NEVER

21

Profile Questionnaire for Rating Communicative Performance in a Home Environment*

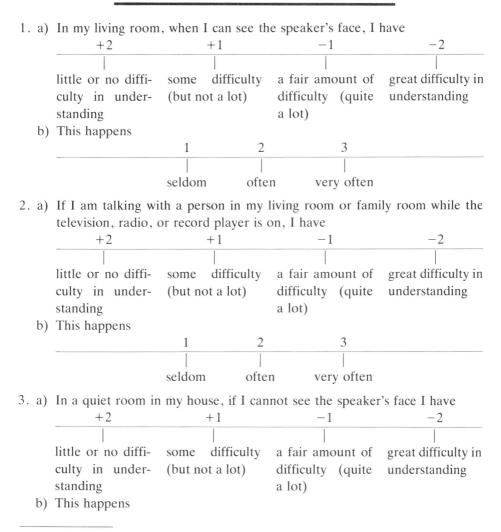

1. a) In my living room, when I can see the speaker's face, I have

+2	+1	−1	−2
little or no diffi-culty in under-standing	some difficulty (but not a lot)	a fair amount of difficulty (quite a lot)	great difficulty in understanding

b) This happens

1	2	3
seldom	often	very often

2. a) If I am talking with a person in my living room or family room while the television, radio, or record player is on, I have

+2	+1	−1	−2
little or no diffi-culty in under-standing	some difficulty (but not a lot)	a fair amount of difficulty (quite a lot)	great difficulty in understanding

b) This happens

1	2	3
seldom	often	very often

3. a) In a quiet room in my house, if I cannot see the speaker's face I have

+2	+1	−1	−2
little or no diffi-culty in under-standing	some difficulty (but not a lot)	a fair amount of difficulty (quite a lot)	great difficulty in understanding

b) This happens

---

* Reprinted by permission from Sanders: Hearing aid orientation and counseling. In M. C. Pollack (Ed.), *Amplification for the Hearing Impaired,* © 1975, Grune & Stratton.

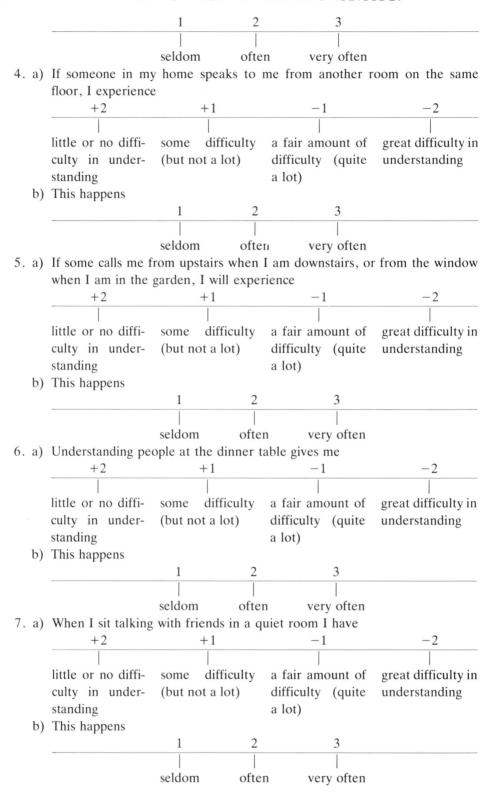

	1	2	3
	seldom	often	very often

4. a) If someone in my home speaks to me from another room on the same floor, I experience

+2	+1	−1	−2
little or no diffi-culty in under-standing	some difficulty (but not a lot)	a fair amount of difficulty (quite a lot)	great difficulty in understanding

b) This happens

	1	2	3
	seldom	often	very often

5. a) If some calls me from upstairs when I am downstairs, or from the window when I am in the garden, I will experience

+2	+1	−1	−2
little or no diffi-culty in under-standing	some difficulty (but not a lot)	a fair amount of difficulty (quite a lot)	great difficulty in understanding

b) This happens

	1	2	3
	seldom	often	very often

6. a) Understanding people at the dinner table gives me

+2	+1	−1	−2
little or no diffi-culty in under-standing	some difficulty (but not a lot)	a fair amount of difficulty (quite a lot)	great difficulty in understanding

b) This happens

	1	2	3
	seldom	often	very often

7. a) When I sit talking with friends in a quiet room I have

+2	+1	−1	−2
little or no diffi-culty in under-standing	some difficulty (but not a lot)	a fair amount of difficulty (quite a lot)	great difficulty in understanding

b) This happens

	1	2	3
	seldom	often	very often

8. a) Listening to the radio, record player, or watching TV gives me

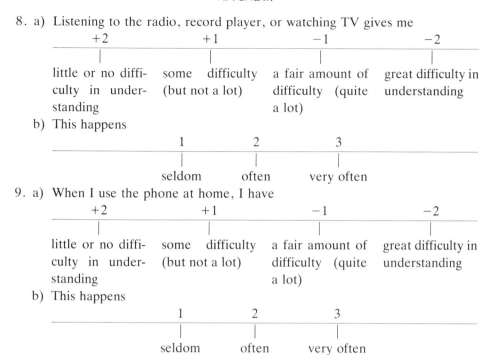

+2	+1	−1	−2
little or no difficulty in understanding	some difficulty (but not a lot)	a fair amount of difficulty (quite a lot)	great difficulty in understanding

b) This happens

1	2	3
seldom	often	very often

9. a) When I use the phone at home, I have

+2	+1	−1	−2
little or no difficulty in understanding	some difficulty (but not a lot)	a fair amount of difficulty (quite a lot)	great difficulty in understanding

b) This happens

1	2	3
seldom	often	very often

2J

Profile Questionnaire for Rating Communicative Performance in an Occupational Environment*

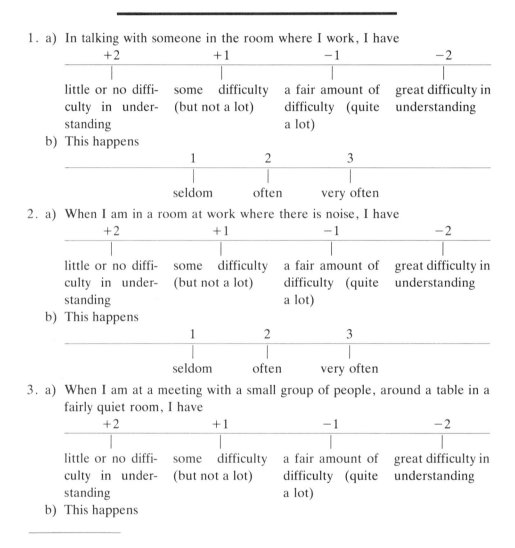

1. a) In talking with someone in the room where I work, I have

+2	+1	-1	-2
little or no diffi-culty in under-standing	some difficulty (but not a lot)	a fair amount of difficulty (quite a lot)	great difficulty in understanding

   b) This happens

1	2	3
seldom	often	very often

2. a) When I am in a room at work where there is noise, I have

+2	+1	-1	-2
little or no diffi-culty in under-standing	some difficulty (but not a lot)	a fair amount of difficulty (quite a lot)	great difficulty in understanding

   b) This happens

1	2	3
seldom	often	very often

3. a) When I am at a meeting with a small group of people, around a table in a fairly quiet room, I have

+2	+1	-1	-2
little or no diffi-culty in under-standing	some difficulty (but not a lot)	a fair amount of difficulty (quite a lot)	great difficulty in understanding

   b) This happens

---

* Reprinted by permission from Sanders: Hearing aid orientation and counseling. In M. C. Pollack (Ed.), *Amplification for the Hearing Impaired,* © 1975, Grune & Stratton.

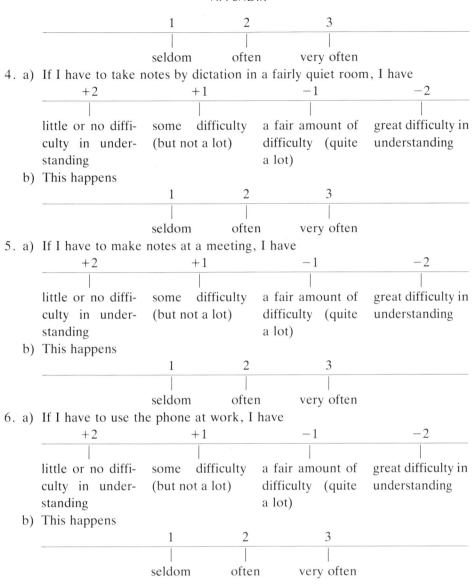

	1	2	3
	seldom	often	very often

4. a) If I have to take notes by dictation in a fairly quiet room, I have

+2	+1	−1	−2
little or no difficulty in understanding	some difficulty (but not a lot)	a fair amount of difficulty (quite a lot)	great difficulty in understanding

b) This happens

	1	2	3
	seldom	often	very often

5. a) If I have to make notes at a meeting, I have

+2	+1	−1	−2
little or no difficulty in understanding	some difficulty (but not a lot)	a fair amount of difficulty (quite a lot)	great difficulty in understanding

b) This happens

	1	2	3
	seldom	often	very often

6. a) If I have to use the phone at work, I have

+2	+1	−1	−2
little or no difficulty in understanding	some difficulty (but not a lot)	a fair amount of difficulty (quite a lot)	great difficulty in understanding

b) This happens

	1	2	3
	seldom	often	very often

APPENDIX

2K

Profile Questionnaire for Rating Communicative Performance in a Social Environment*

1. a) If we are entertaining a group of friends, understanding someone against the background of others talking gives me

+2	+1	−1	−2
little or no diffi-culty	some difficulty (but not a lot)	a fair amount of difficulty (quite a lot)	great difficulty

b) This happens

1	2	3
seldom	often	very often

2. a) If we are playing cards, understanding my partner gives me

+2	+1	−1	−2
little or no diffi-culty	some difficulty (but not a lot)	a fair amount of difficulty (quite a lot)	great difficulty

b) This happens

1	2	3
seldom	often	very often

3. a) When I am at the theater or the movies, I have

+2	+1	−1	−2
little or no diffi-culty in under-standing	some difficulty (but not a lot)	a fair amount of difficulty (quite a lot)	great difficulty in understanding

b) This happens

* Reprinted by permission from Sanders: Hearing aid orientation and counseling. In M. C. Pollack (Ed.), *Amplification for the Hearing Impaired,* © 1975, Grune & Stratton.

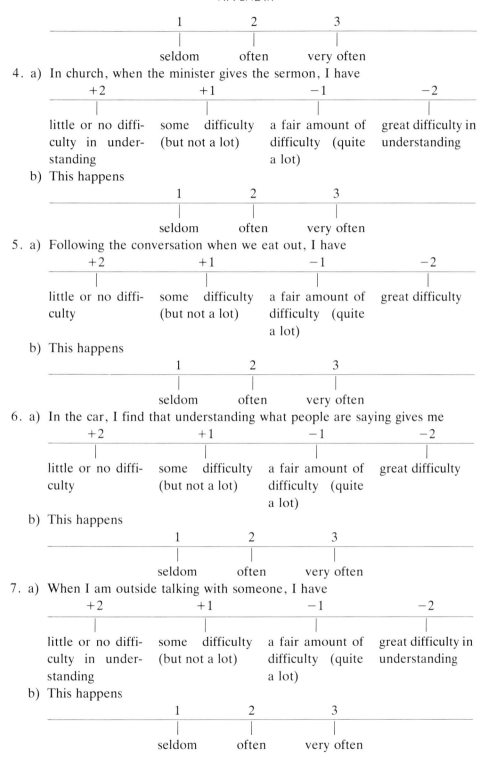

```
              1          2          3
              |          |          |
            seldom     often    very often
```

4. a) In church, when the minister gives the sermon, I have

```
        +2              +1              -1              -2
        |               |               |               |
```

little or no diffi- some difficulty   a fair amount of   great difficulty in
culty in under-   (but not a lot)   difficulty (quite understanding
standing   a lot)

   b) This happens

```
              1          2          3
              |          |          |
            seldom     often    very often
```

5. a) Following the conversation when we eat out, I have

```
        +2              +1              -1              -2
        |               |               |               |
```

little or no diffi- some difficulty   a fair amount of   great difficulty
culty   (but not a lot)   difficulty (quite
                                        a lot)

   b) This happens

```
              1          2          3
              |          |          |
            seldom     often    very often
```

6. a) In the car, I find that understanding what people are saying gives me

```
        +2              +1              -1              -2
        |               |               |               |
```

little or no diffi- some difficulty   a fair amount of   great difficulty
culty   (but not a lot)   difficulty (quite
                                        a lot)

   b) This happens

```
              1          2          3
              |          |          |
            seldom     often    very often
```

7. a) When I am outside talking with someone, I have

```
        +2              +1              -1              -2
        |               |               |               |
```

little or no diffi- some difficulty   a fair amount of   great difficulty in
culty in under-   (but not a lot)   difficulty (quite understanding
standing   a lot)

   b) This happens

```
              1          2          3
              |          |          |
            seldom     often    very often
```

2L

California Consonant Test*

Name_____   Date_____

List 1

Test Items

1 GAVE ___	11 PAGE ___	21 SHIN ___	31 VALE ___	41 KIT ___
GAME ___	PAID ___	SIN ___	DALE ___	KICK ___
GAZE ___	PAYS ___	THIN ___	JAIL ___	KISS ___
GAGE ___	PAVE ___	CHIN ___	BALE ___	KID ___

2 PAIL ___	12 KICK ___	22 MUFF ___	32 PEACH ___	42 PIN ___
SAIL ___	PICK ___	MUCH ___	PEAT ___	KIN ___
FAIL ___	TICK ___	MUSH ___	PEAK ___	TIN ___
TAIL ___	THICK ___	MUSS ___	PEEP ___	THIN ___

Sample Items

1 BACK ___	3 CUFF ___	13 LAUGH ___	23 REACH ___	33 RACK ___	43 BUS ___
BAG ___	CUP ___	LASH ___	REAP ___	RASH ___	BUT ___
BATCH ___	CUSS ___	LASS ___	REEF ___	RAT ___	BUCK ___
BATH ___	CUT ___	LAP ___	REEK ___	RAP ___	BUFF ___

2 RICE ___	4 MUSS ___	14 SHEEP ___	24 BACK ___	34 HAG ___	44 GATE ___
DICE ___	MUCH ___	SEEP ___	BAT ___	HAD ___	BAIT ___
NICE ___	MUSH ___	CHEAP ___	BATCH ___	HAVE ___	DATE ___
LICE ___	MUFF ___	HEAP ___	BATH ___	HAS ___	WAIT ___

3 SEEN ___	5 FAKE ___	15 GAVE ___	25 TAME ___	35 TICK ___	45 LAUGH ___
SEED ___	FATE ___	GAME ___	SHAME ___	SICK ___	LASS ___
SEAL ___	FACE ___	GAGE ___	FAME ___	THICK ___	LASH ___
SEAT ___	FAITH ___	GAZE ___	SAME ___	PICK ___	LAP ___

4 BAIL ___	6 TILL ___	16 BEACH ___	26 CORE ___	36 CHAIR ___	46 HIP ___
TALE ___	CHILL ___	BEEP ___	PORE ___	CARE ___	HIT ___
SAIL ___	PILL ___	BEAK ___	TORE ___	SHARE ___	HISS ___
DALE ___	KILL ___	BEET ___	SORE ___	FAIR ___	HITCH ___

5 LEAVE ___	7 LEASE ___	17 MASS ___	27 RAGE ___	37 BEACH ___	47 HICK ___
LEASH ___	LEASH ___	MAP ___	RAISE ___	BEAK ___	SICK ___
LEAN ___	LEAF ___	MAT ___	RAVE ___	BEET ___	THICK ___
LEAGUE ___	LEAP ___	MATH ___	RAID ___	BEEP ___	CHICK ___

6 RAIL ___	8 SEEP ___	18 PATH ___	28 FILL ___	38 BEAK ___	48 LEAF ___
JAIL ___	CHEAP ___	PATCH ___	PILL ___	BEEP ___	LEASE ___
TAIL ___	SHEEP ___	PACK ___	KILL ___	BEAT ___	LEASH ___
BALE ___	HEAP ___	PAT ___	TILL ___	BEEF ___	LEAK ___

9 FACE ___	19 GAZE ___	29 CHOP ___	39 CHEEK ___	49 CHEEK ___
FAITH ___	GAGE ___	POP ___	CHIEF ___	CHEAP ___
FATE ___	GAVE ___	TOP ___	CHEAT ___	CHEAT ___
FAKE ___	GAME ___	SHOP ___	CHEAP ___	CHIEF ___

10 BAYS ___	20 SICK ___	30 MUCK ___	40 CUP ___	50 RID ___
BABE ___	CHICK ___	MUTT ___	CUT ___	RIB ___
BALE ___	THICK ___	MUSS ___	CUSS ___	RIDGE ___
BATHE ___	TICK ___	MUFF ___	CUFF ___	RIG ___

* Reprinted by permission from *California Consonant Test*, Auditec of St. Louis, 330 Selma Ave., St. Louis, MO 63119.

51	THIN ____	61	TAN ____	71	THAN ____	81	MATCH____	91	HIP ____
	TIN ____		CAN ____		VAN ____		MAT ____		HICK ____
	SIN ____		FAN ____		BAN ____		MATH ____		HIT ____
	SHIN ____		PAN ____		PAN ____		MAP ____		HISS ____
52	HIT ____	62	TORE ____	72	SHEATH____	82	PATCH____	92	TIN ____
	HIP ____		CORE ____		SHEEP ____		PAT ____		KIN ____
	HISS ____		PORE ____		SHEIK ____		PASS ____		PIN ____
	HITCH ____		CHORE ____		SHEET ____		PATH ____		THIN ____
53	PAYS ____	63	SIS ____	73	TAN ____	83	FAITH ____	93	CASH ____
	PAVE ____		SIP ____		PAN ____		FATE ____		CAT ____
	PAGE ____		SIT ____		CAN ____		FAKE ____		CAP ____
	PAID ____		SICK ____		FAN ____		FACE ____		CATCH____
54	HIT ____	64	CUSS ____	74	BATCH____	84	RID ____	94	HATCH____
	HICK ____		CUP ____		BAT ____		RIB ____		HAT ____
	HITCH ____		CUT ____		BACK ____		RIG ____		HACK ____
	HIP ____		CUFF ____		BATH ____		RIDGE ____		HALF ____
55	SICK ____	65	RAP ____	75	PAIL ____	85	CHEAP____	95	DIVE ____
	SIP ____		RACK ____		TAIL ____		CHEAT____		DIED ____
	SIT ____		RASH ____		SAIL ____		CHEEK____		DIES ____
	SIS ____		RAT ____		FAIL ____		CHIEF ____		DINE ____
56	BEET ____	66	KILL ____	76	BUG ____	86	SORE ____	96	SIN ____
	BEEP ____		PILL ____		BUDGE____		CHORE____		FIN ____
	BEACH____		TILL ____		BUZZ ____		SHORE____		THIN ____
	BEAK ____		FILL ____		BUD ____		FOR ____		SHIN ____
57	HATCH____	67	SICK ____	77	SAIL ____	87	POP ____	97	RODE ____
	HACK ____		TICK ____		PAIL ____		TOP ____		ROBE ____
	HALF ____		PICK ____		TAIL ____		CHOP ____		ROVE ____
	HAT ____		THICK ____		FAIL ____		COP ____		ROSE ____
58	CHIN ____	68	PAGE ____	78	ROBE ____	88	MAP ____	98	BAIL ____
	SHIN ____		PAYS ____		RODE ____		MATCH____		JAIL ____
	THIN ____		PAVE ____		ROSE ____		MATH ____		DALE ____
	PIN ____		PAID ____		ROVE ____		MAT ____		GALE ____
59	HAIL ____	69	TORE ____	79	LASS ____	89	DIES ____	99	LEAF ____
	TAIL ____		PORE ____		LAUGH____		DIED ____		LEASE ____
	FAIL ____		CORE ____		LATCH ____		DIVE ____		LEACH____
	SAIL ____		SORE ____		LASH ____		DINE ____		LEASH____
60	SHUN ____	70	LEASH ____	80	FIN ____	90	PEAK ____	100	RAISE ____
	PUN ____		LEAK ____		PIN ____		PEACH____		RAID ____
	SUN ____		LEASE ____		KIN ____		PEAT ____		RAGE ____
	FUN ____		LEAF ____		TIN ____		PEEP ____		RAVE ____

2M

Central Institute for the Deaf (CID) Everyday Speech Sentences*

LIST A

1. Walking's my favorite exercise.
2. Here's a nice quiet place to rest.
3. Our janitor sweeps the floors every night.
4. It would be much easier if everyone would help.
5. Good morning.
6. Open your window before you go to bed!
7. Do you think that she should stay out so late?
8. How do you feel about changing the time when we begin to work?
9. Here we go.
10. Move out of the way.

LIST B

1. The water's too cold for swimming.
2. Why should I get up so early in the morning?
3. Here are your shoes.
4. It's raining.
5. Where are you going?
6. Come here when I call you!
7. Don't try go get out of it this time!
8. Should we let little children go to the movies by themselves?
9. There isn't enough paint to finish the room.
10. Do you want an egg for breakfast?

LIST C

1. Everybody should brush his teeth after meals.
2. Everything's all right.
3. Don't use up all the paper when you write your letter.

* Reprinted by permission from Davis and Silverman: *Hearing and Deafness,* © 1970, Holt, Rinehart and Winston, Inc.

4. That's right.
5. People ought to see a doctor once a year.
6. Those windows are so dirty I can't see anything outside.
7. Pass the bread and butter please!
8. Don't forget to pay your bill before the first of the month.
9. Don't let the dog out of the house!
10. There's a good ballgame this afternoon.

LIST D

1. It's time to go.
2. If you don't want these old magazines, throw them out.
3. Do you want to wash up?
4. It's a real dark night so watch your driving.
5. I'll carry the package for you.
6. Did you forget to shut off the water?
7. Fishing in a mountain stream is my idea of a good time.
8. Fathers spend more time with their children than they used to.
9. Be careful not to break your glasses!
10. I'm sorry.

LIST E

1. You can catch the bus across the street.
2. Call her on the phone and tell her the news.
3. I'll catch up with you later.
4. I'll think it over.
5. I don't want to go to the movies tonight.
6. If your tooth hurts that much you ought to see a dentist.
7. Put that cookie back in the box!
8. Stop fooling around!
9. Time's up.
10. How do you spell your name?

LIST F

1. Music always cheers me up.
2. My brother's in town for a short while on business.
3. We live a few miles from the main road.
4. This suit needs to go to the cleaners.
5. They ate enough green apples to make them sick for a week.
6. Where have you been all this time?
7. Have you been working hard lately?
8. There's not enough room in the kitchen for a new table.
9. Where is he?
10. Look out!

LIST G

1. I'll see you right after lunch.
2. See you later.

3. White shoes are awful to keep clean.
4. Stand there and don't move until I tell you!
5. There's a big piece of cake left over from dinner.
6. Wait for me at the corner in front of the drugstore.
7. It's no trouble at all.
8. Hurry up!
9. The morning paper didn't say anything about rain this afternoon or tonight.
10. The phone call's for you.

LIST H

1. Believe me!
2. Let's get a cup of coffee.
3. Let's get out of here before it's too late.
4. I hate driving at night.
5. There was water in the cellar after the heavy rain yesterday.
6. She'll only be gone a few minutes.
7. How do you know?
8. Children like candy.
9. If we don't get rain soon, we'll have no grass.
10. They're not listed in the new phone book.

LIST I

1. Where can I find a place to park?
2. I like those big red apples we always get in the fall.
3. You'll get fat eating candy.
4. The show's over.
5. Why don't they paint their walls some other color?
6. What's new?
7. What are you hiding under your coat?
8. How come I should always be the one to go first?
9. I'll take sugar and cream in my coffee.
10. Wait just a minute!

LIST J

1. Breakfast is ready.
2. I don't know what's wrong with the car, but it won't start.
3. It sure takes a sharp knife to cut this meat.
4. I haven't read a newspaper since we bought a television set.
5. Weeds are spoiling the yard.
6. Call me a little later!
7. Do you have change for a five-dollar bill?
8. How are you?
9. I'd like some ice cream with my pie.
10. I don't think I'll have any dessert.

3

The Hearing Aid as Related to Rehabilitation

Roger N. Kasten, Ph.D. and
Robert L. McCroskey, Ph.D.

The major thrust of this chapter is to provide a base of information that will permit effective utilization of amplification in the rehabilitative process. The goal is to identify and discuss some critical elements that affect optimal use of amplification.

The target population is the adult segment of society, but adulthood does not remain consistent across the wide age range that it encompasses. The word "adult" is considered, not in the chronological sense or in the legal sense but, rather, in terms of the maturity of the auditory system. Auditorily, adulthood is reached at approximately 10 years of age. The system remains highly stable through the next four decades of life, after which there are changes that cause the system to perform in a manner similar to that during the time period from 9 years of age backward to 0 years.

This chapter will include discussions relating to both the adult and the aging populations. Within each of these groups—but particularly for the aging group—attention will be given to the internal and external forces that help determine the effectiveness with which amplification can be worn. Much of the following is appropriate for both groups of hearing-impaired individuals, but additional information relating primarily to the aging population and their unique abilities and disabilities will be added.

FDA REGULATIONS

The Food and Drug Administration regulations dealing with hearing aids became effective in August of 1977 (FDA, 1977). This document mandated for the first time that certain information had to be made available to the hearing aid user.

Physical Examination Prerequisite

A physician who specializes in diseases of the ear should have examined the prospective hearing aid user within 6 months of the actual selection of the aid. It is the obligation of the hearing aid dispenser and of the audiologist—if the audiologist has first contact with the person—to ensure that the client is informed of the need and the reason for the medical examination and to inform the client of the advantages and disadvantages of exercising the option to waive the medical examination. Persons under 18 years of age are generally required to have this examination but the person over age 18 may sign a waiver that can be obtained from the hearing aid dispenser.

It is difficult to fault the wisdom of the required physician examination. The purpose of the examination is to detect and remediate medical conditions that may contraindicate the use of amplification or that may negate the necessity for amplification following treatment. An informal poll of hearing aid sellers in our geographical area, however, reveals that approximately 85% of hearing aid purchasers are choosing to waive the required medical examination. This high rejection rate for the medical examination does not appear to be unique to any one geographical area. Discussions with those individuals involved with the sale of hearing aids in many parts of the United States consistently produce estimates that 85 to 90% of hearing aid buyers opt to sign the medical waiver in lieu of a medical examination.

The reasons given for this curious turn of events appear to be 3-fold. First, many repeat hearing aid purchasers feel they have experienced no medical problems during their previous hearing aid use and fail to see the need for a medical examination to confirm their own belief that no medical problems exist. Second, many hearing aid purchasers see the requirement for a medical examination as being nothing more than one more governmentally imposed regulation that will increase the price of an already expensive purchase. With the price of physician office visits becoming more and more costly, the purchaser is frequently willing to take the word of the seller that nothing appears to be grossly abnormal. Third, in the past few years many medical ear specialists have elected to add the sale of hearing aids to the range of services offered to their patients. With these physicians now in the business of selling hearing aids, many nonmedical hearing aid sellers see a referral to the ear specialist as the loss of a customer. They report instances of referring potential customers for medical examination and never seeing the customer again.

It is unfortunate that the above circumstances serve to diminish greatly the effectiveness of this worthwhile and important requirement. Care should be taken, with all hearing aid purchasers, to encourage medical examination for the well-being and safety of the hearing aid user.

Labeling Requirements

Instructional brochures accompanying hearing aids contain illustrations that indicate the location and use of operating controls, user adjustments, and battery compartment. Descriptions of accessories to the hearing aid are included so that the user can understand and take advantage of specialized provisions for listening to television or the telephone. According to Castle (1978), the National Technical Institute for the Deaf has available a structured course in telephone communication for the profoundly hearing-impaired. This program lends itself to modification for use with less severely hearing-impaired users of hearing aids.

Instructional information must also include statements for general maintenance and care of the hearing aid. It is not practical to include extensive trouble-shooting procedures, but it is very helpful to include maintenance checks that will identify the most commonly occurring malfunctions and provide suggested steps in the remediation of the problem.

Hearing Aid Repair Service

Informational brochures accompanying hearing aids identify one source of hearing aid repair service. In many instances the instructions are that the hearing aid must be returned to the manufacturer or sent to a regional repair service. Unfortunately, the average hearing aid user has no means of verifying the quality of repairs made to the aid. While one might consider that the user's ear is sufficient to determine whether the aid is functioning properly, there are technical aspects that can influence perception without obvious or gross qualitative differences in the signal delivered to the hearing-impaired user. Users' awareness of their own hearing impairments make them less likely to trust their own judgments of the effectiveness of the repair. A complete electroacoustic analysis following service, however, might reveal that the aid either did not meet its original specifications or that the cause of the original complaint still had not been corrected. In a later section of this chapter, attention will be given to the possible effects of subtle variations in attack/release time on Automatic Gain Control (AGC) Instruments as well as some possible effects of relatively minor levels of distortion.

Warren and Kasten (1976) used a relatively limited sample of hearing aids to determine the quality of hearing repair. Their data indicate that only 39% of repaired hearing aid systems could be considered as acceptable when they were returned to the owner as repaired. The concern for the quality of repair lies not just with audiologists but represents a feeling expressed by many hearing aid dispensers. With the advent of microprocessor hearing aid test boxes (systems) it is possible to verify whether a hearing aid meets the manufacturer's specifications at the time of the sale and to verify the quality of any subsequent repair, with very little time investment. These microprocessors are generally available at university audiology clinics and are increasingly available among hearing aid dispensers. The ability to verify the original specifications and the quality of subsequent repairs should lead to improved service to the hearing-impaired consumer.

Rehabilitation Techniques

Instructional brochures accompanying hearing aids include a general statement indicating that the hearing aid is a first step in the rehabilitative process and that it may need to be supplemented with auditory training and speechreading instruction. The intent is to let the user know that there are factors other than the simple increase in intensity that contribute to the effectiveness of the hearing aid. It should be noted that the user who is aware of the adverse effects of reverberation in a room or theater, or is aware of the factors that make difficult the identifying of a target signal from among many competing signals, will use the hearing aid more effectively than an individual who does not understand why incoming messages are not as clear as they need to be. These elements will be discussed in more detail later.

Many new users of hearing aids appear to be totally unaware that help with communication exists beyond the uninformed use of a hearing aid. Speechreading (lipreading) is viewed as a skill that is to be taught only to "deaf" individuals. They tend to assume that since they have been communicating successfully throughout their lives, they have all the communicative skills that are needed. They are not aware of any additional skills that might serve to make the communication process easier. Indeed, until they are made aware of the potential for improved communication through an educational program, they cannot take advantage of this kind of help. Hearing-impaired persons must be made aware that a complete program of rehabilitation includes more than amplification, and it is the respon-

sibility of everyone involved in the diagnosis and selection of a hearing aid to inform these people not only of the need but of the availability of programs in areas where they live.

Warning Statements

The primary warning is a statement that the hearing aid dispenser should advise the potential hearing aid user to seek medical attention before purchasing the hearing aid if the user has experienced any of the following conditions.

1. Visible congenital or traumatic deformity of the ear
2. History of active drainage within the previous 90 days
3. Sudden or rapidly progressing hearing loss within 90 days
4. Acute or chronic dizziness
5. Unilateral hearing loss of sudden onset within the previous 90 days
6. Audiometric air-bone gap of 15 dB or greater at 500 Hz, 1000 Hz, and 2000Hz
7. Visible evidence of significant cerumen accumulation or foreign body in the ear canal
8. Pain or discomfort in the ear (FDA, 1977)

The awareness of the implications of these conditions is not universal and it is important that the consumer be informed so that appropriate health practice is more likely to occur—particularly where neither the disciplines of otology nor audiology have had previous input into the rehabilitation effort. The need for medical assessment prior to hearing aid fitting is accepted by persons with a background in otology or audiology.

The second warning statement deals with the risks involved in providing high intensity amplification. The statement is:

Special care should be exercised in selecting and fitting a hearing aid whose maximum sound pressure level exceeds 132 dB because there may be risks of impairing the remaining hearing of the hearing aid user. (Note: This statement is required only on brochures accompanying hearing aids capable of producing sound pressure levels greater than 132 dB.)

The relationship between high intensity sound and hearing impairment is well documented in industrial settings. The fact that a high intensity signal is being fed through a device that is supposed to contribute to one's health and well-being does not prevent it from causing damage. Concern over the possible adverse effects of high level amplification upon residual hearing has been expressed a number of times (Harford and Markle, 1955; Kinney, 1961; Macrae, 1968; Kasten and Braunlin, 1970; Jerger and Lewis, 1975). The particular decibel level identified in this second warning statement came from a report by Briskey and Kasten (1973) to the Amplification Committee of the Academy of Rehabilitative Audiology. The specific recommendation to the Food and Drug Administration for the inclusion of that statement was made following unanimous approval by the Academy of Rehabilitative Audiology (Hardick, 1975).

The statement on the maximum allowable limits was aimed primarily at the protection of children, but recent work by Weber (1979) carries the implication that long term fatiguing effects can occur in adults who wear amplification that is set at relatively high intensity levels. Indeed, he has recommended brief periods of rest from amplification during each hour of the day.

Humes and Bess (1981) view potential over-amplification as a specialized area within the general field of noise research. They describe a strategy that involves experimentally induced temporary threshold shift. This relates very closely to the work of Weber (1979) but offers a more stringent criterion of measurement. They propose not a single measure of temporary threshold shift (TTS) but measures of the whole pattern of TTS growth and recovery. This involves calculating a time integral of TTS for the period extending from the onset of noise exposure to complete recovery. They have developed a conversion chart for calculating critical output levels for a 4000-Hz tone for various durations of use of amplification. It is a theoretical construct worth considering. However, other variables appear to be related to the extent of temporary and permanent threshold shift as a function of noise exposure; for example, Carlin and McCroskey (1980) have demonstrated a relationship between eye color (the presence of melanin in the eye and in the inner ear) and noise-induced permanent threshold shift among industrial workers.

The normal expectation for hearing levels

in children is that they will remain stable with the passage of time. If over-amplification occurs and there is a decrement in hearing, it is more easily recognized. However, in that portion of the adult population who are over 18 years of age, the usual gradual decline in hearing sensitivity represents a confounding factor that must be considered. There are several assumptions here that need to be identified, even if they cannot be explained or related fully to the topic at hand. For example, the extensive work of Eagles *et al.* (1963) with school-aged children demonstrated that the auditory sensitivity was far better than the standard audiometric procedures could measure. Thus, it is possible that the gradual decline in auditory sensitivity that is recognized clearly in the middle years of life actually represents a continuum that begins by the time a child is in elementary school. Thus, a child whose true auditory threshold is zero at age 15 may already have sustained a substantial hearing loss as a function of disease, noise, or medication.

The other assumption is that hearing loss is normal as a product of advancing age. Certainly the two occur together but the situation is not universal. Such assumptions tend to steer researchers away from the very questions that need to be asked. There are whole frontiers of research in areas of nutrition, biological factors, environmental forces, and even psychologic factors that may relate to the so-called normal decline in hearing as a function of age.

Trial-Rental-Purchase Option

These options are very beneficial to the potential adult hearing aid user. The referral program at Wichita State University, involving a trial-rental-purchase option, has resulted in approximately a 98% success rate for those who have tried the program. This option allows experience with the amplification system in a pressure-free environment and gives time for either the hearing aid dispenser or the audiologist to help make adjustments in settings or configurations of the hearing aid, which has resulted in greater satisfaction by the user.

Electroacoustic Data

The FDA regulation now requires that the accompanying brochure include electroacoustic characteristics for the hearing aid, as measured in accordance with the American National Standards Institute Standard for the Specification for Hearing Aid Characteristics (ANSI, S3.22-1976). Unfortunately, the mode of presentation is often esoteric and defeats the purpose of providing information to the consumer. Users do not need a great deal of technical information about the decibel as long as there is appreciation of it as a unit of measure that relates to their perception of loudness. Indeed, a simple chart showing decibel values for common and meaningful sound sources may be sufficient. A potential user needs to be aware of the decibel value at which sound becomes uncomfortable, intolerable, or even dangerous to them and then they can relate the saturation output values (SSPL90 or HF-Average SSPL90) of the amplification system to their own needs. It may be adequate to describe the saturation output value in relation to an individual's own tolerance ceiling for intensity.

Frequency Response: The Ear *Versus* The Aid

The general population is more aware of the function of the human ear today than it has been at any time in the past. Units on human audition are regular parts of elementary and secondary education and this may lead the potential hearing aid user to question why there is a discrepancy between the upper limit of normal hearing and the upper limit passed through a hearing aid. The general feeling has been that once an individual has acquired his language and has developed facility with listening to spoken communication, the degree of redundancy in the language allows understanding to take place even when the full range of information in the original signal is not available to the listener. Indeed, some individuals appear to feel that there is some fortuitous relationship between the frequency range that can be amplified conveniently through a hearing aid and the so-called speech frequencies, and this combination gives justification to the restricted frequency range normally available in hearing aids. Professional workers, particularly, should stay cognizant of the kind of information that is available from the work of Guberina (1964) and from Berlin (1980).

Guberina has been concerned with eliminating dialects from the spoken language of individuals who have acquired a second language and, in the process, has found that there are certain optimal frequency bands that make some sounds maximally intelligible—regardless of the linguistic background of the listener. In many instances, the optimal frequency bands lie well above the frequency range available through common amplification systems; for example, the optimal frequency range for /s/ is in the 10,000- to 12,000-Hz range.

Berlin has demonstrated that not only speech production but speech comprehension can be significantly altered by providing profoundly hearing-impaired individuals with amplification in the neighborhood of 10,000 Hz. These data indicate audiologists and otologists must be sensitive to the particular needs of a given listener in making recommendations for amplification. Appreciation for the limitation of the aid is as significant as knowledge of its potential.

Harmonic Distortion

In general, one looks for amplification systems that have as little distortion as possible; however, it must be pointed out that a modest amount of harmonic distortion may have no adverse effect upon the usefulness of the hearing aid. Parker (1979) demonstrated that moderate amounts of harmonic distortion (not over 10%) actually enhanced the ability of a listener to identify certain acoustic events.

CHARACTERISTICS OF POPULATIONS

The incidence of hearing loss is also related to the aging process. Metropolitan Life Insurance Company (1976) statistics clearly demonstrate this pattern. Prior to age 45, the incidence of hearing loss in the general population is less than 4%. Between 45 and 64 years of age, the incidence rate more than doubles and reaches a value of approximately 11.5%. In the decade from 65 to 74 years, another significant increase occurs and the overall incidence reaches 23%. Beyond age 75, the incidence rate again shows a significant increase and reaches a level of 39.9% of the population.

In addition to these rather alarming statistics, consideration should also be given to that portion of the aging population who

reside in nursing homes. Schow and Nerbonne (1976) reported an incidence rate of
hearing loss of nursing home residents of
between 54 and 80%. This range in incidence
values reflected the application of either a 40-
dB or 25-dB cut-off value to represent the
beginning of a hearing loss. Hull (1980) has
reported consistently encountering incidence
rates of 85 to 90% among nursing home residents. Without entering into a controversy
over what constitutes a hearing loss for these
individuals, it should be clear that the prevalence of hearing loss in this restricted population is well in excess of that found in their
non-institutionalized counterparts.

As stated earlier, this chapter addresses two
unique segments of the general population.
When the adult population is mentioned, the
term "adult" will refer to auditory age, not
chronological age. The adult population,
therefore, will range from a chronological age
of approximately 10 years to approximately
55 years of age. Ten years was selected as the
lower age limit based upon the reports of
Willeford (1978) and McCroskey and Kasten
(1980) in which they demonstrated a maturational effect in the auditory system that
appears to stabilize by 10 years of age. Age
55 was selected as the upper limit of the adult
population and the beginning of the *aging*
population. This age was selected on the basis
of reports by Jerger and Hayes (1977) and by
McCroskey and Kasten (1980). Jerger compared speech discrimination performance of
monosyllabic words and synthetic sentences
and found that, beyond the age of 55 years,
subtle changes appear to occur in the auditory
system that result in poorer performance on
the synthetic sentence task; Jerger refers to
this as the "central effect." The difference in
performance becomes more pronounced with
advancing age. McCroskey and Kasten reported a series of investigations designed to
examine temporal auditory processing, and
one must conclude that from age 10 to approximately age 55, the auditory system remains quite stable with regard to auditory
timing functions; however, it is also in the
fifth decade of life that one begins to notice
that the auditory system requires more time
for the performance of a temporal task. This
tendency toward a slowing of temporal processing ability also increases systematically
with advancing age.

GENERAL CONSIDERATIONS FOR ADULT REHABILITATION

While it is important to provide the new or
continuing hearing aid users with all of the
information previously discussed regarding
their amplification systems, it must be borne
in mind that amplification is only a first step
in the total counselling process. From this
point in time—with the realization that all of
this information can be provided prior to the
actual hearing aid fitting—the essential characteristics of the counselling program should
be carried out with the hearing aid user and
with those who interact regularly with the
user. It is essential that we view the process
of counseling not as dealing only with a
hearing-impaired individual, but rather as
dealing with family, social, and vocational
units that have in them a hearing-impaired
individual.

Hearing aid users can be given the information and insights they need to cope with
their new acoustic environment, but it is ex-
ceedingly difficult for these same hearing aid
users to convince those closest to them that
they really know what they are talking about.
For example, imagine a 70-year-old woman
with a new hearing aid who is living in the
home of her daughter along with the daughter's husband and three teenage children. We
can do our best to teach this 70-year-old
hearing aid user how to cope with daily communicative problems, but we encounter real
obstacles as she attempts to relate her insights
into her hearing problem to those in her
family. It is easy to picture this grandmother
in the process of preparing an evening meal.
One of the teenagers runs through the kitchen
and shouts as he passes that he will be having
dinner at a friend's home and will return at
9:30 that evening. Our aided grandmother,
engrossed in her task and partially masked
by the noise of the kitchen, misses the entire
message but does not have time to have it
repeated because the teenager is already out
of the house. When dinner time arrives, the
parents are mildly annoyed because this one
particular child is late for the meal. By 7
o'clock, they are beginning to be concerned
because it is not like this child to be gone
without saying anything. By 8 o'clock, the
parents are beginning to become genuinely
alarmed at the absence of this child. By 9

o'clock the parents are ready to call the police to report a missing child and are also ready to initiate an all-out search in an attempt to determine what has happened. When the child finally arrives home at 9:30, the parents are beside themselves and, out of concern, verbally attack the child for being gone without saying anything. The child immediately retaliates by indicating that he had been home after school and he had told his grandmother exactly where he was going and when he was due to return. The entire family now turns upon grandmother, who might as well be considered as being senile, and another avoidable and unfortunate communicative situation has turned into a major family disaster.

Imagine, if you will, how much success this particular grandmother would have under these circumstances, in trying to convince her family that she could have gotten the message if she had been given a chance. Imagine how much success this grandmother would have in trying to (a) convince the family that their appreciation and understanding of the communicative environment could have changed the whole situation; (b) make the family believe that she could have heard and she could have understood if she had just received a little help from those who were trying to communicate with her; and (c) convince the family that she is not potentially dangerous to have around the house. The irony of this situation is that the family is probably convinced that grandmother should be able to hear because she is wearing a hearing aid— and they are equally convinced that the cause for this unfortunate situation is undoubtedly grandmother's rapidly deteriorating mental condition. The example is somewhat involved but it illustrates that an orientation program is likely to be only marginally successful if it includes just the hearing aid user. Obviously, the family constellation and possibly the vocational setting must achieve some degree of understanding and insight in order to optimize the success with a hearing aid.

States in Personal Adjustment

Prior to any specific discussion of counselling or a hearing aid orientation program, it seems advisable to consider some of the stages of realism that may be encountered by many potential hearing aid users. These stages are presented, not just to help understand the hearing aid user, but to understand the feelings and the biases of those most closely associated with the hearing aid user who have witnessed the progression through these various stages. To begin with, potential hearing aid users experience a period of denial. They are fully aware of the fact that the world is not as loud as it used to be, but the problem centers with the world and not with themselves. They readily acknowledge the fact that they are having more and more difficulty hearing and understanding spoken communication, but the reason for this problem is that people are not talking as loud or as clearly as they used to, or that they are talking faster than ever before. This first line of defense generally gives the hearing aid user an extended period of time during which the existence of the hearing loss is denied or rationalized so as to place the blame for miscommunication on someone else.

Following the denial stage generally comes a stage of anger. Potential hearing aid users begin to acknowledge (but only to themselves) that they may be part of the problem but they righteously chastise those around them when communication fails. It does not seem fair to them that they should be having this kind of problem; they cannot see why they have been selected to bear such a burden. When they are unable to hear or understand the rapid conversations of their children, they may become infuriated; they may seethe within themselves when they either miss or misunderstand instructions or directions in the occupational setting; they become deeply resentful of friends and associates whose comments and quick asides are lost as a result of their hearing disorder; and finally, they display overt anger and annoyance at whispered comments or low level statements that are no longer intelligible.

When denial is futile and anger only aggravates the situation, it is only a short psychologic journey into a state of depression where feelings of self-pity and embarrassment are rampant. The depression stage is probably the most debilitating of all stages and is frequently the most obvious to those who interact with hearing-impaired individuals. The symptoms are not unlike those that characterize the depression stemming from organic or chemical disorders. They finally are confronted with the reality that life style has been affected and dreams for the "good life" may need to be altered. They recognize the fact that they are at a genuine disadvantage in many communicative environments and their attempts to participate in the give-and-take of verbal communication may cause them to appear foolish. Feelings of self-pity and embarrassment are often coupled with deliberate efforts to avoid social settings that require communicative participation. Unfortunately, they not only exclude themselves, but they impose the isolation upon their spouses and their families. Not only do they withdraw from former activities, but they begin to resent those who continue to participate.

Acceptance of the problem and the attendant responsibility may emerge from a variety of experiences. It may come from observing other hearing aid users who have developed skills in coping with difficult listening situations or it may come from direct statements by family and friends. Regardless of the source, the acceptance stage generally lifts an enormous burden from potential hearing aid users. They begin to accept the fact that they are having difficulty only with their hearing and that this is certainly not the end of the world for them. As a general rule, the acceptance stage allows potential hearing aid users to return to their former personalities and signals to family and friends that a severe problem has been averted. Unfortunately, acceptance may not get translated into action. The regained interaction is so well received that the original causative factor—the hearing loss—is masked and rarely mentioned. Our affected individual, now accepting the cause of the problem, again takes an interest in family and friends and begins to interact with the world around him. Unfortunately, the acceptance stage is all too often viewed as the ultimate answer to the problem that precipitated the entire situation. Potential hearing aid users—almost euphoric over the acceptance of the situation and their new found interaction with family and friends—now enter a stage which can best be described as "the stall."

Once engulfed in "the stall," potential hearing aid users are in danger of reentering the cycle syndrome that started with the denial of the hearing loss. It is comforting to know what has been wrong and to realize that they have reentered the mainstream of activity. They are enjoying new, but still imperfect, relationships and there is self-satisfaction in facing and accepting the problem. All of this, unfortunately, has done nothing to alleviate the problem; it has given an opportunity to delay any action that might compensate for the problem. At this point in the evaluation of the hearing loss syndrome, the adult potential hearing aid users have two choices: (a) they can continue in the present stage and risk denying once again the existence of a hearing problem, and (b) they can make the decision consciously to attempt a form of remediation by obtaining a hearing aid. The significance of the decision must be recognized. The first alternative places them back into the syndrome and may lead to many agonizing and uncomfortable periods before they achieve a second stage of acceptance.

The reader who wishes to examine the reaction process in greater detail is referred to an excellent article by Shontz (1965). This presentation discusses the five major phases of shock—realization, defensive retreat, acknowledgment, and adaptation or change. While Shontz deals with crises in general, his concepts and theories are particularly appropriate as they relate to the adult with a gradually progressive hearing loss who may have to face the reality of hearing aid use.

Should the potential hearing aid user opt for a hearing aid fitting, it must be assumed here that the specific instrument recommended and fitted will be one that is appropriate to the loss and will provide maximum useable auditory input. Specific philosophies for hearing aid evaluations with adults and specialized techniques and procedures that are appropriate for adults have been discussed in detail elsewhere, and the reader is invited to study these discussions carefully in order to determine appropriate procedures for use with any given adult client (Alpiner, 1975; Hodgson, 1977).

Predicting Potential for Success

Prior to recommending amplification, judgment of the individual's potential for successful hearing aid use must be made. Determine the stage of adjustment at which the individual is performing. Be aware of the effect that the various stages of the hearing loss syndrome may have on an individual's potential for success. Until recently, this type of decision has been rather subjective and based on the assumption that changes in behavior are to be initiated after the acquisition of the hearing aid. Kasten and Miller (1981) discuss eight primary factors that will influence the degree of success in using a hearing aid. These factors are motivation, adaptability, personal appraisement, money, social awareness, milieu, mobility, and vanity. It is significant to note that they did not include magnitude or severity of hearing loss as one of their factors. They recognize that potential for success decreases with increased magnitude or severity of hearing loss, but they are of the belief that most hearing-impaired individuals can achieve meaningful hearing aid use with careful selection and comprehensive counseling.

Rupp *et al.* (1977) have presented a measurement scale designed to help predict successful hearing aid use. While their scale was primarily designed for use with older individuals, it also is appropriate for use with all adult clients. It provides information relative to individuals' suitability for amplification, and it elicits diagnostic information—in terms of programs to be carried out with a specific client. This feasibility Scale for Predicting Hearing Aid Use involves the following 11 prognostic areas.

1. Motivation and mode of referral to professional services
2. Self-assessment of the individual's communicative difficulties before amplification
3. Verbalization on the client's part as to "help" for the communicative difficulties
4. Magnitude of the hearing loss and understanding difficulties, in audiological units, before and after amplification
5. Informal verbalizations during the hearing aid evaluation
6. Estimate of patient's general state of adaptability and flexibility
7. Age of patient
8. Manual finger and hand dexterity
9. Visual ability
10. Financial resources
11. The presence of a person who is important to the client and is willing to assist in a rehabilitative program

The evaluation form for this feasibility scale, along with an interpretation of results, is shown in Table 3.1. Note that each of the 11 predictive items is rated on a 0 to 5 scale and each of the ratings is multiplied by a weighting factor in order to provide a percentage score for the contribution of that factor. Each of the factors requires some degree of explanation and this is given in Table 3.2. It should be noted that the factors of motivation, self-assessment, flexibility and adaptability, and magnitude of loss are the most heavily weighted factors. Also, careful perusal of the information in Table 3.2 reveals that the scoring of the flexibility scale, while primarily subjective in nature, does have a basis upon which comparative measurements can be made. Clearly, the information gleaned from this type of feasibility scale can provide some clear-cut data on which to predict success with an amplification system and upon which to base counseling or orientation sessions designed to modify the behavior or the thinking of the potential hearing aid user. Another evaluation scale that has both predictive and therapeutic value is the McCarthy-Alpiner Scale of Hearing Handicap (see Appendix 2G) (1980). This scale, designed for administration before and after rehabilitative procedures, can be used to provide insight into the factors, beliefs, or biases of potential hearing aid users and their families. The scale consists of 34 questions that the individual rates on a five-point scale and permits pre- and post-testing of the effectiveness of a rehabilitation program. The 34 questions sample the individual's feelings regarding psychologic, social, and vocational aspects of daily living.

The scale appears to be particularly appropriate in that it provides a mechanism for individuals to rate their reactions prior to amplification and again after the acquisition of amplification and the experience of a hearing aid counselling program. In this regard, the clinician receives valuable input relative to the immediate needs of the potential hearing aid user and to the perceived gains following initial hearing aid use and hearing aid counseling. Although Rupp and his colleagues did not intend for the feasibility scale to be used as a before and after evaluation measurement, it should be obvious that the scale could also be used in this fashion if tester biases were controlled. Whether or not

Table 3.1

Audiology Area, Section of Speech and Hearing Sciences
The University of Michigan Medical School, Ann Arbor, Michigan

FEASIBILITY SCALE FOR PREDICTING HEARING AID USE (FSPHAU):
An analytic approach to predicting the probable success
of a provisional hearing aid wearer

Ralph R. Rupp, Ph.D.   2-76

PROGNOSTIC FACTORS/DESCRIPTIONS (continuum, high to low)	ASSESSMENT 5-High: 0-Low	WEIGHT	WEIGHTED SCORE (Possible) Actual
1. Motivation and referral (self . . . . family)	5 4 3 2 1 0	x 4	(20)_____ 1.
2. Self-assessment of listening difficulties (realistic . . . . . . denial)	5 4 3 2 1 0	x 2	(10)_____ 2.
3. Verbalization as to "fault" of communication difficulties (self caused . . . projection)	5 4 3 2 1 0	x 1	(5)_____ 3.
4. Magnitude of loss: amplification results.			4.
A. Shift in spondaic threshold: ____	5 4 3 2 1 0	x 1	(5) _____
B. Discrimination in quiet:_____ at _____dBB HTL	5 4 3 2 1 0	x 1	(5) _____
C. Discrimination in noise:_____ at _____dB HTL	5 4 3 2 1 0	x 1	(5) _____
5. Informal verbalizations during Hearing Aid Evaluation Re: quality of sound, mold, size (acceptable . . . awful)	5 4 3 2 1 0	x 1	(5) _____ 5.
6. Flexibility and adaptability versus senility (relates outwardly . . . self)	5 4 3 2 1 0	x 2	(10) _____ 6.
7. Age: 95 90 85 80 75 70 65 ⋜ (0 0 1 2 3 4 5)	5 4 3 2 1 0	x 1.5	(7.5) _____ 7.
8. Manual hand, finger dexterity, and general mobility (good . . . . limited)	5 4 3 2 1 0	x 1.5	(7.5) _____ 8.
9. Visual ability (adequate with glasses . . . limited)	5 4 3 2 1 0	x 1	(5) _____ 9.
10. Financial resources (adequate . . . very limited)	5 4 3 2 1 0	x 1.5	(7.5)_____ 10.
11. Significant other person to assist individual (available . . . none)	5 4 3 2 1 0	x 1.5	(7.5)_____ 11.
12. Other factors, please cite	?	?	? 12.

Client _____   FSPHAU: Very limited   0 to 40%
Age _____   Limited   41 to 60%
Date _____   Equivocal   61 to 75%   _____%
Audiologist _____   Positive   76 to 100%   Total Score

(Reprinted by permission from The Journal of the Academy of Rehabilitative Audiology, X: 1, Spring, 1977.)

one chooses to use the above mentioned scales or elects to rely primarily upon subjective reactions to individual and family needs, a baseline of behaviors and attitudes is needed before an appropriate counselling or orientation program can be developed.

One communication questionnaire that incorporates the feelings and attitudes of both the user and the family is the Hearing Performance Inventory (Giolas et al., 1979). This approach identifies a variety of areas that can create problems for the hearing-impaired person. It identifies a large number of everyday situations in which people find themselves and the user is asked to react to those situations. This can be particularly useful in individualizing the counselling for a recent or a potential user of a hearing aid.

The X Factor

A less understood factor that influences the use of amplification seems to stem from a misinformed public or a mistrust of hearing aid systems, or to human inertia. Recently, Hearing Industries Association (1980) commissioned the Gallup organization to conduct a survey that dealt with hearing problems and hearing aids. The results of that survey are interesting and somewhat difficult to understand. They report that, of the respondents who admitted that they had a hearing problem, approximately 18% actually owned a hearing aid. This figure is not out of line with informal estimates based upon hearing aid sales figures and estimated numbers of hearing-impaired persons in the general population. It is difficult to explain why less than one in five hearing-impaired individuals seek help by way of a hearing aid system. This figure is even more difficult to understand in relation to another aspect of the survey in which it was found that 80% of those who reported having a hearing problem also indicated that they would purchase a hearing aid if they found one that would help.

Some companion data from Australia provide an interesting comparison. Cameron (1978) pointed out that approximately 20% of those Australian adults who reported having a hearing problem actually owned hearing aids. This figure is in relative agreement with the results of the Gallup survey, but it should be pointed out that slightly over 50% of the hearing aids sold in Australia cost the consumer $30 or less, due to governmental assistance. In fact, only 12–13% are sold at a cost comparable to that of a hearing aid in the United States. In spite of this sizeable cost differential, only 20% of those adults in Australia reporting a hearing loss actually possessed a hearing aid. Cameron also points out that almost one-quarter of those adults possessing hearing aids never use the instruments, or use them less than once a week. The data on hearing aid usage by hearing aid owners in the United States from the Gallup survey indicates a considerably higher success rate in this country.

It is fascinating to realize that in these two major countries only about one out of five adult hearing-impaired individuals possess a hearing aid. We appear to be faced with some nebulous reluctance to make use of this prosthetic device. It would appear that those individuals involved with the fitting and selling of hearing aids need to invest more effort in

public education and in the counselling process, if these sources of hesitation are to be eliminated. Apparently, it is not sufficient to wait for the hearing-impaired person to arrive at the realization that amplification can be useful; rather, renewed effort must be made to bring this information before the public.

Method of Rehabilitation

The method of accomplishing aural rehabilitation should not be a diluted introductory course to the profession of audiology. The audiologist may be comfortable with the academic model, but experience shows that this method of educating (not rehabilitating) persons with hearing impairments is more gratifying to the audiologist than it is to the client. It has been found that interactive meetings are ranked substantially higher than those meetings wherein the director teaches a great deal. On the other hand, when the aural rehabilitation is conducted by several instructors, each of whom has expertise and interest in a particular phase, the ratings of the lecture-like sessions are much higher than the ratings of the interactive ones. The question, of course, is whether one should respond to the clear preference of the clients, or not.

There is technical information about the auditory system, the hearing aids, the effects of room acoustics, and competing messages that must be conveyed to the potential user of a hearing aid. It is strongly recommended that these bits of information be provided through a demonstration process rather than a lecture process. Where the client has an opportunity to participate in the experience, his retention will remain high.

The length of a given session and the total duration of the rehabilitation program must be related to the age, the perceived condition, and the general circumstance of the person to be served. Obviously, the duration of sessions would be different for persons living in retirement centers than it would be for a group of hearing-impaired high school students. It is altogether possible that counselling sessions might continue for an entire semester with young people and be highly productive, but with individuals living in retirement centers, the interest, ability, and motivation for long term investment of time may be quite minimal. In a recent survey of elderly persons who participated in an aural rehabilitation

Table 3.2
Scoring the FSPHAU factors

1. Motivation/Referral	5. Completely on own behalf
	4. Mostly on own behalf
	3. Generally on own behalf
	2. Half self; half others
	1. Little self; mostly others
	0. Totally at urging of others
2. Self Assessment	5. Complete agreement
	4. Strong agreement
	3. General agreement
	2. Some agreement
	1. Little agreement
	0. No agreement
3. Verbalization as to "fault" of communicative difficulties	5. Clearly created by hearing loss
	4. Usually by loss
	3. Loss and others
	2. Environments and others
	1. Mostly of others
	0. Others totally at fault

4. Magnitude of loss; and results of amplification*	ST shift	Understanding in quiet at —dB HTL	Understanding in noise at —dB HTL
	5. 30+dB	90%	70%
	4. 25	80-88	60-68
	3. 20	70-78	50-58
	2. 15	60-68	40-48
	1. 10	50-58	30-38
	0. 5	48	28

5. Informal verbalizations during hearing aid evaluation re: quality of sound, mold, size, weight, look	5. Completely positive
	4. Generally positive
	3. Somewhat positive
	2. Guarded
	1. Generally negative
	0. Completely negative
6. Flexibility and Adaptability	5. 90th percentile
A. Questionnnaire and observation	4. 70
	3. 50
B. Raven's Progressive Matrices	2. 25
	1. 10
C. Face/Hand Sensory Test	0. 5

program, it was found that they were willing to invest a relatively concentrated period of time (2 hours per day to a maximum of 8 hours) but the group indicated an unwillingness to continue into a second week of training (Britten, 1981). This view was expressed after having participated in a program that combined lecture, discussion, and participation in drill exercises.

It is tempting to say that if some creative use of modern technology had been included, the interest in a longer program may have been higher; however, modern technology can be highly confusing for the older person, and can serve to reinforce feelings of inadequacy rather than building an improved self-respect.

One creative application of common laboratory technology to the task of aural rehabilitation is illustrated by the work of Montgomery et al. (1981). In brief, they describe a procedure for enhancing the integration of

Table 3.2 *continued*

7. Age	5. 65 years
	4. 70
	3. 75
	2. 80
	1. 85
	0. 90+
8. Manual/Hand Dexterity via Purdue Peg Board and Symbol Digit Modalities Test	5. Superior
	4. Adequate
	3. Slow but steady
	2. Slow and shaky
	1. Slow and awkward
	0. "Arthritic"
9. Visual Ability (with glasses)	5. Very good—no problems
	4. Corrected, adequate
	3. Adequate but safeguarded
	2. Limited visibility
	1. Very limited
	0. Blind
10. Financial Resources	5. Unlimited resources
	4. Generally unrestricted
	3. Adequate
	2. Adequate but close
	1. Dipping into savings
	0. Poverty level, on assistance
11. Significant other person	5. Always available
	4. Often
	3. Sometimes
	2. Occasionally
	1. Seldom
	0. Never

*Alternate scoring scheme for factor 4 in cases where the ST shift was minimal due to loss in high frequencies only.

(Average threshold shift at 2000 and 3000 Hz)	5. 25+ dB
	4. 21-25 dB
	3. 16-20 dB
	2. 11-15 dB
	1. 6-10 dB
	0. 0-5 dB

(Reprinted by permission from The Journal of the Academy of Rehabilitative Audiology, X: 1, Spring, 1977.)

auditory and visual components of a spoken event. The technique involves a voice-actuated switch which is set to a sensitivity level that causes it to be activated only when higher intensity sounds (vowels) are spoken. The effect is to delete the consonants and when the client is presented with a video tape of the speech, there must be an integration of the visual (deleted consonants) with the vowels which are presented both visually and auditorily. Montgomery *et al.* report that their subjects showed marked improvement in audio-visual sentence recognition and they conclude that the technique may be of significant benefit to mildly-to-moderately impaired adults when it is employed as part of a comprehensive aural rehabilitation program.

Some of the problems associated with improving receptive communication is illustrated by the work of Dancer *et al.* (1980).

They studied 20 elderly persons who had received hearing aids during their hospitalization at a Veterans Administration Medical Center. They found that 85% could do no better than 70% discrimination and all achieved a 0% speechreading score (vision only) in a face-to-face setting. As a group they felt that they were too old to learn lipreading although 70% showed improved scores on a combined audiovisual task—over that performed on the auditory task alone—in spite of their poor lipreading skills.

In a Family Way

Devine (1981) has pointed out that there are 14 million hard-of-hearing individuals who are surrounded by at least 60 million spouses, children, cousins, and friends—all of whom are trying to help them hear. Unfortunately, a lot of the assistance is misguided and for this reason family members *et al.* should be included in the rehabilitation program. This information is significant and for this reason some paraphrasing of Devine's recommendations are presented in this chapter.

Family members should practice lipreading, too. When they attempt to read lips they develop a higher appreciation for the difficulty of the task and for the need to maintain good visibility when communicating with the affected member of the family. Devine even suggests mimicking mannerisms of family members that tend to make lipreading difficult (a pipe in the mouth, fingers partially covering the mouth, etc.).

Family attitudes create a climate that either helps or hinders the communication as well as the expression of personality. Family members should feel free to make direct and open corrections at the moment a misunderstanding occurs, rather than engaging in dramatic displays (rolling the eyes upward in dismay, or glancing impatiently at another member of the group). In the absence of direct but kind corrections, the hearing-impaired person develops feelings of inadequacy and resentment—neither of which helps future efforts at communication.

Families can give considerable help to the hearing aid user by keeping in mind that just being close to the hearing aid helps it to do its job. Even being mindful of the side on which the microphone of the hearing aid is located will make things easier.

The hearing aid user knows that there are some rooms and some settings in which speech is much more difficult to understand. The user has a responsibility to inform family members of these settings.

The acoustic characteristics of the space in which communication takes place has a profound effect upon the success of that communication. In a highly reverberant room, even normal hearing individuals may have difficulty understanding speech, but those with hearing aids have particular difficulty. The hearing aid amplifies everything and does not distinguish the source from all of the background noise that is entering the microphone. Both the family and the user should try to converse in rooms that contain carpets, drapery, and other sound-absorbent surfaces in order to help the speech signal stand out more distinctly. Even in these settings, the presence of a competing television set or a radio from another room will tend to mask out the frequencies that may be in common with the music frequencies. The hearing aid amplifies everything.

The absence of reverberation is most noticeable when one is talking outdoors. One may eliminate reflected sounds by talking outdoors, but wind, airplanes, power motors, lawn mowers, neighborhood air conditioners, traffic, children, and other common sounds compete for the limited frequency range that can be amplified by the hearing aid. There is a real problem where surrounding noises are too close or too intense relative to the conversation that is taking place. The short commentary by Devine (1981) entitled "Some Tips for the Family of the Hearing-Impaired" would make an excellent handout for an aural rehabilitation program.

THE AGING ADULT

In this chapter, the critical age between the adult listener and the aging listener is considered to be age 55 years (Jerger and Hayes, 1977; McCroskey and Kasten, 1980). The many auditory infirmities associated with the aging process is generally viewed as the inevitable consequence of aging. This is an attitudinal set that can interfere with the creative application of information and technology to the solving of problems with listening in later years of life. It has been too easy to attribute all disabilities of the aging adult to the aging process. The fact that the over-65 segment of the population is expected to grow to 32 million by the year 2000 (Special Report on Aging, 1979) is beginning to have its impact on the various health professions. Programs in gerontology are emerging in universities and the various health professions are giving increased attention to the quality of life that the aging person can expect.

This section of the chapter will identify and discuss both the internal and the external factors that influence the effectiveness with which communication can take place among elderly persons.

Internal Factors

The process of tissue aging appears to lead to a functional decline in sensory and motor activities. Such changes lead to a slower speaking rate, lower vocal intensity, and poorer pitch control (Bloomer, 1978). Accompanying decreases in the precision of articulation, as well as decreased ability to understand spoken messages, may reflect the changes that tissues have undergone. It is well understood that there is a loss of brain weight that occurs with advancing age and that there is a decrease in blood flow to the brain. Although altered performance with verbal material may reflect impaired metabolic and neurological control, it must be remembered that many of the conditions can be arrested or reversed, if appropriate diagnosis and treatment are instituted.

The concept of a team approach for the resolution of auditory problems among the aged is not common at this time, but as audiologists become more conversant with the bases of aberrant auditory behavior, the change will occur. Interactions among health professions must go beyond otolaryngology and include nutrition, biology, and neurology. Is it useful to know that the amount of melanin in the system is related to both temporary and permanent threshold shifts as a function of noise exposure? Is it useful to know that critical alpha rhythms decline with age and that some of that decline is attributable to vascular changes? Since blood supply and oxygen supply are interrelated, and in

some cases the vascularity is already reduced, is it possible that treatment procedures using high oxygen concentration (not only breathed in the normal manner but absorbed under conditions of pressurized oxygen) would have a positive effect upon auditory reception and also speech production?

External Factors

It is not possible to speak of internal and external factors as if they existed independently of one another. They interact inevitably and it is out of the combination that perception evolves. Unfortunately, there is a long history of relatively little concern with the amount or quality of communication among elderly individuals, as Lubinski (1979) has pointed out. Just as the field of gerontology has experienced gratifying growth in recent years, so has the interest in the exploration of communicative characteristics among the aging population. Howell (1971) has stated that those aged individuals most likely to be placed in nursing homes have hearing or speech deficits that are sufficient to make communication difficult. To help eliminate this communicative deficit, more specific research describing communicative attributes is needed. Elias and Kinsbourne (1974) compared a group of young persons with a group of elderly persons on the basis of processing (response) time. The older group was significantly slower than the younger group, but it is of interest to note that men and women performed differently on the verbal and nonverbal processing tasks. Men seem to be equally proficient with both verbal and nonverbal information but the women (in both groups) exhibited less proficiency with the non-verbal data. This discrepancy in processing time becomes more apparent with advancing age.

If one is going to consider amplification or give serious attention to communication problems among the aging, then the work of Kasten and McCroskey (1980) and that of Schmitt and McCroskey (1981) must be incorporated in the overall analysis of the interacting internal and external factors. Perhaps this is illustrated by the work of Weiss (1959) in which it was pointed out that the ear analyzed time as well as frequencies and it was suggested that the aging individual may have an impairment of temporal functions along with reduced sensitivity to various frequencies. Externally, there is a real temporal relationship among the frequencies and intensities that comprise a speech event, but internally the processing time fails to keep pace and the intensity pattern across frequencies is altered by the loss of sensitivity to certain frequencies. Adaptation to the new time-frequency-intensity patterns may be difficult because of the 50 years' experience with comprehending speech. Listener expectations do affect perceptions and habits are difficult to change.

During the adult auditory years which may stem from age 10 to age 55, the auditory feedback system has grown accustomed to particular temporal relationships between the airborne and the bone-tissue borne sounds that reach a speaker's ears. The auditory loop is certainly coordinated with a tactile-kinesthetic loop that assists in both auditory comprehension and in speech production. Not only has auditory processing slowed, but tactile information is also reduced. Thus, internal alterations, which seem to become clear around age 55, disrupt the familiar balance among the input and feedback systems. Signal intensity affects transmission time and elderly listeners have reduced sensitivity to sounds. Speech is composed of frequency patterns—in addition to time and intensity patterns—and elderly listeners do not have all of the frequencies available. The duration of silent interphonemic intervals and the duration of interphonemic transitions contribute to the discrimination of speech sounds and the predictive qualities of our language, and at approximately age 55 listeners begin to have reduced temporal integrity of the auditory system and the rapid recognition of short duration transitions is affected. When these interacting internal and external factors are combined with the additional time-intensity-frequency alterations (Danaher and Pickett, 1975) that occur with the addition of an amplification system, it becomes obvious that there is more to successful amplification than simply supplying a hearing aid.

The rate at which people speak to an aging listener may be as important as the frequency range available or the exact amount of amplification provided a hearing aid. The data are not entirely consistent but there is general agreement that the slower speaking rates are the more understandable to the aging listener (Schmitt and McCroskey, 1981). One must be careful of the interpretation of various studies because some have used single words as the stimuli while others have used sentences and connected discourse. The effects of rate of speaking become more pronounced as the length and complexity of the utterance increases. Intuitively, or through some subtle shaping process, most adults know that they should speak slower to the elderly listener.

Other features of the environment can have significant impact on the aging listener. Spatial distribution of sound is not easily accomplished with most amplification units. The hearing aid user attempts to give primary attention to the source that contains the most pertinent information, but this selectivity is difficult for adult listeners and very difficult for the aging listener. The problem of age-related impairments to auditory selectivity has been studied by Maule and Sanford (1980) but it is an area where considerable additional research is required.

SPECIAL AUDITORY AIDS

Traditionally, texts dealing with amplification for the adult hearing-impaired have not identified some of the special instrumentation that is available and more commonly used with adults who have severe to profound hearing impairments. It seems appropriate to identify some of these in order to help the reader be aware of the range of possibilities that might be utilized for a given client.

Cochlear Implants

Work in this area began in the United States in the 1960s but it was not until 1971 that an implant was accomplished. Australian workers have led the way in multiple-electrode implants and more recently a similar expansion has taken place in the United States. The quality of the signal delivered through cochlear implants, with respect to speech clarity, still leaves a great deal to be desired but technological advances are steady and one can anticipate that highly functional systems can be implanted in the future. For additional information on this type of auditory aid, the reader is referred to the American Hearing Research Foundation (55 East Washington Street, Chicago IL 60602).

Tactile Hearing Aids

Human skin has rather limited frequency response and tactually presented information would seem to need assistance from some other channel; however, there has been limited success with the transmission of vowel information (Goult and Crane, 1928; Guelke and Huyssen, 1959; Pickett, 1963). There has been virtually no success with consonants. Fortunately, some of the linguistic information relating to consonant production can be perceived on the basis of the detection of interphonemic pause time and the duration of voice onset times. The combination of the two may provide a solution for some listeners.

Optic Sound Displays

The aging individual experiences reduced sensitivity in several sensory avenues and it is for this reason that the audiologist should be familiar with alternatives to the delivery of speech via the auditory system only. Where both auditory and tactile sensory systems have reduced sensitivity, the aging individual may still have good functioning visual information. In this instance, the audiologist might consider recommending a device similar to the Upton Eyeglass Speech Reader (Upton, 1968; Pickett et al., 1974). The eyeglass hearing aid takes advantage of the ease with which specific features such as voiced/unvoiced, and stop/fricative sounds can be detected and displayed as distinctive light patterns. These light patterns are built into the lenses of regular eyeglasses and are visible to the wearer but not to persons with whom communication is taking place.

Electrical Stimulation

Electrical stimulation of the auditory nerve is a relatively recent advent (Kiang and Moxon, 1972; Neff et al., 1975). Some experimental models utilize actual electrical shock applied to any surface of the body. The rationale is that all of the information in a speech signal can be converted to a voltage display that can be felt in the form of electrical shock. The advocates suggest that the discomfort associated with patterned electrical shock is more psychologic than physiologic and with the proper orientation there would be no reluctance on the part of the user. For a discussion of electrotactile and vibrotactile stimulation, the reader is referred to the work of Scott (1979).

SPECIAL PROCEDURES

Noise-Cancelling Microphones

A directional hearing aid with a noise-cancelling microphone might be very useful. In this arrangement, two microphones facing in opposite directions would receive room noise equally and, since they would be 180 degrees out of phase, theoretically the noise would be essentially cancelled. Since the microphone would have directionality (at least in one direction) the speech signal coming from in front of the listener would be stronger than the speech signal received by the microphone facing in the opposite direction. This would give a signal advantage while cancelling ambient noise. It is entirely possible that some minor delay circuitry would be needed for the second microphone in order to adjust the time relationships of the signals entering the two microphones.

Theater Systems

With the advent of FM transmitters, it now becomes possible for hearing-impaired individuals to use FM receivers and sit any place in a theater or church without the problems faced in "distance hearing." Some companies currently making FM Auditory Trainers for use in classrooms have adapted the systems for use in theaters and auditoriums. One of the more recent innovations is a new German Sennheiser System that is being used in a variety of public places. Basically, individuals with severe hearing impairments are able to have an enjoyable experience with musical productions and other theatrical forms by way of a system that converts audio sounds into invisible infrared light which is beamed to headphone receivers that have lenses for reconverting the rays to audible sounds. This system not only is good for public installations but has application to home television sets or stereo systems (National Hearing Association, 1010 Jorie Boulevard, Suite 308, Oak Brook, IL 60521).

Portable TTYs

For those adults and aging individuals who cannot function adequately on a telephone with standard amplification, there are portable devices (about the size of a standard telephone) that permit messages to be typed and transmitted over telephone lines to any location where a similar unit has been installed. To use the device, one simply places the receiver of a cradle-type telephone into a receptacle on the TTY and carries out the normal functions via the keyboard rather than by voice. Messages are displayed in normal printed form utilizing LED displays or similar visual systems. These devices can work on regular house current, on rechargeable batteries, or on regular alkaline batteries in an emergency.

The discussion of graphic displays rather than auditory displays in communication by hearing-impaired persons may seem a bit out of place, but if one is concerned with providing guidance and counselling that will lead to effective communication, not only in face-to-face situations but via long distance where the demand on the auditory system, the hearing aid, and the telephone circuitry is greater because there are no visual supplements, then audiologists must assume responsibility for providing guidance on communication that goes beyond the use of an amplifier. Perhaps it is unfortunate that when we think of hearing-impaired individuals we do not think of persons whose impairment is so extensive that telephone communication is either unsatisfactory or so questionable as to constitute a hazard to health and life.

It is a fortunate circumstance that emergency numbers, such as fire department, police department, and emergency centers, have begun to install TTYs for use by the hearing-impaired. This alternative has been identified as service to the deaf population but it is clearly an alternative that must be kept in mind for persons who have acquired severe hearing losses and are not categorized as deaf. The use of these teletype systems offers a secure basis for giving and getting information by many hearing aid users. The audiologist should be aware that there are toll-free numbers that are available and could be very useful to the hearing aid user. The following is a partial list just to illustrate the kinds of services that are available.

Nationwide Crisis Center	1–800–446–9876
Greyhound Bus Line	1–800–345–3109
United Airlines	1–800–323–0170
American Airlines	1–800–543–1586
Social Security	1–800–325–0778
Internal Revenue Service	1–800–428–4732

Information regarding types of communicative devices can be obtained from such companies as the following.

Telephone Pioneers of America
406 East Monroe Street
Springfield, IL 62721

American Communication Corp.
180 Roberts Street
East Hartford, CT 06108

Krown Research, Inc.
10331 West Jefferson Boulevard
Culver City, CA 90230

General Communication Systems
1020 East English
Wichita, KS 67211
(316) 262-0612

Specialized Systems, Inc.
11558 Sorrento Valley Road
Building 7
San Diego, CA 92121

Audiologists would do well to keep the Telephone Pioneers of America in mind as a source of assistance. This group has a special interest in communication via the auditory system and it has a history of providing inexpensive, if not free, service to persons with special hearing problems.

References

ALPINER, J. G., Hearing aid selection in adults, In M. Pollack (Ed.), *Amplification for Hearing Impaired.* New York: Grune & Stratton, 1975.

ANSI (AMERICAN NATIONAL STANDARDS INSTITUTE), *Specification of Hearing Aid Characteristics.* American Standard S3.22-1976. New York: ANSI, 1976.

BERLIN, C. I., Electrophysiological developments in central auditory evaluations. A paper presented at the Symposium on Current Trends and Recent Developments in Speech-Language Pathology and Audiology, University of Kansas, February 15, 1980.

BLOOMER, H. H., Speech and the coming of age. *Perspect. Aging,* 4–7 (September/October 1978).

BRISKEY, R., and KASTEN, R. N., *Subcommittee Report to the Committee on Amplification for the Academy of Rehabilitative Audiology,* 1973.

BRITTEN, C. F., Effects of training upon auditory performance of adults. Unpublished doctoral dissertation, Wichita State University, Wichita, Kansas (1981).

BUTLER, R. N., and GASTEL, B., Hearing and age: Research challenges and the National Institute on Aging. *Ann. Otol. Rhinol. Laryngol.,* **88,** 676–683 (1979).

CAMERON, R. J., *Hearing and Use of Hearing Aids (Per-*

sons Aged 15 Years or More). Canberra: Australian Bureau of Statistics (1978).

CARLIN, M. F., and McCROSKEY, R. L., Is eye color a predictor of noise-induced hearing loss? *Ear Hear.*, **1**, 191–196 (1980).

CASTLE, D. S., Telephone communication for the hearing impaired: methods and equipment. *J. Acad. Rehab. Audiology*, **11**, 91–104 (1978).

DANAHER, E. M., and PICKETT, J. M., Some masking effects produced by low-frequency vowel formants in persons with sensorineural hearing loss. *J. Speech Hear. Res.*, **18**, 261–271 (1975).

DANCER, J., RUDD, A. K., and ABRAMS, H., An aural rehabilitation program for institutionalized elderly patients. *Hear. Aid J.*, **33**, 9, 54 (1980).

DEVINE, E., Some tips for the family of the hearing-impaired. *Am. Hear. Res. Found.*, **10**, 5–7 (1981).

EAGLES, E. L., WISHIK, S. M., DOERFLER, L. G., MELNICK, W. L., HERBERT, S., Hearing Sensitivity and Related Factors in Children. St. Louis, MO: *The Laryngoscope* (1963).

ELIAS, M. F., and KINSBOURNE, M., Age and sex differences in the processing of verbal and non-verbal stimuli. *J. of Gerontol.*, **19**, 162–171 (1971).

EVANS, E. F., The sharpening of cochlear frequencies selectivity in the normal and abnormal cochlea. *Audiology*, **14**, 419–442 (1975).

FDA (FOOD AND DRUG ADMINISTRATION), Food and Drug Administration rules and regulations regarding hearing aid devices. *Federal Register*, 9286–9296 (February 15, 1977).

GIOLAS, T. G., OWENS, E., LAMB, S., and SCHUBERT, E. D., Hearing Performance Inventory. *J. Speech Hear. Disord.*, **44**, 169–195 (1979).

GOULT, R. H., and CRANE, G. W., Tactual patterns from certain vowel qualities communicated from a speaker to a subject's fingers. *J. Genet. Psychol.*, **1**, 353–359 (1978).

GUBERINA, P., The audio-visual global and structural method, *Advances in Teaching of Modern Languages.* Oxford: Pergamon Press, 1964.

GUELKE, R. W., and HUYSSEN, R. M. J., Development of apparatus for the analysis of sound by the sense of touch. *J. Acoust. Soc. Am.*, **31**, 799–809 (1959).

HARDICK, E. J., Letter from the Academy of Rehabilitative Audiology to the Food and Drug Administration (1975).

HARFORD, E. R., and MARKLE, D. M., The atypical effect of a hearing aid on one patient with congenital deafness. *Laryngoscope*, **65**, 970–972 (1955).

HEARING INDUSTRIES ASSOCIATION, *A Survey Concerning Hearing Problems and Hearing Aids in the United States.* Princeton: The Gallup Organization, Inc. (1980).

HODGSON, W. R., Clinical measures of hearing aid performance. In W. Hodgson and P. Skinner (Eds.), *Hearing Aid Assessment and Use in Audiologic Habilitation.* Baltimore: Williams and Wilkins Co. (1977).

HOWELL, S., Advocates for the elderly: A contribution to the reshaping of the professional image. *Hear. Speech News*, 7–9 (1971).

HULL, R., Aural rehabilitation treatment for the older adult—a new look at an old subject. Paper presented before the Aspen Symposium on Communication Problems of the Aging, Aspen, Colorado, 1980.

HUMES, L. E., and BESS, F. H., Tutorial on the potential deterioration in hearing due to hearing aid usage, *J. Speech Hear. Res.*, **24**, 3–15 (1981).

JERGER, J., and HAYES, D., Diagnostic speech audiometry. *Arch. Otolaryngol.*, **103**, 216–222 (1977).

JERGER, J. F., and LEWIS, N., Binaural hearing aids: are they dangerous for children? *Arch. Otolaryngol.*, **102**, 480–483 (1975).

KASTEN, R. N., and BRAUNLIN, R. J., Traumatic hearing aid usage: a case study. A paper presented to the American Speech and Hearing Association, New York, 1970.

KASTEN, R. N., and McCROSKEY, R. L., New dimensions in assessing auditory capabilities of aging individuals, *Audiology*, **7**, 65–81 (1982).

KASTEN, R., and MILLER, W., Considerations for the use of amplification among elderly clients. In R. Hull (Ed.), *Rehabilitative Audiology.* Baltimore: University Park Press, 1981.

KIANG, N. Y.-S., and MOXON, E. C., Physiological considerations in artificial stimulation of the inner ear. *Ann. of Otol. Rhinol. Laryngol.*, **81**, 714–730 (1972).

KINNEY, C. E., The further destruction of partially deafened children's hearing by the use of powerful hearing aids. *Ann. of Otolaryngol.*, **70**, 828–835 (1961).

LUBINSKI, R. B., Why so little interest in whether or not old people talk: A review of recent research on verbal communication among the elderly. *Int. J. Aging Hum. Dev.*, **9**, 237–245 (1978–79).

MACRAE, J. H., Deterioration of the residual hearing of children with sensorineural deafness. *Acta Otolaryngol.*, **66**, 33–39 (1968).

MAULE, A. J., and SANFORD, A. J., Adult age differences in multi-source selection behaviour with partially predictable signals. *Br. J. Psychol.*, **71**, 69–81 (1980).

McCARTHY, P. A., and ALPINER, J. G., The McCarthy-Alpiner Scale of Hearing Handicap. Unpublished study (1980).

McCROSKEY, R. L., and KASTEN, R. N., Assessment of central auditory processing. In R. Rupp and K. Stockdell (Eds.), *Speech Protocols in Audiology.* New York: Grune & Stratton (1980).

METROPOLITAN LIFE INSURANCE COMPANY, Hearing impairments in the United States. *Metropolitan Life Insurance Statistics*, **57**, 7–9 (1976).

MONTGOMERY, A. A., WALDEN, B. E., SCHWARTZ, D. M., and PROSEK, R. A., Training auditory-visual integration in adults with moderate sensorineural hearing loss. Submitted for publication (1981).

NEFF, W. D., DIAMOND, I. T., and CASSEDAY, J. H., Behavioral studies of auditory discrimination: Central nervous system. In W. D. Keidel and W. D. Neff (Eds.) *Handbook of Sensory Physiology.* Vol. V/2. Eidelberg: Springer-Verlag (1975).

PARKER, R., An Investigation of auditory temporal processing under varying conditions of distortion. An unpublished dissertation, Wichita State University, 1979.

PICKETT, J. M., Tactual communication of speech sounds to the deaf: Comparison with lip reading. *J. Speech Hear. Disord.*, **28**, 315–330 (1963).

PICKETT, J. M., GERGEL, R. W., KUINN, R., and UPTON, H. W., Research with the Upton Eyeglass Speech Reader. *Speech Communication Seminar*, **4**, 105–109 (1974).

RUPP, R., HIGGINS, J., and MAURER, J., A Feasibility Scale for Predicting Hearing Aid Use (FSPHAU) with older individuals. *J. Acad. Rehab. Audiol.*, **10**, 81–104 (1977).

SCHMITT, J. F., and MCCROSKEY, R. L., Sentence comprehension in elderly listeners: The factor of rate. *J. Gerontol.*, **36**, 441–445 (1981).

SCHOW, R., and NERBONNE, M., Hearing levels in nursing home residents, *Research Laboratory Reports #1.* Department of Speech and Audiology, Idaho State University (1976).

SCOTT, B. L., Development of a tactile aid for the profoundly hearing impaired: Implications for use with the elderly. In M. A. Henoch, (Ed.), *Aural Rehabilitation for the Elderly.* New York: Grune & Stratton, (1979).

SHONTZ, F. C., Reactions to crisis. *Volta Rev.*, **67**, 364–370 (1965).

Special Report on Aging: 1979, U. S. Department of Health, Education, and Welfare, National Institute on Aging. National Institutes of Health Publication Number 79-1907 (September, 1979).

UPTON, H. W., Wearable eyeglass speech reading aid. *Am. Ann. Deaf*, **113**, 222–229 (1968).

WARREN, M. P., and KASTEN, R. N., Efficacy of hearing aid repairs by manufacturers and by alternative repair facilities. *J. Acad. Rehab. Audiology*, **9**, 38–47 (1976).

WEBER, H. J., An alternative system for the selection and fitting of hearing aids for infants and children. A paper presented to the Kansas Speech and Hearing Association, Kansas City, Kansas, October 19, 1979.

WEISS, A. D., Sensory function. In J. E. Birren (Ed.), *Handbook of Aging and the Individual.* Chicago: University of Chicago Press (1959).

WILLEFORD, J. A., Sentence tests of central auditory dysfunction, In J. Katz (Ed.), *Handbook of Clinical Audiology.* 2nd Ed. Baltimore: The Williams & Wilkins Co. (1978).

4

The Remediation Process

Patricia A. McCarthy, Ph.D. and
Jerome G. Alpiner, Ph.D.

The rehabilitation of hearing-impaired adults remains the area of audiology which has received the least attention and consequently the least research. While technological advances are being made in all aspects of life, little progress has been made in improving the prognosis for better communication skills for the hearing-impaired adult. Yet rehabilitation of the hearing-impaired adult continues, often with methods and procedures designed and adopted decades ago.

While little advancement has been made, the need for effective remediation programs is greater than ever. This can be seen in the frustration felt by both the hearing-impaired individual and the audiologist when traditional aural rehabilitation methods demonstrate little measurable progress. Questions remain as to whether the methods being utilized are truly ineffective or whether our current measuring tools are too insensitive to reflect the change which has actually occurred.

Despite the paucity of research and minimal improvement in rehabilitative procedures, some notable research has been done to demonstrate the reciprocal nature of visual and acoustic cues for speech perception (Binnie, 1973; Garstecki, 1976; Erber, 1974). While much needs to be learned about integration of the senses in information processing, it is clear that communication will be improved only if all sensory input is maxi-

mized. The reader should be cognizant of this while reading about the various components of and approaches to aural rehabilitation presented in this chapter. At present, there is no single mode or approach to remediation. Rather, the state of the art dictates that as many components as possible be incorporated into the remediation process in a meaningful approach. The purpose of this chapter is to present the various components of the therapy process, several approaches to remediation, and the variables involved in the therapy process. The reader is encouraged to experiment with these components and approaches in the remediation process in order to assist hearing-impaired individuals in improving their communication ability.

COMPONENTS OF THE REMEDIATION PROCESS

Aural rehabilitation is a comprehensive process which is comprised of several components. While each component is only one aspect of the total rehabilitative process, for organizational purposes a discussion of each will follow.

Visual Training

The role of vision in speech perception cannot be underestimated. This fact has remained the justification for utilizing lipreading as the basic therapeutic tool in the aural rehabilitation process. As cited in Chapter 1, lipreading practice has been conducted in this country since the early 1900s (Nitchie, 1913; Kinzie, 1918; Bunger, 1924; Bruhn, 1927). And while the emphasis in these early methods was heavily placed on recognition of individual sounds, it is interesting that the audiologists and researchers in aural rehabilitation today are continuing to stress the role of vision in the communication process.

Traditional lipreading has taken on new meaning in recent years so that visual sound training is only one part of the process. The fact that approximately 60% of the speech sounds are either obscure or invisible precludes total reliance on the visual identification of sounds for communication. Therefore, the lipreading process has expanded to include recognition of gestural cues, awareness of facial expressions and observation of environmental cues in addition to visual sound training. A discussion of each of these components of visual training follows.

Lipreading

The purpose of lipreading is to provide visual cues to aid in the perception of speech. Perry (1977) has proposed that the long-term goals for lipreading include the following.

1. Perceptual proficiency—the lipreader perceives speech elements rapidly.
2. Synthetic ability—the lipreader augments words and phrases he can identify with available linguistic and situational cues.
3. Flexibility—the lipreader remains ready to revise his tentative identification of spoken messages when new information necessitates a change.

Perry is critical of the typical exercises found in lipreading manuals which include quotes or state 10 unrelated facts. She argues that these "canned" lessons are not representative of the way adults communicate with each other. Rather she suggests that lipreading exercises should incorporate individuals' interests, occupations, ages, language ability, vocabulary, and hearing loss.

The effects of visual training of consonant sounds has been investigated to determine if lipreading instruction would influence the recognition of visually contrasted English consonants (Walden et al., 1977). The results of this study suggested that the visual recognition of consonants can be improved with a concentrated program of lipreading instruction. The authors report that basic consonant-recognition training was utilized. These findings underscore the importance of developing basic visual sound recognition skills in lipreading before proceeding to more difficult tasks.

Developing these visual recognition skills, however, can often be discouraging for the hearing-impaired adult. The expectations of the hearing-impaired individual when initially attending an aural rehabilitation session are typically quite high and unfortunately often unrealistic. The fact that the majority of sounds in the English language are not fully visible on the lips can be disheartening to even the most enthusiastic client. It is of utmost importance, therefore, that from the beginning hearing-impaired individuals be educated regarding the limitations of lipreading as a complete substitute for the auditory modality. However, the negative aspects of lipreading need not outweigh the benefits. In a study concerning attitude changes following lipreading training, Binnie (1977) noted several positive consequences of group lipreading training offered a hearing-impaired adults. First, the adults in this study reported generally improved communication ability as well as increased confidence and assertiveness in communication, despite the fact that no significant improvement in lipreading was noted. Second, the adult group members responded favorably to class procedures and teaching methods and felt they had a better understanding of their hearing loss. And finally, group dynamics in the rehabilitation sessions were positive and characterized by support, encouragement, and interaction among the members.

In conducting lipreading training, therefore, it is essential that hearing-impaired individuals be made aware that lipreading is but one aspect of the total aural rehabilitation process. Realistic goals can then be set and hopefully achieved. Examples of various approaches to lipreading training will be presented later in this chapter.

Recognition of Gestural Cues

Gestures in communication include not only movement of the hands and arms but also other body parts. Haspiel (1964) encourages watching gestures and body movements in addition to lip movements in the rehabilitation process. Certain gestures have general meaning regardless of language or culture. For example, a student may enter his professor's office to inquire about the results of an examination. Without uttering a word, the professor points his thumbs downward. It becomes apparent to the student that his performance on the examination was less than acceptable. Other examples include nodding the head vertifically to signify "yes" and horizontally to mean "no."

There is little research to evaluate the contribution of gestures in the lipreading process. However, an increasing study was conducted by Berger *et al.* (1970) to determine the value of gestures in providng direct or supplementary meaning to sentences. Results indicated that gestures contributed significantly to understanding sentences.

According to Ruesch and Kees (1956), gestures are used to illustrate, to emphasize, to point, to explain, or to interrupt; therefore, they cannot be isolated from the verbal components of speech. Sanders (1971) describes gestures as having additional symbolic value. He states that meaning is arbitrarily given to a gesture which now "stands for" the object, event, or idea rather than being an "extension" of it. In this situation, the gesture becomes the word. An example of this interpretation is the system of gestures used by bidders at an auction. The auctioneer recognizes that a tug of the ear may mean a bid.

Awareness of Facial Expressions

Facial expressions can frequently give as much information as the verbal content itself (Pauls, 1960). The speaker's facial expression can set the mood or tone of the conversation for the lipreader. Berger (1972) has stated that as a minimum, facial expressions probably offer a clue to the speaker's own psychological state and to his opinion of the subject matter under discussion. Since facial expressions can reveal such emotions as surprise, shock, sorrow, disgust, and happiness, lessons can be designed to train clients to identify these aspects which convey non-verbal communication. For example, a second student may ask his professor about the results of a final examination. Without any verbal response, the professor smiles happily at the student. This student leaves the instructor's office, also smiling because he has apparently been successful on the examination.

Literature regarding the contribution of facial expressions to the lipreading process is extremely minimal and lacks research data. The basis for including facial expressions is clinical experience which indicates that use of all the factors in lipreading appear to help many persons understand speech. This is compatible with the earlier stated contention that communication will be improved if all sensory input is utilized.

Observation of Environmental Cues

Environmental or situational cues can give the hearing-impaired person a set into which the subject matter of the conversation will fit. The physical environment, as well as the participants in the situation, contribute cues. As suggested by Alpiner (1973), environmental cues may also provide information without utilization of speech. A hearing-impaired person, for example, may see a group of his friends at a sporting goods store hovering around bowling balls; interest is centered there and some aspect of bowling is likely to be the topic of conversation. The assumption is that the visual background information has provided a meaningful cue concerning the subject matter.

By assessing situational cues, the hearing-impaired person increases his probability of determining the subject matter while eliminating irrelevant words and subjects. Sanders (1971) summarizes the present concept regarding environmental cues. He states that from the massive amount of stimuli presented, the hearing-impaired individual will select that stimulus which he considers to have a probable relationship to the content of the message signal being received by him. Jeffers and Barley (1971) further postulate that deductive reasoning may help the speechreader in gaining information from non-verbal environmental cues.

Auditory Training

Unfortunately, auditory training is typically considered part of the rehabilitation of hearing-impaired children and not an integral part of the rehabilitation process for adults. Yet improvement in the recognition and discrimination of sounds should be a goal in the rehabilitation of any hearing-impaired individual. Support for inclusion of auditory training in adult therapy was found in the work of Walter and Sims (1978). In a study of the auditory discrimination, speech-reading, and English of young deaf adults, results showed that individuals who had used hearing aids for more than 10 years performed better as a group on all three of these tasks than those who had worn a hearing aid less time or not at all. These findings support the utilization of auditory training procedures for improved discrimination of speech particularly with introduction to the use of hearing aids.

Auditory training has been defined in a number of ways. Carhart (1960) states that auditory training is the process of teaching the hard of hearing to take full advantage of sound cues which are still available to him. This definition can be applied to all ranges of hearing impairment since the majority of even the severe to profoundly hearing-impaired individuals have a great deal of usable residual hearing. In fact, Ross (1972) states that auditory training is actually the systematic training of residual hearing for the improvment of auditory abilities. Kelly (1953) considers the goals of auditory training to be improved awareness, discrimination

and retention of speech sounds. DiCarlo (1948) believes that auditory training for the hearing-impaired adult is not further development, but rather efficient restoration of hearing interactions to permit satisfactory social adjustment. Oyer and Frankmann (1975) indicate that some relearning of auditory cues for speech discrimination may be necessary in auditory training with adults. Based on a synthesis of these definitions and experience, auditory training can be defined in terms of three parameters.

1. Learning to recognize auditorily those sounds which are incorrectly discriminated.
2. Pre- and post-hearing aid orientation including adjustment to amplification.
3. Improvement of tolerance levels.

The type and degree of hearing loss frequently dictate the kinds of sound confusions which may occur. Fletcher (1953) has indicated the phonemes according to frequency and intensity. A wide range of frequencies and intensities is necessary to discriminate the sounds in our language (Fig. 4.1). For example, in a high frequency sensorineural hearing loss, the client may have difficulty distinguishing between the consonants /m/ and /n/, or /ʃ/ and /tʃ/. The clinician must

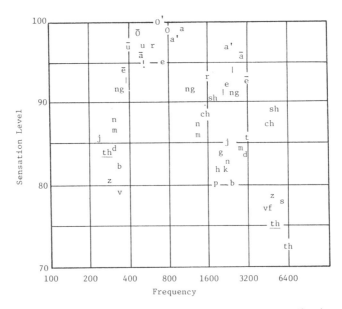

Figure 4.1. Phonemes according to frequencies and intensities. (From Fletcher, H., *Speech and Hearing in Communication.* New York: Litton Educational Publishing, Inc., copyright 1953. Reprinted by permission of Van Nostrand Reinhold Company.)

first identify these sound confusions for the client by using the recommended discrimination test procedures presented in Chapter 2. There is little research to demonstrate that speech discrimination ability can actually be improved. Bode and Oyer (1970), however, in a limited study, compared several procedures for improving discrimination ability of hard of hearing adults. They varied both the types of responses required of the subjects and the background noise used with speech stimuli. Responses were either open set or multiple choice. The background noise, speech babble, remained at the same intensity level or was increased in intensity as the training sessions progressed. The results of 3 hours of practice showed improved scores of CID W-22 words and Rhyme Test words but no improvement for the Semi-Diagnostic Test words. Results also indicated that the two listening conditions were equally effective. Similarly, the two types of training material resulted in about equivalent increases in overall speech discrimination. Finally, listeners who reported the greatest hearing handicap also tended to show the greatest loss in speech reception and speech discrimination in noise. It is interesting to note that the researchers had initially intended to conduct an auditory training program for a 6–10 week period. Due to a lack of enthusiasm on the part of clients, however, the training had to be condensed into a short term program. What improvement might result from a long term auditory training program with continuous high levels of motivation is an interesting question.

The role of the audition in the bisensory perception of speech was studied by Erber (1979). Based on the premise that auditory perception can be improved in a poor acoustic environment with the addition of visual cues, Erber attempted to look at the reverse of this situation. Three studies of the combined auditory-visual perception of speech with systematically reduced optical input were conducted. In past studies of the role of audition and vision, acoustic maskers were typically used to identify the role of visual cues. In Erber's study, a Plexiglas sheet was used to act as a "visual masker." The distance of the Plexiglas was varied resulting in a blurring of the environment and obvious reductions in visual cues. Results were consist-

ent with previous studies which demonstrated the reciprocal nature of vision and audition. Visual cues alone with the Plexiglas resulted in very poor identification of speech. However, with the introduction of auditory cues, identification of speech improved significantly. Erber suggests that the systematic reduction of clarity for visual cues in lipreading during auditory-visual communication exercises be used as a novel approach to auditory training.

Owens (1978) suggests utilizing programmed instruction in the learning or re-learning of consonant recognition. However, prior to implementing any auditory consonant identification training, Owens proposes that an individual analysis of consonantal errors be undertaken. Further, he states that the California Consonant Test can provide a good index of the consonants difficult to recognize for individuals with mild and moderate hearing losses. From the data he has collected on consonant error frequency and substitution, he suggests starting a programmed training approach which initially presents the easiest consonants and progresses to the most difficult. Owens also emphasizes that visual and auditory modalities in consonant recognition generally complement each other. That is, consonants that are difficult to recognize auditorily may be relatively easy to identify visually and vice versa. This is additional confirmation of the role of auditory training in the total aural rehabilitation process.

It is unrealistic to expect that a client will experience no adjustment problems after a hearing aid is fit. In fact, many audiologists believe that the most important part of the hearing aid evaluation is orientation and counselling. Extensive counselling regarding the limitations and advantages of amplification may be necessary. An in-depth discussion of the hearing aid's role in orientation is presented in Chapter 3.

Upon completion of hearing aid orientation procedures, additional auditory training may be required to improve tolerance levels. Often when a person is fit with a hearing aid, the amplified sound will be regarded as unnatural. Even after the client has been made aware of this, amplified sound may continue to annoy the hearing aid user. Kelly (1953) refers to the concept of "tender" and "tough" ears. It has been demonstrated that the "tender" ear may be "toughened" following exposure to loud sounds (Davis *et al.*, 1946). Even reasonably short periods of exposure to amplified sound may improve tolerance levels. It is hoped the hearing aid user will be able to accept greater intensity of sound over a period of time.

Therapy can be approached in terms of dealing with individual sound confusions and general conversational speech both in quiet and in noise conditions. Depending on the client's discrimination difficulties, it may be necessary to proceed with Carhart's (1960) four steps in auditory training: development of sound awareness, development of gross discriminations, development of broad discriminations among simple speech patterns, and development of finer discrimination for speech. Hirsch (1970) indicates that it is unlikely that the hard of hearing adult needs to relearn awareness of sounds. Gradual loss of hearing, however, will be accompanied by a failure to attend to those aspects of sound that become difficult to hear.

Oyer (1966) proposes a sample lesson plan for group auditory training.*

1. Goal: Learning to discriminate monosyllable words in a background of recorded factory noise.
2. Equipment: Two tape recorders and a speaker system.
3. Materials: Taped list of 100 monosyllabic words that use vowels /I/ and /i/, response sheets and pencils, mimeographed lists of the words, and a large score chart.
4. Procedures.:
   a. Have all aids set at most comfortable loudness levels (MCL) for ordinary conversation.
   b. Present list of words at an average level of 50 dB in quiet—adults listen and write them down.
   c. Check accuracy with mimeographed lists.
   d. Introduce factory noise at a level of 50 dB.
   e. Present word list once more in different order—adults listen and write them down.
   f. Check accuracy with mimeographed lists.
   g. Raise noise levels to 60 dB and then 70 dB, repeating above procedures.
   h. Compute average scores for each person

---

* Oyer, H. J., *Auditory Communication for the Hard of Hearing.* Englewood Cliffs, NJ: Prentice-Hall, Inc., copyright 1966. Reprinted by permission of Prentice-Hall, Inc.

and discuss problems associated with listening in noise.

This procedure can easily be adapted for use in individual therapy. An alternative for word lists is the use of lists devised by Kelly (1953) and discussed in Chapter 2. Different formats in which initial, medial, or final phonemes are varied are presented. A typical word list, for example, would include the words crew, grew, and brew.

Pengilley (1973) has proposed general auditory training exercises. The emphasis is directed toward more realistic communication activities. She suggests a broader concept in which single sounds or syllables are not used. The clinician must determine at what level the client is functioning in order to select the appropriate exercises. Sample exercises follow.

1. A client needs to maintain an interest in sounds, voices, and accents. This interest may be stimulated if he is no longer paying attention to auditory signals within his range of hearing. The client may record his own voice and others reading a passage, and then analyze the differences. He may also want to collect interviews to listen to, for example short conversations with other persons. In addition, the client can listen to a repetitive program with the same format each day; that is, either television or radio. Family members can read short passages from the newspaper to the client.

2. Make various noises using common household items (doorbell, vacuum cleaner, alarm clock) where the items cannot be seen by the clients. Each item can then be shown and the sounds repeated. The ultimate intent is to associate the item with the appropriate sound.

3. Play passages which reflect various moods, that is, the same passage with different inflection. For example, have a dialogue spoken three ways: expressing dreariness, anger, and humor. The clients are required to select which inflection is being used. An example for using different inflections is presented.

Husband and Wife Going Out

Husband: We're late again!
Wife: I'll only be a few moments.
Husband: You said that an hour ago.
Wife: I have so much to do in the evenings. Perhaps you could help.
Husband: (Changing the topic) I'll get the car out.

It is obvious that there are a variety of ways in which auditory training materials can be presented, either in group or individual therapy. The important consideration is that the client has been evaluated appropriately to determine at what level auditory training should begin and what goals may be anticipated.

Listening Training

Educating hearing-impaired individuals as to the difference between "listening" and "hearing" is a prime responsibility of the audiologist. Listening training is an essential ingredient in the rehabilitative audiology process for without effective training in listening, all other components can be negated. Due to increased amplification capabilities of hearing aids, listening has taken on increased importance in rehabilitation. Even severely hearing-impaired individuals may benefit from amplification when complemented by audiology training and effective listening.

Hampleman (1958) defines listening "as the act of giving attention to the spoken word, not only in hearing symbols, but in reacting with understanding." The key point to this definition is the difference between the physiologic process of hearing and the psychologic aspect of listening. The emphasis in listening is to train a given individual to be alert, to be attentive, and to be set to receive communication from those who are speaking to him.

Several misconceptions about learning to listen are illustrated by a listening quiz (Barker, 1971), found in Table 4.1. According to Barker (1971), the answer to all of the items is "false." The underlying principle of these statements is not completely understood by most individuals. The important consideration is that listening can be taught and the hearing-impaired adult should be trained to listen. The normal hearing person who is a poor listener is apt to miss much of what is said to him in everyday conversation. The individual with a hearing loss could be doubly handicapped without good listening habits. The underlying principle of Barker's (1971) statements is that listening is not an innate ability but rather a skill which can be learned.

In spite of the fact that we spend 45% of our time listening, Ayers (1978) describes four common faults which lead to ineffective communication. He proposes the faults are as follows.

Table 4.1
Listening quiz [a]

T _ F_1.	Listening is largely a matter of intelligence.
T _ F_2.	Speaking is a more important part of the communication process than listening.
T _ F_3.	Listening requires little energy, it is "easy."
T _ F_4.	Listening is an automatic, involuntary reflex.
T _ F_5.	Speakers can command listening to occur within an audience.
T _ F_6.	Hearing ability significantly determines listening ability.
T _ F_7.	The speaker is totally responsible for the success of communication.
T _ F_8.	People listen every day. This daily practice eliminates the need for listening training.
T _ F_9.	Competence in listening develops naturally.
T _ F_10.	When you learned to read, you simultaneously learned to listen.
T _ F_11.	Listening is only a matter of understanding the words of the speaker.

[a] From Larry L. Barker, LISTENING BEHAVIOR, © 1971, p. xiii. Reprinted by permission of Prentice-Hall, Inc., Englewood Cliffs, New Jersey.

1. Being busy can lead to ineffective listening.
2. Daydreaming can interfere with listening.
3. Close-mindedness in a discussion can lead to ineffective listening.
4. Distraction by someone's personal appearance can detract from effective listening.

Ayers proceeds, however, and suggests that the following techniques supplemented by practice be implemented.

1. Fight off distractions.
2. Try to determine the speaker's main point and supporting reasons.
3. Prepare to listen by being in the right frame of mind.
4. Use non-verbal communication.
5. Keep your eyes on the speaker.

Listening must be separated into constituent parts if it is to be taught, according to Tutolo (1977). He describes these component parts as acuity, discrimination, and comprehension. Acuity and discrimination are common concepts to the audiologist. However, Tutolo further separates comprehension into literal comprehension (factual recall), interpretation (what was meant by what was said), and critical listening (evaluation or judgment about what is heard). A graphic representation of these concepts is presented in Fig. 4.2. Keeping these concepts in mind, it can be seen that listening can have different purposes. In teaching listening skills to hearing-impaired adults, it is suggested that instruction begin with auditory discrimination and move to the more complex cognitive processes involved in literal comprehension, interpretation, and critical listening.

Speech Conservation

The need for speech conservation can best be understood by relating it to the speech servo system model proposed by Fairbanks (1954). Speech difficulties can be caused by a breakdown in the monitoring portion of the speech servo system. Lack of adequate feedback to the control system (brain) causes adjustments in output production. Depending on the severity of the hearing loss and the frequencies affected, the ability of a hearing-impaired person to hear his own speech may be altered. Without auditory self-monitoring, it is possible for an individual to develop misarticulations and inappropriate voice levels.

Oyer (1966) reports that speech errors increase with the severity of the hearing loss. The extent of articulation difficulty caused by a hearing loss is dependent upon the individual's need for an intact monitoring system. For example, the client with a slowly progressing hearing loss maintains a greater monitoring ability than the individual with a marked, sudden impairment. Since most acquired hearing losses are gradual, relatively few adult clients with articulation and voicing problems are seen. Speech conservation, however, can be considered in terms of prevention.

It may appear that there should be a direct relationship between the frequencies affected by the hearing loss and the acoustic composition of auditory speech signals. Fig. 4.1 illustrates how a hearing loss might have some effects on speech perceptions and resultant articulation difficulties. It illustrates further how it may be possible to have a hearing loss which causes difficulty in perception of a sound at the fundamental frequency and still perceive the sound because of the information provided by harmonics. In other words, sounds may not simply become "unheard," they may become distorted.

Griffith (1969) suggests that two principal characteristics, loudness and distortion, may result in feedback disturbance and defective speech output for some persons. As these distorted sounds begin to be perceived, the servomechanism alters the output, resulting in distorted speech. When sounds are not heard accurately, the phonemes will be perceived incorrectly and result, therefore, in incorrect sound production.

The first detectable change occurs in vocal quality, regardless of the type of hearing loss (Bergman, 1952). Bergman's study includes persons possessing mild to severe hearing losses with varying times of onset. He states that quality may become strained and lack resonance because speech is retracted to the back of the mouth. His specific findings were that high frequency hearing loss can cause nasal emission, a dull sounding or omitted /s/, a distorted or omitted /r/, a substitution of /d/ or /t/ for /ð/. Some sounds, /s/, /z/,

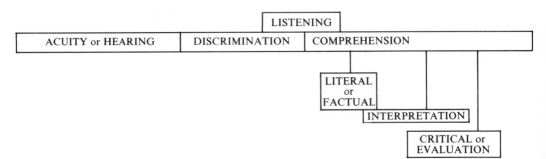

Figure 4.2. The constituent part of listening. (From Tutolo, J., A cognitive approach to teaching listening. *Lang. Arts,* **54,** 262–265 (1977).

/ʃ/, /ʒ/, and /dʒ/ may be omitted since they are not heard when combined with other sounds. This situation may occur when sounds fall within the defective frequency areas due to the low acoustic power and relative invisibility of these sounds.

Because of this difficult situation of low acoustic power and relative invisibility of sounds, several attempts have been made to develop instrumental aids which facilitate the accurate learning of speech gestures. The purpose of these aids is to provide visual or tactile feedback for the acoustic signal to aid in phoneme recognition. Ling (1976) reports that such recognition is a prerequisite to improving articulatory skills which is often a primary part of any speech conservation program. Bargstadt *et al.* (1978) state that these devices generally fall into two categories. The first type provides sensory information relative to general prosodic features of speech (fundamental frequency variations, intensity variations, and temporal factors). The second type provides information for the recognition and production of individual phonemes. These authors attempted to describe the value of a video articulator (visual speech recognition device) by examining the ability of normal hearing adults to identify the visual correlates of phonemes displayed by this instrument. Their results indicated that information transmission via the video articulator was generally low. They noted that video configurations from two speakers may not be the same, making its generalizability for speech recognition very low. The authors conclude that the video articulator appears to have limited value for aiding in phoneme recognition for improved articulatory performance.

The value of speech training as an aid to auditory perception was investigated by Lieberth and Subtelny (1978). Several authors have reported that auditory training results in improved speech production (Asp, 1975; Winitz, 1975). Therefore, Lieberth and Subtelny attempted to test the inverse of this by administering auditory phoneme identification tests to hearing-impaired young adults before and after a 20-week speech training period. A control group who received no speech training was also included. Their results showed significant improvement in phoneme recognition after the intensive speech training, while the control group demonstrated no significant gain. The authors conclude that the speech training had a positive influence on auditory phoneme recognition. These results give further support for a rehabilitation program which capitalizes on all sensory modalities. It would appear that in this study the auditory, visual, and kinesthetic senses were contributing to improved communication for these individuals.

To further investigate the reciprocal nature of the senses, Conklin and Subtelny (1980) investigated the effect of speech training on lipreading skill and the relationships between consonant production and recognition. Articulation and two lipreading tests were administered to hearing-impaired adults before and after individualized speech therapy. Significant improvement was found both in visual-auditory recognition and speech production. The authors conclude that rehabilitative procedures with an emphasis on speech training had a significant effect in reinforcing visual-auditory reception skills. They suggest that therapy planning can be more efficient by combining assessment and rehabilitation of visual-auditory reception with speech production. Further, they discuss the interdependency of perception and production as applied to the rehabilitation process.

Whitehead and Barefoot (1980) investigated the role of oral air flow in plosive consonant production as related to the intelligibility of hearing-impaired and normal hearing adults. Their results showed a significant voiced/voiceless distinction for rate of air flow occurred for normal hearing and intelligible hearing-impaired subjects. However, the semi-intelligible hearing-impaired subjects produced voiced plosives with significantly greater air flow and produced the voiceless plosives with significantly greater air flow in consonant-vowel (CV) context. In the VCV context, semi-intelligible hearing-impaired speakers produced both voiced and voiceless plosives with significantly less air flow. The authors suggest these results can be applied to a speech rehabilitation program. When appropriate, emphasis should be placed on voiced/voiceless distinctions in terms of onset of voicing and the use of the proper amount of air flow.

In terms of therapy, Carhart (1960) suggests four necessary procedures. First, the client must learn to preserve the phonetic elements of speech by becoming fully aware of the kinesthetic characteristics of each element. Second, the client must develop an awareness of the bodily sensations associated with the proper control of melody, rhythm, quality, and emphasis. Third, the client must maintain physical alertness, facial expressiveness, and spontaneous gestures. Finally, the client must learn to maintain effective control of voice loudness.

The reciprocal nature of the senses, as well as the interdependency of perception and production give speech conservation procedures an important place in the total aural rehabilitation process. In the past, speech training has been restricted to individuals with severe to profound hearing impairments and to the congenitally deaf. It appears from the recent research that speech training can have a significant effect on the overall communication abilities of even the mildly hearing-impaired adult. It is recommended that audiologists incorporate speech training into the rehabilitation of all hearing-impaired adults for the purpose of improving auditory-visual perception, as well as speech production when applicable.

Counselling

It is the opinion of these authors that counselling of the hearing-impaired adult is a vital part of the remediation process. The success of all other aspects of rehabilitation are dependent on effective counselling of the hearing-impaired individual, as well as his/her family members. These concepts are discussed in depth in Chapter 5, as well as in the progressive approach later in this chapter.

APPROACHES TO REMEDIATION

The preceding discussion has presented the primary ingredients in an adult aural rehabilitation program. However, the way these components are presented can be very different depending on the philosophy of the audiologist. The following section will present four different approaches to the remediation process. It should be noted that while each approach is distinct and has merits and detractions, there is often overlap in methodologies. The reader should keep in mind that at present, there is no approach which is correct while the others are incorrect. It appears that

different approaches are successful dependent on the instructor and the individual. Flexibility and a knowledge of each of these approaches to the aural rehabilitation process will allow the audiologist to plan the most effective therapy for the hearing-impaired individual.

Bisensory Approach

In rehabilitative audiology, the traditional view has been that acoustic training may retard lipreading. Siegenthaler and Gruber (1969), however, feel that the effectiveness of either audition or vision alone is improved by the use of the other. The idea of coupling the auditory with the visual modality for better overall communication is not new to the field of audiology. Numbers and Hudgins (1948) were among the first to recognize that the reading of manual language or the use of residual hearing are not substitutes for lipreading but may assist an individual to acquire the skill of lipreading. Visual cues seem to provide information for speech development and recognition not perceived through audition while audition provides information not perceived through vision (Whitehurst, 1964). The bisensory approach, encompassing both vision and audition, offers more communication cues even though acoustic components may be distorted and visual components obscure. It seems that this approach would be beneficial in improving overall communicative functioning.

Implementation of the bisensory approach necessitates that the client initially focus on either audition or vision alone. This appears to be contradictory to the ideology of combining them. O'Neill and Oyer (1961), however, purport that only as a result of this initial "sensory isolation" will the hearing-impaired adult be altered to use these two sensory channels alternately, independently, or simultaneously.

Several researchers have found that the auditory-visual presentation of speech will yield the best possible speech discrimination score. Siegenthaler and Gruber (1969) recommended a bisensory auditory-visual presentation of speech materials to obtain a realistic assessment of speech. Dodds and Harford (1968) suggest that a bisensory presentation of sentence material in hearing aid evaluations will yield additional information about the ability of the hearing-impaired to understand general conversational speech. Whitehurst (1964) suggests integrating auditory training and lipreading in audiology therapy. Krug (1960) determined bisensory discrimination scores at various relative intensity levels and found that bisensory reception provided the maximum intelligibility scores.

Recently, several researchers have conducted studies which demonstrate the improvement in communication via the combination of auditory and visual modalities. Steele et al. (1978) studied the effects of bisensory stimulation in the adaptive testing of speech discrimination. The rationale for their investigation was based on the premise that assessment of speech discrimination by audition only is not representative of a hearing-impaired individual's total communication ability. The adaptive or sequential testing method shifts the presentation levels within a test list depending upon the preceding responses and according to a pre-planned strategy. Using this technique, they found that combined auditory-visual presentations resulted in better speech discrimination scores than when the auditory-only stimuli were presented in adverse listening conditions. In addition, they found good agreement between adaptive testing methods and constant level testing for the auditory-visual condition. The authors suggest the use of the adaptive technique in speech discrimination assessment, hearing aid evaluations, and in auditory-visual intelligibility training programs. They propose that the adaptive technique can serve to evaluate the integration of auditory and visual cues and indicate problem areas for the individual such as speech-to-noise ratios which cause a breakdown. For further information regarding this technique, the reader may refer to Steele et al., (1978) and Bode and Carhart (1974, 1973, 1970).

An interesting remediation procedure utilizing a bisensory approach has been developed by Garstecki (1980). Development of the procedure was based on the premise that auditory-visual speech perception is more resistant to competing noise than auditory perception alone and the fact that the auditory versus auditory-visual perception of sentence material has received little study. The experimental procedure which he describes is client-centered and systematically manipulates four parameters: message type, competing noise type, competing noise level, and the use of situational cues. A performance criterion level is predetermined by systematically varying the four parameters to increase message redundancy by increasing message content, changing competing signal type, and decreasing level of presentation and by adding relevant situational cues. Garstecki has outlined a plan to implement this training where M_0 represents the use of unrelated sentences. N_0 represents the use of multispeaker babble, SN_0 represents use of a 0-dB PM/CM (primary message/competing message) ratio, and C_0 represents non-use of a situational cue. The variation progresses as follows.

a. Message content changes from unrelated sentences (M_0) to related sentences (M_1) to paragraphs (M_2) to story material (M_3).

b. Competing noise changes from multispeaker babble (N_0) to single-speaker babble (N_1) to white noise (N_2) to quiet (N_3).

c. Competing noise changes from 0-dB (SN_0) to a positive level (SN_1).

d. Situational cues change from no cue (C_0) to a relevant background (C_1) to relevant auditory and visual background cues (C_2).

The procedure requires that a measure of baseline performance first be obtained and then further probing can be conducted at higher levels where message redundancy is increased (up to level 11) according to the following scheme where message redundancy increases from level 1 to level 11:

Level	a	b	c	d
11	M_3	N_0	SN_0	C_2
10	M_3	N_0	SN_0	C_1
9	M_2	N_0	SN_0	C_2
8	M_2	N_0	SN_0	C_1
7	M_1	N_0	SN_0	C_2
6	M_1	N_0	SN_0	C_1
5	M_0	N_0	SN_0	C_2
4	M_0	N_0	SN_0	C_1
3	M_3	N_0	SN_0	C_0
2	M_2	N_0	SN_0	C_0
1	M_1	N_0	SN_0	C_0
Baseline	M_0	N_0	SN_0	C_0

In this plan, the message content (column a), situational cues (column b), and noise level (column c) remain constant. The point at which the pre-determined performance criterion is achieved is termed the ceiling level. If the individual cannot achieve the pre-determined criterion level, then the scheme can be revised to include an increased primary-to-competing message ratio (SN_0 becomes SN_1). The next step in the process would be to change the noise type where N_0 becomes N_1. A final manipulation would involve eliminating the competing message with N_3 replacing N_2. It should be emphasized that this scheme is devised according to the individual's abilities and needs.

Garstecki suggests that this systematic procedure be used to attain short-term remediation goals by developing improved communication skills at each successive level of redundancy from ceiling (as level 11) to baseline. The program can be terminated when satisfactory baseline performance is achieved or when the individual achieves no additional progress.

The program outlined by Garstecki is experimental and he states that further investigation is needed to define the relative importance of the various message parameters in everyday communication. However, this approach represents an organized, logical procedure for therapy where goals can be set according to the demonstrated needs of the individual. Furthermore, therapy can progress in a logical manner and the process can be terminated based on the achievement of the individual. In addition, the utilization and manipulation of the four message parameters represents a realistic approach to therapy in terms of carry-over to everyday communication. The adult hearing-impaired population has been resistant to participation in aural rehabilitation in the past for several reasons. Whitehurst (1964) contends that the lack of acceptance is due to the fault of the methods or materials used by the clinician. Miller (1970) maintains that the failure to obtain successful participation is due to the lack of a rationale for therapy. Programs such as the one proposed by Garstecki address both of these issues and represent a positive step for the field of aural rehabilitation.

From the preceding discussion and clinical experience, it appears logical to employ both the auditory and visual modalities in any remediation plan. In everyday communication situations, these clients will be faced with both kinds of cues. Remediation therapy, therefore, should emphasize maximum utilization of both auditory and visual cues. In therapy it is appropriate to present materials as visual only or auditory only on occasions. The rationale is that in some communication situations the client may have to be more dependent on one sensory modality than the other. The intent is to prepare the client to communicate in both ideal and difficult listening situations. The bisensory approach can utilize any of the therapy materials presented in this chapter by combining audition and vision.

Traditional Approach

This approach to the rehabilitation of hearing-impaired individuals has changed little since the early days of lipreading therapy where heavy emphasis was placed on the recognition of placement of sounds. Perhaps the most significant addition to the traditional approach is the inclusion of training in listening, recognition of gestural cues, awareness of facial expressions, and observation of environmental cues discussed earlier in this chapter. While this approach has its limitations, it is presented here because of its strong visual orientation. Clearly, visual training is needed in the aural rehabilitation process. It is recommended that the methods employed for visual training in the traditional approach be incorporated into a rehabilitation plan in conjunction with the other methods emphasizing utilization of the other senses.

The ultimate goal of remediation is improvement of communication for hearing-impaired adults. Several approaches within the traditional method are utilized for visual instruction. Two major techniques which have been advocated are analytic and synthetic. There is probably no pure analytic or synthetic method being used, but rather some combination or interaction of the two.

Theoretically, the underlying basis for the analytic approach is that one can learn to lipread more effectively if training stresses the more elemental aspects of speech. With the synthetic approach, it has been advocated that most therapy time should be spent on general speech discourse. Elemental aspects of speech should be taught briefly for purposes of identification or structuring. Both methods have the same goal, improving a

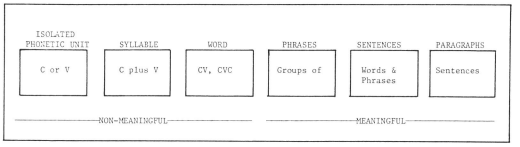

Figure 4.3. Representation of the analytical approach to the teaching of lipreading. (From O'Neill J. J., and Oyer H. J., *Visual Communication for the Hard of Hearing.* Englewood Cliffs, NJ: Prentice-Hall, Inc., copyright 1961. Reprinted by permission of Prentice-Hall, Inc.)

client's ability to understand everyday speech. Figs 4.3 and 4.4 (O'Neill and Oyer, 1961) illustrate these two approaches.

For the traditional approach, both analytic and synthetic procedures are recommended. The program of instruction for hearing-impaired adults is based on eight consecutive weekly sessions of 2 hours duration each. The following procedures are recommended for implementation of this methodology.

1. Audiologic evaluation (pure tone and speech auditometry)
2. Assessment of lipreading functions
3. Planning of group therapy sessions
4. Implementation of therapy
5. Post-therapy evaluation
6. Prognosis and recommendations

When a combined analytic and synthetic approach is used, the procedure is that individual sounds will be presented in isolation for structuring purposes only. The rationale for presenting sounds in isolation is to afford the client an opportunity to learn how individual phonemes appear visually. Experience has shown that many clients, in the traditional approach, have considerable difficulty in phoneme recognition if they have received no prior instruction. It is probably wise to present the phonemes with a carrier vowel, such as /ɑ/, in the initial introduction of the consonant. This practice seems to help hearing-impaired clients differentiate between the alphabet letter and the sound which that letter represents. The layman is usually unfamiliar with the concept of phonemes and often confuses them with alphabet letters. During the 8-week therapy period, sounds are presented according to homophenous categories, proceeding from most visible to least

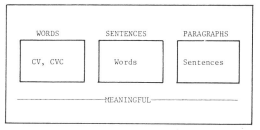

Figure 4.4. Representation of the synthetic approach to the teaching of lipreading. (From O'Neill, J. J., Oyer, H. J., Visual Communication for the Hard of Hearing. Englewood Cliffs, NJ: Prentice-Hall, Inc., copyright 1961. Reprinted by permission of Prentice-Hall, Inc.)

visible. The homophenous sound groups are introduced first so the client has a better opportunity to experience success during his initial therapy exposure. Each homophenous category is presented briefly at the beginning of the therapy session.

The synthetic aspect of therapy is introduced in a progressive sequence in which words and sentences with new sounds are presented. Remediation experience has shown it feasible to present related sentences (theme approaches) to the hearing-impaired adult. This procedure is based on the assumption that most communication situations revolve around a central theme. There are times, however, when unrelated sentences are used, since communication situations are not always predictable. The intent is to prepare the client for the unexpected.

Based on the research data of Binnie *et al.* (1974), it is recommended that homophenous sound categories be taught in the following sequence.

1. Bi-labials /p, b, m/

2. Labio-dentals /f, v/
3. Interdentals /ð, θ/
4. Rounded labials/ ʃ, ʒ/
5. Linguals /s, z/
6. Linguals /t, d, n/
7. Rounded labial /w/ (from Woodward and Barber, 1960)
8. Lingual palatal /dʒ, tʃ/ (from Bunger, 1961)

Sounds are presented to the clients in orthography rather than according to the International Phonetic Alphabet since most lay persons are unfamiliar with the phonetic alphabet.

Few data are available on the utilization of vowels in lipreading therapy. In our opinion, teaching vowels to clients seems to enhance their ability to lipread. It is suggested that vowels be taught since words are made up of syllables of which they are an essential part. Bunger (1961) says, regarding speech movements, that vowels open the mouth. She states that we use lips, tongue, and jaws to shape the opening so our voices produce one vowel or another. Changing the shape of the opening changes the sound. In this way, vowels can assist the client to understand speech through lipreading. The difficulty in identifying the vowels arises because the preceding consonant influences the shape of the vowel. It should also be noted that 60% of the speech sounds are invisible or obscure on the lips; over one-half of the vowels and dipthongs are included in this sound (Jeffers and Barley, 1971).

To understand the traditional process more fully, an example of lesson plans for a beginning term are presented in Appendix 4. It should be noted that the instruction is designed as an 8-week program with each session lasting approximately 2 hours. It should be emphasized that these lessons are intended to serve only as a guide for conducting traditional therapy. It will be necessary for the clinician to use his own intuition and experience, as well as considering individual client situations for modifications of these guidelines. The intent is to indicate that procedures outlined here are only one way in which traditional instruction can be provided.

The underlying principles for the format of these lessons need to be discussed. It is essential that a working rapport be developed between clinicians and clients, as well as among clients themselves, to conduct effective therapy. Established rapport should enhance clients' confidence in the ability of the clinician. Without this confidence, it is not uncommon for the client to discontinue therapy. Rapport is necessary among clients within a group to provide an atmosphere in which they are willing to become active participants, interacting with each other, for example, in sharing and exchanging feelings and experiences. The procedure for establishment of rapport begins in the initial session. Utilization of a question-discussion format including such items as occupation, birthplace, family, interests, hobbies, and referral source for therapy is suggested. Experience has shown that some people are hesitant to interact during the first session. If the clinician, however, is able to create a comfortable and relaxed atmosphere, most clients will participate more actively in subsequent sessions.

Experience has shown that the client begins the group with some misconceptions about lipreading. Often a client will initiate therapy believing that he will be able to understand speech completely through the sole use of the visual sensory modality. It is a disappointment for him to learn that only about one-third of the sounds in our language are visible on the lips. At this point the lipreading process should be explained. Discussion of the components of the lipreading process, listening ability, facial expressions, gestures, and environmental cues, follows. Emphasis is placed on maximizing the other cues to compensate for the limitation of understanding speech through vision only.

Pre-service lipreading tests recommended in Chapter 2 are administered to the clients. The results obtained provide the clinician with baseline data which will be compared with post-service tests given at the conclusion of therapy. These tests attempt to measure the client's improvement in lipreading. They do not measure his improvement in communication ability. Because of problems inherent in lipreading testing, the clinician can only interpret subjectively whether the client's communication has improved.

Unfortunetely, many of the clients participating in therapy have never had the nature and implications of their hearing losses explained to them. During the portion of the session dealing with this aspect, clients receive a brief description of the hearing mechanism, causes of hearing loss, types and degrees of hearing loss, and an explanation concerning the role of hearing aids in aural rehabilitation. This information is interpreted in terms of individual problems and we have found that it has stimulated group interaction and interest, resulting in a greater understanding of hearing problems.

Research has shown that sounds may be differentiated on the basis of homophenous groupings (Binnie *et al.*, 1976; Erber, 1975; Woodward and Barber, 1960). This lends some justification to teaching visual identification of phonemes. Sounds are presented through homophenous groups. One group is presented each week, generally proceeding from the most visible to the least visible.

Experience has shown that some hearing-impaired persons can understand a key word in a sentence because they have been able to identify one of the visible sounds in that word. Perception of that key word may lead to understanding in a difficult listening situation. The implication is that some hearing-impaired people are better able to understand because of an apparent ability to lipread sounds within individual words or continuous discourse.

Many clients report that their most difficult communication situations are those in which there is competing background noise. It is assumed that the visual modality will help to compensate for the masking effect of the background noise. In an attempt to simulate real life situations, various types of background noises are utilized when speech stimuli are presented at normal conversational levels. For this reason, recordings of the noises encountered in a restaurant, in an automobile, on a street, or at a party are used in therapy. The clinician should use realistic signal-to-noise ratios in remediation to stimulate a relatively quiet situation or a very noisy situation.

Infrequently, in therapy, speech stimuli are presented using no voice. The use of this procedure is questionable. Presently there is no justificaiton for presentation of speech under this condition. It is suggested that the no voice condition be used occasionally to emphasize the importance of the visual modality in learning to identify homophenous sound groups and to assist hearing-impaired clients when auditory cues are minimal or unavailable.

It is important to realize that the client is constantly confronted with everyday commmunciation situations. Since lipreading lessons do not always conform to the realities of everyday life, general conversational situations are included in therapy to help the client cope with a variety of real experiences.

Communication is a reciprocal process between speaker and listener; the hearing-impaired person needs to be actively involved in remediation. For this reason, the client assumes both active and passive roles in therapy by presenting stimuli materials to the group as well as receiving them. This technique creates a better understanding of the dynamics of the communication process.

Although primary emphasis is on instruction dealing with the lipreading process, some time during each session is spent on client input. The client is asked to indicate the kinds of situations in which he has difficulty and the clinician and other members of the group suggest ways of overcoming these difficulties. This is a way to incorporate a progressive aspect into a basically traditional approach.

Clients frequently ask clinicians if there is a specific time when they should practice lipreading. Our approach has been to emphasize that lipreading practice is part of all daily communication activities in which clients participate. Specific assignments, however, are given so they may fulfill the objectives of the lesson plans. Prepared homework assignments are also helpful in providing clients with an active role in the presentation of stimulus materials.

The client who has participated in traditional instruction should be aware of the following requisites for improving communication proposed by Erickson (1974).

1. Watch the speaker—not just his lips, but everything he does: expressions, gestures, and so forth.

2. Check the seating arrangement. This is particularly true in group situations. Do not sit where the speaker will have bright lights behind him. The resulting eye strain will make speech-reading hard, and it will also put the speaker's face in a shadow. It is always best to have your back to the light. In small, informal groups, this is also important. If the room is arranged with a sofa faced by two or three chairs, it is better to sit in one of the

chairs in order to have a better view of all the other speakers. If you choose the sofa, the persons on both sides of you will be difficult to speechread. In an auditorium or similar situation, sit close enough to see as well as hear as much as possible.

3. Learn the topic being discussed. When we know what a person is talking about, it is easier to follow the conversation. By following the trend of main ideas, one can contribute to the conversation and avoid making guesses that are far from the topic. When entering a group late, always ask, "What's being discussed?"

4. Learn to look for ideas rather than isolated words. This is the hardest thing a speechreader has to do. With hearing, following ideas is natural. We don't pay attention to any specific words, we just seem to hear and synthesize. The speaker stresses the key words to make them stand out to the listener with normal hearing, an aid to following ideas. While the speechreader may not be able to take advantage of every word a speaker says, with many speakers he can become especially aware of changes in rhythm, stress, timing, and gestures that indicate the words being emphasized and the changes in meaning. By keeping alert for key words in the sentence, the speechreader can follow ideas, even if he misses some of the "verbal filling" from adverbs, prepositions, and other descriptive parts of speech. Nouns and verbs are the most important parts of speech. The other parts of speech embellish or add details that are not vitally essential. To prevent confusion, we are not suggesting that people omit various parts of speech when talking to the hard of hearing, but rather that speechreaders will do better if they do not try to identify every word. As skill advances, more details will become apparent.

5. Use the clues from the situation to help get meanings. The idea is often spelled out by the actual situation. One may also anticipate what vocabulary or phrases will probably be used. The speechreader must recognize and make use of all details in the situation.

6. Stay aware of current events. When we know something about a topic we can more readily recognize the key words, names, and so forth. Because people talk about what is on television and in the news, it will be helpful to read the daily newspaper and to be aware of the programs many people may watch, even if you do not watch television.

7. Keep informed of your friends' interests. Most of our friends have favorite topics. Much as we might desire a change, it is actually a blessing because limited content makes speechreading easier.

8. Try to relax. Do not strain to get every word or syllable. It is not important to understand every word as long as you get the idea. In fact, when you try too hard and get too tense, this will interfere with your ability to speechread.

9. Do not be afraid to guess. Some instructors call it "intelligent guessing." If we know the topic and pick out key words, we can automatically guess the rest of the speech. Some persons will not permit themselves to guess. They have to be sure; consequently, they are constantly getting lost. While they are trying to figure out a word or a phrase, the speaker has continued to talk. Meanwhile, the speechreader who is afraid to guess is concentrating on only one word at a time. By the time he has figured out the introductory remarks, the speaker has completed the story.

10. Be flexible and ready to change your mind when necessary. Because some words may look the same, you will need to get the word clues in the rest of the sentence.

11. Remember you will usually be using your remaining hearing in combination with your speechreading ability. You can get clues from both channels and use them together to understand the speaker. This will vary with each hard-of-hearing person, depending on his hearing loss or how much a hearing aid helps. Also, situations will vary; you may have to rely on speechreading in some situations more than others.

12. Inform your friends that you are studying speechreading. Tell them it will help you if they do not shout or exaggerate their lip movements when they speak. They also might make a special effort not to cover their mouths and to make sure you can see their faces when they are talking.

13. Keep your sense of humor. There are times when you may confuse a word or subject and feel a little foolish. You may have to say "I sure was off on that word!" and then resume the conversation. As speechreading skills increase, this will happen less often.

14. Watch your own speech. If you talk softly, shout at others, or slur your words together, you are not presenting the model of good speech you would like others to use when talking to you.

15. Do not be afraid of speechreading. Let it become a friend. Like all good friendships, let it develop slowly. It is a skill that requires much practice, not just during lessons, but in everyday living.

Progressive Approach

The progressive approach is primarily a counselling-oriented methodology. This approach places heavy reliance on client input obtained through the use of various communication assessment inventories. It attempts to deal with adjustment to and acceptance of problems concomitant with an acquired hearing loss. The emphasis is on coping with communication situations and reducing anxieties in the communication process through counselling rather than through traditional lipreading techniques (Alpiner, 1971). The assumption in the progressive approach is that teaching lipreading and auditory training is not adequate in dealing with communication problems. Advocates support the progressive approach because research proving the benefits of lipreading and auditory training is lacking. In her Communication Therapy Approach, Fleming (1972) indicates that both lipreading and auditory training are excluded from the remediation process. However, the progressive approach can be seen as an extension of the traditional approach where the counselling methodology is employed in conjunction with traditional remediation procedures.

As a variation of the progressive approach, Pengilley (1980) has described a strategy for coping with hearing problems. Pengilley views the progressive approach as a "problem-solving" and "information-giving" approach for which she proposes five tactics.

1. Changing amplification to suit specific occasions. For example, telephone amplifiers or television amplifying devices may be used in place of traditional hearing aids.
2. Supplementary speech. The use of fingerspelling, the Scandinavian Hand-Mouth System, or common gestures can be used to supplement the spoken message.
3. Environmental changes. The environment can be advantageously manipulated to enhance listening and lipreading.
4. Attitude changes. Problem-solving techniques can be presented with situational role-playing used to demonstrate solutions.
5. Changing attitudes in the community. Associates and family members can be counselled in acceptance of and how to deal with hearing impairment.

Pengilley has also developed a model for problem solving and developing hearing tactics. She proposes that the following stages be conducted.

Stage One: The individual *locates* and defines a specific problem.
Stage Two: The problem is *clarified* to avoid peripheral issues.
Stage Three: Possible *solutions* to the problem are generated.

Stage Four: *Experimentation* with solutions is conducted through role-playing.
Stage Five: *Plans* are developed for implementation of the solutions.
Stage Six: *Action* is implemented.
Stage Seven: The first 6 stages are *evaluated* in terms of effectiveness. New problems are discussed.

The problem-solving model proposed by Pengilley as well as the hearing tactics are useful techniques for the counselling-oriented progressive approach.

Inclusion of family member or friends can be a very effective way of improving success with the progressive approach. McCartney and Nadler (1979) have suggested family and/or friends be made aware of *how* to communicate with hearing-impaired individuals in order to minimize frustration. They propose the following guidelines.

1. Talk at a moderate rate.
2. Speak in a normal tone of voice and avoid shouting.
3. Use longer phrases in order to increase redundancy and produce greater understanding.
4. Keep your voice level even and avoid dropping the volume at the end of a sentence.
5. Do not overarticulate because it causes obscuring of natural mouth movements.
6. Be sure that the hearing-impaired person follows changes in the conversation.

Implementation of the progressive approach is perhaps best explained through the presentation of case studies. Personal profiles of three young college students with moderate to severe hearing losses are presented. These are examples of clients for whom traditional therapy alone may not be recommended or should be incorporated with the progressive approach.

The first student's hearing loss was first noticed when she was about 4 years old. Since then, her loss has become progressively more severe. She reported concern about the progression of the loss and an interest in lipreading to improve her communication. Prior to her first year in college, she had no lipreading, auditory training, or speech therapy, although speech therapy had been recommended to improve distorted /s/, /ʃ/, and /r/ sounds. She reported having the greatest difficulty communicating in group situations and when there was music background noise. She stated that she had more difficulty understanding female voices. In addition, she reported that she became tired and nervous in some listening situations. It was stated that she often answered questions inappropriately because she did not understand what was being said. Although she was a candidate for a hearing aid, she said she would never wear one. She also reported that it was her opinion that other people really did not understand what it was like to have a loss of hearing.

The second student's hearing loss was identified when he entered the first grade and he was fitted with a hearing aid at that time. He indicated that he wore the hearing aid most of the time, except in extremely noisy situations. He had lipreading instruction in the first two grades of elementary school. Although the /s/ and /ʃ/ sound were distorted, he indicated that he had never had any speech therapy. He reported considerable difficulty in group situations in which there was background noise. He also reported difficulty when riding in automobiles trying to understand people. In addition, female voices were more difficult for him to comprehend. He reported that communication situations made him tired and nervous and he would respond inappropriately to a comment which he did not understand. He also indicated his belief that other people do not understand how frustrating it may be to have a hearing loss. He reported he is often "up tight" when involved in communication situations.

The third student never wore a hearing aid, although she claimed she always had difficulty hearing. When asked why she had not considered amplification, she stated that she had never known the extent of her hearing loss. She indicated that she never had any lipreading or auditory training. Her /s/ and /ʃ/ sounds were distorted, although during elementary school she had some speech therapy to assist in improving her articulation. She reported that it was most difficult to hear conversation in groups and in noisy restaurants and bars. In addition, female voices were difficult for her to understand. She reported that her hearing loss affected her socially and she tended to withdraw from situations where communication was required. She also indicated feeling left out of situations and would avoid asking people to repeat what they had said.

In analyzing the commonalities among these clients, the following problem areas are evident.

1. All three clients had a need for speech therapy because of the nature of their hearing impairments.
2. The clients all expressed communication difficulty in group situations.
3. Background noise posed a problem in general communication for all.
4. All three clients expressed particular difficulty in understanding female voices.
5. Stress, manifesting itself in withdrawal, nervousness, fatigue, tension, and feelings of isolation, was a result of hearing loss which was felt by all three.
6. Inappropriate responses in conversation, as well as unwillingness to ask for repetition, were experienced.
7. Two of the clients had rejected the use of amplification while the third client had some difficulty with a hearing aid in noisy situations.
8. All three clients expressed the feeling that normal hearing people did not understand what it was like to have a hearing loss.

These three clients presented typical attitudes expressed by hearing-impaired adults seen in therapy groups. Obviously, in each of the above cases, lipreading and auditory training would not be sufficient in dealing with total communication problems. It is suggested that there may be a need for the family and vocational counselling mentioned in the client examples in Chapter 3. The following discussion should explain how these clients benefitted from use of the progressive approach.

There appear to be several reasons why the audiologist should be familiar with counselling procedures. Counselling provides an outlet for meeting the needs of hearing-impaired clients (Alpiner, 1971). Northern and Sanders (1972) have emphasized these needs by outlining three key factors. First, the client's reaction to his hearing loss influences his success in achieving satisfactory communication. Second, the client's psychologic stability may be threatened due to added demands of increased numbers of problems resulting from the hearing loss. Finally, preoccupation with personal problems may hamper the hard-of-hearing client's progress in the aural rehabilitation process. Feelings of anxiety, caused by reaction to his hearing loss, may influence the client's ability to communicate effectively in various environmental situations. Through effective counselling methods, however, a reduction in anxiety and tension may be a major factor in improved communication (Alpiner, 1971). It should be noted that anxiety reduction appeared to be a need shared by the three clients described earlier.

Several authors have considered this problem. The importance of counselling cannot be overemphasized when one considers the potential effects of hearing loss on adults. Meyerson (1963) states that each individual reacts differently to the impact of hearing impairment. Initially, the client may have a great deal of difficulty accepting his loss of hearing (Tuxen, 1972). It is not uncommon for the client to deny the existence of hearing impairment, especially when the loss is small (Alpiner, 1973). According to Rousey (1971), the client may react to his hearing loss by using such defense mechanisms as regression reaction-formation, and isolation. Myklebust (1960) found that hard-of-hearing adults emphasized the problems created by increased stress of everyday life, difficulty in maintaining friends, loss of friends, despondency, social isolation, and the need to identify with other hard-of-hearing individuals.

Various types of counselling may be offered to hearing-impaired adults, ranging from being a willing listener (Northern, 1972) to a psychologic referral (Binnie, 1976). The hard-of-hearing client should be allowed to discuss the implications of his hearing loss and information concerning the nature and type of his loss should be explained (Alpiner, 1971). Sanders (1975) states that counselling may be broken down into informational and personal adjustment guidance. The client should be allowed to get a feeling of how his hearing loss will affect daily life.

Intervention strategies may help the client adjust to specific situations in which communication difficulties occur, especially with family members and in vocational situations. If the client is agreeable, the audiologist may contact his spouse, employer, or friend to discuss the effects of hearing loss. This interview may occur with the client present or in private sessions between the audiologist and those persons who are part of the client's environment. Experience has shown it to be helpful to have family members attend therapy sessions for counselling purposes. It has been found to be beneficial to make personal visits to employers when permission is granted by the client. These contacts with other persons, explaining the ramifications of hearing loss, may help create a more positive environment for the hearing-impaired client.

There are some general guidelines which need to be considered in carrying out the progressive approach. As in the traditional approach, the client receives an audiologic evaluation to determine the amount of his hearing loss. This information allows the audiologist to make an initial judgment regarding the need for remediation, which may include a hearing aid evaluation. In addition to objective audiologic data, client input may be obtained through use of assessment scales of communication function discussed in Chapter 2. Based on the communication scales, some problem areas experienced by the client as a result of his hearing loss will be identified.

The clinician then explores the client's problem areas with him. During this procedure, it will be necessary to establish rapport, a working relationship with the client which is an ongoing process essential for successful therapy. During initial sessions, rapport may be achieved through effective interaction between the clinician and client. In addition to obtaining information, verbal interaction should help the client think constructively about his problem areas. The clinician has the critical task of selecting appropriate questions to encourage meaningful discussion. Seven types of questions may be used in the counselling process. Examples of them and their purposes are included in Table 4.2 (Industrial Relations Center, 1961).

The manner in which a question is posed can be important in eliciting a meaningful response. Some general guidelines suggested by the Industrial Relations Center (1961) are as follows.

1. Be brief.
2. Be sure the question relates directly to the subject discussed.
3. Cover only a single point. Avoid double-barreled questions.
4. Develop thinking from a constructive point of view.
5. Use words that come naturally to you.
6. Use words that are meaningful to the client.
7. In most cases, avoid questions requiring merely a "yes" or "no" response.

Table 4.2
Types of questions used in the counselling process[a]

Type	Purpose is . . .	Examples are . . .
1. Factual	1. To get information 2. To open discussion	1. The 5 "W" questions: who, what, where, when, why? 2. The "H" question: how?
2. Explanatory	1. To get reasons and explanations 2. To broaden discussion 3. To develop additional information	1. "In what way would this help solve the problem?" 2. "What other aspects of this should be considered?" 3. "Just how would this be done?"
3. Justifying	1. To challenge old ideas 2. To develop new ideas 3. To get reasoning and proof	1. "Why do you think so?" 2. "How do you know?" 3. "What evidence do you have?"
4. Leading	1. To introduce a new idea 2. To advance a suggestion of your own	1. "Should we consider this as a possible solution?" 2. "Would this be a feasible alternative?"
5. Hypothetical	1. To develop new ideas 2. To suggest another, perhaps unpopular, opinion 3. To change the course of discussion	1. "Suppose we did it this way—what would happen?" 2. "Another company does this—would this be feasible here?"
6. Alternative	1. To make decisions between alternatives 2. To get agreement	1. "Which of these solutions is best—A or B?" 2. "Is A our choice in preference to B?"
7. Coordinating	1. To get agreement 2. To pave the way for action	1. "Can we conclude that this is the next step?" 2. "Is there general agreement on this plan?"

[a] Reprinted by permission from Industrial Relations Center, The University of Chicago, © 1961 (CD-504-2).

The clinician should have some idea about what he wants to ask the client. He must remain flexible, however, to obtain the maximum possible amount of information. This may mean deviating from the original lesson plan. The key is to remember that the questions asked must be relevant to the development of the discussion.

Information obtained during initial sessions determines the direction the clinician will follow in therapy. The goals of therapy in the progressive approach are to modify either the client's behavior and attitudes or his environment, or a combination of both. In modifying the client's behavior and attitudes, the emphasis is on developing his ability to:

1. Be willing to admit the existence of the hearing loss and its handicapping effects.
2. Be willing to admit the hearing loss to others.
3. Be willing to take positive action to minimize communication difficulties by asking others to repeat, by asking others to speak more clearly, and by asking for selective seating.

Modification of the client's environment places emphasis on educating those persons within his family, vocational, and social environments. Some examples include the following.

1. Encouraging family members to attend therapy sessions in order to gain a better understanding of the limitations imposed by hearing loss.

2. Allowing the clinician to meet with an employer to discuss modifications in the work environment.

3. Allowing the clinician to speak to civic or social groups regarding hearing impairment and its ramifications.

A major benefit of the progressive approach should be the client's realization that his communication problems are not unique. Through interaction with the members of his group, the client becomes aware that other hearing-impaired individuals share his experiences. Suggestions for coping with difficult communication situations may come from other group members. Acceptance of hearing loss is often easier in this situation where others share common problems. Again, it should be stressed that the progressive approach is frequently used in combination with the traditional approach, depending on the needs of individual clients.

Reference is made to the problems common to the three clients cited earlier in this chapter. The first four areas of difficulty indicated the need for traditional therapy. These clients were given individual speech therapy to improve their defective articulation. General communication practice using a bisensory approach (combined vision and audition) with competing background noise was also utilized.

The final four areas of difficulty experienced by these clients indicated the need for progressive therapy. The Denver Scale of Communication Function was administered and the clients' problem areas were identified. In the group session, dialogue was used to explore these problems further. Group interaction followed the format suggested for modifying client behavior, attitude, and environment. Stress and its manifestations were minimized when the clients eventually were ready to admit and accept the reality of hearing loss. Subsequently, they were able to admit the hearing impairment to others and to take positive action to compensate for the auditory deficit. This process took approximately 10 weeks of therapy sessions. Verbal reports and post-test results of the Denver Scale of Communication Function indicated

that stress, as a result of hearing loss, was significantly reduced. Clients also expressed a willingness to ask for repetition in difficult listening situations.

The two clients who had previously rejected the use of amplification agreed eventually to hearing aid evaluations. Individual body type auditory trainers were used as a desensitization process during group sessions. Clients' willingness to try the auditory trainer occurred during the 5th week of therapy. By the time these clients were released from therapy, they had purchased hearing aids and were wearing them regularly. Ultimately the clients realized that they could communicate more effectively. Normal-hearing persons no longer posed a threat to them in communication.

Sequentially, the progressive approach proceeds in the following manner.

1. Audiologic and hearing aid evaluation.
2. Assessment of communication function.
3. Identification of problem areas due to hearing loss.
4. Verbal discussion within the group regarding problems.
5. Admission of hearing loss to themselves and to others.
6. Modification of behavior, attitudes, and environment.
7. Willingness to utilize amplification in nonthreatening therapy sessions.
8. Reduction of stress in communication situations.
9. Willingness to utilize amplification outside of therapy sessions.
10. More effective communication with normal-hearing persons.
11. Termination of therapy.

Linguistic Approach

There is a little information available regarding the linguistic structure of language as it relates to lipreading ability (Hull and Alpiner, 1976). Several authors have recognized and stressed the importance of obtaining knowledge regarding the structure of language and its relationship to visual perception of speech (Jerger, 1968; Lloyd, 1964; Lowell, 1969; O'Neill, 1968; Woodward and Barber, 1960). O'Neill (1968) emphasizes this need, stating that "lipreading training must be aimed at communicative meaningfulness; in other words, not working at the sound or word level, but a units of meaning . . . proceeding on the assumption that we are dealing with a learned form of lingustic behavior."

The use of the linguistic approach attempts to provide a different technique for acquainting clients with visual speech through language understanding. This can be done visually, auditorily, and combined (Hull, 1976). Hull and Alpiner (1976) studied this approach to determine the effects of language syntax on understanding speech. They attempt to answer the question, "What effect will six systematic variations in the presentation of parts of speech have on the identification of sentences?" The three conditions were as follows.

1. Under the condition of visual only at the thought and verbatim levels.
2. Under the condition of auditory only at the thought and verbatim levels.
3. At the thought and verbatim levels of prediction when systematic additions of auditory word cues are combined with intact visual presentation of stimulus materials.

Words were systematically deleted from prepared sentences to determine those parts of speech which might enhance the predictability of sentences. The syntactic combinations abbreviated P for principle words, V for verbs and modifiers, and C for connectives or function words (prepositions, conjunctions, articles, and so forth). Words were randomly varied six ways for presentation to subjects. The syntactic combinations concluded PVC, VCP, PCV, CPV, VPC, and CVP. For example, the syntactic combination of PVC would indicate that the principle words were presented first in random order, the verbs and modifiers second, and the connectives last. The subject's task was to attempt to predict sentence content when words within the sentences were missing. The combinations were given auditory only, visual only, and auditory-visual. Table 4.3 illustrates this approach. In this example, a VCP syntactic word order was used under an auditory-visual mode.

Results of this study indicate that the visual only condition resulted in the poorest scores for all syntactic combinations. No syntactic combination seemed to facilitate sentence prediction. It seems that the low subject scores were not the result of the various syn-

Table 4.3
Word order of presentation for the VCP syntactic word order under the AV mode[a]

	1	2	3	4	5	6	7	8
1	V	V	AV	V	V	V	V	V
	—	—	is	—	—	—	—	—
2.	V	V	AV	V	V	V	V	AV
	—	—	is	—	—	—	—	again.
3.	V	V	AV	AV	V	V	V	AV
	—	—	is	blowing	—	—	—	again.
4.	V	V	AV	AV	V	AV	V	AV
	—	—	is	blowing	—	the	—	again.
5.	V	V	AV	AV	AV	AV	V	AV
	—	—	is	blowing	from	the	—	again.
6.	AV	V	AV	AV	AV	AV	V	AV
	The	—	is	blowing	from	the	—	again.
7.	AV	V	AV	AV	AV	AV	AV	AV
	The	—	is	blowing	from	the	north-east	again.
	AV	AV	AV	AV	AV	AV	AV	AV
	The	wind	is	blowing	from	the	north-east	again.

[a] Reprinted by permission from Hull and Alpiner: The effect of syntactic word variations on the predictability of sentence content in speech reading. *J. Acad. Rehab. Audiology*, **9(1)**, 42–56, © 1976, *Journal of the Academy of Rehabilitative Audiology*.

tax combinations, but of the difficult task of using visual cues only.

Poor scores for all syntactic combinations were obtained in the auditory only condition, also. The wide range of word choices from which the subject could select appeared to be the reason for the relatively low scores for this condition.

Under visual presentation combined with systematic addition of auditory cues, sentence prediction scores at the thought level were better. The results for this condition seem to indicate that high scores were due to complementing audition with vision.

This investigation suggests two important therapeutic implications. First, the value of combining audition with vision in lipreading instruction seems apparent. Remediation should stress both vision and residual hearing in comprehension of language. Thought prediction of sentence content, rather than verbatim identification, should be emphasized.

The second implication suggests that clients should be trained to select words carrying the most information in sentences and in conversational speech. Nouns and pronouns appear to be more difficult to lipread while verbs and modifiers are more easily identified. Connectives seem to be highly predictable but difficult to lipread. These factors appear to facilitate prediction in terms of the reception of continuous discourse. While watching the speaker, clients can acquire the ability to "piece together" messages when they cannot hear every word.

VARIABLES IN REMEDIATION

In designing a remediation plan for the hearing-impaired adult, several factors have to be considered. Often, these elements of the therapy process are dictated by clinical administrative structures or time and money constraints on the clinician and/or the hearing-impaired individual. Ideally, however, decisions regarding these variables should be based on the needs, ability, and progress made by the hearing-impaired individual. The following discussion presents these variables and some of the options available in developing a remediation plan.

Individual *Versus* Group Therapy

One of the decisions an audiologist needs to make is whether therapy should be conducted individually or in groups. Several factors should be considered in making this decision. Oyer (1966) cites obvious advantages and disadvantages for individual therapy. Advantages include more time with the client for repeated trials, better situations in which to discuss adjustment problems, and greater opportunities to make constant checks on performance and practice. Disadvantages in individual therapy include lack of peer evaluation, no psychologic support from peers, no opportunity to compare and contrast individual efforts with others, and no opportunity to perform socially in a practice environment.

In individual therapy, the clinician is able to devote the entire therapy time to only one person. This could result in fewer sessions needed to accomplish the goals of remediation with less interference in the client's everyday responsibilities. The client who is reluctant to devote time to longer term therapy may be willing to attend a short term individualized program. In an individual program, the objectives of a particular lesson allow the client to progress at his own rate. The client can continue to work in areas of difficulty without interfering with the progress of other persons. In addition, the client is free to discuss his communication adjustment problems with the clinician in a more discrete environment. It is often easier for the client to discuss his problems with the clinician on a one-to-one basis than it would be to do so in a group situation. It is possible that the client will feel a certain confidentiality in discussing his communication difficulties with the audiologist alone. From the viewpoint of the audiologist, there is more opportunity to monitor individual progress. Individual therapy also enhances client-clinician interaction.

There are disadvantages to individual therapy. The individual client will not have the benefit of feedback from other hearing-impaired clients. He will also miss the opportunity to discuss communication problems common to hearing-impaired adults. Individual therapy sessions may not allow the client to realize that this communication problems are not unique. The client must depend solely on the clinician for indication of his performance in individual sessions. Lacking is the opportunity to compare his progress in relation to the progress of others in the group. Further, the client has no opportunity to interact socially with others who have hearing problems.

According to Sanders (1971), economics is the most common motivation for group therapy. He states that not all of us are fortunate enough to work in a university or community clinic where individual therapy sessions are conducted by students under supervision or funded by United Way agencies. Other than this economic factor, however, there are additional important considerations which justify group therapy. The group situation allows the hearing-impaired clients to share their problems with empathetic listeners. The adventitiously hearing-impaired adult may never have encountered other persons with hearing loss. A group setting encourages clients to work together in solving common difficulties posed by hearing impairment. Group interaction can encourage positive attitudes toward the therapy process by increasing the client's motivation for self-improvement. Often, emotional support and reinforcement are more meaningful when they emanate from peers. It needs to be emphasized that the group should be composed of members with homogeneous levels of hearing handicap. For example, an individual with severe discrimination difficulties should not be placed in a group where he will impede the progress of others.

Length of Remediation Term

No data exist regarding the optimal duration of a rehabilitative audiology term for either individual or groups. However, Perry (1978) has reported that her clinical experience shows that most adults can absorb lipreading in 10 to 12 weekly sessions lasting 1 hour each. The assumption was made earlier that fewer sessions are necessary in individual therapy because concentrated effort is expended in working with just one client. In university training programs, it appears that the duration of remediation is determined by the length of the academic term. This situation, unfortunately, is due to convenience. Research regarding the optimal time frame has also been neglected.

Length of Therapy Sessions

The length of therapy sessions is dependent primarily upon the attention span of the client. Since listening is one of the elements in the remediation process, it is important to be aware of its components. Barker (1971) believes that there are four interrelated processes involved in listening: attention, hearing, understanding, and remembering. In determining the length of the session, it is necessary to consider attention and its ramifications. Eisenson et al. (1963) state that a listener cannot give continuous attention; even when he tries very hard to attend, he does not hear everything. They indicate further that attention comes in spurts similar to the irregular intervals of waves on a beach. Early experimenters estimated that an attention length unit should be from 5 to 8 seconds. Psychologists today, however, conclude simply that the duration of attention is brief. They believe that it is impossible to determine an absolute time value since that is dependent upon the stimulus intensity. Duration of attention varies with the individual and is influenced by such factors as fatigue and interest in the communication. They also feel that individual attention spans vary. Graham (1951) states that different forms and combinations of stimuli give different attention spans.

The clinician needs to be cognizant of this information when determining the length of the session. Because of the constant intensity of the stimuli, both auditory and visual, our experience has shown that the client in group therapy will realize his maximum benefit in sessions lasting from 1 to 1½ hours. In individual therapy, the client seems to function best in ½- to 1-hour sessions. Consistent with the research mentioned, it is important to vary the materials used in a lesson and to have alternating periods of high and low intensity stimuli. (Intensity here refers to the degree of attention required, rather than the physical attribute of sound.)

Manner of Presentation

In a study of lipreading, Nakano (1960) found that the following factors influenced lipreading performance: familiarity with the speaker, distance between speaker and client, articulation of the speaker, and residual hearing. According to Petkovsek (1961), lipreaders appear to understand speech better when they are familiar with the language, dialect, and speech habits of the speaker. Berger and DePompei (1972) report that lipreaders indicate that it is easier to lipread relatives and close friends.

This information implies that success in communication with close friends and relatives will provide the reinforcement necessary for improvement in overall communication. It provides a transition from communication in less threatening situations to communication with employers, strangers, and others in everyday communication situations. His concept gives support for including family members in the therapy session.

It is preferable in the group situation to use a semi-circular seating arrangement. This arrangement allows clients to experience communication at various angles and distances. Considerable research regarding distance between clinicians and clients has been done, but results have been inconclusive due to the multitude of variables employed. Berger (1972) best summarizes the aspects of distance by indicating that from the available evidence, distances of up to 20 or 24 feet do not have a significant effect on lipreading performance. He advocates distances of between 5 and 10 feet since they are typical of daily conversational situations. The semi-circular seating arrangement suggested above, within the limits of a reasonable distance, allows the client to practice with different conditions he will experience in his environment. In individual therapy, too, the client should be exposed to a variety of distances and angles. It is assumed that the client will have normal or corrected visual acuity.

In a study examining the lipreading performance of vowels and diphthongs, Wozniak and Jackson (1979) determined that no significant differences existed between 0 and 90° angles in lipreading phoneme identification. Interestingly, however, they did determine that diphthong stimuli were easier to read than vowel stimuli at both angles.

The clinician should also be aware of room illumination during the therapy session although ideal lighting conditions are not always present in everyday communication situations. As a guideline for therapy, Thomas (1962) found that lipreading efficiency of trained subjects decreased as room illumination decreased, although not significantly so. This study seems to suggest that if a person is familiar with the content of the message and given some training, he will do well even in poorly lighted environments.

The question often arises whether voice should be used in instruction. The vast majority of clients with acquired hearing loss have some residual hearing and will be receiving both auditory and visual cues under most communication conditions. From a realistic point of view, therefore, it would appear that therapy materials should be presented using both visual and auditory cues. Therapy using no voice has been and is still being used. The historical bias for this practice stems from the lack of good amplification systems in the early days of lipreading. With the advent of more sophisticated amplification systems, focus in therapy has shifted to simulating the difficult listening situations encountered daily.

Clients often complain that they miss parts of communications because of their hearing loss. For this reason, therapy is approached in two ways. The first is to present stimulus materials utilizing related sentences in which some words of each sentence are presented auditorily and others are presented without voice. For example, in the sentence, "Washington, D. C. is the capital of the United States," the words " . . . capital of the United States" would be given voiceless. The client is then able to utilize both auditory and visual cues in understanding the thought or idea of the communication. The second approach is to present stimulus materials auditorily in the presence of competing background noise. This noise should simulate a condition which would create a difficult listening situation for the client. Auditory stimuli should be presented at a normal conversational level. The clinician will have to determine the signal-to-noise ratio dependent upon hearing levels of the individual clients. These levels can be varied to simulate either very easy or very difficult listening conditions.

In the ideal listening situation, the hearing-impaired person prefers listening to one who speaks in a normal conversational manner in a quiet condition. The everyday communication environment, unfortunately, is not ideal. Clients frequently complain about the speaker who articulates poorly, speaks too rapidly or too softly, utilizes minimal lip movements, or has other distracting facial characteristics. For example, clients may complain about one clinician who has a mustache or another who wears excessive lipstick. It may be necessary for the client to explain his hearing loss and ask for clarity and repetition. In addition, the client must realize that everyday communication will involve distractions caused by facial characteristics. Again, the client needs to inform the speaker of his hearing loss so the message may be repeated for more complete understanding. Frequently, it is difficult for a client to admit his hearing loss and ask for repetition. In terms of real life, however, it will be helpful to admit that communication difficulties exist. Failure to do so will only lead to frustration, confusion, and embarrassment.

Ongoing Remediation Sessions

At the conclusion of a beginning remediation term, some clients will feel the need for additional assistance. The rationale for continuing remediation is the need for additional improvement in communication ability or maintenance of acquired effective communication ability. Individual needs vary among clients. In many centers, beginning therapy sessions are given sequentially to achieve predetermined goals. Those clients who need further work to meet established goals, therefore, are referred for further rehabilitation.

The format of the ongoing sessions is designed so that attendance is not required at every session. Clients are informed that sessions will deal with general communication skills as well as providing the client an opportunity to discuss specific problem areas which may occur. Clients are encouraged to attend ongoing sessions when they feel they are having recurring communication difficulties. The important consideration is that clients know assistance is available at a designated time each week. Clients are also encouraged to contact the clinician during intervals between sessions if they are experiencing communication problems.

Rather than establish a formal advanced lipreading group with mandatory attendance, clients with persistent difficulties are placed in individual therapy where their problems can receive highly individualized attention.

Release Criteria

A difficult aspect of adult rehabilitative audiology is determining when therapy should be terminated. This is due, in part, to the wide variability found among individual clients. Clients with apparently similar auditory difficulties reach different levels of communication proficiency. Obviously, there can be no one set of criteria for all hearing-impaired persons. It should be emphasized that remediation does not imply a "cure" but rather an effort to reach maximum efficiency in communication for the individual.

The client's release must be determined by the total remediation process. A review of this process should be helpful in developing release criteria. After the client has been evaluated for both auditory function and communication ability, the clinician identifies individual problem areas for which therapy must be planned. The clinician, in conjunction with the client, establishes understandable and realistic goals appropriate to the level of communication difficulties. During therapy, it is possible that these goals will need modification in terms of the client's successes and failures.

It would appear that release criteria involve three alternatives, related directly to goals which have been established. The most obvious release criterion is fulfillment of these pre-determined goals. The client should be informed that periodic evaluation is desirable. In addition, if he experiences difficulties after termination of therapy, the client is encouraged to return to determine if the need exists for further remediation. A second alternative occurs when the client has not attained the pre-determined goals of therapy. If the clinician feels that further progress can be achieved, the client may be referred for additional therapy, either individual or ongoing group. When this recommendation is made, goals must be re-defined. The third alternative happens when the client has not achieved established goals and it appears unlikely that he will be able to do so. It is possible that he has already achieved his maximum communication effectiveness.

Innovative Variables

With the technological advances that are being made, particularly in the computer field, it is not surprising that innovative approaches to aural rehabilitation are being developed. Technology is allowing traditional tasks like lipreading, auditory training, and speech training to be taught via computer-controlled video and audio systems. One such system called DAVID (Cronin, 1979) was devised at the National Technical Institute for the Deaf (NTID). The acronym stands for Data Analysis in Video Interactive Device and the components consist of the following: a 12-inch color monitor, a specially modified videotape recorder, an audio amplifier, a Wang VP mini-computer, a keyboard, a micro-computer to interface the Wang and the videotape recorder, a disk storage system, and a printer. The DAVID system is currently being used at NTID for controlled self-instruction in lipreading and auditory training (Sims, *et al.*, 1979). Von Feldt (1978) reports that a combination of student interaction (active learning) when combined with motion and audio may provide significant instructional gains in aural rehabilitation. He also maintains that these systems contribute to learning by providing immediate feedback since data indicates that waiting for reinforcement deteriorates learning.

McQuay and Coscarelli (1980) have described a unique, individualized Self-Instruction Lab at NTID. Based on the premise that the more an individual practices under highly structured conditions, the more likely he will achieve success in improving communication skills, this lab provides students with supplemental independent practice in speech, lipreading, auditory training, English skill proficiency, and manual/simultaneous communication. The lab consists of carrels each containing a cartridge storage area, color television monitor, videocartridge player, binaural amplifier, audiocassette unit, headphone, student work area, posture swivel chair, and master power switch.

While it is obvious that the equipment described above is costly and beyond the means of most practicing clinicians, advances in technology may make this equipment more accessible and affordable in the future. Meanwhile, these systems and labs are in a position to research the value of such devices and techniques and which may make a valuable contribution to the field of aural rehabilitation.

References

ALPINER, J. G., Rehabilitative audiology. *Rehabil. Rec.* **14**, 9–13 (1973).

ALPINER, J. G., Planning a strategy of aural rehabilitation for the adult. *Hear. Speech News*, **39**, 21–26 (1971).

ASP, C. W., Measurement of aural speech perception and oral speech production of the hearing-impaired. In S. Singh (Ed.), *Measurement Procedures in Speech, Hearing, and Language.* Baltimore: University Park Press (1975).

AYERS, T. R., You can listen ... if you want to: A structured approach to active listening. *Tennessee Education*, **8(1)**, 23–25 (1978).

BARGSTADT, G. H., HUTCHINSON, J. M., and NERBONNE, M. A., Learning visual correlates of fricative production by normal hearing subjects: A preliminary evaluation of the video articulator. *J. Speech Hear. Dis.*, **43**, 200–207 (1978).

BARKER, L. L., *Listening Behavior.* Englewood Cliffs, New Jersey: Prentice-Hall, Inc. (1971).

BERGER, K. W., *Speechreading.* Baltimore: National Educational Press, Inc. (1972).

BERGER, K. W., and DEPOMPEI, R. A., Speechreaders report on speechreading. In K. W. Berger (Ed.), *Speechreading.* Baltimore: National Educational Press, Inc. (1972).

BERGER, K. W., MARTIN, J., and SAKOFF, R., The effect of visual distractions on speech reading performance. *Teacher Deaf*, **68**, 384–387 (1970).

BERGMAN, M., Special methods of audiological training of adults. *Acta Otolaryng.*, **40**, 336–345 (1952).

BINNIE, C. A., Attitude changes following speechreading training. *Scand. Audiol.*, **6**, 13–19 (1977).

BINNIE, C. A., Relevant aural rehabilitation. In J. L. Northern (Ed.), *Hearing Disorders.* Boston: Little, Brown and Co. (1976).

BINNIE, C. A., Bi-sensory articulation function for normal hearing and sensorineural hearing loss patients. *J. Acad. Rehab. Audiol.* **6**, 43–53 (1973).

BINNIE, C. A., JACKSON, P. L., and MONTGOMERY, A. A., Visual intelligibility of consonants: a lipreading screening test with implications for aural rehabilitation. *J. Speech Hear. Dis.*, **41**, 530–539 (1976).

BINNIE, C. A., MONTGOMERY, A. A. and JACKSON, P. L., Auditory and visual contributions to the perception of consonants. *J. Speech Hear. Res.*, **17**, 619–630 (1974).

BODE, D. L., and CARHART, R., Stability and accuracy of adaptive tests of speech discrimination. *J. Acoust. Soc. Am.*, **56**, 963–970 (1974).

BODE, D. L., and CARHART, R., Measurement of articulation functions using adaptive test procedures. *IEEE Trans Audio* Electro-Acoust., AU-21, 196–201 (1973).

BODE, D. L., and CARHART, R., Sequential testing of speech discrimination. Presented at the Acoustical Society of America meeting, Houston, November 1970.

BODE, D. L., and OYER, H. J., Auditory training and speech discrimination. *J. Speech Hear. Res.*, **13**, 839–855 (1970).

BRUHN, M. E., *Elementary Lessons in Lipreading.* Lynn, MA: Nichols Press (1927).

BUNGER, A. M., *Speechreading—Jena Method.* Danville, IL: The Interstate (1961).

BUNGER, A. M., Appraising progress in speech reading. *Volta Rev.*, **26**, 503–504 (1924).

CARHART, R., Auditory training. In H. Davis and S. R. Silverman (Eds.), *Hearing and Deafness.* New York: Holt, Rinehart and Winston, Inc. (1960).

CONKLIN, J. M., and SUBTELNY, J. D., Effect of speech training upon speechreading in hearing-impaired adults. *Am. Ann. Deaf*, 442–448 (1980).

CRONIN, B., The DAVID system: the development of an interactive video system at the National Institute for the Deaf. *Am. Ann. Deaf*, 616–618 (1979).

DAVIS, H., HUDGINS, C. V., MARQUIS, D. G., NICHOLS, R. H., and PETERSON, G. E., The selection of hearing aids. *Laryngoscope*, **56**, 85–115, 135–163 (1946).

DICARLO, L. M., Auditory training for the adult. *Volta Rev.* **50**, 490 (1948).

DODDS, E., and HARFORD, E., Application of a lipreading test in a hearing aid evaluation. *J. Speech Hear. Dis.*, **33**, 167–173 (1968).

EISENSON, J., AUER, J. J., and IRWIN, J. V., *The Psychology of Communication*. New York: Appleton-Century-Crofts (1963).

ERBER, N. P., Auditory-visual perception of speech with reduced optical clarity. *J. Speech Hear. Res.*, **22**, 212–223 (1979).

ERBER, N. P., Auditory-visual perception. *J. Speech Hear. Dis.*, **40**, 481–492 (1975).

ERBER, N. P., Auditory-visual perception of speech: a survey. *Scand. Audiol.* (suppl.) **4**, 12–30 (1974).

ERICKSON, J. G., *Speechreading: An Aid to Communication*. Urbana-Champaign, IL: University of Illinois, Department of Speech and Hearing Science (1974).

FAIRBANKS, G., Schematic research in experimental phonetics: a theory of the speech mechanism as a servo system. *J. Speech Hear. Dis.*, **19**, 133–139 (1954).

FLEMING, M., A total approach to communication therapy. *J. Acad. Rehab. Audiol.* **5**, 28–31 (1972).

FLETCHER, H., *Speech and Hearing in Communication*. New York: Van Nostrand Company, Inc. (1953).

GARSTECKI, D. C., Adult auditory-visual training. Paper presented at fall meeting of American Auditory Society, Detroit, November, 1980.

GARSTECKI, D. C., Situational cues in visual speech perception in geriatric subjects. *J. Am. Audiol. Soc.*, **2**, 99–106 (1976).

GRAHAM, C. H., Visual perception. In S. S. Stevens (Ed.), *Handbook of Experimental Psychology*. New York: John Wiley & Sons, Inc. (1951).

GRIFFITH, J., *Persons with Hearing Loss*. Springfield, IL: Charles C Thomas (1969).

HAMPLEMAN, R., Comparison of listening and reading ability of fourth and sixth grade pupils. *Elementary English*, **35**, 49–53 (1958).

HASPIEL, G. S., *A Synthetic Approach to Lipreading*. Magnolia, Massachusetts: The Expression Company (1964).

HIRSH, I. J., Auditory training. In H. Davis and S. R. Silverman (Eds.), *Hearing and Deafness*. New York: Holt, Rinehart and Winston, Inc. (1970).

HULL, R. H., A linguistic approach to the teaching of speechreading: theoretical and practical concepts. *J. Acad. Rehab. Audiol.*, **9**, 14–19 (1976).

HULL, R. H., and ALPINER, J. G., The effect of syntactic word variations on the predictability of sentence content in speechreading. *J. Acad. Rehab. Audiol.*, **9**, 42–56 (1976).

INDUSTRIAL RELATIONS CENTER, *Coaching and Developing Individuals*. Chicago: Industrial Relations Center (1961).

JEFFERS, J., and BARLEY, M., *Speechreading (Lipreading)*. Springfield, IL: Charles C Thomas (1971).

JERGER, J., Research—present status and needs. In J. G. Alpiner (Ed.), *Proceedings of the Institute on Aural Rehabilitation*. Denver: University of Denver (1968).

KELLY, J. C., *Clinicians Handbook for Auditory Training*. Washington, D. C.: Alexander Graham Bell Association for the Deaf, Inc. (1953).

KINZIE, C. E., The Kinzie method of speechreading for the deaf. *Volta Rev.*, **20**, 249–252 (1918).

KRUG, R. F., Effects and interactions of auditory and visual clues in oral communication. U. S. Department of Health, Education, and Welfare, Project Number 499 (1960).

LIEBERTH, A., and SUBTELNY, J. D., The effect of speech training on auditory phoneme identification. *Volta Rev.*, 410–417 (1978).

LING, D., *Speech and the Hearing-Impaired Child: Theory and Practice*. Washington, D. C.: Alexander Graham Bell Association for the Deaf (1976).

LLOYD, L., Sentence familiarity as a factor in visual speech perception. *J. Speech Hear. Dis.*, **29**, 409–413 (1964).

LOWELL, E. L., Rehabilitation of auditory disorders. In *Human Communication and Its Disorders—An Overview*. Bethesda: National Institute of Health, Public Health Service, **69** (1969).

MCCARTNEY, J. H., and NADLER, G., How to help your patient cope with hearing loss. *Geriatrics*, 69–76 (1979).

MCQUAY, K. C., and COSCARELLI, L. S., A self-instruction lab for developing communication skills of deaf post-secondary students at NTID. *Am. Ann. Deaf*, 406–412 (1980).

MEYERSON, L., The psychology of impaired hearing. In W. Cruikshank (Ed.) *Psychology of Exceptional Children and Youth*. Englewood Cliffs, NJ: Prentice-Hall, Inc. (1963).

MILLER, J. B., Oralism. *Volta Rev.*, **72**, 211–217 (1970).

MYKLEBUST, H., *The Psychology of Deafness*. New York: Grune & Stratton (1960).

NAKANO, Y., A study on the factors which influence lipreading of deaf children. *Bull. Faculty Educ. Tokyo U.*, **6**, 141–156 (1960).

NITCHIE, E. B., Lipreading, an art. *Volta Rev.*, **15**, 276–278 (1913).

NORTHERN, J. L., Visual and auditory rehabilitation for adults. In J. Katz (Ed.), *Handbook of Clinical Audiology*. Baltimore: The Williams & Wilkins Co. (1972).

NORTHERN, J. L., and SANDERS, D. A., Philosophical considerations in aural rehabilitation. In J. Katz (Ed.), *Handbook of Clinical Audiology*. Baltimore: The Williams & Wilkins Co. (1972).

NUMBERS, M., and HUDGINS, C. V., Speech perception in present day education for deaf children. *Volta Rev.*, **50**, 449–456 (1948).

O'NEILL, J. J., Lipreading—significance and usage for children and adults. In J. G. Alpiner (Ed.), *Proceedings of the Institute on Aural Rehabilitation*. Denver: University of Denver (1968).

O'NEILL, J. J., and OYER, H. J., *Visual Communication for the Hard of Hearing*. Englewood Cliffs, NJ: Prentice-Hall, Inc. (1961).

OWENS, E., Consonant errors and remediation in sensorineural hearing loss. *J. Speech Hear. Dis.*, **43**, 331–347 (1978).

OYER, H. J., *Auditory Communication for the Hard of Hearing*. Englewood Cliffs, NJ: Prentice-Hall, Inc. (1966).

OYER, H. J., and FRANKMANN, J. P., *The Aural Rehabilitation Process*. New York: Holt, Rinehart and Winston (1975).

PAULS, M. D., Speechreading. In H. Davis and S. R. Silverman (Eds.), *Hearing and Deafness*. New York: Holt, Rinehart and Winston (1960).

PENGILLEY, P., Hearing tactics: the strategy of coping with a hearing problem. Paper presented to the Audiologial Society of Australia, 4th National Conference, 1980.

PENGILLEY, P., *By Word of Mouth.* Vermont Victoria, Australia: The Advisory Council for Children with Impaired Hearing (1973).

PERRY, A. L., A lipreading curriculum for adults. *Volta Rev.,* **79,** 86–92 (1977).

PETKOVSEK, M., The eyes have it. *Hear. News,* **29,** 5–9 (1961).

ROSS, M., *Principles of Aural Rehabilitation.* New York: The Bobbs Merrill Company, Inc. (1972).

ROUSEY, C. L., Psychological reactions to hearing loss. *J. Speech Hear. Dis.,* **36,** 382–398 (1971).

RUESCH, J., and KEES, W., *Nonverbal Communication.* Los Angeles: University of California Press (1956).

SANDERS, D. A., Hearing aid orientation and counselling. In M. C. Pollack (Ed.), *Amplification for the Hearing-Impaired.* New York: Grune & Stratton (1975).

SANDERS, D. A., *Aural Rehabilitation.* Englewood Cliffs, NJ: Prentice-Hall, Inc. (1971).

SIEGENTHALER, B. M. and GRUBER, V., Combining vision and audition for speech reception. *J. Speech Hear. Dis.,* **34,** 58–60 (1969).

SIMS, D., VON FELDT, J., DOWALIBY, F., HUTCHISON, K., and MYERS, T., A pilot experiment in computer assisted speechreading instruction utilizing the data analysis video interactive device (DAVID). *Am. Ann. Deaf,* 618–623 (1979).

STEELE, J. A., BINNIE, C. A., AND COOPER, W. A., Combining auditory and visual stimuli in the adaptive testing of speech discrimination. *J. Speech Hear. Dis.,* **43,** 115–122 (1978).

THOMAS, S. L., Lipreading performance as a function of light levels. M.A. thesis, Michigan State University (1962). In K. W. Berger (Ed.), *Speechreading.* Baltimore: National Educational Press, Inc. (1972).

TUTOLO, D. J., A cognitive approach to teaching listening. *Lang. Arts,* **54,** 262–265 (1977).

TUXEN, I., Educational and vocational problems in adolescents with slight and medium loss of hearing. *Scand. Audiol.,* **1,** 111 (1972).

VON FELDT, J. R., *A Description of a Prototype System at NTID Which Merges Computer Assisted Instruction and Instructional Television.* Rochester: National Institute for the Deaf (1978).

WALDEN, B. E., PROSEK, R. A., MONTGOMERY, A. A., SCHERR, C. K., and JONES, C. L., Effects of training on the visual recognition of consonants. *J. Speech Hear. Res.,* **20,** 130–145 (1977).

WALTER, G. G., and SIMS, D. G., The effect of prolonged hearing aid use on the communication skills of young, deaf adults. *Am. Ann. Deaf,* **123,** 548–554 (1978).

WHITEHEAD, R., and BAREFOOT, S., Some aerodynamic characteristics of plosive consonants produced by hearing-impaired speakers. *Am. Ann. Deaf,* **125,** 336–373 (1980).

WHITEHURST, M. W., Interaction of auditory training and lipreading. *Volta Rev.,* **66,** 730–733 (1964).

WINITZ, H., *From Syllable to Conversation.* Baltimore: University Park Press (1975).

WOODWARD, M. F., and BARBER, C. G., Phoneme perception in lipreading. *J. Speech Hear. Res.,* **3,** 212–222 (1960).

WOZNIAK, V. D., and JACKSON, P. L., Visual vowel and diphthong perception from two horizontal viewing angles. *J. Speech Hear. Res.,* **22,** 354–365 (1979).

4

Sample Lipreading Lessons

---

1. Introduction of clients and clinicians: Brief discussion of occupation, place of residence, and general interests.
2. Discussion of referral source and reasons for enrolling in the group.
3. Clinician's interpretation of objectives for the lipreading group.
4. Discussion of what lipreading is, other names used synonymously with lipreading, and advantages and limitations.
5. Administration of tests:
   (a) Lipreading Screening Test (From Binnie, Montgomery, and Jackson, 1974).
   (b) The Denver Quick Test of Lipreading.
   (c) **The McCarthy-Alpiner Scale of Hearing Handicap.**
6. Demonstration of the use of lipreading in everyday situations. Most people do some lipreading without realizing it. For example, the following sentences are usually identified correctly without the use of voice:
   (a) How are you?
   (b) What time is it?
   (c) Good morning.
   (d) Thank you.
   (e) Good-bye, it was nice meeting you.
7. Discussion of any questions or comments by clients.
8. Introduction of first homophenous sound group with description of how sounds are formed on the lips. The sounds are /p, b, m/.
   Key words, using these sounds, are presented to the clients and then used in related sentences:

p	b	m
people	belong	majority
politics	members	women
president	cabinet	men

(a) Many people like to discuss politics.

(b) Most people belong to a political party.

(c) The two major parties in this country are Republican and Democratic.

(d) Both groups like to elect the president from their parties.

(e) In some elections, the majority of people don't vote.

(f) The president picks the members of his cabinet.

(g) Someday, a woman may become president.

(h) More women are joining men in politics.

9. Emphasize that it is important to get the thought or idea — "not every word."

10. Assignment for next session: Note those situations in which you have the greatest communication difficulty. Determine if gestures and facial expressions help you in understanding people. What happens when you turn the volume on your television set down one half when watching your favorite newscaster?

Adult Lipreading Group   *Session 2*

1. Review of assignment from the first session. Discussion of those situations in which you had the greatest communication difficulty. Reactions to observing facial expressions and gestures of other persons. Reaction to reducing the volume on the television set.

2. Presentation of an overview of the hearing mechanism by audiologist. Included are the different kinds of hearing loss and the causes of hearing loss. Also, hearing losses of individual clients are discussed.

3. Review of the sounds /p, b, m/. Practice sentences are presented.

(a) Please pass the butter.

(b) My brother smokes a pipe.

(c) Baseball is a popular sport.

(d) Money has decreased in buying power.

(e) Most people like apple pie.

4. Explanation of other clues that can aid understanding in various communication situations.

(a) Environmental clues: This type of clue suggests that the environment in which a particular speaker communicates may dictate the topic being discussed.

(b) Gestures: Observing the speaker, you may get some idea about what he is saying by watching his movements, particularly hand and arm movements.

(c) Facial clues: Some of the conversation may be understood by watching the expressions on a person's face (look for frowns, smiles, grimaces, and so forth).

   (d) Be a good listener: If we are not watching the other person or are simply not paying attention, we can miss much of the conversation whether there is a hearing loss or not.

5. Introduction of the homophenous sound group /f, v/. Include description of how sounds appear visually.

   Key words, using these sounds, are presented to the clients and then used in related sentences.

<u>f</u>	<u>v</u>
families	vacation
often	visit
fishing	expensive
France	vary
Finland	have

   (a) Families often plan vacations for the summer.
   (b) Vacation plans often vary during different seasons.
   (c) A fun vacation is fishing.
   (d) Fishing can be enjoyed by everyone in the family.
   (e) Foreign vacations are more expensive.
   (f) Have you visited France or Finland?
   (g) Some vacations are just to visit families and friends.

6. Present materials which contrast the two homophenous sound groups: /p, b, m/ and /f, v/.

7. Introduction of vowels: /o/ as in boat and /e/ as in meet. The /o/ is made by the rounding and thrusting forward of the lips. The /e/ is made by the drawing of the lips back and the opening of the teeth is normally small. Examples of words with these sounds are: toe, bow, so, low, foe, beet, seat, feet, treat, and key.

8. Remember, however, the important consideration is to get the "idea" or "thought."

9. Presentation of general conversational sentences, using a theme and key words, without regard to specific sounds.

10. Assignment for next session: Evaluate yourself in terms of all the clues we mentioned today. Have relatives or friends make up sentences with the sounds presented to date. Make up five sentences using these sounds for presentation to the group next week. Let us know how you get along.

Adult Lipreading Group   *Session 3*

---

1. Review of assignment from second session. Discussion of self-evaluation in terms of utilization of clues that help us understand in different kinds of

communication situations, such as environmental clues, gestures, facial clues, as well as being a good listener. How did you react to those difficult communication situations?

2. Presentation of sentences composed by clients using previously presented sounds.
3. Introduction of homophenous sound group /th/, both voiced and voiceless, as in that (voiced) and thimble (voiceless).
   Include description of how sounds appear visually.
   Key words, using these sounds, are presented to the clients and then used in related sentences.

th (voiced)	th (voiceless)
the	theater
bother	thunderstorm
gather	three
rather	month
weather	thermometer

   (a) A tour group gathered at the airport for a trip to New York.
   (b) The group had waited two months for the big day.
   (c) At three-thirty they boarded the airplane.
   (d) The weather was hot and dry on this day.
   (e) The thermometer outside the terminal read 93 degrees.
   (f) The air conditioning inside the plane felt rather good.
   (g) **After the passengers were airborne, the theater screen was lowered for a movie.**
   (h) The thunder storm on the outside didn't bother the passengers; the movie was too exciting.

4. Present materials which contrast the three homophenous sound groups: /p, b, m/, /f, v/, voiced and voiceless /th/.
5. Introduction of vowels: /a/ as in pat and /i/ as in pie. The /a/ is made by drawing the lips back and the opening between the lips is quite noticeable. The /i/ is made in much the same way as the /a/ with the lips slightly drawn back and the opening between the lips noticeable, but as the sound is made, the lips are drawn back in a more gliding motion. Examples of words with these sounds are: laugh, bath, cat, apple, ride, line, die, buy.
6. General discussion of the lipreading process: lipreading per se, listening, facial expressions, gestures, and environmental clues.
7. Presentation of general conversation sentences using a theme and key words without regard to specific sounds.
8. Assignment for next session: Practice the homophenous sound groups learned to date. Have a family member or friend help you. Are you getting more out of communication situations now since you have attended these few lipreading sessions? Make up a sentence for each of the sounds presented to you so far to present to the group next week.

1. Review of assignment from third session. How are you benefitting from the lipreading sessions so far? How do you see yourself as communicator in different sessions? How did you do in lipreading with a family member or friend?
2. Presentation of general conversational sentences using a theme and key words without regard to specific sounds.
3. Introduction of homophenous sound group /sh/ and /zh/ as in "beige." Include description of how sounds appear visually.
   Key words, using these sounds, are presented to the clients and then used in related sentences.

sh	zh
station	garage
shop	vision
windshield	casual

   (a) I took my car to the service station.
   (b) It needed to go through the auto wash.
   (c) The man at the garage noticed an oil leak under the car.
   (d) I guess he had better vision than me.
   (e) The man suggested leaving the car in the shop for a day.
   (f) He also noticed a crack in the windshield.
   (g) All of the repairs should cost about one hundred dollars.
   (h) I looked at him in a casual manner and said, "That's the way it goes."
4. Presentation of sentences composed by clients using previously presented sounds.
5. Present materials which contrast the three homophenous sound groups: /p, b, m/, /f, v/, voiced and voiceless /th/, and /sh, zh/.
6. Review of vowels: /o/ as in boat, /e/ as in meat, /a/ as in pat, and /i/ as in pie. Practice contrasting the four vowel sounds in isolation and proceed to sentences using these vowel sounds.
7. Remember the importance of maintaining good listener-speaker rapport. You must show sincere interest in what the speaker has to say. By explaining your hearing difficulty, you give the speaker something positive to deal with by showing that you are interested in what is said.
8. Assignment for next session: Pick any topic and make up three or four related sentences using those sounds discussed so far. Think about the environment in which you live and work. How do the setting itself, the people you are involved with, and other environmental factors aid or detract from your effectiveness as a communicator?

1. Review of assignment from fourth session. How do you see yourself, interacting with others in communication with the use of environmental factors? What kind of communication rapport do you establish with those who are not aware of your hearing loss?
2. Introduction of homophenous sound group /s/ and /z/. Include description of how sounds appear visually.
   Key words, using these sounds, are presented to the clients and then used in related sentences.

<u>s</u>	<u>z</u>
stamps	Arizona
postal	cards
scenes	zip
first class	relatives
post office	those

   (a) I would like to buy some post cards.
   (b) They will be sent to my relatives in Arizona.
   (c) First class is the best way to send the cards; they now go by air.
   (d) We'd better mail the gift package by parcel post.
   (e) On the way to the hotel, we will stop at the post office.
   (f) I'd better register the package.
   (g) Those new stamps are very attractive with the mountain scenes.
   (h) I need to look up the zip code in the postal directory.
3. Remember that the important consideration is to get the "idea" or "thought." It is not necessary to get every word in order to understand a communication.
4. Presentation of general conversational sentences using a theme and key words without regard to specific sounds.
5. Review of vowels and sounds through contrast of groups.
6. Presentation of sentences composed by clients using previously presented sounds.
7. Practice identifying words with the category given as a key word.
   Teams: New York Jets, Denver Broncos, Chicago Bears
   Equipment: football, catcher's mitt, homeplate, goalpost
   Baseball: home run, foul ball, umpire, shortstop
   Players: Joe Namath, Babe Ruth, Hank Aaron, Knute Rockne
   Places: playing field, tennis court, stadium, baseball diamond
   Positions: quarterback, goalie, center, catcher
   Games: baseball, hockey, basketball, soccer

8. Assignment for next session: Evaluate yourself in various types of listening situations. Are you a good listener? Do you think people speak clearly or mumble? What can you do when people don't speak clearly? Make up four or five sentences about your work or hobby.

Adult Lipreading Group   *Session 6*

1. Presentation of general conversational sentences using a theme and key words without regard to specific sounds.
2. Introduction of homophenous sound group /t, d, n/. Include description of how sounds appear visually.
   Key words, using these sounds, are presented to the clients and then used in related sentences.

t	d	n
television	daytime	night-time
today	dramas	news
contests	documentaries	children
cartoons	comedies	shown

   (a) Television today differs from its early days.
   (b) Today, television has functions other than entertainment.
   (c) News can be seen throughout the day.
   (d) Documentaries have become an important part of television.
   (e) Day-time television is mostly game shows and contests.
   (f) Night-time television has dramas, comedies, and sports.
   (g) Cartoons are shown on Saturday mornings for children.
3. Practice using the cues in the following situation. In a doctor's office, we may express the following emotions facially: sorrow, concern, anger, anticipation, and relief.
4. Presentation of sentences by clients about work or hobbies. Discussion of self-evaluation about listening. Did you encounter people who did not speak clearly during the past week? If so, how did you deal with the situation?
5. Practice contrasting sounds between the various homophenous groups: /p, b, m/, /f, v/, voiced and voiceless /th/, /sh, zh/, /s, z/, and /t, d, n/.
6. Practice contrasting vowels previously presented.
7. Presentation of short story or anecdote followed by questions. Story will be presented with voice and questions will be presented without voice.
8. Assignment for next session: Prepare three or four sentences about a certain television show to present to the group. See if the members of the group can guess what show it is. Be prepared to discuss the one most difficult communicative experience you encountered during the week. Explain what you did and what you could have done.

---

1. Presentation of short story or anecdote using background noise (such as speaker or cafeteria noise). Questions are also asked with background noise.
2. Discussion of any sound group causing particular difficulty to any individual member of the group.
3. Presentation of sentences by clients about television shows. Discussion of the most difficult communication situations encountered during the last week.
4. Presentation of general conversational sentences using a theme and key words without regard to specific sounds.
5. Introduction of new sound: /w/. Include description of how it appears visually. Key words, using these sounds, are presented to the clients and then used in related sentences.

<u>w</u>

winter	water
window	wood
weather	redwood
warm	walk
warning	worker

   (a) The new home will be finished by winter.
   (b) We ordered tinted windows to minimize the summer heat.
   (c) When the weather turns warm, the lawn will be planted.
   (d) The house will have a new fire warning system in it.
   (e) An underground sprinkler will make it easier to water the lawn.
   (f) The wood for the outside patio will be redwood.
   (g) The walk to the garden area is very pretty.
   (h) The construction workers are doing a fine job.
6. Practice contrasting sounds between the various homophenous groups: /p, b, m/, /f, v/, voiced and voiceless /th/, /sh, zh/, /s, z/, /t, d, n/, and /w/.
7. General communication practice: What people say at a service station.
   (a) Fill it up?
   (b) Regular, premium, or unleaded?
   (c) Check the oil?
   (d) Engine sounds fine.
   (e) Windshield washed?
   (f) Check your tire pressure?
8. Assignment for next week: What has the lipreading group meant to you? Do you feel that you are becoming a better communicator? Are there other things that you think should have been covered in this group?

---

1. Presentation of final homophenous sound group: /ch, j/. Include description of how the sounds appear visually.
   Key words, using these sounds, are presented to the clients and then used in related sentences.

<u>ch</u>	<u>j</u>
checked	jury
chamber	journalist
chief	charge
charted	judge

   (a) The jury has been selected for the trial.
   (b) Each member of the jury had to be checked carefully.
   (c) The journalists were there to cover the case.
   (d) The charge against the defendant was fraud.
   (e) At nine o'clock A.M., the judge entered the chambers.
   (f) He presented his charge to the people of the jury.
   (g) The local police chief was present to keep order.
   (h) The defense attorney charted his plan of action.
2. Practice contrasting sounds between the various homophenous groups: /p, b, m/, /f, v/, voiced and voiceless /th/, /sh, zh/, /t, d, n/, /w/, and /ch, j/.
3. Review of vowels by contrast and within sentences.
4. Presentation of general conversational sentences using a theme and key words.
5. Review of the lipreading process: lipreading per se, listening, facial expressions, gestures, and environmental clues.
6. Administration of lipreading tests as post-therapy measures:
   (a) Lipreading Screening Test (from Binnie, Montgomery and Jackson, 1976)
   (b) The Denver Quick Test of Lipreading
   (c) **The McCarthy-Alpiner Scale of Hearing Handicap.**
7. Discussion of what the lipreading group has meant to each member. Do you feel that you are a better communicator? What other things do you think should have been covered in this group?
8. Discussion of future options, such as enrollment in an Ongoing lipreading group.
9. Arrangement of individual appointments to discuss future audiological needs of clients.

5

The Remediation Process: Psychologic and Counselling Aspects

Margaret A. Wylde, Ph.D.

Sound is that countryside speeding by your car window you know you will never see again. It is an instantaneous event. Unlike a visual image, a sound cannot be studied or held for future reference. Part of the frustrations of being hard-of-hearing is knowing that what you just missed will never be heard.

Perhaps the stage can be set for this chapter if we try to recall some experiences that may be akin to those encountered by the hard of hearing. For those with normal hearing the ordeal may last but a moment; for those with the sensorineural hearing loss it is perpetual.

Does a hearing loss make someone feel the way you did when the winning play of a tied game was obliterated by the giant who leapt to his feet in front of you? Or is it like the way it felt to realize you have just missed the punch line of a joke and everyone else is laughing hysterically around you? Is it like the time of aggravation when you were trying to listen to a speaker (or hear the soundtrack in a movie or get lost in your favorite album) when someone created just enough noise to rob you of the pleasure of the activity?

A hearing loss can be emotionally and physically draining. Being unable to understand the conversations flowing around you can be annoying, aggravating and unnerving. Having to ask someone to repeat himself not

once or twice, but maybe three or four times and then still not understand what was said can be tantamount to open warfare between both parties. Responding to a simple question with a totally inappropriate answer is a frequent occurrence. The miscommunication leaves the hearing-impaired respondent shaken and unsure of himself because of the startled, skeptical look on the questioner's face.

The frustrations and uncertainties which accompany hearing loss are readily apparent. Many chapters and articles which address the psychologic implications of hearing loss state that the hearing-impaired population has emotional problems, withdraws from family and friends, no longer is allowed to make decisions, and probably should be receiving psychologic counselling. An alarming number of publications on this subject have been written, however, without the assistance of either empirical evidence or comparable study of a control group of normal-hearing individuals.

Hearing loss is not a picnic. Few hearing-impaired adults, however, would fit the common descriptions of their psychologic problems. None of us with normal hearing are tolerant of conditions that create a temporary loss of hearing (masking or decreased volume). If faced with such a situation we often display anger, immature emotions, and efforts to remedy it by eliminating the noise or increasing the volume. It is understandable that someone who experiences communicative failure on a regular basis would be unhappy with those circumstances and would seek to improve their communicative conditions. Their adaptive behaviors and feelings of frustration are normal.

To summarize, this chapter is not going to dramatize the problems of the hearing-impaired. Its purpose is 2-fold: first, to outline the psychologic ramifications of acquired hearing loss; second, to offer some suggestions for counselling the hard-of-hearing adult.

Terminology

The audiologist treading in the psychologic realm should use the jargon of that field as carefully as we would wish the psychologist to use the vernacular of our profession. Many authors of accounts of the psychology of the hearing-impaired have been psychiatrists or psychologists. Consequently, the initial use of terms such as despondency, depression, and introversion may have been appropriate descriptors of the individuals they studied. Generalized use of these terms is inappropriate. Using the same line of reasoning, we can argue that the psychiatric investigators used just one descriptor of auditory deficit. Commonly, all degrees, types, and configurations of hearing impairment were lumped into one category, *i.e.*, deaf or hearing-impaired, without studying the potential differences these variations could make in individual adjustment. A glossary of terminology of psychology and counselling has been provided in Appendix 5A.

PSYCHOLOGIC ASPECTS OF HEARING LOSS

Variables Affecting Reaction to Hearing Loss

Table 5.1 presents a partial listing of the variables which could influence an individual's reaction to loss of hearing sensitivity. Many of the initial investigations of the psychology of the hearing-impaired ignored (or at least did not report) the audiologic data for the subjects included in the study. Additionally, few of the other variables that may affect

one's ability to "cope" with hearing loss have been systematically investigated.

One would assume that the degree, type, configuration, and ability to understand speech would be primary ingredients in determining the reaction to hearing loss. Additionally, it seems logical that someone with a temporary loss would react differently than someone with a progressive and/or permanent loss. A fluctuating loss could promote a different outlook altogether.

Etiology and temporal characteristics of onset could cause yet a different reaction. Should we expect the same psychologic profile from the individual with a sudden idiopathic hearing loss as we would from the individual working in a noisy paper mill for the past 25 years?

In addition to the auditory components, to what degree does the individual's age, age at onset of loss, sex, race, religion, intelligence, education, occupation, and general health affect his perception of his hearing deficit? Do individuals with tinnitus and/or vestibular disorders experience greater psychologic trauma? To what extent does visual impairment, chronic illness, or other handicapping conditions influence adjustment?

The individual's compensatory abilities complicate the simple categorization of the hearing-impaired by auditory characteristics. Some use amplification, visual cues, and environmental manipulation tactics more effectively than others. Some live in environments with relatives and friends cognizant of their communicative difficulties and the strategies useful for improving communication. Of course there are those who experience communication failure to a more extreme degree, and with greater frequency and duration than others.

Finally, the methods used in measuring psychologic reaction will be determinants of the difficulties observed. We may study the effects of hearing loss on personality, social competence, fears and/or adjustment. The instrument used may be casual observation, self report scales, or standardized tests. We may assess the individual with the hearing impairment or the people who must communicate with them. It has been said that a hearing loss is more of a handicap to the speaker than to the listener.

There are innumerable interactive vari-

Table 5.1
Variables Affecting Reaction to Hearing Loss

Auditory	Personal	Communicative Disturbance	Compensatory Abilities
A. Degree	A. Age	A. Degree	A. Use of amplification
1. Mild	B. Sex	B. Duration	B. Use of visual cues
2. Moderate	C. Race	C. Frequency	C. Willingness/ability to ask for help
3. Severe	D. Intelligence		D. Environmental manipulation skills
4. Profound	E. Education		
B. Type	F. Occupation	**Interpersonal Support**	**Methods of Measuring Reaction**
1. Conductive	G. Socio-economic status	A. Family	A. Instrument used
2. Mixed	H. Health	B. Friends	1. Observation
3. Sensorineural	1. Tinnitus	C. Business/work associates	2. Self-report scales
4. Central	2. Vestibular disorder		3. Standardized test
C. Configuration	3. Visual acuity		B. Reactions studied
1. Degree of slope	4. Illness		1. Personality
2. Unilateral vs bilateral	5. Other physical problems		2. Social competence
3. Symmetry			3. Fears
D. Speech Perception			4. Adjustment
E. Recruitment/loudness discomfort			C. Respondents
F. Etiology			1. Hearing-impaired person
G. Permanency			2. Spouse, significant other
1. Temporary			
2. Fluctuating			
3. Progressive			
4. Permanent			
H. Temporal factors			
1. Duration of loss			
2. Rate of onset			

ables determining the effect loss of hearing has on people. This chapter will be limited in scope in that all of the remarks provided will be about the adult whose hearing loss has occurred after he acquired normal communicative skills. None of the comments in this chapter will be about the deaf adult.

What We Know

"A cardinal tenet in the orientation of hearing health rehabilitators is that the person who is hearing-impaired is also psychologically impaired" (Rosenthal, 1975). Rosenthal is a hearing-impaired adult, author of *The Hearing Loss Handbook* (1975), who vehemently complains about audiologists ascribing negative characteristics to the individuals they serve. He cited several audiology textbooks that attribute to the hard-of-hearing psychologic difficulties such as despondency, sense of inferiority, maladjustment, introversion, hopelessness, fear, suspicion, apathy, and listlessness, to name a few.

Table 5.2, from Rosen (1979), summarizes the experimental variables of most of the studies of psychologic reactions of the adult with a hearing loss. Of the 7 investigations reported in this table, 4 explored the reactions of male war veterans, 2 investigated the feelings of members of a hard-of-hearing society, and 1 looked at veterans with functional hearing loss. Of the 6 investigations of individuals with organic hearing impairment, only one (Welles, 1932), employed a control group of normal-hearing subjects. Five of the investigations did not determine the characteristics of the hearing loss (degree, type, configuration, etiology, onset, etc.) or at least they were not reported.

Many of the investigations in Table 5.2 are frequently cited as evidence of psychologic difficulties of the hearing-impaired. Barker *et al.* (1956) discussing the results of Welles (1932) and Pintner (1933) (both investigators employed the Bernreuter Inventory to obtain their psychologic information), reported that the general conclusions reached by these investigators was that "persons with impaired hearing tend to be more neurotic, introverted, and submissive than persons with normal hearing, but that the large overlap between the groups is more significant than the differences." Concern with the results of these investigations have been expressed because

the Bernreuter Inventory may not be an appropriate instrument for the hearing-impaired since several questions assume the ability to communicate without difficulty.

Knapp (1948) completed psychologic interviews of 4000 male war veterans at Deshon Army Hospital. Of the 4000 patients, 3.7% had a hearing loss with no psychiatric disease or with psychiatric disease unrelated to hearing loss, 5.5% had a neurotic reaction to physiologic hearing loss, 2.8% had a psychogenic increase of hearing deficit, and 5.7% had psychogenic hearing loss.

The first and second groups of patients that Knapp interviewed are of interest. The first group apparently had some degree of hearing impairment without any psychiatric disorder occurring as a result. The second group of patients described in Knapp's report are those whom he determined through psychiatric interviews had a neurotic reaction to physiologic hearing loss. Their comments in the interview sessions and Knapp's study of their social history led him to the conclusion, "The population of this study showed no one "psychology of deafness," but the psychology of many individuals defending themselves against a sensory handicap which led primarily to difficulty in communication."

The finding of "neurotic reaction" in Knapp's study cannot be generalized to any other population because his subjects were hospitalized male war veterans, his audiometric and otologic data imprecise, his research merely a categorization of elicited comments and histories from the veterans, and his final conclusion a statement that one cannot categorize the hearing-impaired into a psychologic pattern.

Myklebust (1964) administered the Minnesota Multiphasic Personality Test to 44 males and 53 females who were in attendance at a hearing society. The individuals belonging to such a society may not be representative of the adult hard-of-hearing population as a whole. The mean hearing loss of the members was severe (68 dB for males, 66 dB for females). The mean age of the males was 39.37 years and the mean age of the females was 49.66 years, yet 57% of the males and 47% of the females had never been married. Almost 50% of the males and 25% of the females continued to live with their parents. These characteristics suggest that this group

Table 5.2
Summary of Studies of the Psychology of Hearing Impairment in Adults[a]

Author and Date	Subjects	Source	Controls	Audiological Information	Psychological/Psychiatric Information
Welles, 1932	225, both sexes; 87% female	Hard-of-Hearing Society	148 friends of subjects; 89% female	None	Bernreuter Inventory; questionnaire
Ramsdell, 1947	Male war veterans	Deshon Army Hospital	None	None	Personal analysis based on observation and experience
Ingalls, 1946	1100 male war veterans	Bordon Army Hospital	None	None	None specified; 31.47% reported to have nervous or mental illness
Knapp, 1948	4000 male war veterans	Deshon Army Hospital	None	"Majority 30–50 dB"	Psychiatric interviews
Myklebust, 1964	44 male 83 female	Hard-of-Hearing Society	None	Mean loss; males, 68 dB females, 66 dB	MMPI; questionnaire; self-report
Nett, 1960	252 male 126 female	Clinic referrals	None	Pure tone and speech audiometry	MMPI; WASI; direct interview
Chaiklin and Ventry, 1965	64 veterans with functional hearing loss	Veterans Hospital	36 veterans with organic hearing loss	Full audiological evaluation	Psychiatric and psychological evaluation; ENT, neurology and physical examination

[a] Reprinted by permission from Rosen, J. K., Psychological aspects of the evaluation of acquired hearing impairment. *Audiology* **18**, 249 (1979).

may be more representative of a minority group of hard-of-hearing adults who may have attended the hearing society for companionship as well as assistance in communication. Myklebust (1964) did identify some deviation in personality characteristics from the "normal." The performance of this one small group, however, should not be used to draw conclusions about the effects of hearing loss on personality.

Nett (1960) compiled the most comprehensive audiologic and psychologic data for his 378 subjects. One of his major conclusions was that the kind of handicap reported by the hard-of-hearing is a function of associations between the hard-of-hearing individual and the persons in different role relationships to him, the size and function of the group, and the frequency of auditory (communication) failure. In essence, he said it is not hearing loss alone that determines the extent of the concomitant problem.

When looking at all of the psychologic studies completed in the 33 years between 1932 and 1965 one could believe that hearing loss will cause "people who suffer from it to develop certain characteristic emotional reactions including: depression, unreasonable suspicion, undefined fears and withdrawal from social contacts" (Helleberg, 1979). These generalizations attributed to the hard-of-hearing population have been *derived* from observations of hospitalized World War II veterans and members of hard-of-hearing societies. Few of the variables listed in Table 5.1 have been systematically explored or controlled, particularly those describing the hearing deficit.

A recent investigation (Frankel, 1981) has attempted a more orderly assessment of the handicap experienced by the population with adult-onset hearing loss who are still within the work force and have not yet attained senior citizen status. She assessed the adaptation of her adult subjects in "terms of their educational and occupational attainments, personal characteristics, interpersonal relationships, communication patterns, social interactions, perceived hearing handicaps and hearing loss patterns." Frankel (1981) found that "the relationship between experienced handicap and actual hearing impairment was not as strong as had been suggested by the literature" for the 421 adult participants in her survey.

Frankel (1981) has provided us with a realistic view of a cross-section of the hard-of-hearing population. Her subjects, who were between the ages of 18 years and 50 years (mean 39.8 years), were selected from audiology clinics at three teaching hospitals in London, Canada. Although the average hearing-related characteristics of her subject group appeared to be representative of a population with fairly good hearing, her sample did include participants with significant hearing impairment. "The better ear pure tone averages ranged from 0 to 87 dB, with a mean of 17.1 dB. For the poorer ear, the range was 2 dB to 88 dB, with a mean of 34.3 dB." Her sample was comprised of individuals with both conductive and sensorineural and temporary, permanent, and fluctuating hearing loss. These variables were apparently not taken into consideration in the analyses of the data.

The importance of Frankel's work is that it demonstrated "understanding adjustment to hearing impairment requires consideration of all classes of variables—sociodemographic, hearing-related, social, and psychological." She found that psychologic and social variables were more strongly related to measures of adjustment than to the actual severity of impairment.

What we know about the psychologic implications of hearing impairment is that we don't know. The review of the research conducted since 1932 has suggested there are more similarities (overlap) between the normal and the hearing-impaired groups than there are differences. The reports of the psychologic reactions of hard-of-hearing individuals should not be casually discarded, but they should be viewed with the knowledge that their reactions may not be solely a result of their hearing loss.

What We Think

Apparently we think that there is more to a hearing loss than just the inability to hear and that the audiologist should provide more than just technical assistance to the hearing-impaired. We, at least in the literature, have begun to increase the attention paid to the rehabilitative needs of our hearing-impaired clients.

The research literature does not support a specific psychology of the hearing-impaired, yet at times we see clients who do not appear to be appropriately adjusting to and/or compensating for their hearing loss. Their reaction to their communicative difficulties seems to be getting in the way of improving their ability to communicate.

Frankel (1981) found that almost two-thirds (270) of the 421 hearing-impaired respondents wanted to talk to someone about their hearing loss. They cited reasons such as the following.

Trouble at home	49.3%
Trouble at work	42.6
Wanting information	74.1
Wanting hearing aid information	19.6
Wanting lipreading information	4.8
Interpersonal problems related to hearing loss	31.9

Many hearing-impaired patients express thoughts and feelings that suggest they would like to talk to someone about the way they feel. Some of these comments follow.

That others do not understand what it is like to have a hearing loss.

That the hearing loss makes them nervous.

That they do not wish to wear a hearing aid.

That they do not wish to wear a hearing aid under any circumstances, ever.

That they do not like to go places (functions) where they will be unable to hear because of the noise.

That hearing individuals are inconsiderate toward the hearing-impaired.

That they feel left out.

That they think others consider them retarded (slow, dim-witted, senile) when they respond inappropriately to something said.

That they can hear fine, people just don't enunciate anymore.

That they can hear better than Mrs. Jones up the street.

That the noises in their head make them nervous (are annoying, distracting).

That their friend just had surgery and can hear normally now and won't this work for them too.

That they were going to go to this specialist they heard about.

That they had a hearing aid before (or a friend or relative did) and it didn't do them any good.

That even though mother, three uncles, and two sisters have a hearing loss that began about the same age, they don't think their hearing loss was inherited.

Many of the comments just listed suggest that those uttering them (or something similar) may be trying to deny the existence of the hearing loss, reduce the severity of it and/or appear as if they had normal hearing. These attitudes towards their hearing impairment may be the result of the attitude of our society toward the handicapped.

Societal Attitudes

Wright (1960) describes this attitude as "You are (or I am) less good, less worthy because of the disability. It is something to be hidden or made up for." When we see an individual with a handicap, we usually don't see the person first and the handicap second. We see the handicap first and expect certain behaviors because of it. The adult with a hearing loss may find it difficult to accept the loss because of the attitudes he has held towards others whom he knows with hearing difficulties or whom he has seen wearing hearing aids.

Throughout history, the hearing-impaired have been discriminated against. How many reading this chapter would employ the individual wearing two ear-level hearing aids? How many would have dated (and/or married) the classmate in high school or college with the hearing aid? How often have you been surprised by the severely hearing-impaired adult who functions quite well in a busy work and social environment, who is matter of fact about the hearing loss and hearing aids, and who just didn't fit your expectations of the way one should react to the hearing loss?

Wright (1960) suggests that the handicapped feel the need to behave "as if" they are normal for a variety of reasons. First, they are reluctant to be identified as one of a population (minority group) that is discriminated against in employment and marital opportunities. Many among the "normal population" are disturbed when a handicapped individual performs tasks that are considered to be outside his capabilities. The handicapped are expected to "know and keep their place" (Wright, 1960).

The hard-of-hearing have had several characteristics attributed to them, a group stereotype. Probably one of the more common is that they are "suspicious" of others when they cannot hear what is being said. They are considered suspicious when they merely may be wondering what was said. They are "compensating" when perhaps they were merely interested, and they are "feeling inferior" when maybe they are just realizing their own limitations (Wright, 1960).

We expect the hearing-impaired to be troubled by their hearing loss. Many (perhaps most) are not. We proliferate this misconception by making general statements similar to the following. "Even though there is no such thing as a typical hard-of-hearing personality, the nature of hearing loss is such that people who suffer from it do tend to develop certain characteristic emotional reactions, including: depression, unreasonable suspicion, undefined fears, and withdrawal from social contacts" (Helleberg, 1979).

Those of us with normal hearing may never understand what it is like to have a hearing loss. We may overreact to the hearing-impaired because of this lack of understanding and because frequently the hearing loss is a greater problem for the speaker than the listener.

What we should think of the psychology of the hard-of-hearing adult, then, is the following. Each hearing-impaired adult is an individual with different communicative demands and strategies of compensating and adjusting to them. Each person brings to us a different developmental, social, psychologic, and oto-audiologic profile and if we are to be of service to the hard-of-hearing adult we will not develop a certain set of expectations about his emotional make-up and psychologic needs. We should develop our skills in listening to the hard-of-hearing adult and learn to provide the supportive services he wants from us.

What We Do Not Know—What We Need To Know

We do not know if there is a certain psychologic reaction (or complex of reactions) that occurs as a result of adult-onset loss of hearing sensitivity. Returning to Table 5.1, we realize that we really do not know how any of these variables affect adjustment to or acceptance of loss of hearing sensitivity.

What we need to know then, or better yet, what must be done if we are going to find out

what we need to know is to conduct systematic, tightly controlled investigations on both hearing-impaired and normal-hearing adults. Audiometric data, otologic, and aural rehabilitation history should be reported and should be representative of the adult hard-of-hearing population. The control group should be matched with the hearing-impaired group on all variables including age, gender, occupation, socioeconomic status, etc. Ideally, psychologic data could be obtained on individuals prior to their loss of hearing and at various intervals thereafter.

COUNSELLING THE HARD-OF-HEARING ADULT

Aural rehabilitation is an outgrowth of our desire to be helpful to people. It is satisfying when you have helped someone. It is disconcerting and uncomfortable when you realize you have failed to help someone. Frequently, our standard audiologic procedures (hearing evaluation, hearing aid evaluation, hearing aid fitting) do not produce the results we had hoped for. We have recognized that our technical methods of assistance sometimes fall short of the mark, not necessarily because they were inadequate, but because the individual was not ready for them.

The first section of this chapter did not necessarily demonstrate a need for providing counselling assistance to the hard-of-hearing adult. This portion will demonstrate the need for counselling. The following parts will address the realm of counselling, the role of the audiologist as counsellor, tools and techniques of counselling, and suggestions as to when referral to a clinical psychologist, licensed psychologist, and/or psychiatrist is appropriate.

Need for Counselling

The word "counselling" conjures up several thoughts, some positive and some negative. We have traditionally thought of counselling as the sole function of the psychologist or psychiatrist and we may think that we are trespassing into their professional territory if we adopt the role of counsellor. We may rationalize against the idea of audiologists providing counselling with the following thoughts.

First, the client came for a hearing test, not to be psychoanalyzed.

Second, few professionals in our field have received formal training in counselling.

Third, the time spent in counselling the client could be spent more profitably since we customarily do not charge by the hour but by the service (hearing evaluation, hearing aid evaluation, etc.).

If we accept these ideas, then it is apparent that there is no need for the remainder of this chapter. Not quite.

Whenever we give advice or a judgment to direct the opinion or conduct of another individual, we are counselling. Each time we recommend to a client that he seek additional evaluation, medical services, a hearing aid, or rehabilitation services, we are counselling.

The hard-of-hearing adult frequently requires additional information; confirmation of a thought, belief, or attitude; and the opportunity to discuss something bothering him. Any of these activities we engage in with him can be referred to as counselling.

Many clients (66%) attending audiology clinics in London, Ontario, stated they wanted to talk to someone about a variety of concerns related to their loss (Frankel, 1981). Brooks (1979) found that the experimental subjects who received pre- and post-hearing aid fitting counselling wore their hearing aids significantly longer, were more adept in handling their hearing aids, and had a greater reduction in social hearing handicap than the non-counselled, matched, control group of hearing aid recipients.

It is apparent the desire and need for counselling exists among the individuals we serve.

Role of Audiologists as Counsellors

No need to rush out and buy a new degree or boards and paint for a new shingle. It's all right to counsel (be helpful) without a degree in clinical psychology or psychiatry. We must recognize when the counselling we are providing is within our realm of expertise and when we should refer our clients to another agency. Some suggestions of when, how, and where to refer will appear later in this chapter.

Audiologists, because of their information on hearing, hearing loss, and the communicative dysfunction it creates, and of aural rehabilitation methods are the appropriate specialists to provide helpful consultation to the hard-of-hearing adult. The audiologist is appropriate as long as the hearing impair-

ment is the primary caustic agent in the difficulties experienced.

Many will argue that the audiologist is trained in technical skills and consequently would be inept in the counsellor's role. This "button-pusher" citation is rather archaic in light of the increased emphasis placed on aural rehabilitation in the training programs, literature, and field. Additionally, members of the traditional counselling profession advocate the use of lay counsellors in the mental health field (Carkhuff, 1968; Carkhuff and Truax, 1965; and Rioch, 1966). They cite a shortage of professionals available to counsel and the demonstrated effectiveness of lay counsellors (such as ward attendants, community volunteers, and college students) as two primary reasons why lay counsellors should be trained and put to work.

THEORIES, TOOLS, AND TECHNIQUES OF COUNSELLING

Theories

A Psychiatric Glossary, Fifth Edition, produced by the American Psychiatric Association (Werner *et al.*, 1980) lists more than 30 schools of psychiatry. The schools are divided into two groups: (1) reconstructive, (2) re-educative and supportive. Some of the theories among the schools considered reconstructive are Psychoanalysis (Sigmund Freud), Analytical Psychology (Carl Jung), Cognitive (Jean Piaget), and Transactional Analysis (Eric Berne). The re-educative and supportive schools include Client-centered (Carl Rogers), Behaviorism (John B. Watson), Operant Conditioning (B. F. Skinner), and Psychobiology (Adolf Meyer), among others.

The purpose of this chapter is not to discuss all of the garden varieties of counselling, nor is it to discuss counselling in general. The intent is to offer the reader some guidelines in developing his own theory of counselling hearing-impaired adults and their families. Although it is not absolutely necessary that one adopt or form a theory of counselling, having a rationale for what you call counselling should help you decide when and what type of counselling is necessary, when your counselling has been effective, and when you need to revise your counselling procedures.

The guidelines offered by this author have as their origin the theory of counselling attributed to Carl Rogers (1961, 1951) often referred to as client-centered, non-directive, and/or the human potential philosophy. Additionally, the words and works of Luterman (1979, 1976), Brammer (1973), Chermak (1979), and Wright (1960) have shaped the philosophy and approach used by this author when counselling hearing-impaired adults.

The basic theory underlying this chapter, then, is first that human beings are inherently motivated to grow, improve their existence, and to realize their maximum potential. They may meet stumbling blocks in their growing process as a direct result of their hearing impairment; their fears, emotions, and misconceptions about it and their inability to find solutions by themselves. Provided with appropriate information and an atmosphere of trust and acceptance, the hearing-impaired adult will determine the course of action best suited for him.

Tools of Counselling

There are four basic tools of counselling: information, assessment scales and indices, the environment, and the counsellor.

Information—Information can be divided into two categories: content and affect. Information is available to the patient in a variety of ways: talking, demonstration, written literature, movies, videotapes, and any other media form. Content information assists the client in understanding the specifics about his hearing loss, the rehabilitation process, hearing aids, etc. Effect information looks at the feelings associated with a hearing loss. Appendix 5B presents a list of sources for informational brochures and/or media packages that are written for the hearing-impaired adult.

Dreher and Baltes (1973) recommended bibliotherapy as a supplement to counselling. Books and pamphlets can be used both for informative reading (aimed at the intellect) and emotional release. Biography and fiction may provide empathy and catharsis. Reading of someone else's problems and reactions to them, finding that someone else has had the thoughts and feelings you have had, and seeing the communication disorder from another's perspective can be of significant benefit. Individuals reluctant to discuss the way they feel may find the assistance they need in the pages of a book.

Assessment Scales—The counsellor may use different approaches to obtain information about the client's reaction to his hearing loss and the effect it has had on his social and emotional well-being. One method is through the use of self-assessment scales. Chapter 2 contains a discussion of several of these scales. The reader is referred to that chapter for a more thorough discussion of their use.

Questions such as "Do you ever get the feeling of being cut off from things because of difficulty hearing?" and "Does this feeling upset you at all?" from the Hearing Measurement Scale (Noble and Atherly, 1979) pry the emotional door open for discussion. Similarly, scaled items from the Denver Scale of Communication Function (Alpiner *et al.*, 1971) such as: "People sometimes avoid me because of my hearing loss"; "Other people do not realize how frustrated I get when I cannot hear or understand," and "I tend to be negative about life in general because of my hearing loss" provide the clinician with the patient's rating of his emotional status. This information can be used to begin discussion on the issues the client expresses the greatest concern about.

Environment—Counselling can be effective in a variety of environments. It is not so much that the environment is a tool in the counselling process, but that the environment can completely preclude counselling from beginning.

Counselling a hearing-impaired client and his normal-hearing family can lead to logistical problems. Counselling is stilted and disjointed if the client cannot understand what is being said or if the client automatically turns to the spouse for an interpretation after each comment by the counsellor.

The clinician should instruct the counselling participants where to sit and should take the opportunity to explain why this seating arrangement was chosen. Fig. 5.1 shows four seating arrangements for counselling sessions. The first, referred to as the Ping Pong (*A*) placement, puts the patient between the clinician and the spouse. If the client is dependent on visual clues then this arrangement will keep his head turning back and forth between clinician and spouse. It has the advantage that the client will always be able to see the speaker's mouth so long as he is quick enough to turn his head.

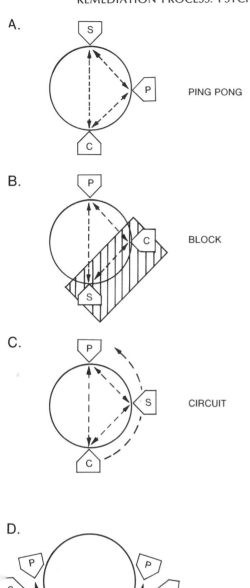

A. PING PONG

B. BLOCK

C. CIRCUIT

D. COMMUNICATION

Figure 5.1. Seating arrangement influence on communication. C, clinician or counselor; P, patient or client (hearing-impaired); S, spouse or significant other.

In setting *B*, the patient's view of the clinician's mouth is blocked every time the clinician turns to say something to the spouse. It is a natural seating arrangement for the clinician to sit between the client and his

spouse, but it will also cut the patient out of the flow of the discussion.

The third seating arrangement (*C*), with the spouse seated closest to the clinician enhances the chance of the counselling session turning into a session of talking about the hearing-impaired individual or of having the spouse act as an interpreter for the counsellor's comments. It puts distance between the patient and clinician which may lead the patient to the well-worn phrase, "Wha'd she say?" This set-up blocks the view of the spouse's face when speaking to the clinician.

The primary consideration should be on having the client situated so that it will be easy for him to communicate with both spouse and clinician (*D*). In this arrangement the spouse sits on the patient's "good ear" or "aided ear" side. The patient is always able to see both the clinician's and spouse's face. The distance between speaker and listener is reduced.

This may have seemed to be a rather lengthy discussion of where to sit, but too frequently we ignore this simple adjustment which will facilitate communication. In addition to the seating arrangement, the clinician should ensure that the patient is not looking into a light source (glare) to try and see the clinician's face, and that any extraneous noise (room air conditioners for example) is eliminated. If more than one hearing-impaired person is present and/or if there are more hearing relatives and friends present, then the clinician will need to think through the seating plan again.

The environment should be as free of distractions as possible. This includes both physical and psychologic distractions. If the parent of a young child is concerned about what the child is getting into while you are trying to talk with them, they will be unable to attend to the conversation. Some patients are reluctant to discuss their feelings about their hearing loss because they often involve the spouse and/or other relatives. The clinician should be sensitive to the effects of others on the hearing-impaired client and should escort the distractors to the waiting room or schedule the counselling session for another day.

Counsellor—The counsellor is the primary tool in the helping relationship. What are the traits that make up a good counsellor? Who will make a good counsellor? How do we know if we possess the qualities to provide good counselling?

There are no specific set of traits that we can study and assimilate to become expert counsellors. Each of us will provide our clients with a different counselling experience, just as each client will provide us with different experiences. Most texts suggest, however, that to be a people helper we must first begin with ourselves. We must decide what our values are, what we believe in, what our expectations are for ourselves and for humanity, how we perceive others to learn, why we want to help others, and why they might seek our help. Of the many questions we need to ask ourselves and discover an answer for, the one that asks us why we want to help others is probably the most important.

The helping relationship should develop so that the client is gaining increased independence from the clinician. We may begin by providing our clients with a large amount of information and opinions about what course of action would be best for them, but if we have provided them with the appropriate form of help they will soon no longer need us for information or assistance in decision-making.

Motivation to help people so that we will feel needed, or so that we will be important in the eyes of others will lead us to put our needs before theirs. No one is purely altruistic. We each have some motivating reason for providing assistance, and we should each realize that when we help we are helping ourselves. I will unashamedly admit that some of the finest times of my life have been when I realized that I helped someone. When you realize that you have made a difference in someone's life you feel good all over.

There are three qualities or conditions considered to be the core dimensions of helping (Wallston and Weitz, 1975; Rogers, 1961 and 1951). The first is accurate empathy. This term refers to the counsellor's ability to be able to understand the patient's emotions, to experience the emotion with him, to feel the way he does. Accurate empathy means the clinician is aware of the client's feelings, understands why the client feels that way and responds to these emotions appropriately. The skill underlying accurate empathy is listening. Several statements often made by hearing-impaired clients were listed earlier in

this chapter. Each of these statements and their many variations may be responded to on either the content or affective level—our response will depend on our accuracy of empathy. For example:

Client: I had a hearing aid 5 years ago. It made me so nervous I just threw it away.

Content response: Hearing aid technology has really improved in the last 5 years. We can adjust your new hearing aid so that it will fit your hearing loss to a "T."

Empathetic response: Many patients feel the way you do. How did you feel when the hearing aid made you nervous? What made you nervous?

or: You must have been pretty frustrated to have thrown away such an expensive item. I'm sorry it didn't help you. How did it make you nervous?

The second core dimension of helping is unconditional positive regard. This attribute means you believe in the inherent worth and value of your client. You will accept your client as he is regardless of his attitude toward you or his willingness to accept your recommendations.

Frequently, we work with clients who have decided that there is nothing wrong with their hearing, they do not have any trouble communicating and all this talk of hearing aids is a bunch of rubbish. We can adopt two different attitudes when working with these people. The first can be crudely summarized by saying that they are ignorant fools—let them live with their own misery. The second is that each person knows what is best for himself. We can present the options available to the client, provide support to the client regardless of the decision he makes and believe in his ability to do what's right for himself.

If it is difficult to envision investing time (under the assumption time is money) in someone who is unlikely to purchase your product or service, try considering this time as an investment in the future. The very person you felt was a lost customer becaue you didn't sell him a hearing aid or because you didn't enroll him in your aural rehabilitation class, may be your best advertisement because he believes you are interested in what's best for him and because he feels you will not push him into anything he doesn't want. What may seem to have been lost revenue initially may benefit your coffers many times over.

The third dimension of counselling is genuineness, self-congruence. The client must believe he is in an atmosphere of trust, where his thoughts and feelings will be respected. We cannot present the client with confusing signals (our mouths saying one thing and our attitude another), nor can we play games with his emotions. Should the client perceive incongruence (intentional or not), your effectiveness as a counsellor will be diminished. The client will play his own game, and in essence use you until he has gotten the benefits he expected or wanted from your service. He is the primary initiator and terminator of the counselling services and will simply not show up if displeased or convinced he is not receiving benefit.

The role of counsellor is one that we must continually review. We must judge our effectiveness against our theory of helping and determine if we have benefitted our patient in accordance with it. If we believe our effectiveness as a counsellor was diminished because of a problem in relating to a specific client then we must bolster our counselling skills.

Luterman (1976) listed five conditions that must be present if both helper and helpee are to grow and benefit from their relationship. He stated that counselling proceeds best when:

1. We understand what constitutes the helping relationship.
2. We learn to listen.
3. We trust the wisdom within the individual.
4. We cease being judgmental.
5. We are real.

Of these five conditions, I find that I must continually remind myself to listen to what the patient says. Frequently, I will be well into my dissertation on the numbers of people who first experience nervousness while wearing hearing aids and how you can break into wearing the hearing aids, etc., etc., etc., when I realize that perhaps the client wanted to talk about his nervousness to have someone understand how he felt. The second area in which I have had the greatest difficulty matching my practice with my philosophy is in always accepting the client's decision about what is right for himself with regard to a hearing aid. I have finally been able to accept the feelings of those who do not even want to try a hearing aid and no longer feel as if I had failed if I cannot compel the client to at least try a hearing aid. When and if the client is ready, he will present himself to try the hearing aid.

We may be unable to subjectively determine if we have the qualities that make a good counsellor. Wallston and Weitz (1975) did not find a significant correlation between self-report scales on the core dimensions of helping and actual assessment of counselling skills through behavioral assessment. They found that people who obtained high scores on self-assessment scales of empathy, acceptance of others, and genuineness were not necessarily the ones who conveyed these attributes during video-taped observations of their counselling performance.

Our best assessment of utility as a counselling tool will be the growth of our clients and of ourselves. Brammer (1973) devotes a significant portion of his book to learning specific skills of counselling. It is not in the scope of this chapter to try and duplicate the excellent work he has completed. The reader is referred to his text to learn additional, specific skills to enhance his counselling effectiveness and efficiency.

Techniques of Counselling

The counselling relationship should be allowed to develop naturally as we work with our hearing-impaired clients and families. We should not attempt to plug them into a program for counselling just because it is the only means by which we are comfortable providing them with "counselling." Yet, if we have a basic understanding of how we expect the counselling to progress and if we have developed certain counselling skills, we can facilitate our client's growth, use our time efficiently, and provide ourselves the opportunity for self-evaluation of our counselling skills.

The balance of this section is an adaptation of parts of the book *The Helping Relationship: Process and Skills* by Lawrence Brammer (1973). Brammer's book is written primarily to assist the individual developing skills devoted primarily for psychologic counselling. I have attempted to couch his ideas into the framework that we as audiologists are not providing assistance to those whose primary problems are psychologic, but that we are providing help to individuals who are experiencing problems because of their hearing impairment. I also have attempted to mold his ideas so that they will be usable for the audiologist wishing to provide his client with content assistance, *i.e.* the acclimation of a hearing aid; with training assistance, *i.e.* in the development of new skills as a result of communication training and in emotional support in the realm of adjusting to the limitations of a hearing impairment and developing a positive attitude towards the requirements for remediation.

Fig. 5.2, also adapted from Brammer (1973, p. 48) depicts the helping relationship. At first glance, it is apparent the only difference between the helper and helpee is that the helper happens to have expertise, if you will, that the client does not. The client has a problem (hearing impairment) for which the audiologist possesses a variety of remediation skills. The importance of this figure is that it should remind the audiologist that there is very little difference between himself and the patients. On many occasions we will find that we are

the helpee and another the helper. We must base our every action in the manner that we would have it done unto us.

Audiologists sometimes have difficulty realizing how much of their time is actually spent in counselling clients and thus possibly believe that attention paid in developing these skills would be better spent in other areas of training. If we define counselling as providing help so that the hearing-impaired adult can determine the course of action best suited for himself, then we see that all of the items listed in Table 5.3 fall within this domain.

There are three levels or realms of counselling that audiologists provide. These are informational, rational acceptance or adjustment, and emotional acceptance or adjustment. The three realms are inextricably intertwined, yet frequently we will interact with a client totally within one level. With some clients we will only provide counselling at the informational level, with others perhaps only the emotional, and with many (I hope) we will progress through all three.

Eight stages of the helping relationship are

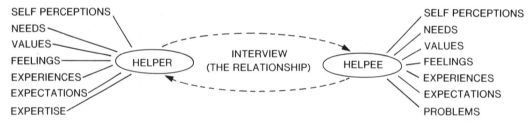

Figure 5.2. The helping relationship. Reprinted by permission from Brammer, L., *The Helping Relationship: Process and Skills,* Englewood Cliffs, NJ: Prentice-Hall, Inc. (1973).

Table 5.3
Counselling Responsibilities of Audiologists

Informational	Rational Acceptance/Adjustment	Emotional Acceptance/Adjustment
Hearing loss	Hearing loss	Effect of hearing loss on self
Description	Permanency of	Feelings
Comparison with normal	Need for treatment	Attitude
Cause	Need for additional testing	Image
Anatomy/function of ear	Need for hearing aid(s)	Ability to communicate
Availability of medical assistance	Need to conserve residual hearing	Ability to work
Hearing aids	Aural Rehabilitation	Effect of hearing loss on relationships
Costs	Need to learn new communication skills	Family
Where to purchase		Friends
Advantages/disadvantages	Need to improve communication habits	Associates
Care/use/function	Family	
Availability of other technical devices	Friends	
Availability of other services	Work place	

Table 5.4
Eight States of the Helping Relationship

Stage	Goals
Entry	1. Open the avenue for assistance from the audiologist. 2. Lay the groundwork for trust. 3. Enable the patient to define his problems related to his hearing impairment.
Clarification	1. Define the client's specific problems as related to his hearing impairment. 2. Get a better feel for how the client sees his hearing impairment and its effect on his general life situation.
Structure	1. Determine if the audiologist has the skills necessary to meet the client's needs. 2. Identification of the agency and the type of help offered, the qualifications and limitations of the audiologist. 3. Acknowledgement of the time to be involved, any fees to be charged and any restrictions to be imposed.
Relationship	A turning point in the process. The client and audiologist either continue to build the relationship through mutual agreement or the relationship is terminated by either party.
Exploration	1. The strategies for intervention are outlined. 2. The client's feelings are explored. 3. The alternatives of action are outlined.
Consolidation	1. The client will decide on a course of action. 2. The client's feelings are clarified. 3. The client will practice new skills.
Planning	1. Plans for termination and continuing alone are formulated. 2. Plans for referral are completed (agencies are contacted, applications completed).
Termination	1. Accomplishments are summarized. 2. The helping relationship is ended through: a. Termination. b. Referral. c. The promise of follow-up. d. The offer of "stand-by" help.

presented in Table 5.4. These stages, as outlined by Brammer (1973) have been applied to the hearing-impaired adult client. The first stage, entitled "Entry," is our first step with a client. The manner in which this stage is begun will be dependent on the level (or realm) of counselling the client desires. This step would normally occur after we have discovered that the client has a hearing impairment. This could be when we have heard from the client that he suspects he has a hearing impairment or at the conclusion of a hearing evaluation. We begin the counselling process by outlining some of the possibilities of assistance for this individual.

The client's trust is gained by answering his questions honestly and without reservation. The audiologist should present the availability of his services simply and without aggrandizement.

One of the most important aspects of the Entry stage is that we let the patient define his problem. We should, if at all possible, curb our tongues and let the patient tell us why he has come to see us, what his problems are and what he is currently prepared to do about them. A frequent mistake committed by a number of professionals is to tell the patient what they think about their rehabilitative plans during the first few moments of discussion. As one patient told me after I recently committed this error, "I wish you professionals would decide what you think. I go one place and they tell me one thing; I go someplace else and they tell me the opposite."

The second stage, "Clarification," allows us to help the client focus on the specific aspects of his communicative disorder that are causing him difficulty. For instance, on the rational level, the client may describe his problem as being unable to understand speakers in the noisy environment because he has been unable to focus on the individual speaking. He finds that he immediately tunes out everyone to avoid having to deal with the confusion. On the emotional level, the client may describe that his hearing difficulties have caused problems when he attempts to communicate with his wife because she does not attempt to speak plainly, and deliberately obscures her face and/or speaks to him while she is working at the stove or kitchen sink. He feels she knows that he can never understand her when she speaks to him from these locations, but still she continues to do so.

In Stage 3, "Structure," the audiologist and the client should determine if the audiologist has the requisite skills to provide the patients the services he needs. At times the decision will be academic; the client is in need of medical treatment and consequently must be referred to a physician for appropriate care. At other times, conversely, the decision of whether to refer or to whom to refer may not be readily apparent.

The decision of whether or not the audiologist possesses the skills required by the patient may be answered when the audiologist explains the nature of his facility and the type of services he is prepared to provide. Sometimes we have helped a patient make a decision about whether or not to continue under our service when we have outlined the length of time we would take in providing him the service and/or told him that we do charge for the services we provide.

In Step 4, "Relationship," we either go ahead with the plans as they have been developing, or one or both of the parties decide that the service is not warranted. If counselling is to continue, there will be a mutual agreement between the audiologist and the client. Brammer (1973) states, "The relationships should be firmly established by the end of Stage 4, with the helpee ready to go to work specifically toward goals announced upon his arrival and as clarified and amplified in Stages 2 and 3."

During Exploration, "Stage 5," we get down to work. The specifics of the rehabilitative plan are outlined and the patient is presented with all available options. If the patient is working at the emotional level, he will begin to outline what it is he must do to resolve the problems he is having. The audiologist is able to take a more active part in assisting the client to determine how he can

be helped because the audiologist should have a definite idea of who the patient is, what he wants, and how he can be helped.

The "Consolidation" stage begins when the patient has a firm idea of what he is going to do. He will decide on a specific course of action. For some (again depending on the level) this may mean that they will agree to a hearing aid evaluation. For others this may mean that they will begin practicing new communication strategies at home to eliminate the silent struggle that says you don't understand what it is like to have a hearing loss or, you don't care enough about me to be sure that I understand what you say or, I know you can hear what I'm saying, you just don't want to talk with me.

In Stage 6, "Planning," we begin planning for the end. We decide the specific goals and objectives that must be met for the client to be able to function completely without our assistance. We review the previous steps and ensure that the plan selected wil move our client towards increased independence. We incorporate the learning of skills so the client will be able to identify potential problems (on any of the three levels) and can remedy them on his own. An example of planning skills on the informational level would be that we would teach our client troubleshooting skills for identifying sources of malfunction of his hearing aid. We would ensure that he learned to identify the problems and the resources to alleviate them so that he would not have to be dependent on our skills and time for minor problems he could take care of himself.

On the emotional level, we could, for example, help the client learn to discern when the noise in his environment was causing him to become unduly nervous. We could help him discover the methods to use to alleviate this nervousness and suggest practical ways for him to monitor his progress.

The final stage is "Termination." We have completed our work with this client. The goals that he has outlined he has met. We assist him in summarizing his accomplishments and say good-bye. For some we will need to ease out of our relationship. We may need to tell them that we will schedule an appointment in 6 months or a year (or less if needed); or we can given them the open invitation to call us if they should experience difficulty.

For some, the termination stage will mean referral to another agency. The final section of this chapter discusses the referral process.

WHEN TO REFER

Our counselling should be hearing-loss related. When we delve into areas of interpersonal relationships where the hearing loss, methods to resolve the communicative difficulties, and the interpersonal problems concomitant to communication failure are not the focal point, then we are overstepping our professional bounds.

There are three basic categorizations of "when to refer." First, we should refer our clients to counselling specialists when they present indications of psychologic, emotional, mental, and/or physical distress, regardless of whether or not the distress is hearing-loss related. Even though a person's difficulties are apparently caused by a hearing loss, this does not give us sole jurisdiction for counselling and rehabilitation. Maintain a list of referral agencies (private and publicly supported) that you can present routinely to your clients. Provide them with this list and the information that these are sources available for medical and psychologic consultation. State that you provide all clients with this information and should they wish additional information you will be happy to provide it for them.

Be prepared for "faint-knocking" at this point in time. A faint-knocking question may be, "I've heard that the psychologists at the Mental Health Center just perform a lot of tests, but never really talk to the clients." You can follow this faint-knocking question with a variety of responses.

"Yes, I've heard that complaint before."
"Who told you that? The psychologists at the MHC are well-trained and are vitally interested in the welfare of their clients."
"That may be true, I don't know. Are you interested in talking with someone?"

The second major categorization of when to refer is when you are aware that the person's emotions and reactions are out of line with his hearing-loss caused communicative difficulties, when you become aware that the client is not receiving benefit (is not improving) as a result of the services you provide, or

when a dependent relationship is developing between the client and clinician. The referral recommendation should be specific, and the client should be urged to seek additional help elsewhere.

The third and obvious category of when to refer includes all clients whose behaviors are not normal. As my clinical psychology associates have said on numerous occasions, "You can tell when someone is not behaving normally." We have fairly rigid guidelines inherent in our societal expectations that signal to us a person is not normal. Some abnormalities (such as claustrophobia) are not as interruptive to our helping relationship with our clients as are the behaviors that suggest to us the client is dangerous to himself or other people. Clearly, these behaviors are abnormal, cannot be remedied solely by aural rehabilitation and should be handled by a specialist.

When you refer a client for counselling by a specialist you should be ready to relinquish your counselling relationship with him. After making a referral to a specialist you should not make the appointments for the individual or complete any other arrangements for him. If your client believes that the recommendation is "right," then it will be pursued. If you have worked with the client for sometime and have developed a professional friendship, it is appropriate and desirable for you to follow up your referral with a phone call or short note to say "Hello" and to wish him well.

References

ALPINER, J. G., CHEVRETTE, W., GLASCOE, G., METZ, M., and OLSEN, B., The Denver Scale of Communication Function. Unpublished study, University of Denver (1971).

BARKER, R. G., WRIGHT, B. A., and GONICK, M. R., *Adjustment to Physical Handicap and Illness: A Survey of the Social Psychology of Physique and Disability.* Bull. 55. New York: Social Science Research Council (1956).

BRAMMER, L. *The Helping Relationship: Process and Skills,* Englewood Cliffs, NJ: Prentice-Hall, Inc. (1973).

BROOKS, D. N., Counselling and its effect on hearing aid use. *Audecibel* **28,** 194–206, (1979).

CARKHUFF, R., Differential functioning of lay and professional helpers. *J. Counseling Psychol.* **15,** 117–126 (1968).

CARKHUFF, R., and TRUAX, C., Lay mental health counseling. *J. Consult. Psychol.* **29,** 426–431 (1965).

CHAIKLIN, J. B., and VENTRY, I. M., The efficiency of audiometric measures used to identify functional hearing loss. *J. Aud. Res.* **5,** 196–211 (1965).

CHERMAK, G. D., Audiologists and the counseling process, *Audiol. Hear. Educ.* **5**, 13, 16 (1979).

DREHER, B. B., and BALTES, L., Bibliotherapy for the communication disordered: rationale and materials. *ASHA* **15**, 528–534 (1973).

FRANKEL, B. G., Adult-onset hearing impairment: social and psychological correlates of adjustment. Ph.D. dissertation, The University of Western Ontario, London, Ontario (1981).

HELLEBERG, M. M. Emotional needs of the hearing impaired. *Hear. Aid J.* **34**, 7, 44–45 (1981).

HELLEBERG, M. M., Emotional needs of the hearing impaired: guidelines for counseling clients. *Hear. Aid J.* **32**, 6, 34–37 (1979).

INGALLS, G. C., Some psychiatric observations on patients with hearing defects. *Occup. Ther. Rehabil.* **25**, 62–66 (1946).

KNAPP, P. H., Emotional aspects of hearing loss. *Psychosom. Med.* **10**, 203–222 (1948).

LUTERMAN, D., *Counseling Parents of Hearing-Impaired Children.* Boston: Little, Brown and Co. (1979).

LUTERMAN, D., The counseling experience. *J. Acad. Rehab. Audiol.* **9**, 62–66 (1976).

MYKLEBUST, H., *The Psychology of Deafness: Sensory Deprivation, Learning and Adjustment:* New York: Grune & Stratton (1964).

NETT, E. M., *The Relationship between Audiological Measures and Handicap, Project No. RD-0167.* Washington, D. C.: United States Department of Health Education and Welfare, Office of Vocational Rehabilitation (1960).

NOBLE, W. G., and ATHERLY, G. R. C., The hearing measurement scale: a questionnaire for the assessment of auditory disability. *J. Aud. Res.* **10**, 229–250 (1970).

PINTNER, R., Emotional stability of the hard of hearing. *J. Genet. Psychol.* **43**, 293–311 (1933).

RAMSDELL, D. A., The psychology of the hard-of-hearing and the deafened adult. In H. Davis and S. R. Silverman (Eds.), *Hearing and Deafness.* New York: Holt, Rinehart and Winston (1970).

RAMSDELL, D. A., The psychology of the hard-of-hearing and the deafened adult. In H. Davis and S. R. Silverman (Eds.), *Hearing and Deafness.* New York: Holt, Rinehart and Winston (1947).

RIOCH, M. Changing concepts in the training of therapists. *J. of Consult. Psychol.* **30**, 280–292 (1966).

ROGERS, C., *On Becoming a Person.* Boston: Houghton Mifflin (1961).

ROGERS, C., *Client Centered Counseling.* Boston: Houghton Mifflin (1951).

ROSEN, J. K., Psychological and social aspects of the evaluation of acquired hearing impairment. *Audiology* **18**, 238–252 (1979).

ROSENTHAL, R., Audiologists: Analysts without portfolio. *Hear. Speech Action,* **44**, 5–8 (1976).

ROSENTHAL, R., *The Hearing Loss Handbook.* New York: St. Martin's Press, Inc. (1975).

WALLSTON, K. A., and WEITZ, L. J., Measurement of the core dimensions of helping. *J. Counseling Psychol.* **22**, 567–569 (1975).

WELLES, H. H., Measurement of certain aspects of personality among hard of hearing adults. *Contributions to Education, No. 545.* New York: Teacher's College, Columbia University (1932).

WERNER, A., CAMPBELL, R. J., FRAZIER, S. H., and EDGERTON, J., *A Psychiatric Glossary.* 5th Ed. Boston: Little, Brown and Co., Boston (1980).

WRIGHT, B. A., *Physical Disability—A Psychological Approach,* Harper and Row, New York (1960).

5A

Glossary*

---

adaptation Fitting one's inner needs to the environment, typically by a combination of autoplastic maneuvers (which involve a change in the self) and alloplastic maneuvers (which involve alteration of the external environment).

adjustment Functional, often transitory, alteration or accommodation by which one can adapt himself better to the immediate environment.

anxiety Apprehension, tension, or uneasiness from anticipation of danger, the source of which is largely unknown or unrecognized. Primarily of intrapsychic origin, in distinction to fear, which is the emotional response to a consciously recognized and usually external threat or danger. May be regarded as pathologic when it interferes with effectiveness in living, achievement of desired goals or satisfactions, or reasonable emotional comfort.

denial A defense mechanism, operating unconsciously, used to resolve emotional conflict and allay anxiety by disavowing thoughts, feelings, wishes, needs, or external reality factors that are consciously intolerable.

depression When used to describe a mood, depression refers to feelings of sadness, despair, and discouragement. As such, depression may be a normal feeling state.

fear Emotional and physiologic response to recognized sources of danger, to be distinguished from anxiety.

grief Normal, appropriate emotional response to an external and consciously recognized loss; it is usually time-limited and gradually subsides. To be distinguished from depression.

guilt Emotion resulting from doing what is conceived of as wrong, thereby violating superego percepts; results in feelings of worthlessness and, at times, the need for punishment. See also shame.

introversion Preoccupation with oneself and accompanying reduction of interest in the outside world; the reverse of extroversion.

---

* Reprinted by permission from Werner, A., Campbell, R. J., Frazier, S. H., and Edgerton, J., *A Psychiatric Glossary*. 5th Ed. Boston: Little, Brown and Co., Boston (1980).

mood

A pervasive and sustained emotion that, in the extreme, markedly colors one's perception of the world. Common examples of mood include depression, elation, and anger.

mourning

A process of emotional detachment from an important person, object role, status, or anything considered part of one's life which frees one to find other interests and enjoyments.

neurosis

In common usage, emotional disturbances of all kinds other than psychosis. It implies subjective psychologic pain or discomfort beyond what is appropriate in the conditions of one's life.

psychiatrist

A licensed physician who specializes in the diagnosis, treatment, and prevention of mental and emotional disorders. Training encompasses a medical degree and four years or more of approved residence training.

psychologist

A person who holds a degree in psychology from an accredited program. Providers of psychologic services are licensed under applicable state law, whereas those who teach or do research are usually exempt from licensure requirements.

psychologist, licensed

A psychologist who generally holds a doctoral degree from an accredited graduate program in psychology and has two years of supervised work experience. Psychologists provide a wide range of services in a variety of settings from the evaluation and amelioration of mental disorders to consultation with industry.

psychosis

A major mental disorder of organic or emotional origin in which a person's ability to think, respond emotionally, remember, communicate, interpret reality, and behave appropriately is sufficiently impaired so as to interfere grossly with the capacity to meet the ordinary demands of life.

shame

An emotion resulting from the failure to live up to self-expectations.

withdrawal

A pathologic retreat from people or the world of reality, often seen in schizophrenia.

5B

Information Resources

Books

CALKINS, E. E., *And Hearing Not*. New York: Doubleday (1969).

CANFIELD, N., *Hearing, a Handbook for Laymen*. Garden City, NY: Doubleday (1959).

CORLISS, E., *Hearing Aids*. Monograph 117. Washington, D.C.: U. S. National Bureau of Standards (1970).

FRANKEL, G., *Let's Hear It: Confessions of a Hard-of-Hearing Doctor*. New York: Stratford House (1953).

HEINER, M. H., *Hearing is Believing*. New York: World Publishing House (1949).

HELLEBERG, M. M., *Your Hearing Loss: How to Break the Sound Barrier*. Chicago: Nelson-Hall (1979).

O'NEILL, J. J., *The Hard-of-Hearing*. Englewood Cliffs, N.J.: Prentice-Hall (1964).

ROSENTHAL, R., *The Hearing Loss Handbook*. New York: St. Martin's Press, Inc. (1975).

WARFIELD, F., *Cotton in My Ears*. New York: Viking (1957).

WARFIELD, F., *Keep Listening*. New York: Viking (1957).

Articles

As I see it—Dr. Mark Ross candidly answers . . . questions on hearing aid evaluation. Hear. Instruments, **25(3)**, 12–15, 23 (1974).

CAMPANELLI, P. A., Audiological perspectives in presbycusis. *Eye Ear Nose Throat Mon.*, **47**, 3–9, 81–86 (1968).

Deafness—The silent epidemic. Condensed from R. Tunley, *The Lion. Reader's Digest*, **104**, 143–146 (March 1974).

Hearing aids. *Consumer Reports*, **31**, 30–39 (January 1966).

Hearing aids: I. What the buyer should know. II. What audiologists and otologists should know. *Consumer Reports*, **36**, 310–320 (May 1971).

Hearing loss: Ways to avoid it—or live with it. Interview with R. E. Jordon. *U. S. News and World Report*, **76**, 48–50 (January 21, 1974).

RATCLIFF, J. D., I am Joe's ear. *Reader's Digest*, **99**, 131–134 (October 1971).

JENSEN, P., When your mate can't hear. *NRTA Journal*, **25**, 26–27 (1974).

KNOX, G. N., How to handle a hearing loss. *Better Homes and Gardens*, **47**, 38, 40, 108 (June 1969). Also available as a reprint from Sonotone Corporation, Elmsord, NY 10523. Free.

RHODES, L. M., What you should know about hearing aids. *Today's Health* **47**, 40–42, 61–64 (August 1969).

ROSENTHAL, R., Do you need a hearing aid? *Prevention*, **26**, 155–156 (January 1974).

RUPP, R. R., and KOCH, L., How to choose a hearing aid. *Modern Maturity*, **11**, 65–66 (April–May 1969).

Simple courtesy and the hard of hearing. *Good Housekeeping*, **53**, 145 (November 1957).

Pamphlets

ASHA Publications List, 1979–1980. American Speech-Language-Hearing Association, 10801 Rockville Pike, Rockville, MD 20852.

Choosing a Hearing Aid. Children's Bureau Folder No. 55-1965 770-874. Superintendent of Documents, U. S. Government Printing Office, Washington, D. C. 20402.

A Doctor Learns to Hear Again, Jason B. Wells. Dahlberg Electronics, Inc., Golden Valley, MN 55427.

Facts about Hearing Aids. Better Business Bureau Consumer Information Series (1973). Publications No. 03-250-73, A 250873. Council of Better Business Bureaus, 1150 17th Street, N.W., Washington, D. C. 20036.

Have You Heard? Have You Heard! (1968). Hearing Aid Industry Conference, Suite 1400, 221 LaSalle Street, Chicago, IL 60601.

Hearing Aid Care, The Human Ear, and additional educational materials. Starkey Laboratories, Inc., P. O. Box 9457, Minneapolis, MN 55440

Hearing Aids and Their Components. Zenith Hearing Aid Sales Corporation, 2510 West Grand Avenue, Chicago, IL 60635.

Hearing Health Care Series. Oticon Corporation, 29 Schoolhouse Road, Somerset, NJ 08873.

Hearing Loss Can Be Permanent. Tracor Medical Instruments, 6500 Tracor Lane, Austin, TX 78721.

Hearing Loss—Hope through Research. Health Information Series, No. 53 (reprinted 1971). U. S. Department of Health, Education, and Welfare. Superintendent of Documents, U. S. Government Printing Office, Washington, D. C. 20402.

Helpful Hearing Aid Hints, Elizabeth Dodds and Earl Harford. Alexander Graham Bell Association for the Deaf, 3417 Volta Place, Washington, D. C. 20007.

Here's Information of Hearing Alert! Hearing Alert, Alexander Graham Bell Association for the Deaf, 3417 Volta Place, N.W., Washington, D. C. 20007.

How to Buy a Hearing Aid. Information Bulletin 37 (July 1964). Detroit Hearing and Speech Center, 19185 Wyoming Ave., Detroit, MI 48221.

Learning to Hear Again, Sidney Blackstone. Reprint No. 565. Volta Bureau, 1537 35th Street, N.W., Washington, D. C. 20007.

25 Most Often Asked Questions about Hearing Aids and Their Answers. Maico Hearing Instruments, Minneapolis, MN 55435.

Noise Pollution—Now Hear This! U. S. Environmental Protection Agency, Office of Public Affairs (1972). No. 5500-0072. Superintendent of Documents, U. S. Government Printing Office, Washington, D. C. 20402.

Practical Suggestions for Persons with a Hearing Impairment, S. J. Barranco. Charles J. Novak, Suite 204, Medical Arts Buildings, 1417 Lakeland Hills Boulevard, Lakeland Hills, FL 33801.

Recommended Procedures when a Hearing Loss is Suspected. Detroit Hearing and Speech Center, 19185 Wyoming Ave., Detroit, MI 48221.

Ten Danger Signs of a Hearing Loss. Maico Hearing Instruments, Minneapolis, MN 55435.

They Overcame Hearing Loss/12 Success Stories. (Order in quantities of 100 or more). Better Hearing Institute, Suite 632, 1001 Connecticut Avenue, N.W., Washington, D. C. 20036.

Tinnitus Educational Materials. American Tinnitus Association, P. O. Box 5, Portland, OR 97297.

Audio-Visual Materials

Hearing: The Forgotten Sense. Film (color, sound) 19 min. University of Michigan Audio Visual Education Center, 416 South Fourth Street, Ann Arbor, MI 48103.

The Glass Wall. Film (color, sound) 28 min. National Association for the Hearing and Speech Action, 814 Thayer Avenue, Silver Springs, MD 20910.

Lifeline to the World of Sound. Film (color, sound) Public Information Department, Beltone Electronics Corporation, 4201 West Victoria Street, Chicago, IL 60646.

To Conserve and Protect. Film (color, sound) 15 min. Public Information Department, Beltone Electronics Corporation, 4201 West Victoria Street, Chicago, IL 60646.

The Ears and Hearing. Sound, 10 min. Education Section Graphic Presentation and Film Loan, Michigan Department of Health, Lansing, MI, 48933.

Audio Materials

Getting Through—A Guide to a Better Understanding of the Hard of Hearing, Aram Glorig (1971). 33⅓ rpm (stereo). Zenith Radio Corporation, 6501 West Grand Avenue, Chicago, IL 60635.

How They Hear . . . The Sounds of Abnormal Hearing, Earl Harford (1964). 33⅓ rpm. Gordon Stowe and Associates, P. O. Box 233, Northbrook, IL 60062.

6

Rehabilitation of the Geriatric Client

Jerome G. Alpiner, Ph.D.

The extent of speech and hearing loss among older people is much greater than traditionally thought by medical experts, according to testing conducted through demonstration projects at the University of South Dakota and Northern State University (Carstenson, 1978). It is only recently that interest in working with the older population has emerged. Schow *et al* (1978) have cited possible explanations for this developing awareness. One major factor deals with a realization that each of us will grow old at some time and we wish to improve the living conditions of the elderly, avoiding some of the adverse conditions which presently exist. Another factor cited is that the number of persons over age 65 is 23 million, about one-tenth of the population of the United States (U. S. Bureau of Census, 1977). It is projected that by the year 2000, there will be more than 31 million individuals in this category.

The majority of older Americans reside within their own residences (Hull, 1980). According to the Office of Human Development (1978), most of these persons are generally healthy. Chronic health conditions, however, do effect about 41% of those persons over age 65. Another 1.2 million persons live in a variety of extended health care facilities and possess more serious health problems which affect their everyday living activities, including the ability to communicate adequately. It appears that the rehabilitation process for the majority of those persons living in their own residences is comparable to those adults who are younger.

A major problem area in rehabilitative audiology continues to exist for those individuals in extended care facilities. Little quantified data are available regarding the results of therapy in these settings. This is not surprising when we consider that our rehabilitation interest in the older population is so recent. As interest increases, it is anticipated that data will be forthcoming. In the first edition of this book, this author cited several personal experiences in nursing homes regarding the resident's lack of "interest" in communication. It is felt that certain questions and comments are still applicable with regard to this non-communication attitude.

These questions are as follows.

1. What approach could be used with residents who appeared not to care whether they spoke to one another?
2. Was there something else wrong with these persons?
3. Were there some aspects of this particular home for the aged that inhibited communication?
4. Were there techniques that could be used to change this situation?

At one of the facilities, a physician conducted an in-service lecture for all staff. He said medical science had given more years to life. We now had a responsibility to put more life into the years of our senior citizens, a statement meaningful to all of us who work with older persons. How can we put more life into those years? Communication is an integral part of life for most people. This chapter will discuss those aspects of communication relative to hearing loss which may assist us in making the quality of life more meaningful and productive for more than 23 million persons in the United States who are past the age of 65 years.

TERMINOLOGY

The age of 65 years has been stereotyped as the beginning of the senior years, ignoring the great variability that exists among individuals. On a daily basis, we have contact with persons older than 65 years who appear to have more vitality and energy than some much younger individuals. Economic conditions, population growth, and other factors often force the retirement of individuals at age 62 or 65 years, even though they may not be ready or willing to leave the work force. The inference that "old age" begins at 65 years refers to an arbitrary designation for medical-legal purposes rather than to factual evidence that people in this age group can no longer function vocationally. It is also important to be aware that the geriatric client may be younger than this arbitrary age of 65 years, but classified as geriatric because of a general physical condition.

Geriatrics may be defined as the study and treatment of physiological and pathological aspects of old age. Presbycusis is progressive loss of auditory acuity as a result of the aging process (Nicolosi et al., 1979). Medical confirmation of presbycusis is made by the physician. The audiologist is concerned with audiologic evaluation and remediation procedures which may be implemented to improve deficient communication.

INCIDENCE OF HEARING LOSS

Several estimates of the prevalence of hearing impairment in the over-65 population exist. It is estimated that approximately 35 to 40% of all persons over 65 years of age possess some degree of hearing impairment (Glorig and Roberts, 1965; Metropolitan Life Insurance Company, 1976; Radcliffe, 1978). It has also been estimated that between 60 and 97% of extended care facility residents have significant hearing impairment (Alpiner, 1964; Miller and Ort, 1965; Schow and Nerbonne, 1980).

The variability in the data reported is due to the difficulties in sampling the aged population since they reside in thousands of homes for the aged, nursing homes, and care centers, as well as in private residences. The implication, however, is that a significant number of older persons have serious hearing impairment and need rehabilitative assistance.

PROFILE OF THE SENIOR CITIZEN

Audiology students seeing their first senior citizen for therapy often do not understand why the client may not readily accept the services we wish to offer him. When we realize that hearing loss is only one problem with which the senior citizen has to contend, the need to understand the psychology and physiology of the geriatric individual becomes apparent. There is probably no other age group which possesses so many associated problems needing consideration in the overall rehabilitation process.

According to Kimmel (1974), those persons who are concerned with management of the aged see five broad areas of concern: income, health, housing, transportation, and nutrition.

1. Income. In 1971, 1 of every 4 senior citizens lived in poverty as compared to 1 of 9 younger persons (U. S. Senate Special Committee on Aging, 1971).
2. Health Care. Kimmel (1974) states that changing health insurance provisions make adequate protection doubtful. He cites the problems related in insufficient health coverage for prescription drugs, eyeglasses, dentures, and hearing aids.
3. Housing. Living quarters should meet health and aesthetic needs. They should be located where senior citizens want to live and where they can easily visit those places which interest them. The same is true for those who live in extended care facilities and are still physically and mentally able to participate in the activities of everyday living.
4. Transportation. It is a critical need for senior citizens to be mobile within their environment. Transportation must be geographically available and economical, as well as safe and convenient.
5. Nutrition. Kimmel (1974) explains that poor nutrition may be caused by inadequate income, but it can also result from social isolation, physical inability to eat or to shop, or from loneliness and

depression. Senator Muskie (1971) summarized, "dry economic statistics can never convey the emotional meaning of growing old in poverty, often in dangerous urban neighborhoods, and of having to choose between money for food or money for desperately needed medical care."

To appreciate these implications, it seems appropriate to describe some of the characteristics of the older American as indicated by the Office of Human Development (1978).

1. In 1976, 1 out of every 9 persons in the United States was 65 years of age or older, comprising 22.9 million persons.
2. Over 5% of these persons, 1.2 million persons, reside in various extended care facilities.
3. At 65 years of age, life expectancy for men is 14 years and for women it is 18 years.
4. The older population is expected to increase 39% by the year 2000.
5. About 30% of all older persons live alone or with non-relatives. Those older persons living in family settings decreases rapidly with advancing age.
6. One out of every 7 couples received incomes of less than $4000 in 1975. The median income of those living alone was about $3300.
7. Over 40% of older Americans were limited in their activities due to chronic health conditions in 1975.
8. Older persons have about 33% more physician visits during a year than those individuals under age 65.
9. About 92% of these persons wear eye glasses and 5% wear hearing aids.

It continues to be appropriate to summarize data from the President's Council on Aging (1963) since it provides a good generalization of characteristics which exist for the older American.

1. He may be between 65 and 70 years, but is probably older.
2. He may have an adequate income, but probably does not.
3. He may be working, but it is unlikely.
4. He may be in good health, but probably is not.
5. He would like to have more to do, but the opportunities do not exist.
6. He may have adequate health insurance, but probably does not.

The Council goes on to say that certain adjustments are necessary for the older citizen for the following reasons.

1. His income is cut at least in half.
2. Leisure time replaces the hours he once worked.
3. Regularity of work no longer exists.
4. Association with co-workers ends.
5. He no longer has work to occupy his mind.

The characteristics which have been profiled may explain why many senior citizens do not wish to engage in hearing rehabilitation. They are preoccupied with too many other factors. The psychologic, physiologic, and social difficulties accompanying a deficient auditory system create serious and challenging problems for audiologists reaching out to help senior citizens.

PATHOLOGY OF PRESBYCUSIS

Considerable research has been done to determine the nature of hearing loss associated with presbycusis. According to Yarington (1976), the pathophysiology of presbycusis is complex and controversial. He points out that while research has been conducted on temporal bones from older patients, the wide variety of pathologic processes common to or related to aging makes correlation of a discrete pathology to hearing loss somewhat difficult.

Pestalozza and Shore (1955) state that the lesions responsible for presbycusis may be located in different parts of the auditory mechanism, namely, in the hair cells of the organ of Corti, in the nerve fibers, in the spiral ganglion cells, or in the central pathways. Hinchcliffe (1962) states that although a number of degenerative changes throughout the auditory mechanism must contribute to the development of presbycusis, it seems more likely that changes in the brain are primarily responsible for the overall audiologic picture of presbycusis. Kirikae *et al.* (1964) indicate the following.

1. There is no question that presbycusis is caused, in part, by lesions of the inner ear; however, senile changes of the nerve cells of the central auditory pathway must also be considered an important factor in the origin of presbycusis.
2. Elevation of auditory threshold, especially at higher frequencies, lowering of speech discrimination, and diminished binaural hearing synthesis in the aged may be due to senile changes of the auditory nervous system, such as the reduction and atrophy of ganglion cells from the level of the spiral ganglion to the auditory cortex.

Schuknecht and Igarashi (1964) emphasize that deafness of aging is caused by independent, degenerative changes in the auditory neural pathways and in the cochlea. The neural type of prebycusis, resulting in reduced discrimination ability, is due to senile changes in the brain and auditory nerve. Cochlear-type presbycusis results in a loss of threshold sensitivity, described as a progressive hearing loss, primarily affecting the higher frequencies.

Another type of presbycusis has been considered by Johnsson and Hawkins (1972). It is characterized by loss of the small vessels supplying the spiral ligament, stria vascularis, and the tympanic lip. This type of presbycusis may be related to the metabolic etiology.

Four basic processes leading to presbycusis have been classified by Schuknecht (1974): sensory, neuronal, strial, and atrophy of the spiral ligament. Sensory presbycusis is characterized by degeneration of the organ of Corti, mainly of the basal coil. There may be associated degeneration of the cochlear neurons in the spiral ganglion. Neuronal presbycusis results in a loss of neurons in the spiral ganglion and their fibers. All of the coils of the cochlea may be affected. It is often characterized by poor speech discrimination. Strial presbycusis results in pathological changes in the stria vascularis, the source of nutritive supply to the organ of Corti. Discrimination ability may be good in cases of stria vascularis presbycusis but it can become poor as the hearing loss increases. Atrophy of the spiral ligament may result in atrophy of this supporting element of the cochlear duct affecting the vibrating mechanics of the cochlear partition. This fourth type of presbycusis currently is in the speculative stage.

Not every elderly individual has presbycusis. Willeford (1971) cautions that it is important to avoid over-generalization regarding hearing loss in the aged due to presbycusis. He states that it is not unusual for audiologists occasionally to see an elderly person exhibiting little or no abnormality in auditory function. It is reasoned that these persons have incurred only minimal structural changes in their auditory mechanism or that the damage is restricted to anatomic structures which do not elevate the auditory threshold.

It is generally agreed that degenerative changes occur at all levels of the auditory system, although there is no concurrence regarding specific lesion sites. Hull and Traynor (1977) state that whatever the cause of presbycusis, the effect on the elderly person is the same, with some differences from individual to individual. Self-isolation, depression, and withdrawal from family and society are the common consequences of severe auditory dysfunction in the elderly. In addition to the difficulties posed by auditory impairment, when remediation is considered it is also necessary to be cognizant of such other physiologic and psychologic factors as impairment of memory, deterioration of intellect, changes in personality, affective disorders, and focal neurologic symptoms such as cerebral atrophy (Pearce and Miller, 1973).

AUDIOLOGIC IMPLICATIONS

In the routine audiologic evaluation, presbycusis is usually indicative of either a sharply sloping or progressive, slightly sloping sensorineural hearing loss depending on whether the etiology is sensory or neuronal presbycusis. A descending high frequency hearing loss may also be due to atrophy of the spiral ligament. Exceptions may exist for strial presbycusis in which the audiogram will appear as a flat sensorineural hearing loss. Yarington (1976) indicates the need to differentiate between high frequency configurations of hearing loss caused by presbycusis and noise-induced hearing loss. A noise-induced loss is generally a pure tone loss occurring from 4000 to 6000 Hz with return to near normal hearing at higher levels. In presbycusis, the loss in the higher frequencies increases as the frequency scale is ascended. The loss in the high frequencies due to presbycusis gradually spreads to the lower frequencies, which can then affect the entire speech spectra. Pure tone air and bone conduction results are essentially equal (Sataloff, 1972).

Speech reception thresholds are generally in agreement with the pure tone speech frequency average for 500, 1000, and 2000 Hz. Clinical experience has shown that this agreement exists in most cases of presbycusis. In some instances, however, it is necessary to repeat the test words to allow sufficient time for the person to respond to the audiologist. This procedure helps to compensate for what appears to be a slow reaction time on the part of some aged clients.

Another routine measure considered to be extremely critical in evaluation is discrimination testing. Reduced discrimination function, referred to as phonemic regression, appears to have become a classic symptom of presbycusis for many persons. Gaeth (1948) first described phonemic regression as possessing the following features.

1. Audiometric findings which indicate a sensorineural hearing loss.
2. Threshold scores for connected speech which agree well with pure tone averages.
3. Low scores for discrimination tests which do not always agree with the type and severity of the loss.
4. General mental capacities which do not appear to be deteriorated.
5. Phonemic regression appears more common among older patients but a substantial number of older patients with impaired hearing do not display this syndrome.

The aged person with reduced discrimination function almost invariabily complains that he hears the speakers, with or without amplification, but the words are not clear. During hearing aid evaluation, the initial tendency is to blame the instrument rather than the deficient auditory system.

Threshold of discomfort and possible recruitment problems are also considered in the audiologic evaluation. Recruitment, of course, can play a very important role in terms of amplification. Hinchcliffe (1959) states that recruitment is not characteristic of presbycusis. Supporting his contention is a study on Bekesy audiometry tracings (Jerger, 1960). It should be noted, however, that the majority of tracings for presbycusis in this study are of the Type I and Type II tracings, which tend to be indicative of cochlear lesions in which recruitment is more apt to occur. In a study by Goetzinger et al. (1961), 27 ears showed complete recruitment, 41 incomplete recruitment, and 12 ears had no recruitment for the males tested. Of 40 female ears tested, 7 had complete recruitment, 16 incomplete recruitment, and 17 had no recruitment. On the basis of this information, the recruitment phenomenon in presbycusis appears to be an individual matter that should be considered in hearing aid evaluation.

Only minimal information is available regarding the threshold of discomfort. It has been our subjective impression that loud sounds and speech are more a psychologic problem creating nervousness and annoyance than a physical problem of discomfort.

Yarington (1976) indicates that the Short Increment Sensitivity Index (SISI) test is entirely unpredictable in presbycusis. According to Jerger et al. (1959) the SISI score is usually low at frequencies below 1000 Hz. Above 1000 Hz, three different patterns may emerge.

1. The score may continue to be low.
2. The score may rise gradually to an intermediate value.
3. The score may rise sharply to a high level of 90–100%.

According to normative data for the SISI, scores between 0 and 20% are indicative of possible retrocochlear lesions, conductive hearing losses, or normal hearing. Scores between 50 and 100% are indicative of possible cochlear involvement. A gray area would include the range of scores between 20 and 50%. It is interesting to note that some of the SISI scores have occurred in this indeterminate area. No consistent pattern for presbycusis has yet emerged with the SISI test.

Degeneration may also occur in the eighth cranial nerve and the central nervous system. Primary degeneration in the nuclei of the auditory system in the brain stem, the midbrain, and the cortex may produce disorders in hearing which primarily involve disturbances of complex interpretive skills (Cohn, 1981).

Other major effects are imposed by aging of the central auditory and vestibular mechanisms. Antonelli (1978) has indicated, for example, that as the number of neural units decreases, the rate at which they die increases, central blood flow decreases, and brain metabolism is altered. For these reasons, we may observe slower reaction to communication demands with reduced concentration ability.

Bergman et al. (1976) found that listeners' performance on a comprehensive speech test battery showed an abrupt decline in test scores for persons in their forties and a sharper decline in individuals in their sixties for all complex speech measured.

General Observations

Older clients with presbycusis who are being seen at a speech and hearing center for audiologic evaluation have complaints which fall into a general pattern (Alpiner, 1965). The client may state that he became aware of gradual difficulty with his hearing during the past 5 years which appears to be getting worse. He reports that loud sounds and noise may not hurt his ears, but they tend to make him nervous at times. He is bothered by tinnitus, which is particularly disturbing at bedtime or when he is alone in a quiet environment. Although he may turn up the television or radio volume or ask people to speak more loudly, he has considerable difficulty in understanding clearly what is said by most persons and even greater difficulty when background noise is present. This frustration prevents him from participating in movies, church, lectures, and other social activities he previously enjoyed.

Extended Care Facility Services.

Fifty nursing home administrators in Colorado and Mississippi were interviewed regarding aural rehabilitation programs. Seven questions regarding their interest in hearing conversation programs comprised the interview. The first question dealt with the kinds of rehabilitative programs presently operating in their facilities. Activity or social directors were hired by all facilities on a full-time basis. Occupational and physical therapists were available on a consultant basis. Speech therapy was available in 60% of the facilities on an on-call basis, usually in conjunction with a university training program for free service; private practitioner services were available when they would be paid for by the residents, an insurance company, or an agency such as Easter Seals. Residents receiving speech therapy were generally stroke victims with concomitant speech and language difficulties.

The second question asked the administrators if they were familiar with hearing conservation programs. Ninety percent of the administrators were aware of these programs even though the vast majority of facilities were without the service.

The third question posed to the administrators was whether or not they were familiar with the services provided in a hearing conservation program. Ninety percent of the administrators responded affirmatively, indicating that a hearing conservation program involved either a hearing screening of some kind, the sale of hearing aids, or some kind of therapy such as lipreading.

The fourth question asked the administrators if they were interested in a hearing conservation program for their particular facility. The responses were divided equally, with 50% responding favorably and the remaining 50% stating that they were unaware of what a hearing conservation program was.

The fifth question dealt with the most significant factor regarding the establishment of a hearing conservation program. All 50 administrators responded that funding of a formal program was not possible at this time. Only resident fees could subsidize such a program and that was not feasible. Residents could not financially support a hearing conservation program.

Question six asked if a hearing conservation program could be an attractive feature for prospective residents since it would improve the residents' communication ability. The responses were the following.

1. It would be a drawing card to get more funding from the state social service department.
2. Yes, especially in a small community.
3. Not really.
4. The individual program itself would not be a drawing feature, but physicians would be favorably influenced to recommend this facility to their hearing-impaired patients.
5. It would be a minimal part of the approach because many residents and their families would not know what hearing rehabilitation was.

The final question asked the administrators if they felt that a hearing conservation program would be an essential program to have in an extended care facility. An affirmative response was given by 40% of the respondents. Ten percent said no and the remaining 50% indicated that they really did not know.

Generally, it appears that administrators were aware of hearing conservation programs but not all were ready or able to implement them. A need still exists to promote aural rehabilitation programs in extended care facilities. The major obstacle at this time is financial; the funds for service will need to be paid for by residents, family members, insurance companies, families, or agencies.

PSYCHOLOGIC AND SOCIAL IMPLICATIONS

Considerations

Physical problems of the senior citizen may have serious implications regarding hearing rehabilitation but it is also necessary to consider the psychologic and social adjustment problems which may be related to the person's physical condition. Individuals may not openly welcome hearing remediation since physical disabilities, which may be a threat to life itself, are of greater concern. Audiologists need to be aware of this situation in which some clients may simply reject rehabilitative audiology.

Some negative reactions to therapy may be due to the client's inability to view the future positively. He may feel that he is just too old to "fool around" with hearing aids and hearing rehabilitation. Lack of client motivation to do something about the problem needs full consideration so that attempts may be made to reverse negative thoughts about the future. The ramifications of this matter may indicate a need to create a favorable environment in which communication is both mandatory and rewarding. The older adult must be made aware of the importance of communication. We all communicate because, hopefully, there is a need to communicate. This fact is critical in planning therapy for senior citizens.

We must also be aware of the behavioral characteristics the client exhibited before he entered into the time period designated as "old age." Many previously independent clients may refuse therapy. An example is the person who may have owned his own business, was involved almost totally in decision making, and relied very little on others in his social environment. Conversely, clients who were outgoing, enjoyed being around people, and were socially active with others throughout their lives may seem more willing to engage in therapy to maintain their previous interactive life style. Every effort should be made by the audiologist planning therapy to determine the early personality characteristics of clients. If the client has a family, it is often possible to obtain additional information from them. Communication assessment

scales for senior citizens, discussed later in this chapter, may also be helpful in this area.

An important consideration affecting the factors just discussed has to do with the mental stability of individuals. If certain stages of senility have been reached, any type of therapy may be meaningless. It is not uncommon to find inexperienced clinicians attempting to work with senile clients when physiologic conditions preclude therapy. Caution regarding this matter, however, is important.

Individuals have been inappropriately labeled "senile" because of serious discrimination problems which made adequate communication impossible. Since an individual responds inappropriately or not at all to communication, he may be judged mentally incompetent by his family and/or by staff members of an extended care facility who are not familiar with the ramifications of hearing impairment. In-service training and family education is crucial in dealing with this problem of "pseudo-senility."

Psychologic-Social Model

Not all older citizens undergo the same social and emotional difficulties. Some individuals find that being older can be fun and challenging. The key to these feelings seems to relate to the ability to remain active and participate in the activities afforded by the community. Active participation can relate to the prevailing attitudes of the senior citizen.

It seems that there are four significant factors which may ultimately lead to the emergence of significant attitudes. These four factors are communicative status, physiologic problems, environmental constraints, and economic limitations. Their collective relevance leads to psychologic interactions which occur in the individual. It is a time of sorting out and processing the impact caused by the four factors; it may be a time of confusion and frustration. These interactions ultimately lead to a psychologic set. It is that stage in the structure in which a person begins to develop, if possible, a means by which he can view himself and how he thinks others consider him. Fig. 6.1 depicts how attitudes can emerge. As audiologists, we will encounter the feelings of individuals with regard to the remediation process. The attitude that eventually emerges may be one of either acceptance, rejection, or uncertainty. Our hope is

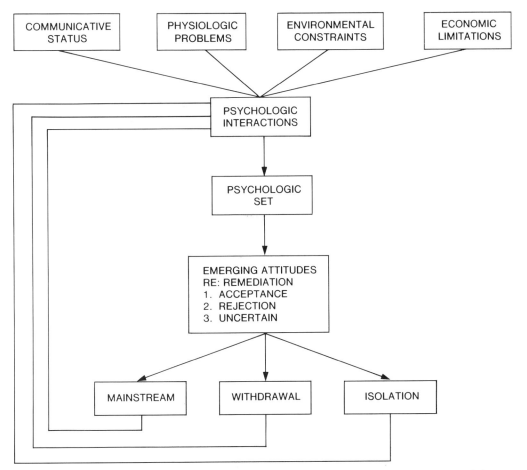

Figure 6.1. Proposed psychologic structure of attitudes emerging in geriatric clients with hearing loss. (Reprinted by permission from Alpiner, J. G., The psychology of aging, in M. Henoch (Ed.), *Aural Rehabilitation for the Elderly*. New York: Grune & Stratton (1979).)

that the client will enter a mainstream in society. He may, however, choose withdrawal or isolation. These three options probably relate to the psychologic interactions based on the four factors. What becomes apparent is that the audiologist has to be aware of all affecting factors in the rehabilitation process. We do not create the factors found in hearing-impaired persons, we inherit them. Although the mission is to remediate, we do not remediate alone because there may be little our efforts can accomplish regarding physiologic problems, environmental constraints, and economic limitations. The attitudes of these adults may already be firmly established.

If rehabilitation of this population has any potential for success, we will find ourselves working with other professionals and individ-uals who have some control over the factors indicated in this psychologic-social model (Alpiner, 1979). Communication assessment scales can be helpful in determining client attitudes. Various considerations affecting psychologic-social attitudes are discussed next.

Maintenance Therapy

Rehabilitation for the geriatric client may be viewed in terms of maintenance therapy (Rudd and Margolin, 1968). This therapy concept developed from the needs of handicapped veterans after World War II. Maintenance therapy involves the use of therapy procedures which may retard the deterioration of chronically ill patients by either slowing or arresting the process, even though it may be only temporary. The concept is significant, according to Rudd and Margolin (1968) because: (1) the disorders of the older person are more likely to be chronic; (2) it may be necessary to return for treatment periodically because old pathologies tend to recur; (3) rehabilitation and medicine are geared toward improvement and recovery; (4) geriatric clients and veterans need prolonged, frequent treatment with positive results; and (5) treatment for persons requiring extended care is an essential adjunct to the total process provided by specialists concerned with the geriatric individual.

Therapist Attitudes

In long term therapy, it is important to consider the attitude of personnel providing therapy (Rudd and Margolin, 1968). Enthusiasm about remediation may be difficult to maintain when little or no progress is observed over extended periods of time. Frequently the therapist becomes hostile and his attitude jeopardizes the client's progress. Stanton and Schwartz (1954) demonstrate that the negative attitude of the therapist affects therapy adversely and hostile attitudes can be recognized by clients even if they are not expressed openly. The importance of therapist-patient reciprocal need satisfaction for effective therapy is emphasized.

Some clinicians do not enjoy working with older clients. They may have difficulty with individuals who exhibit the profile characteristics of senior citizens described earlier in this chapter. Negative attitudes can emerge when clients do not show quick and significant progress, often the case with geriatric clients. This author regards patience as a mandatory virtue for clinicians working with older clients. The clinician's own emotional stability is equally important.

Emotional Stress

Braceland (1962) states that in old age sensory equipment is becoming defective and reduction in perceptual stimuli tends to isolate the individual. This isolation is a potent source of emotional stress. Altered body image is a serious threat to the aged person. Personality characteristics determine whether rebellion, overcompensation, or regression may be the response. Deficits of vision or hearing may also ignite previous conflicts

resulting in the onset of paranoid tendencies.

It is difficult to discuss psychologic and physiologic aspects of aging independently (Alpiner, 1965). The interaction between them is almost certain to be in continual operation and the result is a vicious circle. Physiologic disorders may cause emotional stress and since the ailments associated with the aging process are usually irreversible, stress only increases. If the aged person is concerned about high blood pressure, heart disease, arteriosclerosis, and so forth, the audiologist is not apt to find himself welcomed with "open arms" when attempting to engage in auditory rehabilitation. The possible threat to life itself almost invariably will supercede the desire to acquire better hearing.

Emotional Problems

Prevention could be the best approach to psychologic problems which may occur in senior citizens. The essence of this statement is that individuals should be appropriately prepared for their later years, not in a negative way, but in terms of the advantages afforded by old age. If prevention is not possible, Mead (1962) indicates that emotional problems resulting in certain behavioral characteristics may occur.

1. "Turning to childish superficial satisfaction." This type of reaction may exist because the older person cannot look ahead to the future. A number of clients attempt to evade focusing on the planned therapy lesson by telling jokes about their childhood during sessions. Clinicians are sometimes accused of treating elderly clients like children: "Hello, Honey, how is my girl today?" "Now, now, that is all right. Don't feel bad. You will understand it next time." These statements are complemented by vocal intonations which might be used with pre-school children.

2. "Denial mechanism." The person denies old age by resorting to such things as "health fads." Some clients have insisted that vitamins or various liquid supplements will reverse the hearing loss. They claim that hearing loss is due not to aging, but rather to a dietary deficiency caused by eating inappropriate foods.

3. "Non-acceptance of the aging process." The person does not accept the idea that disability is the result of aging and, subsequently, seeks other causes for the existing disorders. Clients have stated that hearing difficulties exist because they fell as a child, had some serious unknown illness or that their parents had hearing loss (heredity).

Although these factors may very well be true, the outright refusal to consider the aging process as a possible cause seems to be the pattern for this category.

4. "Inability to accept the changes of old age." The person falls into a state of apathy or depression. This is not due solely to the hearing loss but is seen as only one traumatic aspect of a broad range of such disorders as diabetes and heart disease. The client tells the clinician that hearing is not important to him; there are simply too many other problems which cannot be reversed. The client feels so burdened by problems that he gives up. Even though many medical problems can be controlled, the client cannot seem to adjust to them.

5. "Senility." The final reaction may result from actual cortical deterioration resulting in senility. This condition precludes the audiologist from engaging in therapy.

Stotsky (1970) reported on the wide range of abnormal behaviors seen in nursing homes. These behaviors were categorized as follows.

1. Depressed patients. These patients were withdrawn, retiring, and compliant. Some were apathetic and lacked interest in people and activities.

2. Passively uncooperative patients. Patients in this category were often quiet, sullen, negativistic, stubbornly seclusive, and often refused to follow routine. They frequently wandered off and became lost.

3. Disturbed, aggressive patients. They were threatening and assaultive to others, destructive to property, overactive, restless, aggressive, and unpredictable in behavior.

4. Agitated patients. These patients were tense, jittery, anxious, and often were observed wringing their hands.

5. Deteriorated patients. Such patients were confused, disoriented, and suffering from severe intellectual impairment. They were unable to bathe, feed, or dress themselves.

Since so many of these characteristics are seen in older clients regardless of their place of residence, we will attempt to categorize some of the psychologic-social aspects of old age which may be helpful in planning realistic remediation programs. According to Hunter (1960), these center around three categories. The first has to do with changes in needs. Certain basic needs in operation throughout life include good physical health, affection and love, expression of interests, and emo-

tional security. The way a person meets these needs changes as he grows older and loved ones die or move, health deteriorates, and activities decrease. If these needs are not met, motivation will suffer in therapy.

The second category focuses on changes in mental capacity. A decline in mental capacity may not be noted until the onset of senility. The change is gradual. Therapists, while not talking down to clients, should realize that memory, logic, and awareness are gradually diminishing and presentation of material should be paced more slowly for the aged than for other groups.

The third category concerns changes in personality. It has been stated that most personality changes are likely to be caused by disease rather than old age. Increases in neuroticism and introversiveness are often noted. It is difficult for the client in pain to be enthusiastic about communication and interaction in social situations. We may speculate that if individual needs are being fulfilled, if mental capacity is functioning "adequately," and if personality characteristics are normal and adequate, rehabilitative procedures have a much better potential for success.

Two major problems arise which may affect successful rehabilitation. The first, discussed above, involves the aged person whose many other psychologic and physiologic problems negate interest in audiologic procedures. The second concerns older citizens who are initially agreeable to audiologic evaluation and therapy. Disappointing results with amplification and seemingly overwhelming difficulties of learning how to lipread may cause subsequent rejection. Anticipation of these problems and preparation for handling them should be given serious consideration in a concentrated team effort.

REHABILITATIVE AUDIOLOGIC IMPLICATIONS

Normal Aging Process

Gilmore (1980) attempted to determine if there is such a thing as a normal aging process. A variety of communicative functions were investigated such as pitch, rate, expressive language, speech motor function, and so forth. Of interest to audiologists in providing rehabilitation was the aspect dealing with social, solitary, and interpersonal activities.

The performance of a baseline group of 30 females and 20 males, living independently, was determined. The purpose of Gilmore's study was 3-fold:

1. To develop a screening procedure for senior citizens.
2. To develop normative baseline data.
3. To apply the results to the remediation process.

There were 20 solitary activities and 15 interpersonal activities used in this study (Table 6.1). The total mean number of activities engaged in by subjects was 17.1 out of 35. The average hours spent in activities each week was 78.4. Subjects participated in 5.6 solitary activities for an average of 41.1 hours per week. The total average number of interpersonal activities for the group was 11.5 with an average of 37.3 hours per week spent in these activities. Although the data is preliminary, it is hoped that it will be possible to be more definitive in determining what older persons do with their time. The rehabilitation implication would be to capitalize on the interests of older persons in planning and conducting therapy.

Several studies report hearing-rehabilitation programs for the aged. Gaitz and Watshow (1964) evaluated 40 residents in a home for the aged. All but 4 persons agreed to be tested. Of the 4, 1 wore a hearing aid and the other had no apparent loss of hearing. Fourteen of the remaining 36 subjects were found to have serious hearing impairment. Hearing evaluations were recommended for the 14 with serious loss. Three refused. The remaining 11 were given additional tests. Discrimination ability was markedly reduced for 3 subjects and hearing aids were not recommended. Eight of the 11 received recommendations for amplification, but only 3 of these followed the suggestion. The other 5 reported the following reasons for rejecting hearing aids:

1. Lack of money (even though the home agreed to pay for the aid).
2. Denial of hearing impairment.
3. A feeling of being too old to learn to use a hearing aid.

The authors felt that lack of motivation was the main reason for rejection of amplifi-

Table 6.1
Activity Checklist

When answering the following items, think back on last week's activities.*

Solitary Activities

1. Hobbies (list):   Yes ___   No ___
   _____
   Amount of hours/week   _____

2. Go to park: Yes ___   No ___
   Amount of hours/week   _____

3. Go to library: Yes ___   No ___
   Amount of hours/week   _____

4. Go to movies: Yes ___   No ___
   Amount of hours/week   _____

5. Take rides or walks: Yes ___   No ___
   Amount of hours/week   _____

6. Go shopping: Yes ___   No ___
   Amount of hours/week   _____

7. Go out to dinner: Yes ___   No ___
   Amount of hours/week   _____

8. Reading: Yes ___   No ___
   Amount of hours/week   _____

9. Listen to radio/TV: Yes ___   No ___
   Amount of hours/week   _____

10. Sit and think about things: Yes ___   No ___
    Amount of hours/week   _____

11. Write letters: Yes ___   No ___
    Amount of hours/week   _____

Interpersonal Activities

1. Hobbies (list):   Yes ___   No ___
   _____
   Amount of hours/week   _____

2. Go to park: Yes ___   No ___
   Amount of hours/week   _____

3. Go to library: Yes ___   No ___
   Amount of hours/week   _____

4. Go to movies: Yes ___   No ___
   Amount of hours/week   _____

5. Take rides or walks: Yes ___   No ___
   Amount of hours/week   _____

6. Go shopping: Yes ___   No ___
   Amount of hours/week   _____

7. Go out to dinner: Yes ___   No ___
   Amount of hours/week   _____

8. Visit with friends: Yes ___   No ___
   Amount of hours/week   _____

9. Visit with relatives: Yes ___   No ___
   Amount of hours/week   _____

10. Go to classes at school/center: Yes ___   No ___
    Amount of hours/week   _____

11. Play cards, chess, checkers, bingo:
    Yes ___   No ___
    Amount of hours/week   _____

Table 6.1 *continued*

12. Belong to clubs (list): Yes ___ No ___

Amount of hours/week _____

13. Serve as officer in clubs: Yes ___ No ___

14. Participate in service projects (list):
Yes ___ No ___
_____

Amount of hours/week _____

15. Participate in church work: Yes ___ No ___
Amount of hours/week _____

16. Work for money: Yes ___ No ___
Amount of hours/week _____

17. Have people visit you: Yes ___ No ___
Amount of hours/week _____

18. Voted in last election: Yes ___ No ___

19. Campaigned for an election: Yes ___ No ___

20. Run for office: Yes ___ No ___

* Participation in an activity receives one point, with each additional listing under hobbies, clubs, and projects receiving an additional point each. Information can be obtained from family member, attendant, or any person familiar with subject if the subject cannot respond to the orally presented checklist.

cation. They suggested that examination for hearing impairment by an otologist and an audiologist should not be a part of the routine examination in homes for the aged. They felt that evaluation should be reserved for situations in which either the residents ask for assistance or the staff becomes concerned that a resident's adjustment is being affected by possible loss of hearing. Exception may be taken to the above recommendation since most staff members in extended care facilities are not usually acquainted with the problems of hearing impairment and its ramifications.

Another study showing a lack of acceptance of hearing aid recommendations was done by Grossman (1955). In the homes for the aged he studied, only 6 of 181 residents wore hearing aids when 21 might have profited from them.

Alpiner (1964) administered hearing conservation programs in two residential homes for the aged and in a Golden Age Center. At the Golden Age Center, where residents lived in their own apartments and were self-sustaining, 22 had hearing losses which would merit the consideration of a hearing aid. Nine were wearing hearing aids and the remaining 13 agreed to evaluation. Despite the stated willingness of clients to engage in hearing aid

evalatuion, only 5% of residents in all facilities did so. Feelings of rejection and lack of motivation were noted in the subjects who did not want to wear hearing aids. Three general attitudes emerged: (1) a definite denial that a problem was present, (2) an attitude of hopelessness (some residents said they were going to die soon and the time should be spent with younger persons), and (3) a recognition of the hearing loss but no desire for rehabilitation.

Alberti (1977) conducted a study at a center for geriatric care which encompasses a chronic care hospital, a residential home, and an active day-care program for non-residents. The aim of the staff employed for the study was to undertake an audiometric evaluation of all day-care participants and residents in the home, combined with an otologic examination and to make recommendations concerning hearing aids. There were 560 people tested, almost equally divided between residents and day-care participants. The former were largely disinterested while the latter became enthusiastic after their initial apprehension was resolved. Most of the participants ranged in age from 70–90. The most common otologic finding in the 466 people examined was wax in the ear canals. Twenty percent had marginal hearing, almost 45% had a hearing loss that was socially inadequate and 40% had abnormally low speech discrimination. Impedance testing was done to rule out middle ear pathology. Other purposes of the study were to identify those who might benefit from a hearing aid, to provide aural rehabilitation, and to evaluate those subjects who were satisifed with their aids. Sixty-four percent of the total group were considered potential hearing aid users; however, only 34 owned their own aid. The following factors were relevant in providing satisfied hearing aid use: good speech discrimination wearing an aid, younger age, a non-resident of the facility, and the ability to manage the aid without much help. The subjects did not want to pay anything toward the hearing aid. Those who did not obtain aids were usually too proud to use welfare and they did not want to ask their children for help. Aural rehabilitation was found to be of limited value for those who were senile. For those subjects who were still active, the program was of great benefit. Facilities for hearing tests should be provided in all large residential homes so that potential aid users can be screened.

Ego Considerations

McCauley *et al.* (1959) report an interesting approach which may be considered in dealing with amplification and follow-up rehabilitation. Twelve clients were studied through psychiatric interviews, psychologic testing, and social service interviews with members of the clients' families. The ego problem, in adjustment to amplification, was studied. Three sets of factors were described: positive motivation factors, negative motivation factors, and the nature of the ego function in a particular client.

The positive motivation factors contain four categories:

1. Utilitarian. The necessity of the hearing function as a tool for dealing with the external environment. The authors noted that the desire for this function varies within the individual. For example, the need for auditory perception in the young adult is different from that of the same person whose activities have been restricted by growing older.
2. Cultural values and expectations. If a culture values a maximum auditory function for communication, this may influence an individual to seek benefit from amplification.
3. Social pressure. If highly regarded persons in the individual's environment value auditory perception and accept the wearing of a hearing aid, the person with a hearing loss is also likely to want an aid.
4. Intra-psychic aspect. A person who has developed the characteristic of being alert to stimuli may be more positively motivated than the person who tends to avoid stimuli.

Negative motivating factors are similar to the positive ones but operate in reverse. The implications of this study relate to the environment in which the senior citizen lives. Family members or extended care facility staffs must provide an environment in which communication is essential. An equally important consideration, which is discussed in detail later, is that evaluation of the environment prior to initial therapy contact with the client should be the first step in planning and conducting therapy.

Motivation

Studies on the aged regarding therapy procedures are limited. The general feeling is that these procedures are not too successful. More relevant is the speculation that we have not been able to motivate this population even to attempt therapy. This in itself is a considerable problem. Punch and McConnell (1969) state that the aging process can be a factor which reduces effective mastery of such rehabilitative procedures as lipreading, auditory training, and amplification. Willeford (1971) stresses that the elderly person presents himself for professional assistance only after considerable urging by family and friends. Campanelli (1968) suggests that reluctance of this population is due to feelings that hearing deficiencies must be accepted as part of the process of growing old. He states that audiologists must change the attitude that nothing can be done to offset the breakdown in communication. He suggests that when the physician states that no medical treatment is available, the client interprets the statement to mean that there are no ways to help at all.

Harless and Rupp (1972) describe a hearing rehabilitation program for elderly persons under the sponsorship of the University of Michigan Speech Clinic. The program was designed to reach a maximum number of elderly persons with hearing loss. The Audiology Division of the Speech Clinic provided speechreading and hearing counseling classes at a community service center and at two retirement centers in the Ann Arbor area. Services were provided for 10 weeks and included hearing screening, speechreading practice, review of tips and helpful hints, group discussions, overview of service availability, and a therapy report to each participant.

When significant hearing deficits were identified, one or more of the following suggestions were made.

1. Ear specialist's review. A careful medical evaluation constituted the first step in the rehabilitation program. All otologists in the Ann Arbor area were listed, and the elderly person was encouraged to make an appointment with the physician of his choice.
2. More complete audiologic review. The audiologic evaluation provided knowledge not only about the nature and degree of hearing impair-

ment but also about the communicative disability of the individual. In every case, this recommendation accompanied the first suggestion.

3. Investigation into a personal hearing aid. If the otologic and audiologic findings indicated the need for a hearing aid, the elderly person was encouraged to make an appointment at the clinic for a hearing aid evaluation.

4. Speechreading instruction. This recommendation reviewed the proposed 10-week class and suggested that such training would help improve listening and attending abilities.

Harless and Rupp (1972) cite several unique factors about the program. One deals with transportation. This program was taken to the client. In one of the facilities, more than half of the clients said that they would not participate if the classes were held elsewhere. By going to the clients, the audiology staff demonstrated its interest and concern.

Services were provided free or for a minimal charge. There was no charge for the screening part of the project. The fee for the entire rehabilitation program was 10 dollars for each participant.

The program also enabled the audiology staff to initiate research projects with the elderly. One was a study comparing the speechreading skills of the aged with those of a younger population. A second was to deal with the use of amplification with special modification of the instruments. The authors conclude that the goals of this particular program were fulfilled. Further, they stress that the audiologist must assume the responsibility in educating, guiding, and providing a program of therapy for elderly clients.

This model is worthy of consideration by audiologists who assume the responsibility for providing service to senior citizens. It is important, however, to be aware of the mechanics of funding. Most audiologists could not provide remediation services without outside support. Financing of programs should not inhibit the development of models for delivery of services to older citizens. At the same time, however, we need to seek ways to provide the necessary funds for rehabilitative services.

Two factors are prominent in consideration of hearing rehabilitation programs. One deals with the psychologic aspects of aging, with motivation being a probable key factor. The second is concerned with the actual benefits received from amplification and therapy. We have not determined which factor is the more important; perhaps both are equally important. There is a need, however, to increase our success rate with the aged.

THE OLDER CITIZEN AND THE ENVIRONMENT

An atmosphere which stimulates communication is an essential ingredient for the senior citizen receiving hearing rehabilitation. There is always concern about carryover from therapy into everyday communication. The effects of therapy would be meaningless if an individual spends most of his time in a setting which does not afford the opportunity to communicate with others. Put another way, the older person needs someone to talk to and share experiences with and others who care about him. He needs empathy and understanding and he needs to know that others are willing to participate with him in the activities of daily living.

In private residences family and friends take on increased importance for providing an atmosphere which lends itself to communication. Senior citizens who live in extended care facilities depend on the staff to create a stimulating living environment. The challenge of making life meaningful is both important and necessary. The first step in hearing rehabilitation may well be the need to modify the client's living environment so that communication becomes recognized as a necessity for the mentally alert.

Extended Care Facility Environment

The extended care facility has become an important focal point for audiologic services due to the incidence of hearing impairment in the older population. Chapter 1 stated that many extended care facilities provide only the necessities for living, that is food, clothing, and shelter. Any additions to these basic needs could be regarded as luxury features of the residence. Nevertheless, the development of a favorable environment cannot be ignored, regardless of financial limitations on other services.

Dominick et al. (1968) investigated the variables related to successful adjustment of residents living in 23 extended care facilities. Two registered nurses independently rated each resident's overall adjustment on the basis of how well the individual had become acclimated to the facility. The individuals were divided into two groups, successfully adjusted and poorly adjusted. There were 20 subjects in each group. Open-ended questions were used. Examples of the 31 questions are presented.

1. Cognition
   a. Expectations: What did you know about the home before you came?
   b. Orientation: What is today's date? What did you eat for breakfast?
   c. Restrictions: What are some of the rules and regulations you must follow?
   d. General attitudes: What do you like about living in the home?
2. Physical needs: What do you do when you do not feel well?
3. Interaction
   a. What are your roommates like?
   b. What are their names?
   c. Do you eat in the dining room with other residents?
   d. How often do you talk with your nurses?

A positive relationship was found between increased activity and successful adjustment. The successfully adjusted group perceived itself to be better oriented, more friendly, and more active. They also had a better overall attitude toward the home and toward their own health. The greatest differences between successfully and poorly adjusted residents were in the area of interpersonal relationships. Successfully adjusted persons were better informed than the poorly adjusted, and they were outgoing in all of their everyday encounters. The successfully adjusted individuals indicated a need for increased communication with the nurses and initiation of more activities for the residents of the home.

"If most homes are proprietary in nature, can these facilities simultaneously provide adequate care for residents and still return a financial profit to the owners?" (Kosberg and Tobin, 1972). Additional staff, facilities, and services needed for improving and modifying the environment increase operating expenses. These factors will influence the administrator of a facility in determining if changes can be made. Kosberg and Tobin (1972) note that larger facilities offer more programs than smaller ones. Extra charges were made to the residents for additional services but fees were

necessary to enable the home to offer the services. Although most of us would prefer to avoid the monetary issue, it cannot be overlooked in terms of planning rehabilitation programs.

In addition to the problem of hearing loss, two other reasons may be cited to explain the lack of personal interaction among residents. Burnside (1969) states that one reason for minimal communication is that residents probably come from very different backgrounds and may have little in common to talk about. A second reason is that no one else in the environment encourages residents to make new friends, and without encouragement they will not make the effort. They regard themselves as being at the end of their social careers.

Environmental Modification

We need to view ways in which communication can be encouraged. One method is to examine the residents' physical environment. McClannahan (1973) cites ways of increasing interaction among individuals in homes. Higher social interaction was noted in heterogeneous rather than homogeneous age settings. Seating areas located in lobbies and high use areas, such as outdoors by the front entrance, promoted social interaction more than the usual outdoor seating enclosed by some kind of barrier, such as shrubs, in the rear of the building. It is also better than the usual indoor seating in quiet peripheral areas. Verbal interaction was shown nearly to double when chairs were placed around square tables as opposed to placement in neat rows along the walls.

Table 6.2
Mean noise levels from two extended care facilities

Location	Ambient Noise Levels	
	dBA Scale	dBC Scale
1. Quiet halls	50	65
2. Noisy halls	55	75
3. Front TV room (TV on)	70	75
4. Front lounge	65	70
5. Cafeteria (with people)	65	75
6. Pay telephone (by coke machine)	65	75
7. Ice machine	60	70
8. Back TV room (TV on)	60	70

Table 6.3
Physical Environment Check List

Area	Noise Level	Obstructions	Internal Correction	External Correction
1. Lounge no. _____				
2. Lounge no. _____				
3. Lounge no. _____				
4. Dining area no. _____				
5. Dining area no. _____				
6. Outdoor area no. _____				
7. Hallway area no. _____				
8. Hallway area no. _____				
9. Hallway area no. _____				
10. Hallway area no. _____				
11. Telephone area no. _____				
12. Telephone area no. _____				
13. Personal room				
14. Kitchen				
15. Living room				
16. Dining room				
17. Family room				
18. Patio area				
19. Recreation room				
20. Basement area				
21. Other: _____				
22. TV viewing				

Noise measurements were made in two of the extended care facilities served by this writer (Table 6.2). It was found that noise levels were excessively high in many areas of the facilities used by residents for socialization. Even if residents wanted to communicate, the noise levels would have made it very difficult. A number of our clients reported the greatest problem in communication was in the presence of background noise.

We have attempted to correct some of these situations. For example, it was recommended that soft drink and ice machines be relocated in non-lounge type areas of the building. It also was recommended that the schedule for waxing the floors be changed so as not to interfere with social activities as well as dur-ing the times of aural rehabilitation therapy. It is not as easy to effect changes when air conditioning and heating systems are the cause of noise interference. Put another way, the lower the cost factor for physical change, the easier to have the recommendation accepted by the administrator.

In order to evaluate noise and other environmental factors, check lists were designed to allow us to view problem areas in an organized manner (Table 6.3 and 6.4). These check lists also can be used to evaluate the physical environments of those persons living in private residences. We have found these checklists to be useful in planning therapy and establishing the most optimal environment possible.

Table 6.4
Physical Environment Check List: Obstruction Code

		dB Level
1. Excessive ambient noise from: _____		

  a. Vending machines
  b. Intercom system
  c. Cleaning apparatus
  d. Traffic
  e. Staff activity
  f. Kitchen activity
  g. Heating and cooling systems
  h. Television or radio
  i. Appliances
  j. Other _____

2. Personal safety
  a. Stairways
  b. Lighting
  c. Floor covering
  d. Wheelchair mobility
  e. Hand rails for walking
  f. Telephone and electric switch access
  g. Other _____

3. Furniture arrangement
  a. Conducive to communication (placement)
  b. Accessible for television and radio
  c. Levels of furniture (for tuning in at eye level)
  d. Shades or curtains for controlling light
  e. Communication areas separate from game areas and television-radio areas.

4. Other (specify)
  a.
  b.
  c.
  d.
  e.

Another technique to increase communication requires involving staff in positive interaction with residents. Staff must communicate on a social basis, providing an appropriate climate which stimulates interaction.

A study by Arthur *et al.* (1973) found that residents who received "voluntary companionship therapy" (systematically supervised by volunteers) showed improved morale which enhanced communication. Differences in the amount of improvement were found to be dependent on the type of resident-volunteer interaction. The greatest improvement was seen in residents who were visited by different volunteers each week. Smaller levels of improvement were seen in residents who saw the same volunteer for 10 weeks. The larger improvement in the first group was explained by the fact that each week the session had to be a different and novel experience because two different people were interacting.

It is important to provide a variety of experiences when planning group or individual interactions with residents to keep interest levels high. A major advantage to this approach is that it can result in carry-over for communication from hearing therapy. Working with the Activity Director of the facility will probably afford the best opportunity for effecting changes that lead to increased communication. This employee is the one primarily responsible for planning and conducting the social activities in a home.

A wide variety of activities can be suggested for implementing modifications in those homes appearing to inhibit communication. There are many volunteer groups within a community whose mission is to assist others. Girl and boy scouts, civic organizations such as the Lions and Kiwanis Clubs, church auxiliaries, school groups, and others can provide different kinds of programs to give residents an opportunity for personal interaction on varying topics. Logistically, it means that the facility must continually be involved in scheduling these visits.

Within the resources of a home, social activities can be incorporated into the meal service. For example, a "meal of the month" may be based on a particular theme like Thanksgiving, Valentine's Day, or Hallow-een. This approach may stimulate communication by providing the residents with something to talk about. Captioned (sub-titled) Hollywood movies which enable hearing-impaired residents with adequate vision to understand the film are made available to groups of hearing-impaired by the Department of Health and Human Resources. This author has participated in these activites and has found them to be helpful in the communication management of many residents.

Posner (1974) examined the matter of benefits provided for residents. He indicates that the primary purpose of an extended care facility is to shelter and take care of mentally and physically incompetent elderly individuals and that administrative planning was in this direction. The residents were being rewarded for their problems with primary attention through maintenance care. Socially able residents, needing minimal personal maintenance, were more or less left on their own, in effect, being punished by being denied attention.

It is the author's personal feeling that this concept is rather narrow. The limited resources of many homes appear to be the primary reason the majority of time must be devoted to those not readily able to care for themselves. The matter of which services are available within the existing resources of a home is an important and interesting issue which must be dealt with realistically. Philosophic differences exist about ways to provide optimal services and whether the priority should be to provide total care for the senile individual or meaningful life experiences for those who can benefit from them. Direct exposure to the nursing home environment seems to help students gain a greater insight into understanding the ramifications of aging, realizing that hearing loss is only one aspect of the process.

One nursing home administrator told audiology students that they must be realistic in facing the issue that most homes have both mentally competent and incompetent residents. He said that persons who are mentally able become emotionally depressed when living in an environment with senile individuals.

The philosophy of this administrator was to create an atmosphere, an environment, a milieu which would add to the happiness, health, and lives of the residents. He said that more than at any other time in life, the alert senior citizen requiring care needs interactions, associations, tranquility, friendships, sharing, and comfort. Emphasis in his facility was on relatively homogeneous placement. Only the mentally alert are accepted as residents. This is a matter of great sensitivity and not an easy topic to deal with. It affects residents, family members, staff, and others who provide service.

Private Residence Environment

The majority of older citizens in the United States live in their own homes or in the homes of family members. Many are extremely self-sufficient, in relatively good physical and mental condition, and financially able to provide for all of their needs. Some continue to work part- or full-time and are able to function within their communities. There are many, however, who feel useless, unfulfilled, and isolated from the mainstream of life. Although they are capable of activity, their isolation may have been created by themselves or by members of their family with whom they reside. In addition, they may prefer to withdraw from the mainstream whether or not a hearing loss exists. In either case, communication is diminished due to the particular life style of the person.

This population is difficult to locate for purposes of hearing conservation. They may know little about audiology services. If, as suggested in Chapter 1, we make our services known to physicians, we may be able to reach more individuals who have hearing loss and need rehabilitation. There are also organizations, discussed below, which we can approach.

According to Wolff (1959), badly managed retirement is the most frequent cause of emotional upset in older people. He feels that everybody should allow himself at least 10 years to create and test a plan of retirement.

Too many people begin in the 30s and 40s to invest in annuities or to build up financial investments for their retirement, but neglect, until the day they retire, planning what they are going to do with their retirement years. Effective planning may reduce the social and emotional problems of the senior citizen, minimizing his tendency to avoid the mainstream if hearing loss is present.

The older individual should be helped, when necessary, to participate in community activities. Leadership roles should be encouraged. Employment should be sought if desired. Sports, crafts, and other talents should be maintained or rediscovered. Church groups, bridge clubs, fund-raising groups, discussion groups, and garden clubs are examples of organizations with which the older individual can become affiliated to enrich his life. Since contact may be made with groups rather than individuals, the task of reaching senior citizens for hearing conservation may be simplified.

ORGANIZATIONS FOR SENIOR CITIZENS

There are specific groups for older people which foster integration into the mainstream. One such group was started several years ago by older persons facing the common problems of retirement. These individuals had worked for different church and social service organizations and they desired to continue working for social changes within society. The group called in students from a nearby college to share their concerns, and a coalition called the Consultation of Older and Younger Adults was organized. A New York radio announcer suggested "Gray Panthers" as a more exciting name. The Gray Panthers presently has a loose network of groups and individuals throughout the country. They work against all forms of age discrimination. They promote respect and dignity for older persons and work for constructive social change. Some resolutions from their convention in 1975 (Gall, 1976) are the following.

1. The Gray Panthers will consider collecting and disseminating information on actions for comprehensive community care and other alternatives to institutions for the elderly in their communities.
2. Older citizens should have every sort of housing alternative, from living in their own homes to communal living, from complete independence to quasi-dependent or entirely dependent living.

There should be supportive services for every lifestyle so that a choice is available.
3. Endorsement of the Equal Opportunity for the Displaced Homemaker's Act to provide necessary training, counseling, and services for displaced homemakers.
4. Urging the Association of American Medical Colleges to require geriatrics courses in all medical schools.
5. Opposing compulsory retirement in the United States on the basis of age.

Another major group for senior citizens is the American Association for Retired Persons (AARP) (Simpkins, 1976), organized in 1958. It is not confined, however, only to retired persons. The purpose of AARP is to help older Americans to meet their problems more realistically and economically. Some of the services provided by this organization are as follows.

1. Consumer Information Program. The AARP makes available consumer consultation and acts as a clearing house for information on consumer affairs. It conducts consumer education programs and acquaints members with basic economic principles, budgeting, price comparisons, installment purchasing, and consumer frauds.
2. Publications. A publication, *Modern Maturity*, provides information on health, food, travel, sports, books, humor, and legislation. The AARP News Bulletin provides information about national developments, local AARP activities, and other practical information.
3. Health Education Program.
4. The Institute of Lifetime Learning. Courses in music appreciation, psychology, creative writing, government, and literature are among those which are offered.
5. Tax-Aid Programs.
6. The Ethel Percy Andrus Gerontology Center. This center, built by AARP, offers training facilities for graduate students and faculty for age-related studies.
7. Travel Service Program.
8. Consulting Service. The AARP consults with private and government groups on pre-retirement and retirement programs.
9. Automobile Insurance and Driver Improvement Programs.
10. Life and Group Health Insurance Programs.
11. Placement Service. This organization has a project to place members in community housing, public service, and private employment.

Audiologists should acquaint themselves with available programs in order to make hearing rehabilitation known to older citizens. A problem widely experienced by senior citizens is the sense of isolation resulting from forced or chosen detachment from the world of work, from uninterested family and acquaintances, or from activities formerly pursued. We have an opportunity, through these organizations, not only to reach the senior citizen, but to make hearing rehabilitation meaningful by encouraging participation in the activities of daily living. Therapy carryover would then become more realistic since it is far easier to emphasize the value of communication when people have something to communicate about.

EVALUATION OF COMMUNICATION FUNCTION

Now that we have a broad overview of the senior citizen and the factors that affect his life style, we may begin to focus on the communication function related to problems of hearing loss. For the older person living in his own residence, we recommend the assessment scales described in Chapter 2. The clinician may be able to utilize only parts of these scales. For example, those items pertaining to employment would be excluded if the client is no longer working.

A variety of assessment scales of communication function have been developed to determine the handicapping conditions resulting from hearing loss. Only a few of these scales have specifically addressed themselves to use with the elderly. In attempting to assess the effects of hearing loss on communication function, it becomes important to try to evaluate individuals according to their unique living situations. Not all scales can apply to all individuals and all items within a given instrument may not be appropriate.

Blumenfeld *et al.* (1969) used the Hearing Handicap Scale to observe the relationship between scores on the Rhyme Test and the HHS for geriatrics. The results of their study indicated that, for persons with sensorineural hearing loss, performance on the Rhyme Test agreed substantially with the individual's self-estimates of hearing handicap as measured by Form A of the HHS. Berkowitz and Hochberg (1971) studied the relationship between the HHS and a battery of audiologic tests in a geriatric population whose age range was from 60 to 87 years. They found a relationship between the HHS and pure tone average and speech reception threshold for persons between 70 and 79 years. For persons between 80 and 87 years, no significant relationship emerged. It was indicated that the HHS has clinical application as a screening device for the elderly when an audiologic evaluation cannot be done for use in interpreting the implications of hearing loss. McCartney, Maurer and Sorenson (1974) compared the HHS with the Hearing Measurement Scale (Noble and Atherley, 1970) using a geriatric population. Significant correlations were found for both scales when compared to the audiologic test battery. The authors indicated that the two scales should not be used interchangeably. The internal bias of the HHS is towards the patient and his ability to answer each question appropriately. The HMS is interview-biased allowing the interviewer to pursue more reliable answers. One of the author's conclusions was that both scales should be compared to other self-assessment measures.

Manzella and Taigman (1980) devised a questionnaire to identify those elderly persons with hearing loss who need audiologic services including hearing aid evaluation. A 16-item self-assessment questionnaire was developed (Appendix 6A). Their results indicated that subjects with 40 dB or worse hearing in the better ear gave three or more positive indicators of hearing loss; those subjects with good hearing (less than 30 dB average) gave less than three positive indicators of hearing loss; and those subjects with mild hearing losses (30 to 39 dB) demonstrated no discernible pattern of response. The authors of this questionnaire believe that it is both simple and quick, as well as predictive. It was indicated that the questionnaire can be given easily in a variety of settings, including senior citizen's centers, board and care facilities, acute hospitals, and medical offices.

The Denver Scale of Communication Function for Senior Citizens Living in a Retirement Center (DSSC) was developed by Zarnoch and Alpiner (1977) (Appendix 6B). The DSSC was developed from the original Denver Scale of Communication Function. It is designed for presentation through an individual interview with residents. Clinical experience indicated that self-scoring scales are not feasible for many persons in extended care facilities. Residents seem to understand the task better when they are interviewed by the audiologist and allowed to respond verbally. The DSSC consists of 7 major questions which cover the following general areas of communication: family, emotional, other persons, general communication, self-concept, group situations, and rehabilitation. Included under each of the main questions is a "Probe Effect," and an "Exploration Effect." The Probe Effect determines the specific problem areas related to the general question and the Exploration Effect tries to determine how applicable the general question is to the individual client. For example, question 1 asks, "Do you have trouble communicating with your family because of your hearing problem?" The probe questions determine if there are specific areas related to the family which are creating problems for the individual. The exploration questions help determine the full impact of the problem, if one does exist. There may not be a family or they may live so far away that the client never sees them. In those cases, the question would be irrelevant and could be eliminated from future therapy goals. The scale does not attempt to compare one individual's success with another, but rather to evaluate the client's impression of his communication performance prior to and following any rehabilitative procedures. A scoring form is utilized to help in the interpretation of the responses (Appendix 6C). For each category, appropriate scoring boxes are included for the main questions and probe effects. A + or − is placed in each of the boxes to indicate a response of yes or no. Adjacent to the score boxes is a section for writing the responses to the exploration effects. Finally, there are two additional boxes for each category, labeled as "Problem" or "No Problem." After examining all of the responses in a particular category, one of the boxes should be checked depending on the clinician's final decision on whether or not a client's responses indicate a problem area.

The original Denver Scale of Communication Function was modified by Kaplan *et al.* (1978). One of the purposes of their study was to modify it so that it would be more usable for senior citizens living in retirement settings or with their families (Appendix 6D). Three basic modifications were made.

1. The interview technique was adopted.
2. The seven-point scale was reduced to five points, with each point defined for the client, to reduce confusion.
3. In this revision, all items concerned with vocational adjustment were eliminated since most senior citizens are not employed. The category "family," was changed to "peer or family attitudes" since many senior citizens do not live with families. The categories "self" and socialization," were combined into a single category, "socialization," which was designated to probe degrees and feelings of participation in social activities. A new category, "specific difficult listening situations," consisting of 11 new items was added. This category was added because, to understand a client's communication problems, it was considered important to have some assessment of his specific problem situations.

The authors indicated that the Modified Denver Scale was a reliable tool for the elderly population. However, individual test-retest reliability was found to be extremely variable. It was stated that audiologists must be cautious in using the scale as a pre- and post-therapy evaluation tool.

Schow and Nerbonne (1977) developed two hearing handicap measures for use with a geriatric institutionalized population, the Self and Staff versions of the Nursing Home Hearing Handicap Index (NHHI) (Appendices 6E and 6F). The indices were administered to 105 residents of four different nursing homes in conjunction with pure tone threshold tests. Data indicated that when using pure tone average as a standard, some nursing home staffs are better than others in identifying hearing handicaps. Staff NHHI scores generally correlated better ($r = 0.62$) with pure tone averages than did Self NHHI scores ($r = 0.49$). The conclusion was that staff personnel are more objective in such evaluations. Additional information indicated that pure tone averages of 40 dB or greater are likely to result in a substantial hearing handicap in a nursing home setting.

To the present available instruments, we add the Communication Assessment Procedure for Seniors (CAPS) (Alpiner and Baker, 1980). It is the intent of this procedure to evaluate communication status in terms of both attitudes and specific communication situations. CAPS (Appendix 6F) is designed to enable clinicians to evaluate subjectively how a person living in an extended care facility reacts to his hearing loss. This evaluation can be used as a pre- and post-test measure for planning and evaluating aural rehabilitation. Questions are provided for five communication areas: general communication, group situations, other persons, self-concept, and family to assess the individual's communication status. A sixth section on rehabilitation is included to determine whether the individual is interested in and could benefit from remediation. CAPS is administered in an interview format and is interpreted subjectively. There is no numerical classification based on client results. The elderly person is compared with himself; he is his own control.

The communication assessment battery will increase the time expended by audiologists in aural rehabilitation evaluation. It appears appropriate, however, to obtain as much information as possible to deal appropriately with specific problems of each individual. It is important to give relevance to aural rehabilitation for the elderly. For the senior citizen whose activities are not limited, assessment scales for adults, as cited previously, can be utilized by the audiologist.

THE REMEDIATION PROCESS

Several models for rehabilitation programs have been reported. A mobile audiology service for senior citizens has been in operation through Portland State University since 1972 (McCartney et al. 1974). The program, Project ARM (Auditory Rehabilitation Mobile), was implemented because of the need for hearing services for older persons. This project considered the problems of reduced financial resources and the lack of mobility of senior citizens. Project ARM includes: (1) identification and rehabilitation of the hearing-impaired; (2) development and initiation of specific intervention procedures appropriate for the older hearing-impaired; (3) assessment of the impact of this intervention on the life-styles of older adults; and (4) investigation of social, economic, and psychologic problems associated with physically and mentally debilitating forms and degrees of hearing handicap.

A typical program schedule allows time for 1 day of screening, 3 days of mobile van testing, and 1 day of follow-up for meetings, staff reports, and phone calls. The van is driven to the test site on a Tuesday morning and left until Friday afternoon, at which time it is driven back to the university. Primary entry into the service program is through hearing screening conducted at senior citizen centers. If an otologic referral is recommended, the client is requested first to contact his family physician. If he has none, a list of otologists in the area is provided. Two handouts are given to those persons attending the screening. The first is a series of 10 hints for understanding hearing problems more fully. The second, an explanation of Project ARM, contains five questions concerning hearing loss with the answers provided for each question. The name of a contact person is also provided so the senior citizen knows someone with whom to discuss his hearing problem.

Each client considering a hearing aid is given the Better Business Bureau Consumer Information Series brochure, Facts About Hearing Aids (1973). Instruments used in the evaluation are limited to low cost aids. These are supplemented by used and reconditioned aids which have been donated to the project by individuals and local hearing aid dealers. Remediation includes hearing aid counselling, lipreading instruction, and auditory training in both individual and group sessions. The average amount of therapy time spent in the project is 5½ hours per individual. It was reported that most persons came to therapy sessions as a result of "word of mouth" from other individuals. Frequently, initial intervention for hearing loss was obtained during interviews in the screening program. Nearly half of the individuals interviewed indicated that they had never sought assistance for their hearing problems. For the other individuals, hearing aid salesmen were the most frequent form of initial intervention.

McCartney et al. (1974) summarize some of the implications of their program.

1. The project would not have been possible without additional support from the university in terms of manpower and finances. Assistance from graduate students helped to provide sufficient staff for the program.

2. Use of mobile vans in metropolitan areas may be obsolete due to economical and ecological considerations. Funds spent for the mobile unit may have been better spent in providing transportation funds for senior citizens to go directly to

established audiology centers or clinics. Use of mobile units should be confined to rural areas where no established facilities are available.

3. The single most effective and substantial contribution of Project ARM has been public education through the screening process.

4. The greatest response to hearing screening occurred at senior citizen centers which serve hot meals. The meal program provides a captive audience and a climate for socialization and participation in other activities prior to and following hearing tests.

5. There is a need for better professional publicity concerning who an audiologist is and what he does. Effective and renewed communication between hearing aid dealers, audiologists, and otologists remains of paramount importance. One might consider a provision within a comprehensive health care system that would provide dentures, glasses, and hearing aids. The senior citizen is no less vulnerable than the child when considering ultimate hearing aid recommendations and audiologic management.

Colton and O'Neill (1976) report on a lipreading program provided for the elderly by the University of Illinois in conjunction with the Champaign County Office on Aging. Hearing screening centers were established at six different locations in the county. Public health nurses trained by the university audiology staff conducted the screening. Following the screening program, a series of lectures on hearing was given at senior citizens' meetings. Topics included descussions of the basic parts and functions of the ear, types and causes of hearing loss, and therapy approaches that could be utilized. As a result of this, 65 senior citizens were enrolled in lipreading classes. Eight persons from the community who had been recommended as potential teachers by the Office on Aging were trained to function as instructors for these groups. They received 17 hours of training from an audiologist. Lectures and demonstrations provided for them included the following.

1. Historical perspectives of lipreading: how long used, primary proponents
2. Basic approaches to lipreading: analytic, synthetic, and combined
3. Basic organization of a lipreading lesson
4. Lesson plans
5. Source of materials
6. Types of materials.

It was stressed that clients should use their residual hearing maximally. Modification of materials and lessons for clients, as well as ways to keep a lesson alive and moving, were emphasized. At least one graduate student from the university was assigned to each aide. Students taught every third lesson, provided additional resource materials for the lay teacher, and saw clients who were experiencing specific difficulties on an individual basis. The students also did pure tone audiometry to determine which clients should be seen for complete audiologic assessment and possible hearing aid evaluation.

Colton and O'Neill (1976) cite the strengths and weaknesses of their program. Weaknesses included the inability of university personnel to be at each lipreading class, the transiency of the lay teachers, the emphasis on a unisensory rather than a multisensory approach, the logistics of getting senior citizens to the audiology clinic, the lack of funds for purchasing hearing aids, the difficulty in establishing homogeneous therapy groups, and the lack of funds for auditory training equipment.

Strengths of the program included the opportunity for student clinicians to be exposed to the hearing problems of older persons, the opportunity to be involved in a new community project, and the provision of a needed service to the community on a consistent basis. In addition, the senior citizens were able to learn a new skill allowing for increased socialization. They were also exposed to persons who had a concern for their well-being.

Figure 6.2 presents a geriatric aural rehabilitation program proposed by Hull and Traynor (1977). This program, under the auspices of the University of Northern Colorado, consists of seven stages. Hearing screening and audiologic evaluation are the first stage. The second provides for hearing aid evaluations. A conservative approach to remediation for amplification for the elderly is suggested. The need to evaluate benefits from amplification for an individual is crucial. Inability to adjust to amplification may result in further negative attitudes toward other rehabilitation procedures. Speechreading and auditory training constitute the third stage in this program. Analytic approaches to speechreading are discouraged due to the extreme

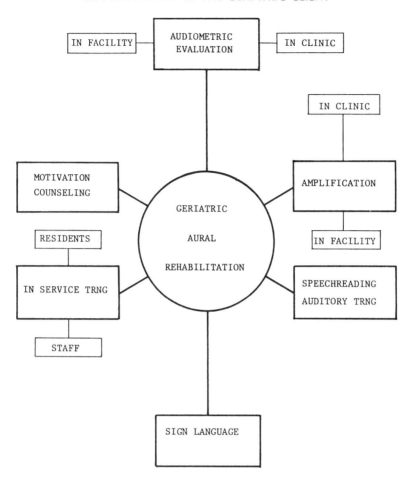

Figure 6.2 A proposed geriatric aural rehabilitation program. (Reprinted by permission from Hull, R. H., and Traynor, R. M., Hearing impairment among aging persons in the health care facility: their diagnosis and rehabilitation. *Am. Health Care Assoc. J.*, **3(1)**, 17, copyright 1977, *American Health Care Association Journal.*)

difficulty encountered in identification of individual phonemes. Language-oriented approaches such as the Linguistic Approach to Speechreading Instruction (Hull, 1976) are recommended.

Motivation counseling, the fourth stage, is regarded as one of the most important aspects of the geriatric aural rehabilitation program. Confidence that one can with concerted effort function adequately again is the key to the rehabilitation effort. It is essential for the audiologist and the retirement center staff to be confident that individual clients in the program can indeed regain some degree of communication capability.

The fifth stage deals with carry-over into the relationships between family and resi-

dent. Family counseling regarding hearing problems can be important to the family's understanding of the ramifications of presbycusis. It may help create a more empathetic relationship and enhance communication.

Stage six is in-service training for the extended care facility staff. Instructions should include lectures on presbycusis, psychosocial impact of hearing loss, the use and misuse of hearing aids, hearing aid troubleshooting techniques, methods of communication, and procedures for therapy carry-over. The seventh stage involves teaching manual communication to those senior citizens who have lost all measurable bilateral hearing and are unable to communicate. The use of signs can allow the resident at least the opportunity to express basic needs without resorting to written messages. For this procedure to be effective, the staff also needs to be taught manual communication.

Kaplan (1979) describes a geriatric aural rehabilitation program in the Washington, D. C. area. The program served clients living in independent retirement apartment communities and in nursing homes. Both assessment and rehabilitation were included in this program. Rehabilitation procedures consisted of hearing aid evaluations, lipreading, auditory training, discussion and counselling, and in-service training.

Hearing aid evaluations were normally performed in the audiology clinic. For those unable to travel, however, informal assessments were conducted in the client's residence. Hearing aids were always issued on a trial basis with follow-up hearing aid orientation provided on a weekly basis for as long as needed.

A part of all therapy sessions was devoted to lipreading practice. Kaplan reports that a majority of clients entering the program consider lipreading their major goal. Lipreading in this program is primarily synthetic in nature, including work on homophenes, idiomatic expressions, dialogues, and so forth. Much emphasis is placed on the use of linguistic and situational redundancy in the language. Clinicians may use any techniques and materials they feel appropriate, but all materials must be relevant to the life situations of group members.

Auditory training includes practice sessions to aid the clients in adjusting to reduced or distorted auditory signals, training in improving habits of auditory attentiveness, and illustration of environmental manipulation to maximize use of audition. Auditory training with the group is synthetic, often using the same materials as in lipreading. It can be performed in quiet, in competing noise or speech, and using live voice or taped materials.

In the nursing home, in-service training of nursing aides, volunteers, office staff, and nursing staff is essential. This is the one aspect of aural rehabilitation that most nursing home administrators find valuable. Two or three one-hour training sessions are sufficient for a group. Since there is considerable turnover of personnel in nursing homes, however, in-service training sessions need to be repeated frequently. It is well to use visual aids, particularly in the discussions of hearing aids, and allow some hands-on experience. In addition to information about hearing aids, nursing home personnel need information about earmolds. They need to understand the importance of proper fit, what causes feedback, how to help residents insert molds properly, and routine cleaning and care.

In the non-institutionalized setting, concern is with peer counselling rather than in-service training. In order to minimize communication difficulties for the hearing-impaired, it is important that the people with whom they live understand the problems associated with hearing loss. In the apartment communities, these people are neighbors. The information shared with them is essentially the same as that which is discussed during in-service training at the nursing home.

Attempt is made to reach non-group members in a number of ways. First, all group members have been encouraged to bring friends to class. These friends may have hearing losses themselves. Invitations also have been extended to families of residents. Second, the program is advertised within the facility in which it is being held. Many people who have not joined the classes have taken advantage of the testing and counselling services. Another way of reaching peers is to use the weekly or monthly newspaper that is printed in most retirement apartments and in many nursing homes.

Kaplan (1979) states that peer counselling has been perhaps the most successful part of the aural rehabilitation program. She has been able to reach far more people than those who have actually attended classes on a continuing basis.

It is interesting to note that many hearing rehabilitation programs for senior citizens are under the auspices of university speech and hearing departments. If the need to expose students to geriatric audiology did not exist, it is doubtful that there would be many meaningful programs for our older citizens in the United States.

There is no central coordinating unit for case management of older citizens with hearing loss. This author suggests that state departments of health should assume this responsibility. Financial limitations exist at the present time, but we hope that a start could be made to provide for eventual nationwide programs. It is not unreasonable to expect that some form of national health mandate may ultimately exist. In the interim, however, each state should do what it can within its existing resources. In addition, university training programs in speech pathology and audiology should receive increased support from federal health agencies to develop programs in conjunction with state health departments within their communities.

The effort must be made to reach as many persons as possible. The ideal goal, of course, would be to reach all senior citizens.

A SUGGESTED HEARING REHABILITATION PROGRAM

Location of Program

It is suggested that clients who reside in their own homes should receive therapy at a speech and hearing center. In larger metropolitan areas, the center used should be the one closest to their home for convenience in transportation. It is also feasible to consider conducting therapy in various facilities throughout a metropolitan area if financial support is available. Churches and banks frequently have space available for community activities. Senior citizen centers also are possible sites. As indicated previously, Harless and Rupp (1972) emphasize the importance of taking therapy to the client to alleviate the difficulties caused by inadequate transportation. After evaluations have been completed, there is no particular reason why therapy must be conducted in a speech and hearing center.

If an extended care facility is able to provide transportation and the residents are physically able, it is beneficial to have these clients receive therapy at a speech and hearing center or other facility. We have observed positive motivation in senior citizens who have been able to leave their facility for therapy. Being able to go to a different location helps to convince these individuals that they do have a certain amount of independence. In most cases, however, this is not possible, and therapy must be conducted in the facility.

Pre-Therapy Considerations

In-service training is a requisite to any aural rehabilitation program. The chances for successful programs are enhanced when concerned individuals understand what hearing loss means to affected persons and what procedures are available to help the client. Hull (1980) has stated that for family members or others who are a part of the client's aural rehabilitation program, education regarding the impact of hearing impairment, hearing aids, and methods of more efficient communication with the elderly hearing-impaired person are essential ingredients for their supportive role. In addition to in-service training for family members, we can add the staffs of extended care facilities including their administrators, other individuals who may have contact with senior citizens, and those in the community who may be influential in program development (such as service clubs).

Hull (1978) has suggested topics for in-service training. He stresses that sessions include the involvement of the older client. It is suggested that the topics could also be included as an integral part of aural rehabilitation therapy. The topics are as follows.

1. What is presbycusis?
   a. How it affects the elderly person's ability to communicate.
   b. The resulting frustrations on the part of the elderly person and those with whom he attempts to communicate.
2. Hearing aids
   a. Why some elderly people cannot utilize amplification on a day-to-day basis even though they appear to be hearing-impaired.
   b. The benefits of amplification as part of a total aural rehabilitation program.
   c. How the hearing aid works.
   d. Hearing aid care and maintenance.
3. How to communicate more efficiently with the hearing-impaired family member.
   a. Speaking at a slightly greater than normal intensity.
   b. Speaking at a normal rate but not too rapidly.
   c. Speaking to the elderly client at a distance no greater than 6 feet, but no less than 3 feet.
   d. Concentrating light on the speaker's face for greater visibility of lip movements, facial expressions, and gestures.
   e. Not speaking to the elderly person, unless you are visible to him (i.e. not from another room), while he is reading the newspaper or watching TV.
   f. Not forcing the elderly person to listen to you when there is a great deal of environmental noise. That type of environment can be difficult for a younger, normal-hearing person, let alone an elderly individual with presbycusis.

A typical agenda for an initial in-service session with extended care facility staffs might include any or all of the following.

1. An overview of hearing loss and incidence.
2. Hearing loss as related to presbycusis.
3. Brief overview of the anatomy of hearing.
4. The measurement of hearing loss related to communication ability.
5. The hearing aid in the rehabilitation process.
6. Therapy procedures for improving communication.
7. The need for interpersonal communication in therapy carry-over.

Screening the staff's hearing has been found to make them more cooperative and allows them to become more intimately involved in the therapy process. On occasion, staff members with hearing loss have been identified through this procedure.

After the staff and the family have been made aware of the ramifications of hearing loss and their responsibilities in the rehabilitation process, the audiologist can begin to identify individual client problems. It is suggested that information be obtained through the use of appropriate communication scales. A subjective interpretation can then be made about conducting remediation in a group, individually, or in a combination setting. Our preference is for a group setting, which permits greater interaction and socialization. Specific individual problems can be dealt with on an individual basis as they are identified.

For clients wearing hearing aids, the first consideration is hearing aid orientation. An in-depth discussion of hearing aids related to rehabilitation is found in Chapter 3. In general, the audiologist needs to make certain that a hearing aid is in good working condition and the ear mold fits properly. If the client is experiencing difficulty with an aid in good mechanical condition, a recommendation for a hearing aid evaluation should be made.

The hearing aid user should be informed about what can be expected from amplification. Both the advantages and the limitations of the aid should be discussed. Troubleshooting procedures, including battery testing, should be explained to the client as well. We have found that numerous clients need to be trained to place the ear mold in the ear

properly. Many clients have difficulty understanding how to use the controls on the hearing aid. Due to physical limitations such as arthritis, it may be difficult to operate the volume controls and on-off switches of ear level aids. The body aid is more convenient for persons with these physical limitations. Ear level aids, however, seem to be preferred. For many individuals it may take weeks before they can adjust their aids properly. There are some who are never able to appropriately adjust controls. This situation places responsibility on staff and family if maximum utilization is to be obtained from hearing aids.

It is our belief that therapy sessions for most older individuals living in private residences can be similar to those of younger adults. For those clients living in extended care facilities, it is proposed that emphasis in therapy should be on general communication, utilizing theme approaches. These remediation sessions could be called discussion groups. Efforts are directed toward maintaining or re-introducing the importance of communication as essential for existence in the environment. For example, successful lessons have dealt with such topics as holidays, politics, religion, and hobbies. In extended care facilities, residents have brought items they have made in the activities program, such as paintings, and sculptures. They seem to take considerable pride in their own accomplishments. Sharing them with other members of the group as well as with clinicians enhances motivation. If lipreading and auditory training seem to be feasible, they can be incorporated into the above activities. For clients living in extended care facilities, we emphasize adjustment to amplification (if a hearing aid is used), improved listening ability, awareness of facial expressions, gestures, environmental clues, and counselling.

Table 6.5 indicates an initial sample therapy lesson used in an extended care facility. It is intended to provide an idea of how a lesson may be planned. The intent is to make the resident an active participant in the group.

There appears to be no generally accepted method utilized in the actual presentation of therapy materials at present. We believe it is important to present an experimental procedure which has been investigated. This procedure can be helpful to us in developing ideas for planning and implementing therapy.

Table 6.5
Sample Initial Therapy Lesson Plan for Use in an Extended Care Facility

The University of Mississippi Speech and Hearing Center

Session Number 1

I. Introduction of clinicians and residents
   A. To achieve rapport
   B. To obtain information about residents: where they lived, what kind of work they did, how long they've been at the facility, and so forth.
II. Objectives of the lipreading group
   A. To become better communicators in all activities and environments (such as in the lounge, at social gatherings, at meal time, etc.)
   B. To become aware of the communication process
      1. Attempt to improve listening ability
      2. Improve awareness of gestures and body language
      3. Train awareness of facial expressions
      4. Increase awareness of environmental cues
      5. Lipreading per se
III. Discussion of resident's activities
IV. General communication activity: tell about your first romance
V. Theme approach with sentences
   A. Theme: weather
   B. Key words: weather, cold, rain, spring, temperature, humidity
   C. Specific sentences
      1. It did not snow this year until January.
      2. Tomorrow will be sunny and warm.
      3. It always rains in the spring.
      4. It is always cold until March.
      5. I like the spring weather best.
      6. The humidity makes it seem even hotter.
      7. The weather this week has been beautiful.
      8. There is a gentle breeze from the South.
      9. If it's too cold for rain, it will hail.
      10. A cold front is moving in from Tennessee.
VI. Homework assignment: Ask the clients to note the most difficult and easiest communication situations in the facility.

It deals with relevant and non-relevant visual and auditory background information. The influence of this background information on visual perception of everyday sentences was measured in geriatric subjects using video-taped material (Garstecki, 1976). The strategy was to observe the effects of speechreading sentences presented with relevant situational cues, non-relevant situational cues, and no situational cues.

Ten sentences were constructed using words selected from Thorndike and Lorge (1944). Sentences averaged 7.2 words in length; proper nouns and names were not used. There were six declarative, three rising interrogative, and one falling interrogative sentence (Table 6.6). Sentences were recorded under three situational background conditions.

1. Without situational cues in the traditional speechreading test format.
2. With a non-relevant visual background scene and a non-relevant audible signal. (For example, the sentence "Do you like to fly at night?" was presented against a city skyline with dogs heard barking in the background.
3. With a relevant visual and audible background cue. (This situation simulated a theoretically optimal condition in which all background cues are relevant to the sentence topic).

Visual background scenes were made by videotaping slides of everyday situations and they appeared alongside the speaker's presentation. Auditory cues were dubbed onto the videotape. The speaker always appeared on a split-half screen. When auditory and visual cues were incorporated, the viewer first saw the background scene and heard the auditory

Table 6.6

Sentences	Situational Cues			
	Visual		Auditory	
	Relevant	Non-relevant	Relevant	Non-relevant
1. Do you like to fly at night?	Jet	Skyline	Jet noise	Dogs barking
2. Some ducks swim in freezing water.	Ducks	Bank	Quacking	Railroad crossing
3. My neighbor goes to church on Sunday.	Church	Seagull	Carillon	Lawn mower running
4. Would you rather swim in a lake or pool?	Swimming pool	Hallway	Children driving	Applause
5. Children entertain themselves with rides and games.	Carousel	Shopping center	Carousel music	Gear stripping
6. Is there a lot of traffic at 5 o'clock?	City traffic	Flower garden	Traffic noise	Chimes tolling
7. Birds fly over the fishing boats.	Harbor	Woods	Boat whistle	Mooing
8. The building on my corner is a fire trap.	Fire engines	McDonald's restaurant	Sirens blaring	Jackhammer noise
9. I enjoy an evening at home.	Living room	Street	Door chimes	Crowing
10. Did you ever ride a horse?	Horse	Home	Neighing	Vacuum cleaner

cue. After five seconds, the audible signal stopped and the speaker appeared on the left side of a split screen. The sentence identification number appeared and was followed by the speaker's presentation of the sentence. When visual and auditory background cues were not used, the visual background was blank and the audible signal was absent.

Twenty-four subjects, ranging in age from 61 to 87 years, were used in the study. Each subject demonstrated sensorineural or mixed hearing impairment. The subjects were administered 10 everyday sentences for speechreading under one of the three conditions. They were asked to relate all or any part of the perceived message to the examiner. Taking enough time and guessing were encouraged.

Responses were scored correct (10%) if the full meaning of each sentence was understood. Partial credit (5%) was allowed for correct speechreading of essential key words or partial understanding of sentence meaning.

The average geriatric subject demonstrating a functional language system, meaningful experimental background, and the ability to process sensory information, used relevant cues to facilitate visual speech perception. The study suggests that situational cues define a category of information that has strong influence on visual speech perception, activating certain expectations. The majority of the subjects demonstrated low speechreading ability when the message was presented without situational cues, and slightly poorer performance when non-relevant cues were provided. Considerably improved performance was observed when relevant cues were provided.

It appears that group sessions have an effective duration of about 1 hour. The rehabilitation program for senior citizens does not have the same time frame reported for younger clients. Instead, it is a continuing program. Residents without hearing loss are encouraged to attend therapy sessions. This procedure seems to have the effect of successfully mainstreaming the residents into the environment in which they live. It is important to restate that carry-over activities must be a part of the process if therapy is to be effective.

The emphasis on communication-oriented therapy is to give the client a feeling that life is still worthwhile. As stated by Routh (1968), we give the client emotional support through certain basic experiences which include the following.

1. A close personal relationship with at least a few other human beings.

2. Opportunities to keep in touch with what is going on in the world at large: the plans, projects, and achievements of the community.

3. Opportunities to make personal decisions to select one's own goals and the means of achieving them.

Reflecting on her experiences in working with older persons in an extended care facility, a graduate student offered the following suggestions.

1. Being at the facility at a set time on a certain day of the week seemed highly significant to the residents. It was an event they could depend upon. It appeared to enhance the building of trust and rapport with the residents, and eventually they began to anticipate the sessions.

2. A morning therapy time might attract more persons, since many residents appear to nap after the noon meal.

3. Making individual personal contacts with group members both before forming a group and on the day of group meetings was felt to contribute significantly to the high retention rate in the group.

4. It is possible to explore and sometimes satisfy some of the personal needs or interests of the residents with relatively little effort. For example, we were able to secure a talking book machine from the library for a resident with cataracts who formerly enjoyed reading.

5. A good relationship with the Activity Director is essential. This staff member must be "sold" on the need for communication if any significant environmental changes are to be made.

6. Much time is wasted getting residents to therapy. It may be wise to instigate a three-member "buddy system" to have members remind each other about the session. If a group member does not show up, try to find him. Chances are that he has just forgotten about the meeting.

7. If homework is assigned, it should be photocopied. Reminder notes should be sent to each member of the group about 2 days before the next meeting.

8. Try to arrange a therapy time which does not conflict with any other major activities in the home such as Bingo.

9. Use name tags for the first few meetings. Remember that it is disrespectful to use first names without permission.

10. When you recommend hearing evaluation and hearing aid evaluation, it is important that you personally explain the situation to the client.

11. Be as alert as possible to the personal needs of each member of your group. The personal attention and recognition you give them may be the only attention they get.

This author views rehabilitative audiology with older adults as a major challenge. A key point to remember is that patience is one of the greatest virtues we can possess in working with this population. There is no easy way to accomplish our goals, but our chances for success can be greatly enhanced by understanding more fully the complexities of the aging process.

References

ALBERTI, P. W., Hearing aids and aural rehabilitation in a geriatric population. *J. Otolaryngol.*, **6**, 1–50 (1977).

ALPINER, J. G., Psychological and social aspects of aging as related to hearing loss. In M. A. Henoch (Ed.), *Aural Rehabilitation for the Elderly.* New York: Grune & Stratton (1979).

ALPINER, J. G., Diagnostic and rehabilitative aspects of geriatric audiology. *ASHA Rep.* **7**, 455–459 (1965).

ALPINER, J. G., Audiologic problems of the aged. *Geriatrics*, **18**, 19–26 (1964).

ALPINER, J. G., and BAKER, B., Communication Assessment Procedures in the Aural Rehabilitation Process. *Semin. Speech Lang. Hear.*, in press.

ANTONELLI, A., Auditory processing disorders and problems with hearing aid fitting in old age. *Audiology*, **17**, 27–31 (1978).

ARTHUR, G. L., DONNAN, H. H., and LAIR, C. V., Companionship therapy with nursing home aged. *Gerontologist*, **13**, 167–170 (1973).

BERGMAN, M., BLUMENFELD, V., CASCARDO, D., DASH, B., LEVITT, H., and MARGUILES, M., Age-related decrement in hearing for speech. *J. Gerontol.*, **31**, 533–38 (1976).

BERKOWITZ, A. and HOCHBERG, I., Self-assessment of hearing handicap in the aged. *Arch. Otolaryngol.*, **93**, 25–33 (1971).

BETTER BUSINESS BUREAU, INC., *Facts About Hearing Aids*, Washington, D. C. (1973).

BLUMENFELD, V. M., BERGMAN, M., and MILLNER, E., Speech discrimination in an aging population. *J. Speech Hear. Res.*, **12**, 210–217 (1969).

BRACELAND, G. J., Psychopathology of aging. *Postgrad. Med.*, **32**, 278–283 (1962).

BURNSIDE, I. M., Sensory stimulation: an adjunct to group work with the disabled aged. *Ment. Hyg. (Arlington, VA)*, **53**, 381–388 (1969).

CAMPANELLI, P. A., Audiological perspectives in presbycusis. *Eye Ear Nose Throat Mon.*, **47**, 3–9, 81–86 (1968).

CARSTENSON, B., Speech and hearing problems among older people. *Aging*, 24–27 (1978).

COHN, A., Etiology and pathology of disorders affecting hearing. In F. N. Martin (Ed.), *Medical Audiology*. Englewood Cliffs, NJ: Prentice-Hall, Inc. (1981).

COLTON, J. C., and O'NEILL, J. J., A cooperative outreach program for the elderly. *J. Acad. Rehab. Audiol.*, **9**, 38–41 (1976).

DOMINICK, J. R., GREENBLATT, D. L., and STOTSKY, B. A., The adjustment of aged persons in nursing homes: the patients' report. *J. Am. Geriatr. Soc.*, **16**, 63–77 (1968). (Copyright 1968, *Journal of the American Geriatrics Society*.)

GAETH, J., A study of phonemic regression in relation to hearing loss. Unpublished doctoral dissertation, Northwestern University (1948).

GAITZ, C., and WATSHOW, M. F., Obstacles encountered in correcting hearing loss in the elderly. *Geriatrics* **19**, 83–86 (1964).

GALL, D., Personal communication (1976).

GARSTECKI, D. C., Situational cues in visual speech perception by geriatric subjects. *J. Am. Audiol. Soc.* (1976).

GILMORE, S., Paper presented at a workshop at the University of Mississippi, March, 1980.

GLORIG, A., and ROBERTS, J., *Hearing levels of adults by age and sex: United States, 1960-62. Public Health Service Publication 770. 1000, Series II, No. II.* Washington, D. C.: U. S. Government Printing Office (1965).

GOETZINGER, C. P., PROUD, G. O., DIRKS, D. D., and EMBREY, J. A., A study of hearing in advanced age. *Arch. Otolaryngol.*, **73**, 662–674 (1961).

GROSSMAN, B., Hard-of-hearing persons in a home for the aged. *Hear. News*, **23**, 11, 12, 17, 18, 20 (1955).

HARLESS, E. L. and RUPP, R. R., Aural rehabilitation of the elderly. *J. Speech Hear. Disord.*, **37**, 267–273 (1972).

HINCHCLIFFE, R., The anatomical locus of presbycusis. *J. Speech Hear. Disord.*, **27**, 301–310 (1962).

HINCHCLIFFE, R., The threshold of hearing as a function of age. *Acoustica*, **9**, 303–308 (1959).

HULL, R. H., Aural rehabilitation for the elderly. In R. L. Schow and M. A. Nerbonne (Eds.), *Introduction to Aural Rehabilitation*. Baltimore: University Park Press (1980).

HULL, R., Assisting the elderly client. In J. Katz (Ed.) *Handbook of Clinical Audiology*. Baltimore: The Williams & Wilkins Co. (1978).

HULL, R. H., A linguistic approach to the teaching of speechreading: theoretical and practical concepts. *J. Acad. Rehab. Audiol.*, **9**, 14–19 (1977).

HULL, R. H., and TRAYNOR, R. M., Hearing impairment among aging persons in the health care facility: their diagnosis and rehabilitation. *Am. Health Care Assoc. J.*, **3**, 14–18 (1977).

HUNTER, W. F., The psychologist works with the aged individual. *J. Counsel. Psychol.*, **7**, 120–126 (1960).

JERGER, J., Bekesy audiometry in analysis of auditory disorders. *J. Speech Hear. Disord.*, **3**, 275–287 (1960).

JERGER, J., SHEDD, J., and HARFORD, E., On the detection of extremely small changes in sound intensity. *Arch. Otolaryngol.*, **69**, 200–211, (1959).

JOHNSSON, L., and HAWKINS, J. E., Sensory and neural degeneration with aging as seen in microdissections of the human ear. *Ann. Otol. Rhinol. Laryngol.*, **81**, 179 (1972).

KAPLAN, H., FEELEY, J., and BROWN, J., A modified Denver scale: test-retest reliability. *J. Acad. Rehab. Audiol.*, **11**, 15–32 (1978).

KAPLAN, H., Development, composition and problems with elderly aural rehabilitation groups. In M. A. Henoch (Ed.), *Aural rehabilitation for the elderly*. New York: Grune & Stratton (1979).

KIMMEL, D. C., *Adulthood and Aging*. New York: John Wiley and Sons, Inc. (1974).

KIRIKAE, I., SATO, T., and SHITARA, T., A study of hearing in advanced age. *Laryngoscope*, **74**, 205–220 (1964). (Copyright 1964, *Laryngoscope*).

KOSBERG, J. I., and TOBIN, S. S., Variability among nursing homes. *Gerontologist*, **12**, 214–219 (1972).

MANZELLA, D. S., and TAIGMAN, M., A hearing screen test for the elderly, *J. Acad. Rehab. Audiol.*, **13**, 21–28 (1980).

MCCARTNEY, J. H., MAURER, J. F., and SORENSON, F. D., A mobile audiology service for the elderly: a preliminary report. *J. Acad. Rehab. Audiol.*, **7**, 25–36, (1974). (Copyright 1974, *Journal of the Academy of Rehabilitative Audiology*).

MCCAULEY, J., FRASER, C., MILLER, A., and CUBERT, C., Psychological factors in adaption to hearing aids. *Am. J. Orthopsychiat.*, **29**, 121–129 (1959).

MCCLANNAHAN, L. E., Therapeutic and prosthetic living environments for nursing home residents. *Gerontologist*, **13**, 424–429 (1973).

MEAD, B., Emotional struggles in adjusting to old age. *Postgrad. Med*, **31**, 156–160 (1962). (Copyright 1962, *Postgraduate Medicine*.)

METROPOLITAN LIFE INSURANCE COMPANY, Hearing impairment in the United States, *Metropolitan Life Insurance Statistics*, **57**, 7–9 (1976).

MILLER, M., and ORT, R., Hearing problems in a home for the aged. *Acta Otolaryngol.*, **59**, 33–44 (1965).

MUSKIE, E. S., Some perspectives on the problems of the elderly. *Hear. Speech News*, **39**, 3–5 (1971).

NICOLOSI, L., HARRYMAN, E., and KRESHECK, J., *Terminology of Communication Disorders*. 2nd Ed. Baltimore: Williams & Wilkins Co. (1979).

NOBLE, W. G., and ATHERLEY, G. R. C., The hearing measure scale: a questionnaire for the assessment of auditory disability. *J. Aud. Res.*, **10**, 229–250 (1970).

OFFICE OF HUMAN DEVELOPMENT, ADMINISTRATION OF AGING, DEPARTMENT OF HEALTH, EDUCATION, AND WELFARE, *Facts about older Americans. National Clearing House on Aging Report. Publication No. (OHD) 78-20006*. Washington, D. C.: U. S. Government Printing Office (1978).

PEARCE, J., and MILLER, E., *Clinical Aspects of Dementia*. Baltimore: The Williams & Wilkins Company (1973).

PESTALOZZA, G., and SHORE, I., Clinical evaluation of presbycusis on the basis of different tests of auditory function. *Laryngoscope*, **65**, 1136–1163 (1955).

POSNER, J., Notes on the negative implications of being competent in a home for the aged. *Int. J. Aging Hum. Dev.*, **5**, 357–364 (1974).

PRESIDENT'S COUNCIL ON AGING, *Profile of the Older American*. Washington, D. C.: U. S. Government Printing Office (1963).

PUNCH, J. L., and MCCONNELL, F., The speech discrimination function of elderly adults. *J. Aud. Res.*, **9**, 159–166 (1969).

RADCLIFFE, D., The aging of America: impact on hearing health. *Hear. Aid J.*, **32(8)**, 44 (1978).

ROUTH, A., *Nursing Homes, a Blessing or a Curse?* Springfield, IL: Charles C Thomas (1968).

RUDD, J. L., and MARGOLIN, R. J., *Maintenance Therapy for the Geriatric Patient*. Springfield, IL: Charles C Thomas (1968).

SATALOFF, J., Presbycusis: air and bone conduction thresholds. *Laryngoscope*, **82**, 2079 (1972).

SCHOW, R. L., and NERBONNE, M. A., Hearing levels among elderly nursing home residents. *J. Speech Hear. Disord.*, **45**, 124–132 (1980).

SCHOW, R. L., and NERBONNE, M. A., Assessment of hearing handicap by nursing home residents and staff.

J. Acad. Rehab. Audiol., **10,** 2–12 (1977).

SCHOW, R. L., CHRISTENSEN, J. M., HUTCHINSON, J. M., and NERBONNE, M. A., *Communication disorders of the aged.* Baltimore: University Park Press (1978).

SCHUKNECHT, H., The pathology of presbycusis. Paper presented at a workshop on Geriatric Aural Rehabilitation, Denver (1974).

SCHUKNECHT, H. F., and IGARASHI, M., Pathology of slow progressive sensorineural deafness. *Trans. Am. Acad. Ophthalmol. Otolaryngol.,* **68,** 222–242 (1964).

SIMPKINS, J., Personal communication (1976).

STANTON, A. H., and SCHWARTZ, M. S., *The Mental Hospital,* New York: Basic Books (1954).

STOTSKY, B. A., *The Nursing Home and the Aged Psychiatric Patient.* New York: Appleton-Century-Crofts (1970).

THORNDIKE, E., and LORGE, I., *The Teacher's Work Book of 30,000 Words.* New York: Columbia University Press (1944).

U. S. BUREAU OF CENSUS. *Current Population Reports.* *Series P-25, No. 704, Projections of the Population of the U. S.: 1977–2050.* Washington, D. C.: U. S. Government Printing Office (July 1977).

U. S. SENATE SPECIAL COMMITTEE ON AGING, *A Pre-White House Conference on Aging: Summary of Development and Data.* Washington, D. C.: U. S. Government Printing Office (1971).

WILLEFORD, J. A., The geriatric patient. In D. E. Rose (Ed.), *Audiological Assessment.* Englewood Cliffs, NJ: Prentice-Hall, Inc. (1971).

WOLFF, K., *The Biological, Sociological and Psychological Aspects of Aging.* Springfield, IL: Charles C Thomas (1959).

YARINGTON, C. T., JR., *Presbycusis.* In J. Northern (Ed.), *Hearing Disorders.* Boston: Little, Brown and Company (1976).

ZARNOCH, J. M., and ALPINER, J. G., The Denver Scale of Communication Function for Senior Citizens Living in Retirement Centers. Unpublished study (1977).

6A

Self-Assessment of Hearing*

Please answer YES or NO to the following questions.

1. Do you find that people fail to speak clearly? _____
2. Do you find that people speak too softly? _____
3. Do you find that people tend to speak too quickly? _____
4. Do you think you have a problem with your hearing? _____
5. Have you ever owned a hearing aid? _____
6. Do you hear better when you can see the speaker's face? _____
7. Has your hearing been getting worse over the last five to ten years? _____
8. Do you have a ringing or buzzing in your ears which bothers you when you are in a quiet place? _____
9. Do people tell you that you speak too softly? _____
10. Do people tell you that you speak too loudly? _____
11. Do you feel that any difficulty with your hearing limits or hampers your personal or social life? _____
12. Can you carry on a telephone conversation without difficulty? _____
13. Can you hear when somebody speaks in a whisper? _____
14. Can you carry on a conversation with one other person when you are in a noisy place such as a restaurant or at a party? _____
15. Does any problem or difficulty with your hearing upset you at all? _____
16. Can you hear when someone rings the doorbell or knocks on the door? _____

* Reprinted by permission from Manzella, D. S., and Taigman, M., A hearing screen test for the elderly, *J. Acad. Rehab. Audiol.*, **13**, 21–28 (1980).

6B

The Denver Scale of Communication Function for Senior Citizens Living in Retirement Centers*

NAME: _____ DATE OF PRE-TEST: _____

ADDRESS: _____ DATE OF POST-TEST: _____

AGE: _____ EXAMINER: _____

SEX: _____

1. Do you have trouble communicating with your family because of your hearing problem? Yes___ No___

Probe Effect I

a. Does your family make decisions for you because of your hearing problem? Yes___ No___

b. Does your family leave you out of discussions because of your hearing problem? Yes___ No___

c. Does your family get angry or annoyed with you because of your hearing problem? Yes___ No___

Exploration Effect

a. Do you have a family? Yes___ No___

b. How often does your family visit you? _____

b. How far away does your family live? In a city_____ Other _____

d. How often do you visit your family? _____

2. Do you get upset when you cannot hear or understand what is being said? Yes___ No___

Probe Effect I (to be used only if person responds yes)

a. Do your friends know you get upset Yes___ No___

b. Does your family know you get upset? Yes___ No___

c. Does the staff know you get upset Yes___ No___

Probe Effect II (to be used only if person responds no)

a. Do your friends realize you are not upset? Yes___ No___

b. Does your family realize you are not upset? Yes___ No___

c. Does the staff realize you are not upset? Yes___ No___

Exploration Effect (to be used only if person responds yes)

a. How does your behavior change when you become upset?

* Reprinted by permission from Zarnoch, J. M., and Alpiner, J. G, *The Denver Scale of Communication Function for Senior Citizens Living in Retirement Centers* (1976).

3. Do you think your family, your friends, and the staff understand what it is like to have a hearing problem?   Yes___ No___

   Probe Effect
   a. Do they avoid you because of your hearing problem?   Yes___ No___
   b. Do they leave you out of discussions?   Yes___ No___
   c. Do they hesitate to ask you to socialize with them?   Yes___ No___
   Exploration Effect
   a. Family   Yes___ No___
   b. Friends   Yes___ No___
   c. Staff   Yes___ No___

4. Do you avoid communicating with other people because of your hearing problem?   Yes___ No___

   Probe Effect
   a. Do you communicate with people during meal times?   Yes___ No___
   b. Do you communicate with your roommate(s)?   Yes___ No___
   c. Do you communicate during the social activities in the home?   Yes___ No___
   d. Do you communicate with visiting family or friends?   Yes___ No___
   e. Do you communicate with the staff?   Yes___ No___

   Exploration Effect
   a. Is your roommate capable of communication?   Yes___ No___
   b. What are the social activities of the home? _____
   c. Which ones do you attend?   _____

5. Do you feel that your are a relaxed person?   Yes___ No___

   Probe Effect
   a. Do you think you are an irritable person because of your hearing problem?   Yes___ No___
   b. Do you think you are an irritable person because of your age?   Yes___ No___
   c. Do you think you are an irritable person because you live in this home?   Yes___ No___
   Exploration Effect
   Do you have to live in this home?   Yes___ No___

6. Do you feel relaxed in group communicative situations?   Yes___ No___

   Probe Effect
   a. Do you get nervous when you have to ask people to repeat what they have said if you have not understood them?   Yes___ No___
   b. Do you feel nervous if you have to tell a person that you have a hearing problem?   Yes___ No___

   Exploration Effect
   a. Do you watch facial expressions?   Yes___ No___
   b. Do you watch gestures?   Yes___ No___
   c. Do you think you are a good listener?   Yes___ No___Why?
   d. Do you have a hearing aid?   Yes___ No___
   e. Do you wear your aid?   Yes___ No___

7. Do you think you need help in overcoming your hearing problem?   Yes___ No___

   Exploration Effect I
   a. A person can improve his communication ability by using lipreading (or

speechreading) which means watching the speaker's lips, facial expressions, and gestures when he's speaking to you.

b. Do you agree with that definition of lipreading?

Probe Effect

a. If lipreading training was available, would you attend?   Yes___   No___

b. Do you think this home provides adequate activities to make you want to communicate?   Yes___   No___

Exploration Effect II

a. Is your vision adequate?   Yes___   No___

b. Are you able to get around unassisted?   Yes___   No___

THE DENVER SCALE OF COMMUNICATION FUNCTION FOR
SENIOR CITIZENS LIVING IN RETIREMENT CENTERS
by
Janet M. Zarnoch, M.A. and Jerome G. Alpiner, Ph.D.

NAME _____
ADDRESS _____
AGE _____

EXAMINER _____

DATE OF PRETEST _____
DATE OF POSTTEST _____

SEX _____

INITIAL EVALUATION _____
FINAL EVALUATION _____

CATEGORY	MAIN QUESTION	PROBE EFFECTS	EXPLORATION EFFECTS	PROBLEM	NO PROBLEM
Family	1. + □ – □	a □ b □ c □	a. b. c. d.		
Emotional	2. + □ – □	I a □ b □ c □ ; II a □ b □ c □	a.		
Other Persons	3. + □ – □	a □ b □ c □	a. b. c.		
General Communication	4. + □ – □	a □ b □ c □ d □ ; e □	a. b. c.		

Reprinted by permission from Zarnoch, J. M., and Alpiner, J. G., unpublished study, The University of
Denver, copyright 1976.

CATEGORY	MAIN QUESTION	PROBE EFFECTS	EXPLORATION EFFECTS	PROBLEM	NO PROBLEM
Self Concept	5. + ☐ − ☐	a ☐ b ☐ c ☐	a. _____		
Group Situations	6. + ☐ − ☐	a ☐ b ☐	a. _____ b. _____ c. _____ d. _____ e. _____		
Rehabilitation	7. + ☐ − ☐	a ☐ b ☐	Ia. _____ b. _____ IIa. _____ b. _____		

Key + = person responded yes to question

 − = person responded no to question

Additional Client Comments: 1. _____

2. _____

3. _____

4. _____

5. _____

6. _____

7. _____

Examiner _____ Date _____

197

APPENDIX

6D

The Denver Scale of Communication Function— Modified*

PRE-THERAPY _____ POST-THERAPY _____

DATE _____

NAME _____ AGE _____ SEX _____

ADDRESS _____

_____

AUDIOGRAM (Examination Date _____

Pure Tone

	250	500	1000	2000	4000	8000	Hz
RE	___	___	___	___	___	___	dB (re:
LE	___	___	___	___	___	___	(ANSI)

Speech

SRT   Discrimination Score (%)

				Quiet	Noise (S/N =)
RE	_____	dB	RE	_____	_____
LE	_____	dB	LE	_____	_____

Hearing Aid Information

Aided _____ For How Long _____ Aid Type _____

Ear _____ Satisfaction _____

_____

Examiner _____

INSTRUCTIONS

I am going to say some statements relating to hearing loss. For each statement, I want you to tell me if you: (1) definitely agree, (2) slightly agree, (4) slightly disagree, or (5) definitely disagree. If you consider the statement to be irrelevant or unassociated to your communication problem, please tell me.

Scoring

(1) Definitely agree   (2) Slightly agree   (3) Irrelevant
        (4) Slightly disagree   (5) Definitely disagree

---

* Reprinted by permission from Kaplan, H., Feeley, J., and Brown, J., A modified Denver scale: test-retest reliability. *J. Acad. Rehab. Audiol.*, **11**, 15–32 (1978).

Attitude Toward Peers

1. The people I live with are annoyed with my loss of hearing. Comments:

____1. Definitely agree
____2. Slightly agree
____3. Irrelevant
____4. Slightly disagree
____5. Definitely disagree

2. The people I live with sometimes leave me out of conversations or discussions. Comments:

____1. Definitely agree
____2. Slightly agree
____3. Irrelevant
____4. Slightly disagree
____5. Definitely disagree

3. Sometimes people I live with make decisions for me because I have a hard time following discussions. Comments:

____1. Definitely agree
____2. Slightly agree
____3. Irrelevant
____4. Slightly disagree
____5. Definitely disagree

4. People I live with become annoyed when I ask them to repeat what was said because I did not hear them. Comments:

____1. Definitely agree
____2. Slightly agree
____3. Irrelevant
____4. Slightly disagree
____5. Definitely disagree

5. Other people do not realize how frustrated I get when I cannot hear or understand. Comments:

____1. Definitely agree
____2. Slightly agree
____3. Irrelevant
____4. Slightly disagree
____5. Definitely disagree

6. People sometimes avoid me because of my hearing loss. Comments

____1. Definitely agree
____2. Slightly agree
____3. Irrelevant
____4. Slightly disagree
____5. Definitely disagree

Socialization

7. I am not an "outgoing" person because I have a hearing loss. Comments:

____1. Definitely agree
____2. Slightly agree
____3. Irrelevant
____4. Slightly disagree
____5. Definitely disagree

8. I now take less of an interest in many things as compared to when I did not have a hearing problem. Comments:

____1. Definitely agree
____2. Slightly agree
____3. Irrelevant
____4. Slightly disagree
____5. Definitely disagree

9. I am not a calm person because of my hearing loss. Comments:

____1. Definitely agree
____2. Slightly agree
____3. Irrelevant
____4. Slightly disagree
____5. Definitely disagree

10. I tend to be negative about life in general because of my hearing loss.

_____1. Definitely agree
_____2. Slightly agree
_____3. Irrelevant
_____4. Slightly disagree
_____5. Definitely disagree

11. I do not socialize as much as I did before I began to lose my hearing. Comments:

_____1. Definitely agree
_____2. Slightly agree
_____3. Irrelevant
_____4. Slightly disagree
_____5. Definitely disagree

12. Since I have trouble hearing, I do not like to participate in activities. Comments:

_____1. Definitely agree
_____2. Slightly agree
_____3. Irrelevant
_____4. Slightly disagree
_____5. Definitely disagree

13. Since I have trouble hearing, I hesitate to meet new people. Comments:

_____1. Definitely agree
_____2. Slightly agree
_____3. Irrelevant
_____4. Slightly disagree
_____5. Definitely disagree

14. Other people do not understand what it is like to have a hearing loss. Comments:

_____1. Definitely agree
_____2. Slightly agree
_____3. Irrelevant
_____4. Slightly disagree
_____5. Definitely disagree

15. I do not feel relaxed or comfortable in a communicative situation. Comments:

_____1. Definitely agree
_____2. Slightly agree
_____3. Irrelevant
_____4. Slightly disagree
_____5. Definitely disagree

Communication

16. Because I have difficulty understanding what is said to me, I sometimes answer questions wrong. Comments:

_____1. Definitely agree
_____2. Slightly agree
_____3. Irrelevant
_____4. Slightly disagree
_____5. Definitely disagree

17. Conversations in a noisy room prevent me from attempting to communicate with others. Comments:

_____1. Definitely agree
_____2. Slightly agree
_____3. Irrelevant
_____4. Slightly disagree
_____5. Definitely disagree

18. I am not comfortable having to communicate in a group situation. Comments:

_____1. Definitely agree
_____2. Slightly agree
_____3. Irrelevant
_____4. Slightly disagree
_____5. Definitely disagree

19. I seldom watch other people's facial expressions when talking to them. Comments:

_____1. Definitely agree
_____2. Slightly agree
_____3. Irrelevant
_____4. Slightly disagree
_____5. Definitely disagree

20. Most people do not know how to talk to a hearing-impaired person. Comments:

_____1. Definitely agree
_____2. Slightly agree
_____3. Irrelevant
_____4. Slightly disagree
_____5. Definitely disagree

21. I hestitate to ask people to repeat if I do not understand them the first time they speak. Comments:

_____1. Definitely agree
_____2. Slightly agree
_____3. Irrelevant
_____4. Slightly disagree
_____5. Definitely disagree

22. Because I have difficulty understanding what is said to me, I sometimes make comments that do not fit the conversation. Comments:

_____1. Definitely agree
_____2. Slightly agree
_____3. Irrelevant
_____4. Slightly disagree
_____5. Definitely disagree

23. I do not like to admit that I have a hearing problem. Comments:

_____1. Definitely agree
_____2. Slightly agree
_____3. Irrelevant
_____4. Slightly disagree
_____5. Definitely disagree

Specific Difficulty Listening Situations

24. I have trouble hearing the radio or the television unless I turn the volume on very loud. Comments:

_____1. Definitely agree
_____2. Slightly agree
_____3. Irrelevant
_____4. Slightly disagree
_____5. Definitely disagree

25. If someone calls me when by back is turned, I do not always hear him. Comments:

_____1. Definitely agree
_____2. Slightly agree
_____3. Irrelevant
_____4. Slightly disagree
_____5. Definitely disagree

26. If someone calls me from another room I have much trouble hearing. Comments:

_____1. Definitely agree
_____2. Slightly agree
_____3. Irrelevant
_____4. Slightly disagree
_____5. Definitely disagree

27. When I sit talking with friends in a quiet room, I have a great deal of difficulty hearing. Comments:

_____1. Definitely agree
_____2. Slightly agree
_____3. Irrelevant
_____4. Slightly disagree
_____5. Definitely disagree

28. When I use the phone, I have much difficulty hearing. Comments:

_____1. Definitely agree
_____2. Slightly agree
_____3. Irrelevant
_____4. Slightly disagree
_____5. Definitely disagree

29. When I play cards, understanding my partner gives me much difficulty. Comments:

_____1. Definitely agree
_____2. Slightly agree
_____3. Irrelevant
_____4. Slightly disagree
_____5. Definitely disagree

30. At lectures or discussions I have much difficulty hearing the speaker, Comments:

_____1. Definitely agree
_____2. Slightly agree
_____3. Irrelevant
_____4. Slightly disagree
_____5. Definitely disagree

31. In church, when the minister gives the sermon, I have much difficulty. Comments:

_____1. Definitely agree
_____2. Slightly agree
_____3. Irrelevant
_____4. Slightly disagree
_____5. Definitely disagree

32. When a movie is shown, I have much difficulty hearing what is said. Comments:

_____1. Definitely agree
_____2. Slightly agree
_____3. Irrelevant
_____4. Slightly disagree
_____5. Definitely disagree

33. I have difficulty understanding announcements sent through the loudspeaker even when the speaker is in the same room. Coments:

_____1. Definitely agree
_____2. Slightly agree
_____3. Irrelevant
_____4. Slightly disagree
_____5. Definitely disagree

34. I have trouble understanding messages sent over the intercom. Comments:

_____1. Definitely agree
_____2. Slightly agree
_____3. Irrelevant
_____4. Slightly disagree
_____5. Definitely disagree

6E

Nursing Home Hearing Handicap Index (NHHI): Self Version for Resident*

	Very Often				Almost Never
1. When you are with other people do you wish you could hear better?	5	4	3	2	1
2. Do other people feel you have a hearing problem (when they try to talk to you)?	5	4	3	2	1
3. Do you have trouble hearing another person if there is a radio or TV playing (in the same room)?	5	4	3	2	1
4. Do you have trouble hearing the radio or TV?	5	4	3	2	1
5. (How often) do you feel life would be better if you could hear better?	5	4	3	2	1
6. How often are you embarrassed because you don't hear well?	5	4	3	2	1
7. When you are alone do you wish you could hear better?	5	4	3	2	1
8. Do people (tend to) leave you out of conversations because you don't hear well?	5	4	3	2	1
9. (How often) do you withdraw from social activities (in which you ought to participate) because you don't hear well?	5	4	3	2	1
10. Do you say "what" or "pardon me" when people first speak to you?	5	4	3	2	1

Total _____ × 2 = _____

$$\frac{-20}{\underline{\hspace{2cm}}} \times 1.25 = \underline{\hspace{1.5cm}}\%$$

* Words in parentheses are optional when items are read to the resident. Reprinted by permission from Schow, R. L., and Nerbonne, M. A., Assessment of hearing handicap by nursing home residents and staff. *J. Acad. Rehab. Audiol.*, **10**, 2–12 (1977).

6F

Nursing Home Hearing Handicap Index (NHHI): Staff Version*

	Very Often				Almost Never
1. When this person is with other people does he/she need to hear better?	5	4	3	2	1
2. Do members of the staff, family and friends make negative comments about this person's hearing problem?	5	4	3	2	1
3. Do they have trouble hearing another person if there is a radio or TV playing in the same room?	5	4	3	2	1
4. When this person is listening to radio or TV do they have trouble hearing?	5	4	3	2	1
5. How often do you feel life would be better for this person if they could hear better?	5	4	3	2	1
6. How often are they embarrassed because they don't hear well?	5	4	3	2	1
7. When they are alone do they need to hear the everyday sounds of life better?	5	4	3	2	1
8. Do people tend to leave them out of conversations because they don't hear well?	5	4	3	2	1
9. How often do they withdraw from social activities in which they ought to participate because they don't hear well?	5	4	3	2	1
10. Do they say "what" or "pardon me" when people first speak to them?	5	4	3	2	1

Total _____ × 2 = _____

$$\frac{-20}{}$$

_____ × 1.25 = _____%

* Reprinted by permission from Schow, R. L., and Nerbonne, M. A., Assessment of hearing handicap by nursing home residents and staff. *J. Acad. Rehab. Audiol.*, **10**, 2–12 (1977).

APPENDIX

6G

Communications Assessment Procedure for Seniors (CAPS)*

NAME: _____ DATE: _____ BIRTHDATE: _____ SEX: ____
ADDRESS: _____
TELEPHONE: _____ PRE-SERVICE: _____ POST-SERVICE: _____

A. General Communication

1. Do you avoid talking to other people because of your hearing problem?

Always _____   Never _____
Sometimes _____   Not applicable _____

2. Do you talk with your roomate?

Always _____   Never _____
Sometimes _____   Not applicable _____

3. Do you talk with people during the social activities of this home?

Always _____   Never _____
Sometimes _____   Not applicable _____

4. Do you talk with people during your meals?

Always _____   Never _____
Sometimes _____   Not applicable _____

5. Do you talk to the staff here?

Always _____   Never _____
Sometimes _____   Not applicable _____

6. Do you have trouble hearing in certain situations? (Example: watching television, listening to the radio, etc.)

Always _____   Never _____
Sometimes _____   Not applicable _____

Comments: Can you tell me more about your listening situations here?

B. GROUP SITUATIONS

1. Do you feel relaxed in group situations?

Always _____   Never _____
Sometimes _____   Not applicable _____

---

* Reprinted by permission from Alpiner, J. G., and Baker, B. R., unpublished study.

2. Do you ask a person to repeat if you don't understand what he says?

Always _____   Never _____
Sometimes _____   Not applicable _____

3. Does it make you nervous to ask a person to repeat what he said?

Always _____   Never _____
Sometimes _____   Not applicable _____

4. Does it make you nervous to tell a person you have a hearing problem?

Always _____   Never _____
Sometimes _____   Not applicable _____

5. Do you think your hearing problem annoys other people?

Always _____   Never _____
Sometimes _____   Not applicable _____

6. Do you get annoyed when people don't speak loudly enough for you to hear?

Always _____   Never _____
Sometimes _____   Not applicable _____

7. Do you feel isolated from group discussions because of your hearing loss?

Always _____   Never _____
Sometimes _____   Not applicable _____

C. Other Persons: Family, Friends, and Staff

1. Do you think other people understand what it's like to have a hearing problem?

Always _____   Never _____
Sometimes _____   Not applicable _____

2. Do others avoid you because of your hearing loss?

Always _____   Never _____
Sometimes _____   Not applicable _____

3. Does anyone ever leave you out of conversations because of your hearing problem?

Always _____   Never _____
Sometimes _____   Not applicable _____

4. Do you mind telling people that you have a hearing loss?

Always _____   Never _____
Sometimes _____   Not applicable _____

5. Do other people understand how frustrated you get when you can't hear them?

Always _____   Never _____
Sometimes _____   Not applicable _____

Comments: Tell me how other people, like your friends, your family, and the staff here react to your hearing loss.

D. Self-Concept

1. Would you describe yourself as a relaxed person?

Always _____   Never _____
Sometimes _____   Not applicable _____

2. Does your hearing loss make you irritable?

Always _____   Never _____
Sometimes _____   Not applicable _____

3. Do you like living here?

Always _____   Never _____
Sometimes _____   Not applicable _____

4. Are you an interesting person?

Always _____   Never _____
Sometimes _____   Not applicable _____

5. Are you a happy person?

Always _____   Never _____
Sometimes _____   Not applicable _____

6. Do you keep busy with hobbies and other activities?

Always _____   Never _____
Sometimes _____   Not applicable _____

Comments: Is there anything else you'd like to tell me about yourself or about living here?

E. Family

Do you have a family? How much do you see your family? Where do they live? (If the person does not have family, do not use this section.)

1. Does your family get annoyed with you when you can't hear them?

Always _____   Never _____
Sometimes _____   Not applicable _____

2. Do they make decisions for you because of your hearing loss?

Always _____   Never _____
Sometimes _____   Not applicable _____

3. Does your family leave you out of discussions because of your hearing loss?

Always _____   Never _____
Sometimes _____   Not applicable _____

4. Do members of your family speak loudly enough for you to hear them?

Always _____   Never _____
Sometimes _____   Not applicable _____

5. Does your family understand what its like to have a hearing problem?

Always _____   Never _____
Sometimes _____   Not applicable _____

Comments: How does your family feel about your hearing loss?

F. Rehabilitation

1. Do you think you need help in overcoming your hearing problem?

Always _____   Never _____
Sometimes _____   Not applicable _____

2. Are you a good listener?

   Always _____   Never _____
   Sometimes _____   Not applicable _____

3. Do you watch facial expressions when someone is speaking to you?

   Always _____   Never _____
   Sometimes _____   Not applicable _____

4. Do you watch gestures, or "body language" when someone is talking to you?

   Always _____   Never _____
   Sometimes _____   Not applicable _____

5. Do you have a hearing aid? (If person responds yes, proceed.)

   Yes _____   No _____

6. Do you wear your hearing aid?

   Always _____   Never _____
   Sometimes _____   Not applicable _____

   Comments: If lipreading training were available, would you be interested in attending?

7

The Adult Deaf Client and Rehabilitation*

Donald D. Johnson, Ph.D. and
Kathleen E. Crandall, Ph.D.

Since communication is a process which involves the whole human person, and since communication is fundamental to normal human development, it becomes priority number one (Denton, 1971).

Denton's statement was made with respect to the needs of deaf children. However, deaf children become deaf adults, and thus, the statement applies to hearing-impaired persons of all ages. His view of the important role communication plays in normal human development is shared by others, including Sanders (1971): "A hearing loss may result in difficulties in emotional and social behavior, in educational progress, or in vocational placement. However, at the core of these problems rests a breakdown in the process of communication."

This chapter will deal primarily with methods for assessing and subsequent remediation of the communication needs of adult deaf clients. However, as both Denton and Sanders have indicated, deafness may have a profound effect on the "whole" person. Thus, any audiologist or speech-language pathologist considering a program of remediation for

hearing-impaired adults should be prepared to deal with other aspects of those persons' lives, including educational status, personal and social development, and employment status. Therefore, preliminary sections of this chapter will be directed at describing the educational and employment status of deaf adults and the personal and social problems that may be encountered during any remediation process. The last portion of this chapter will be devoted to the defining, planning, and remediation of the communication (hearing, English, speech, speechreading, and manual/simultaneous) needs of the deaf adult.

DEFINITION OF TARGET POPULATION

Schein and Delk (1974), in the first national study of the numbers and characteristics of deaf persons carried out in 40 years, delimited their target population by concentrating on the "prevocationally deaf;" that is, those persons whose hearing loss occurred before adulthood and "who could not hear and understand speech and who had lost (or never had) that ability prior to 19 years of age." This definition accounts for both degree of impairment and age of onset. The psychologic and educational effects of deafness differ according to age of onset. The results of the study led to an estimated prevalence rate

*This material was produced in the course of an agreement between Rochester Institute of Technology and the U. S. Department of Education.

of 2 persons per 1,000, "or more precisely, 203 per 100,000 population."

The last formal census of the population (U. S. Bureau of Census, 1970) indicated that there were 125,246,372 persons (approximately 62% of the total population) in the United States between the chronological age (CA) of 15 and 64 years. Thus, according to the Schein and Delk formula presented above, approximately 254,250 of these persons would be predicted to be prevocationally deaf.

For the purposes of this chapter, the concept of prevocationally deaf allows an approximation to be made of the number of persons in the total population who could be expected to exhibit severe or profound hearing impairment. Within this chapter the classification system of the Office of Demographic Studies (ODS) at Gallaudet College (Office of Demographic Studies, 1973) will be utilized to classify deaf individuals in relation to amount of hearing loss. According to this system, 65 to 84 dB ANSI constitutes a severe hearing loss; 85 to 98 dB ANSI, a profound hearing loss; and 99 dB + ANSI, a profound plus hearing loss (Johnson, 1974; Moore, 1975a).

The ODS system expands the lower limit of defined deafness to 65 dB ANSI. However, the utilization of this classification system allows the reader to compare the hearing loss for adult deaf populations with 24,345 deaf children enrolled in approximately 581 schools located throughout the United States. In addition, the National Technical Institute for the Deaf (NTID) at Rochester Institute of Technology (RIT), Rochester, NY utilizes the ODS classification system and thus can be used as a representative model of an adult deaf population throughout this chapter.

The definition of "adult" generally differs according to the concepts of maturation or legality. However, in this chapter, because of the census brackets used by the U. S. Bureau of Census (1970) and those used by the U. S. Bureau of Labor Statistics (1976) to describe the civilian labor force, an adult will be defined as a person who has attained a CA of 15 to 64 years.

Thus, a deaf adult is an individual with a hearing loss of 65 dB ANSI or greater in the better ear and who has attained the CA of 15 to 64 years.

EDUCATIONAL STATUS OF DEAF CLIENTS

Continuing education provides educational opportunities for millions of American adults who seek new skills to adapt to an ever-changing world. However, deaf adults cannot use most existing adult education offerings without unique provisions being made to bridge the communication gap (Costello, 1977).

In considering deaf adults, it is essential to discuss general educational status and the implications that status may have on their overall well-being. This section discusses general principles concerning education which could be applied to most, if not all, populations and, in many cases, other handicapping conditions as well as deafness. General educational principles concern primarily such concepts as (1) treating the "whole" person, (2) individualization of instruction, (3) practice, (4) monitored and instruction-centered self instruction, and (5) learning centers.

General Educational Status

In relation to the NTID student population, Walter (1976) stated, "The evaluation of deaf students' academic skills has consistently revealed that English skills are related to the general educational retardation of the young deaf adult." (By English skills, Walter was referring to reading vocabulary, reading comprehension, and writing intelligibility.) Other authors (Crandall, 1975, 1980a; Donnels, 1976; LeBuffe, 1976; Schein and Delk, 1974; Williams and Sussman, 1971) may not always be in accord with the degree or general problem areas related to the educational deficiencies of the average adult deaf client, but they do agree that they do exist in varying amounts within that population. These authors also agree with Walter that the primary cause of their existence is a general deficiency in English or language skills.

For example, Johnson and Kadunc (1980) reported the results of eight types of communication assessment conducted at two residential schools for the deaf. The population studied ($n = 363$) represented all students at both schools between CA 13.6 and 21.5 years. Their findings demonstrate that, for English reading comprehension, the average grade equivalent score for all CA levels was 4.03. There were no significant differences between mean scores at any CA level. These data were interpreted to mean that the average graduate from these two schools would have achieved fourth grade reading skills.

This information corroborates the statements made by Crandall (1980a). "It is well known that deaf students rarely achieve proficiency in the English language, even though they are educated in programs which typically focus on English language instruction for 12 years or more." She cited other authors dealing with large numbers of deaf persons throughout the United States who expressed the viewpoint that "the average reading skills of deaf 18-year-olds and adults are at the 4th grade level." Thus, the average deaf student at the elementary and secondary levels would be expected to progress approximately 0.2 grade level equivalent points per year in reading comprehension during her/his formal education, a fact that "significantly limits occupational choice and community involvement for deaf individuals."

With respect to her research on continuing education for deaf adults, Donnels (1976) made reference to the results of the 1970 National Census of the Deaf Population (see Schein and Delk, 1974), which indicated that "more than half of the deaf adults contacted had not completed high school and 28 percent had only an eighth-grade education or less." From this and other census information she inferred that probably more than 28% of the adult deaf population were in need of Adult Basic Education (ABE) programs.

Donnels explained that, in 1972, Gallaudet College in Washington, D. C., started a Center for Continuing Education to serve primarily deaf adults in the greater Washington area. By 1974–75, the program had expanded to a seven-location program serving Washington, D. C., Maryland, and Virginia. The CA of the average deaf adult being served in ABE classes within these programs was 27.2 years (the range was between 16 and 48 years). According to Donnels, one very significant finding derived from a formal survey of this ABE population was their overwhelming desire to improve their English skills. "They felt that improving their academic skills especially written English was essential to their future success." Sixty-four percent wanted to improve their English in general, 50% wanted to learn to read better, 36% wanted to improve their writing, and 44%

wanted to learn more math. The Donnels report demonstrates that apparently the desire and motivation of deaf adults to upgrade their academic and other skills is present. However, programs to provide the assistance to improve these skills are in most instances not available.

By 1981, the continuing education program at Gallaudet College had further expanded to include the following components according to achieved English skill levels: (1) Adult Basic Education (grade levels K–3) including such course offerings as basic English, math, and survival skills (counting money, banking, money management, vocabulary, and sign language enrichment); (2) Intermediate Studies (grade levels 3–8) which provides a continuation and further development of basic skills; (3) Preparing for College and General Education Diploma (GED) (grade levels 8–12) which provides an intensive review of English and math for those preparing for college entrance exams or for GED exams; (4) English for College Graduates which provides instruction in English (writing, grammar, reading, and composition for those who need "brush-up" skills such as correcting errors in plurality, subject-verb agreement, punctuation, and vocabulary); (5) English for Foreign Students (thus far, enrollment has included students from 10 countries outside of the United States and representing 10 different foreign languages); and (6) Family Sign Language Class which includes basic sign languages for family members of ABE students.

An update of the Donnels study, Costello (1977), reported the results of the stated needs for continuing education of 574 deaf participants from 15 cities located in various areas around the country including Washington, D. C., New Orleans, Indianapolis, Philadelphia, Charlotte, Tulsa, San Jose, Richmond, Concord, San Francisco, Milwaukee, Oakland, Spartansburg, Baltimore, and Denver. Costello cited and accepted the Knowles and Klevins definition of continuing education to refer to "a process whereby persons who no longer attend school on a regular basis undertake sequential and organized activities with the conscious intention of bringing about changes in information, knowledge, understanding, skills, appreciation, and attitudes." This definition excludes post-secondary and vocational education undertaken specifically to attain a degree or certificate. Utilizing a highly structured priority system approach to study which of 18 needs the deaf population considered most important for their continuing education in order to compete successfully in the fast-changing labor market, Costello found that for all cities the top six needs invariably remained the same. In order of priority the list of needs included (1) improvement of language skills; (2) better management of home, property, and money; (3) increased income through better jobs; (4) improved communication and interactions between deaf and hearing persons; (5) reduction of unemployment; and (6) improvement of family life.

As a result of the Costello report (1977), NTID personnel contacted Gallaudet College, and subsequently, as part of a joint effort, (Johnson et al., 1978) conducted a needs assessment in Rochester, New York. The purposes of the assessment were to determine (1) whether NTID alumni living in the Rochester area and adult deaf Rochester consumers would like to continue their education, and (2) what types of education they would prefer. The 28 deaf NTID alumni and 40 deaf Rochester consumers participating in the needs assessment ranged in age from CA 21 to 36 years (mean = 27 years) and CA 21 to 65 years (mean = 41 years), respectively. Table 7.1 presents some results obtained during the assessment.

As can be seen in the table, the priority assigned to specific items varied considerably according to the perceived need of the population involved except in the case of desire to improve English reading and writing skills. However, in all instances but one, for each group, all items remained within the top ten with respect to need and interest.

As a result of the 1977 needs assessment, NTID, together with an existing consortium made up of 18 Rochester Area Colleges (RAC), Rochester, New York, "developed a delivery system of services for the continuing education of deaf adults. . . . This plan can be adapted to other geographic areas of the country." The program was founded by a Federal Grant, Title I, Special Community and Continuing Education. Further information concerning this program can be obtained by contacting RAC, Cutler Union, 560 University Avenue, Rochester, NY 14607.

Table 7.1
Ranking of Top Six Continuing Education Goals Derived from Needs Assessments Performed on Adult Deaf Consumers in 15 Cities across the Country (Costello, 1977) as Compared to the Ranking for the Same Goals for Rochester NTID Alumni and Rochester Adult Deaf Consumers (Rochester Needs Assessment, October 11, 1977)

15 Cities: Deaf Consumers' Goals in Order of Priority ($n = 547$)		Rank for NTID Alumni ($n = 28$)	Rank for Rochester Adult Deaf Consumers ($n = 40$)
Goal	Rank		
Improve their English reading and writing skills	1	2	1
Manage their homes, money, and property wisely	2	7	9
Earn more income through better jobs	3	7	4
Communicate and interact better with hearing persons	4	3	8
Get and hold a job	5	9	7
Improve family life	6	10	11

The information contained within the preceding paragraphs indicates that college and university programs throughout the country which are training audiologists and speech-language pathologists would find a fertile area for the preparation of a special "breed" of remediation expert; that is, a professional whose expertise lies within the realm of continuing education for the deaf adult. In cities with large populations of deaf adults, satellite continuing education programs such as those described by Donnels (1976) and Costello (1977) should be provided. These types of continuing education programs should be the outcome of a cooperative effort among deaf educators, audiologists, speech-language pathologists, English language specialists, social and clinical psychologists, manual/simultaneous communication instructors, technical experts from industry, and job placement personnel. It is essential that all these professionals (1) be knowledgeable concerning all needs which confront the deaf adult, and (2) possess the skills needed to communicate with all members of this population.

General Educational Concepts and Instructional Strategies

Treating the Whole Person—Numerous authors have attended to the need to deal with or treat the "whole" person, especially with reference to all aspects of instruction and services designed specifically for handicapped individuals (Denton, 1971; Frisina and Williams, 1976; Sanders, 1971; Thoreson and Tully, 1971; Williams and Sussman, 1971). The following examples clarify what is meant by treating the whole person.

In discussing the development of all aspects of human behavior, Frisina and Williams (1976) have contrasted the uneven growth in the special learner to that of the conventional learner ". . . growth in the special learner often proceeds in a relatively uneven manner. The progress of his or her learning is often fragmented; therefore, it is essential when promoting and conducting programs developed to overcome learning deficiencies that these programs be designed to affect the whole person." These authors emphasized that in planning programs for the special learner, both the whole learner and the total environment must be given due consideration. By whole learner, they meant "the cognitive learner, the psychomotor learner, the affective learner, and the communicative learner." They defined the total environment as including "the school, the home, and all other teaching-learning resources and recreational loci that influence learner growth and development."

With respect to the types of services which might be required to help the deaf client meet her/his learning needs, Thoreson and Tully (1971) stated that "vocational rehabilitation service programs require a variety of services to be provided by a variety of professions in a totally integrated plan of action. There are major problems, such as surgical procedures, family and financial problems, physical therapy, speech therapy, psychiatric treatment, etc., to be dealt with by allied professionals."

Thus, the idea of dealing with the whole person embraces both the concept of multivariate personality and behavioral characteristics which may be in need of attention and a variety of services and professionals cooperating to effect a satisfactory remediation process. Because of the great variety of problems which may exist for the adult deaf client, including communication, personal and social, cultural and general educational needs, and marginal employment and underemployment, it is essential to assume an individualized or personalized approach to program planning.

Individualized or Personalized Program Planning and Instruction—Johnson (1976b) described the concept of individualized or personalized instruction as it relates to the development of communication skills within a young adult deaf population. Inherent in this approach to instruction are (1) the need to evaluate various aspects of human behavior including the motivation of the client, (2) determination of how the instruction can best be accomplished, and (3) a need to assess the results of the instruction on a continuous basis. Carroll (1975) defined personalized education as ". . . an attempt to achieve a balance between the characteristics of the learner and the learning environment. It is a match of the learning environment with the learner's information, processing strategies, concepts, learning sets, motivational systems achieved, and skills acquired. It is a continuous process." According to Noar (1972), individualized instruction can no longer be considered a luxury. Because of the great number of people to be taught, the great variety in their backgrounds, and finally, the necessity to provide instruction when the learner needs it, ". . . the traditional classroom model will have to be replaced. The learner must be able to begin when the need occurs and at the place and pace most appropriate for him."

Although by the time the deaf client reaches adulthood, he should be only in need of refinement of basic educational, personal, social, and communication skills, such is not always the case. Some deaf adults display various behavioral traits and mannerisms which have not developed much past those which would be expected of the average child or adolescent, while others typically display a surprising amount of mature behavior in all aspects of their development. It is precisely because of these individual differences that individualized program planning and instructional strategies are essential to the remediation process of the adult deaf client. "Special learners have educational needs which exceed those of conventional learners. Special learners deserve learning opportunities which meet their needs. At times their learning resources may be very different than those used by conventional learners of similar ages" (Frisina and Williams, 1976).

Practice—In addition to personalization of student instruction, a great deal of practice must be provided if the student is to continue to demonstrate progress in her/his attempts at development of all skills. The concept of additional practice is especially valid as it relates to development of the communication skills of the adult deaf client.

Haspiel (1969), Hazard (1971), Streng *et al.* (1967), and other persons involved in communication habilitation and rehabilitation emphasize the need for practice in all aspects of communication development for the deaf child and adult. Berger (1972) stated, "speechreading is a skill requiring much study and practice, proficiency coming perhaps only after some years of determined application." Orlando (1975) has been able to demonstrate that reduction of speech articulation errors in a young adult deaf population is directly related to the amount of time spent in instruction.

Thus, practice is an important aspect of any instructional process planned specifically to meet the needs of the adult deaf client, a fact which is especially applicable to the area of communication skill development. Also, motivation is an important ingredient. Subtelny (1976a) demonstrated that deaf students with outgoing, happy-go-lucky, and venturesome personalities are better candidates for speech therapy because of more positive attitudes and greater motivation toward speech improvement.

The results of a questionnaire administered to all students entering NTID during the Summer Session, 1976 ($n = 296$) indicated that 73% of the population was highly motivated to improve their speech skills while only 7% demonstrated little or no interest in embarking on such an endeavor. These data support Donnel's (1976) contention that development of English and other communication skills was high on the list of priorities for deaf adults enrolled in ABE programs in the Washington, D. C. area.

In summary, practice and motivation are both important components of skill development. A skilled therapist working with the adult deaf client should be able to create the type of atmosphere which is not only interesting and challenging, but demonstrates progress, and thus, inspires motivation.

Self-Instruction and the Learning Center—Individualized or personalized instruction, practice, and motivation have all been described as essential ingredients for success in the educational process of the adult deaf client. Self-instruction is only one teaching strategy through which success may be accomplished.

Johnson (1976b) described both the concepts of self-instruction and learning centers as they relate to communication development. These two concepts cannot be separated since they are parts of the whole; that is, self-instruction is the instructional strategy and the learning center is the physical environment in which the instruction is accomplished.

Two types of learning centers have been described by Johnson. The first is a monitored self-instruction learning center in which the client schedules time for additional practice under the supervision of a trained monitor outside of regularly assigned classroom hours. The second is an instruction-centered learning center which is essentially a classroom setting with special spaces provided for students to receive individualized practice during regularly scheduled class periods. Both types provide the client with much needed practice. The major difference is that, in the latter type, students meet in small groups for short periods of instruction pertinent to the type of skill they are attempting to develop. They then spend the remainder of the class period receiving monitored self-instruction in specially designed carrel spaces. The self-instruction is monitored directly by the classroom teacher.

Fig. 7.1 shows a close-up view of a single carrel complete with storage area and hardware. This carrel has been designed to carry out either type of self-instruction procedure in speech refinement, speechreading, manual/simultaneous reception, and auditory training. The hardware includes, (1) a cartridge storage area, (2) a color television monitor, (3) a modified video cartridge playback unit, (4) a specially designed binaural amplifier developed to provide protection to prevent overdriving the headphones while supplying the students with the required sound pressure levels during listening tasks, (5) an

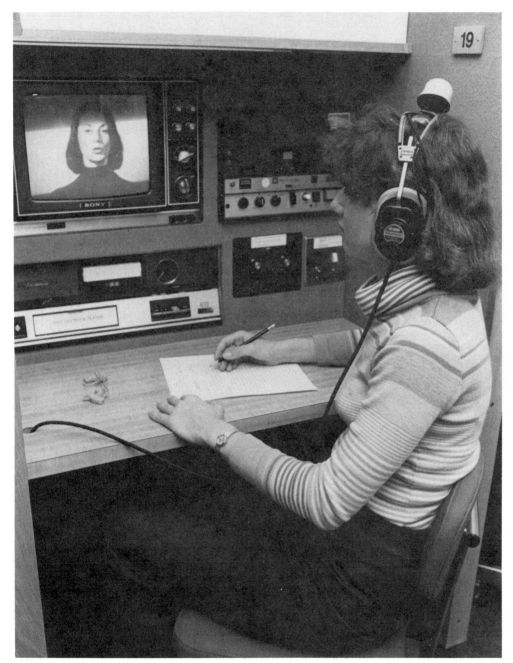

Figure 7.1.   A close-up view of a single monitored self-instructional carrel located within the NTID Communication Self-instruction Laboratory.

audiocassette playback unit, (6) a student headphone with a boom microphone, (7) a student work area, and (8) a secretarial posture swivel chair with carpet casters. Johnson (1976b) and McQuay and Coscarelli (1980) have provided a full description of the special equipment and types of instruction; Snell *et al.* (1976), Snell and Managan (1976), and Jacobs (1975) have described various self-instructional strategies employed within such carrel spaces. Programs providing practice for adult deaf clients can modify both hardware and instructional strategies to meet the needs of their clientele.

Careful analysis of student needs, appropriate media, individual student learning styles, specially trained specialists and aides, and periodic reassessments are all concepts important to the learning center. This type of approach satisfies student needs to begin and continue skill development at their own base level and progress at their own rate. In addition, it is important that all instruction be monitored. Frisina and Williams (1976) stated that in order to ensure productivity and promote a "learner-directed" environment, it is essential that well-informed professional and para-professional staff be continually available to monitor student progress; this is not possible in a non-structured environment. In essence, these authors appear to be of the opinion that exposure to learning materials and situations in an unstructured learning environment will not result in desired outcomes for the learner, but will result in forfeited opportunities and more frustration than the learner can tolerate.

GENERAL PERSONAL AND SOCIAL STATUS OF DEAF CLIENTS

In all the ponderous and opinionated literature on the psychology of the deaf, one astonishing fact stands out beyond dispute: deaf people, on the whole, pass through radically abnormal childhoods and emerge stunningly normal adults. Whatever particular features may distinguish them in general from the hearing, it is their sheer normality, the dazzling ordinariness of their adjustment, that amazes (Benderly, 1980).

Assessment

Potential Problem Areas—Some adult deaf clients may possess psychologic problems which manifest themselves in inappropriate personal and social behavioral traits (Hartbauer, 1975; Levine, 1963; Myklebust, 1950; and Sanders, 1971). Knowledge that certain types of problems of a personal and social nature might exist in a population is of importance to the audiologist, speech-language pathologist and other professionals working with deaf clients from the standpoint of preparation for treatment, counseling/advising, and possible referral. However, it is important to realize that many deaf individuals may not possess any, or perhaps only a few, of the so-called "typical" problems.

Levine (1976) has spoken of "the painful stereotype of 'the' personality of 'the' deaf which has as its principal features emotional immaturity, adaptive rigidity, sociocultural impoverishment, and narrowed intellectual functioning." She speaks of the 30 years of personality studies which have contributed to the making of these stereotypes and the fact that these characteristics would not very well promote 'independent living' for deaf clients. Among other stereotypical traits attributed to the deaf as a group are egocentricity, emotional instability, impulsiveness, tactlessness, low levels of self-esteem, suspicious and narrow-minded natures, self-consciousness, and defensiveness about their inability to hear (Emerton et al., 1979; Garrison et al., 1978a; and Meadow, 1976). These latter authors all stressed, as did Levine, the inappropriateness of stereotyping deaf persons in terms of group personality characteristics.

Some factors which have contributed to the stereotyping of the deaf are (1) inappropriate assessment/evaluation instruments, (2) paper and pencil assessment/evaluation techniques, (3) assessment/evaluation instruments which have been standardized on normal hearing audiences, and (4) inappropriate assessment/evaluation administration procedures (Garrison et al., 1978a; Garrison and Emerton, 1978; Garrison et al., 1978b). For example, Levine (1976) stated that there are those among professional workers with the deaf who view the picture with indignation. "The tests do not tell the true story. There are many who are outraged to find that not even lipservice is given the high heterogeneity known to exist within the deaf population: all deaf persons are stamped with a common personality label." She goes on to state that the deaf personality stereotype continues to persist despite the fact that "no one would argue that it is just as ridiculous to talk of 'the' personality of 'the' hearing as of 'the' personality of 'the' deaf."

Garrison et al. (1978a), for the purpose of comparison, administered the "Tennessee Self Concept Scale (TSCS: Fitts, 1965) to 109 students entering NTID in 1977 and 19 NTID hearing and deaf faculty/staff. This scale was originally standardized on 626 hearing persons from widely differing parts of the country and ranging in age from 12 to 68 years. The general impressions which emerged from analysis of the data for the deaf subjects were those of low self-esteem, confusion and uncertainty in self-perceptions, and the appearance of psychologic stress or maladjustment. When a sample of 30 of the deaf students was retested individually using direct interview techniques and interviewers familiar with the students' preferred mode(s) of communication, the interview data failed to substantiate the findings; and in the case of self-esteem, some evidence was obtained to suggest that there may be a tendency toward slightly inflated self-esteem among this deaf group. As a result of this study, the authors concluded that the deaf students' initial written assessment scores were influenced by both linguistic problems and the paper-and-pencil testing situation, and thus, that the TSCS in its standardized form fails to provide an accurate assessment of the deaf individual's level of self-concept.

The above paragraphs point out the importance of an individualized approach and caution in selection, administration, assessment, and interpretation of test results when attempting to determine the personal and social development needs of deaf clients. Moreover, the authors mentioned above provide evidence in the following paragraphs that "cultural deprivation," and not problems related to inability on the part of deaf persons to develop socially acceptable personality traits is primarily responsible for many of the problems commonly encountered by deaf persons.

To say that there is not a stereotypical deaf personality is not to say that there are not problems which deaf individuals experience in common. However, according to Emerton *et al.* (1979), Layne (1980), Levine (1976), and Meadow (1976), these problems are related to cultural (environmental) deprivation. Levine stressed, moreover, that this cultural deprivation manifests itself in educational and psychologic malnutrition. It is not the outcome of deafness *per se*, but an outcome of failure of those persons in the deaf child's maturational environment to provide enough of those types of experiences necessary for healthy intrapersonal, interpersonal, group, and adaptive societal development.

Emerton *et al.* (1979) came to the conclusion that "Anomalous experience is a source of difficulty for deaf people.... In addition

to not hearing the world around them (for spontaneous or incidental learning), deaf children are often restricted in terms of social environments and experiences.... Experience is a necessary ingredient to social competence."

In an effort to demonstrate the effects of this cultural deprivation on deaf persons, Layne (1980) conducted a year-long ethnographic study in which he interviewed a large number of deaf individuals in a major northeastern city to demonstrate that the manifestations of mental disorders, when they do occur within the deaf community, are culturally bound. These deaf informants described seven problem areas (ranked in order of severity from most to least severe) as being the most prevalent for them and their deaf associates. The problem areas included sex, drinking, dope, money, family, police, and deaf clubs. Table 7.2 shows possible sources of help the deaf informants felt they had available to them when they encounter any of those seven problems mentioned. As can be seen from a review of the table, these deaf persons, often because of problems with communication, feel cut off from many avenues of help typically sought by hearing persons for resolution of their problems. According to Layne, "most primary and secondary sources as listed in the table are deaf people.... Deaf

Table 7.2

Major Problem Areas Envisioned to Exist Within the Deaf Community by Deaf Informants and Primary, Secondary, and Tertiary Sources of Help Elected by Deaf Persons for Problem Resolution [a]

Problem	Primary Help Source	Secondary Help Source	Tertiary Help Source
1. Sex	Deaf friend	Parents	Deaf boy/girl friend
2. Drinking	None [b]	None	None
3. Dope	None	None	None
4. Money	Deaf boy/girl friend	Deaf friend	Parents
5. Family	Deaf boy/girl friend	Deaf friend	— [c]
6. Police	Deaf boy/girl friend	Parents (if deaf)	—
7. Deaf club	Deaf friend	Deaf boy/girl friend	—

[a] The information cited within this table was reproduced directly from a table by Layne (1980).
[b] When the source of help is listed as "None," deaf people will not admit that they have these problems.
[c] —, no tertiary source cited by the informants.

sources offer the comfort of easy communication, even though they may not be able to provide solutions."

Levine (1976) concluded that "cultural deprivation is believed to be an outcome of failure on the part of parents, teachers, peers, etc., to provide information and experiences necessary for human development." As a solution to this cultural deprivation problem that causes many deaf persons to encounter difficulty with the socialization process, Emerton *et al.* (1979) have suggested that professionals working with both deaf children and adults have the responsibility to provide them with as many types of culturally-oriented growth experiences as possible. "It is the responsibility of those involved in the social development of deaf individuals to ensure that the individual has the social competencies needed to move freely within both the hearing and deaf communities." In response to these suggestions, professionals at NTID are in the process of development of courses and supervised, individualized learning experiences which will aid students to develop specific social competencies. These courses and experiences will be discussed in more depth in the following sections.

Comments—The information presented above discusses behavioral trends with respect to personal, social, and cultural development of deaf adults. However, it is necessary to emphasize the fact that one should not conclude that there are stereotypical behavioral traits which are unique to the entire population of deaf individuals. This available information demonstrates the value of an individualized approach toward the assessment of personal and social adjustment. Thus, when counselling is indicated, it should be tailored to meet individual needs. This concept is not in opposition to the value of a small group approach when such appears to be warranted by the homogeneity of the problems of those clients in question.

Instruction Planning

Development of Personal and Social Skills Through Individual Counselling and Therapy—Often the question arises as to who should conduct the counselling sessions when individual guidance or therapy is warranted. Although there does not seem to be any fixed or firm answer to this question, probably it is a matter of the degree or severity of the problem. Under normal circumstances the adult deaf client does not actively seek services directly from a hearing and speech clinic or center. Rather, the need for speech and/or hearing services is determined by a guidance counselor associated with a local office of the State Division of Vocational Rehabilitation (DVR). More often than not, the deaf client does not seek services directly from DVR, but has been referred to them by any one of a number of local sources (Gochnour, 1973; Patterson and Stewart, 1971).

Normally, the DVR counselor will attempt to assess the total needs of the deaf client. When personal or social problems present themselves, DVR makes appropriate referrals to various local organizations such as private family service agencies or various religious organizations or hospital clinics providing such support services. These organizations deal directly with counseling in the areas of intrapersonal/interpersonal and family problems. When the need is related to communication remediation, DVR refers directly to a local hearing and speech clinic, center, or agency and often assumes financial responsibility for services rendered such as purchase of recommended hearing aids and associated accessories. (Note: DVR receives its funding directly from the Federal Government with matching funds from the individual states on an 80/20 basis. One of its primary charges is to promote dependency reduction on the part of handicapped individuals, and, hence help them to become contributing members of society through gainful employment.) In both instances, DVR often maintains management of the client and contact with the organization until such time as remediation has been successfully completed.

During the course of the remediation with an audiologist or speech-language pathologist, the deaf client may disclose a personal or social problem and seek direct guidance from the therapist. When the solution or counselling for the problem(s) is deemed by the therapist to be within her/his realm of skills, there seems to be a growing acceptance that the therapist should provide the counselling or advising services.

For example, a brochure distributed in 1977 by the Teachers Center at the Casa Colina Hospital for Rehabilitative Medicine, located in Pomona, California, announced the forthcoming "Second Annual Workshop on Enriching Counseling Skills with Speech and Hearing Impaired Persons." Quite emphatically (in bold print) the front cover of the brochure read "Counseling Skills An Emerging Necessity for Speech Pathologists and Audiologists."

In addition, Sanders (1971) has emphasized that "a conscientious and concerned therapist will create a suitable climate of mutual trust between herself and the children and adults with whom she is working." Because of the rapport which has been developed, such a client is thus more likely to accept advice and guidance from his therapist than a relative stranger. Sanders also stresses the advantage of periodic guidance from the therapist at the time it may be most effective in lieu of pre-scheduled guidance sessions which may not be readily available when necessary.

When the problem presented is more severe than the hearing or speech clinician can manage, referral for intervention most often is carried out by the DVR counselor with continued support from audiology and speech-language pathology personnel.

It appears that if the audiologist and speech-language pathologist are successfully to involve themselves with communication development and/or guidance counselling with adult deaf clients, it is essential that two conditions exist: (1) they must be skilled and effective simultaneous (speech and manual communication combined) communicators, and (2) they must have preparation in their educational development to recognize personal and social problems when they exist, make an appropriate assessment of the nature and depth of the problem(s), perform guidance and counseling activities when they are within the realm of feasibility, and make appropriate referrals when deemed necessary. These same two conditions pertain to any professional or para-professional persons providing direct services for the adult deaf client.

Concerning the stated need for audiologists and speech-language pathologists to communicate effectively through the simultaneous communication approach, a recent unpublished study conducted by this author at NTID revealed that among those students

entering NTID during the Summer Session, 1976 ($n = 242$), there were essentially three distinct populations with respect to primary mode of information reception: (1) those (approximately 34%) who received information primarily through manual communication (sign language and/or fingerspelling) and had very poorly developed skills for speech-reading with sound (this population increased according to severity of hearing loss); (2) those (approximately 28%) who appeared to be equally facile with both manual communication and speechreading with sound; and (3) those (approximately 24%) who were good at receiving information through speechreading and listening combined, but received very little from manual communication. The remaining 14% were not facile with any mode of information reception. (The techniques for securing this information will be discussed in the section of this chapter dealing with communication assessment.)

The implications to be drawn here are highly supportive of the concept that all persons providing services for adult deaf clients be capable of communicating through all modes of expression and reception including the simultaneous communication approach. This concept of facility with multiple communication modes is also supported by McGowan and Vescovi (1971) as regards counsellors working with the deaf. These authors stated that since deaf people, as a group, use multiple modes of communication expression and reception, ". . .the counselor must be able to understand them all and to apply them himself, as needed, with a deaf individual."

Davis (1976) demonstrated that there is a growing trend for audiologists to attempt to develop skills in manual communication techniques. Questionnaires were forwarded to 70 university programs throughout the country. Of the 36 respondents, 20 indicated that they offer courses in manual communication. Eight of these 20 universities required participation in manual communication courses. Seven of 17 universities offering courses in psychology of deafness required such courses before conferral of the baccalaureate or master's degree in audiology. There is no indication as to whether these courses contained units and/or practicum in personal counselling. However, in a follow-up survey by Garstecki (1978), high on the list of continuing education courses requested by 258 respondent audiologists (37% usable response rate, *n* = 697 questionnaires mailed) were courses in (1) counselling theory and technique, (2) manual communication, and (3) total communication: clinical practicum was desired in the areas of (a) school for the deaf (academic tutoring), and (b) providing counselling services.

The picture for provision of counselling services for the deaf client has been fairly bleak until recently. According to Williams and Sussman (1971), the deaf person is in need of various types of counselling services which have generally not been provided in the past. However, these authors are optimistic that the scene is beginning to change for three reasons. "The first is that deaf people have demonstrated their receptiveness to counselling and their capacities to benefit from it. Second, within the counselling professions there is an increasing awareness of the counselling needs of deaf people. Finally, important progress is being made with respect to the recruitment and training of professional counselors to work with deaf people of all ages." That this claim may indeed be true is no rationale for teacher training programs for speech-language pathologists and audiologists to neglect this important aspect (counselling) of their educational process. It does lend support to the concept that all professionals working with clients should work as a closely integrated team.

Development of Personal and Social Skills Through Courses and Group Counselling—Some therapy or counselling in the areas of personal and social skills development must take place on an individualized basis for obvious reasons. Other problems are not only more amenable to, but require, a group approach. "Problems which arise out of the experience of working together in a training group are examined with the aim of improving the group's effectiveness or the individual's effectiveness as a member of the group. Thus, people learn by their own experience" (Berger and Berger, 1972). Sanders (1971) extols some of the virtues of group learning. "The student also has available to him the comments and reactions of a group of people

who share many of the problems that he experiences." Other virtues of group learning, according to Sanders, include stimulation of motivation through competitiveness, development of mutual sympathy and cooperation, increase in security as a result of shared difficulties, and encouragement of discussion of social experiences. However, Sanders warns that "the success or failure of any kind of group is heavily dependent upon the compatibility of its members."

An excellent example of the type of therapy for the adult deaf client which requires a group approach is called "Interpersonal Communication" (Kelly, 1975; Kelly and Subtelny, 1980). The objectives of this course are (1) to develop skills in attending to the opinions expressed by others, (2) to improve skills in expressing personal opinions and responding to others, (3) to increase confidence and initiative in making introductions within varied social circumstances, (4) to increase competence and provide experience in approaching typical problem situations appropriately, and (5) to familiarize the student with the basic principles of good interpersonal communication and relate these principles to the interview process.

The rationale for development of this course was based upon the results of a 20-item questionnaire administered to 109 students entering NTID during the Summer Session, 1974. The data suggested that approximately 49% of these students could benefit from a basic level course in interpersonal communication while 42% would more appropriately be placed in a more advanced level course. Only 9% of the population demonstrated adequate knowledge of the projected course content. Answers to some of the questions indicated that many students did not choose to introduce themselves in a social situation (53%), attempted communication only after they got to know a person (55%), did not think they should introduce themselves on the first day of employment (61%), did not know how to begin a conversation (22%), did not understand the primary purpose of a job interview (28%), and indicated an inappropriate response when faced with a problem situation (54%).

Group interaction can be used to emphasize special problems which often confront hearing-impaired individuals and other group strategies can provide the deaf client with direct experiences from which to judge his own performance. These strategies include role-playing techniques, group analysis and discussion of problems, lectures, and videotaped demonstrations of good and poor techniques of interpersonal communication. Other examples of lecture and interactive discussion-type courses are exemplified in Table 7.3. These and many other courses not listed in Table 7.3 have been specifically designed to help young adult, deaf, college students at NTID to strengthen and/or develop their personal, social, and cultural skills. Currently, 38 courses are available to NTID students under the following general headings: (1) general education core, (2) personal skills development, (3) social skills development (4) social heritage, (5) career/job development,

(6) creative arts, and (7) independent study. Because of space constraints, the table presents only a few suggested topics for inclusion within each of those courses listed.

It is recommended that professionals involved or interested in providing the adult deaf client with group-type remediation in these and related areas make an assessment of the problems and needs of their respective populations to determine the exact content, instructional strategies, and methods for evaluating progress before proceeding with instruction. Frisina and Williams (1976) emphasized that appropriate planning and management are the processes through which a therapist can substantially increase the probability that optimum growth and development can occur for the handicapped learner. These authors stated that "characteristic

Table 7.3

Course Titles and Descriptors for Group Instruction Designed to Help the Adult Deaf Client Develop Personal, Social, and Cultural Skills Essential for Dependency Reduction and Success on the Job and in the Community

Course Title[a]	Course Description[a]
Dimensions of College Life[b]	Suggested topics: academic settings, living situations, leisure settings, community and academic planning
The Job Search Process[b]	Suggested topics: completing employment application forms, writing and updating personal resumes, the employment interview situation, nature and purpose of the job interview, appearance and responses
Life after College[b]	Suggested topics: marriage and the family, law and the average American, continuing education
The World of Work	Suggested topics: the job search process, co-worker relationships on the job, relationships with the supervisors, understanding job benefits
Leadership Development	Suggested topics: trust building, attending and listening skills, one- and two-way communication, group leadership-fellowship, styles of leadership, leadership roles, formal and informal inclusion
Personal Finance	Suggested topics: budgeting, credit, bank services, sources of income, insurance, taxes, house and apartment expenses, investment
Adjusting to Deafness	Suggested topics: recent research in deafness, deaf clubs and organizations, contributions of deaf persons in education, business, industry, athletics, performing arts, art, literature
Basic Human Sexuality	Suggested topics: human sexuality, pregnancy, birth control, abortion, venereal diseases, hereditary aspects of deafness
Drug and Alcohol Usage	Suggested topics: major drug and alcohol categories, effects of drugs and alcohol, psychologic dependency, State drug and alcohol laws

[a] For a complete detailed description and additional information concerning all course offerings, requests may be directed to the Chairperson, Academic Department for Human Development, NTID, One Lomb Memorial Drive, Rochester, NY 14623.
[b] Courses recommended for all NTID students.

needs of special students demand a particular quality and type of educational system that puts time at a premium and is learner-directed." This is particularly true of the congenitally deaf adult population, as evidenced in a preceding section on educational deprivation.

Audiologists and speech-language pathologists may find themselves directly involved with provision of the type of group instruction or counselling mentioned in the previous paragraphs. However, they may find themselves managing such instruction through intervention with local deaf clubs and organizations or special continuing education programs designed especially for the adult deaf. Again, it is necessary to emphasize that those persons attempting to manage and/or provide instructional programs for the adult deaf must be prepared to communicate with these clients in a flexible manner utilizing those modes of communication expression and reception most conducive to learning. Evidence to support this viewpoint has been cited by Williams and Sussman (1971). These authors speak of the direct and far-reaching consequences that the communication problem imposes on deaf persons. "It affects every aspect of his life. Other problem areas exist principally because of it. His degree of adjustment and achievement in all of his activities is primarily dependent on aspects of his communication skills." Williams and Sussman also stated that transmitting (receiving and sending) deficiencies of the deaf individual are manifested in the written, spoken, and manual aspects of her/his inferior language skills.

Thus, an adequate assessment of all expressive and receptive communication parameters, especially English skills (reading comprehension and writing intelligibility), must be undertaken before determination of any instructional program for these deaf clients.

EMPLOYMENT STATUS OF DEAF CLIENTS

Our Adult Basic Education program this year had about seventy enrollments per semester with a core of about fifty regularly attending students. . . . Many students expressed dissatisfaction with their jobs or wanted to change or advance on the job. They felt that improving their academic skills especially written English was essential to their future success (Donnels, 1976).

The relationship between employment status and the communication skills of the adult deaf client will become more apparent within this section. However, to understand better the employment status of the deaf client, it is essential first to define such terms as the civilian labor force, labor force participation rate, employed, unemployed, primary and secondary employment, underemployment, and marginal employment. Second, it is necessary to explore employment in terms of (1) the general employment outlook, and (2) educational attainment, educational opportunities, and their relationship to employment.

Definitions

Schein and Delk (1974) have explored the employment picture of the adult deaf from the standpoint of most of the following definitions, which were derived from both the U. S. Bureau of Labor Statistics (1974) and U. S. Bureau of Census (1972) reports. An attempt will be made to adhere to these definitions within this section wherever appropriate. Any deviation from the definitions will be duly noted.

Civilian Labor Force—The civilian labor force consists of individuals classified as employed or unemployed in accordance with the criteria described below (minor modification of Schein and Delk, 1974).

Employed—This category is comprised of all civilians 16 years old and over who either (1) were "at work," those who did any work at all as paid employees or in their own business or profession, or on their own farm, or who worked 15 hours or more as unpaid workers on a family farm or in a family business; or (2) were "with a job, but not at work," those who did not work during the reference week but had jobs or businesses from which they were temporarily absent due to illness, bad weather, industrial dispute, vacation, or other personal reasons (minor modification of Schein and Delk, 1974).

Unemployed—Unemployed persons were civilians 16 years old and over and (1) were neither "at work" nor "with a job, but not at work" during the reference week, (2) were looking for work during the past 4 weeks, and (3) were available to accept a job. Also included are persons who did not work at all during the reference week and were waiting to be called back to a job from which they had been laid off (minor modification of Schein and Delk, 1974).

Not in Labor Force—Not in the labor force refers to all non-institutionalized persons 16 years or older who are not actively seeking employment and are not included as part of the labor force according to the above definitions for employed or unemployed. According to the U. S. Bureau of Labor Statistics (1974), this includes persons engaged in home housework, in school, unable to work because of long term physical or mental illness, and other persons who are retired, too old to work, or voluntarily idle whether on a temporary or permanent basis (U. S. Bureau of Labor Statistics, 1976).

Participation Rate—The general participation rate includes that proportion of the non-institutional population that is part of the labor force. It is the ratio between the total labor force and the total non-institutionalized population (U. S. Bureau of Labor Statistics, 1976).

Primary and Secondary Employment—Within the confines of this chapter, a distinction will be made between primary and secondary labor force employment. Primary employment refers to those jobs which have a specific hierarchical structure or career ladders, and thus, the possibility of upward mobility or desirable lateral mobility. Secondary employment refers to those jobs which are lacking in career ladders, and hence, have no potential for mobility of any kind. These jobs are characterized by sporadic employment since they tend to be interim in nature (authors' definition).

Underemployment—"... employment in positions incompatible with the worker's intelligence, skills, and education" (Schein and Delk, 1974).

Marginally Employed—A marginally employed individual is one who, due to lack of opportunity or for reasons of a personal nature, periodically or aperiodically, moves into and out of the labor force. An example would be a mother bearing a child who later returns to the labor force (authors' definition).

When making any comparison between the employment status of the adult deaf population and the general population, it is essential that the concepts imbedded within the above definitions be adhered to rather rigidly. Otherwise the employment characteristics are

apt to be inflated or deflated, as so often happens. Generally, for ease of understanding, the definitions can be aligned according to the following scheme.

Total Civilian Non-Institutionalized Population
1. Total Civilian Labor Force Participation Rate
   A. Employed
      (1) Primary Employment
      (2) Secondary Employment
      (3) Marginal Employment
   B. Unemployed
2. Not in the Civilian Labor Force
   A. Temporary
   B. Permanent

General Employment Outlook

Unemployment—Data resulting from a study conducted to examine the unemployment rate of young deaf adults in a seven-state area in the southwestern United States indicated that an estimated 25% of the population between the ages of 16 and 31 years were unemployed during 1964–1965 (Kronenberg and Blake, 1966). A similar study conducted in the state of Oregon during 1966–1967 found that an estimated 21% of the employable deaf between the ages of 24 and 54 years were unemployed (Berger et al., 1972). A third study (Delgado, 1963), which surveyed the employment status of individuals graduating from the California School for the Deaf at Berkeley from 1959 to 1963, found a 30% unemployment rate among the employable deaf. The inordinately high unemployment rates found in these three studies should be viewed with caution since they appear to be a consequence of population definition as described above and appear to include those persons not in the labor force.

Other authors (Quigley, 1966; Schein and Delk, 1974; Williams and Sussman, 1971) are in agreement that it is not only the unemployment rate, but underemployment which continues to plague the adult deaf population. The Schein and Delk (1974) and Schein (1978) studies are in alignment with the definitions for labor force, rate of employment and unemployment, and total civilian population utilized by the U. S. Bureau of Labor Statistics (1974). Thus, Schein and Delk and Schein information will be utilized herein to summarize the employment status of deaf adults in general.

According to Schein and Delk, in 1972, 2.9% of all deaf males between CA 16–64 years in the labor force were unemployed, as compared to 4.9% of their hearing counterparts. The largest population of unemployed males fell between CA 16–24 years with an unemployment figure of 8.9%. However, even this latter figure compared favorably with the 12.6% unemployment rate for the general population in the same age bracket.

Deaf females in the labor force (CA 16–64 years) fared less favorably when compared with the total female population, with unemployment rates of 10.2 and 6.6%, respectively. Non-white deaf males and females in the labor force showed significantly greater rates of unemployment than did either of their respective white counterparts.

Generally speaking, approximately 80.3% of all deaf males and 50.0% of all deaf females (CA 16–64 years) were considered part of the labor force in 1972. These participation rates were approximately equal for men and 6% higher than for women in the general population with figures of 80 and 44%, respectively. A follow-up study in 1977 performed by Schein (1978) and his colleagues sampled deaf adults from the 1972 census with a subsample of young deaf people who had been in school at the time of the 1972 study. The resulting data ($n = 476$) demonstrated that labor-force participation rates for both deaf males and females declined between 1972 and 1977 by 5.5 and 2.8%, respectively. These declines were contrary to national trends.

According to Schein (1978), unemployment for all deaf labor force participants (CA 16–64 years) increased during this five-year period by 1.3% from 9.6 to 10.9%. Deaf males in this CA category suffered most with a 4.8% decline in employment from 5.4 to 10.2% while the unemployment picture for deaf females improved by 4.5% from 16.5 to 12.0%.

The Schein and Delk (1974) and Schein (1978) studies contain a wealth of additional specific information concerning the employment status of deaf adults. The reader is referred to these sources for more detailed descriptions. The fact is that underemployment rather than unemployment seems to be the greatest problem area for deaf adults. However, the Bureau of Labor Statistics of the U. S. Department of Labor, the government agency that collects the largest amount of data annually on employment and unemployment nationally, has been unable to develop a methodology that would accurately measure underemployment as it concerns the relationship between quality of job and skill of the job holder (Klein, 1973 as cited by Grant et al., 1980). The matter of underemployment as it relates to NTID students will be discussed more throughly in the next subsection.

In an effort to examine the part that advanced education can play in the solution of some of the unemployment problems faced by so many deaf adults, the National Technical Institute for the Deaf (NTID) of Rochester Institute of Technology (RIT) examined the data generated by circulation of a five-page Alumni Feedback Questionnaire (AFQ) through a mail survey. The AFQ was mailed in 1977 to 644 deaf students certified as graduates from RIT through NTID between the the academic years 1968 and 1977 with a 63% response rate ($n = 407$). The AFQ was slightly modified to add a few new questions and was redistributed at the end of the 1978 academic year to 832 certified graduates with a 57.3% response rate ($n = 477$). A comparison of demographic data on those who returned questionnaires during both mailings matches that of the total graduate group indicating that those who returned questionnaires are a representative, non-biased sample. The question addressed was: "Has the education provided by NTID at RIT made any difference for this population of young adult deaf individuals?" Parker and Welsh (1980) made the following general observations as a result of their review of the data.

...Deaf graduates of NTID are highly mobile. Average salary increases for 1978 exceed both the Consumer Price Index and the National Earnings growth. Salaries grow as graduates increase their professional experience.

Graduates have a comparatively low unemployment rate. Those unemployed are only so temporarily and the vast majority of employed graduates are employed full time.

Graduates are employed primarily in occupations which historically have employed few deaf individuals.

The predominent reasons for changing jobs among deaf graduates of NTID at RIT are personal choices for positive professional growth. Unemployed graduates are active in using a wide variety of resources in their job search efforts.

A vast majority of deaf graduates of NTID at RIT are actively involved in furthering their education, primarily for improving their technical skills for their current job.

Graduates chose their place of residence for a variety of reasons, most of which are not related to the fact that they are deaf.

Graduates indicate positive feelings about their jobs and their employers, and the employers and fellow employees seem to be making substantial efforts to accommodate the deaf employees.

Graduates seem to be making strides toward integration into the greater hearing world.

These findings provide good evidence that NTID at RIT does make a difference. It has broken down, for its deaf graduates, many of the historical barriers of entry into a wide range of professional, educational, and personal/social opportunities.

The following two tables illustrate the labor force participation rate of deaf RIT graduates and the types of employment in which they are involved. Table 7.4 shows the labor force participation rate and employment status of 1155 students who graduated from NTID between 1968 and 1980. When these figures are compared with a similar table constructed for 540 students graduating from NTID be-

tween 1968 and 1976, the percentage of labor force participants remains essentially the same (79%). However, the number of graduates within the labor force who are gainfully employed increased from 94 to 98%. Similarly, of those alumni not in the labor force, those who chose to seek higher education before attempting employment rose from 74 to 76%.

Conversely, the percentage of persons not in the labor force who chose homemaking rather than employment dropped from 13 to 9%. Table 7.4 also shows the percentage of persons who elected to take their initial employment in business and industry (82%), government (11%), and education (7%). These figures have remained essentially the same between 1976 and 1980. These latter figures reflect a broadening shift in the types of employment for deaf adults brought about as a result of the increased post-secondary educational opportunities. For example, Stuckless (1980) states that a study conducted by Lunde and Bigman (1959) which examined the occupations of approximately 8000 employed deaf persons reported that "of all professional and technical personnel...50 percent were teachers employed in schools for the deaf."

Table 7.5 allows a comparison of principal occupations in which adult deaf Americans have traditionally been found and examines some of the changes in types of employment which are beginning to take place as a direct result of increased educational opportunities such as those provided by NTID.

Of interest in Table 7.5 is the large number of deaf NTID graduates who have moved into professional and technical employment as a result of their education, in relation to deaf adults in general (Lunde and Bigman, 1959; Schein and Delk, 1974) and the general population (U. S. Bureau of Census, 1977). In addition, it appears that there is a slight increase in the number of NTID graduates who have moved into management positions which may be an indication of upward mobility. At the same time, fewer graduates (23%) have accepted blue collar employment in relation to all other populations studied. For more details concerning the deaf adult and employment, the reader is referred to Grant et al. (1980), Lunde and Bigman (1959), Parker and Welsh (1980), Schein

Table 7.4
Initial Employment Disposition of all NTID Students Receiving Certificates, Diplomas, and Associate, Baccalaureate, and Master's Degrees from 1968 to 1980 (n = 1155)

Employment Disposition for All Program Completers	Number	Percentage	Percentage Total
Not in labor force			
Attending school	172	76	
Homemakers	21	9	
Voluntary idle	22	10	
Unknown	12	5	
Total	227	100	21
In labor force			
Employed	914	98	
Unemployed	14	2	
Total	928	100	79
Employment sector			
Business and industry	749	82	
Government	101	11	
Education	64	7	
Total	914	100	

Table 7.5
U. S. Census Occupational Classifications with Percentage[a] Distribution Comparisons in Principle Occupations

Principal Occupation	Deaf Population				General Population
	Lunde and Big-man (1959)	Schein and Delk (1974)	RIT Deaf Graduates		U. S. Bureau of the Census (1977) Population
			(1977)[b]	(1978)[b]	
	%		%		%
White Collar					
Professional and technical	6.6	8.8[c]	49.0	46.0	15.3
Managers and administrators	3.2	2.2	1.0	3.0	10.4
Clerical and sales	7.2	15.5	26.5	28.0	24.5
Subtotal	17.0	26.5	76.5	77.0	50.2
Blue Collar					
Craftsmen (skilled)	35.9	21.3	8.0	9.0	13.1
Operatives (semi-skilled)	35.2	35.9	13.0	11.0	15.3
Service workers	6.2	9.4	2.0	1.0	13.7
Laborers	2.6	7.0	1.0	2.0	7.7
Subtotal[d]	79.9	73.6	24.0	23.0	49.8

[a] The percentage figures were adapted from tables developed by Stuckless (1980) and Parker and Welsh (1980).
[b] These figures were generated from data collected as a result of the five-page Alumni Feedback Questionnaire (AFQ) mailed to all certified deaf RIT graduates in 1977 ($n = 407$) and 1978 ($n = 477$). The mailing in 1977 was sent to 644 alumni, and that in 1978 to 832 alumni. Thus, the returns include information from 188 new alumni in 1978 and the remainder may in some cases represent returns from alumni who responded during both mailings. However, in the latter case the alumni may have changed employment categories during the year.
[c] Primarily teachers of the deaf.
[d] Totals of more or less than 100% reflect rounding errors.

(1978), Schein and Delk (1974), Stuckless (1980), and Welsh (1980).

Again this information demonstrates that employment rates for deaf adults can be greatly enhanced by provision of suitable educational opportunities. Moreover, underemployment, which is felt to be so endemic among the adult deaf population in general, can be cut drastically through the educational experience.

Underemployment—Berger et al. (1972), Delgado (1963), Donnels (1976), Kronenberg and Blake (1966), LeBuffe (1976), Quigley (1966), Williams and Sussman (1971), and Winakur (1975) have all discussed the deplorable state of underemployment among the adult deaf population. All of these authors have provided support for continuing education programs as having an important role to serve in eradicating these deplorable conditions. According to these authors, the deaf as a group are either marginally employed or underemployed, often do not advance in either responsibility or function, and consequently do not receive salaries commensurate with their technical skill levels.

LeBuffe (1976) stated that "The deaf worker has little opportunity to take on-the-job training which is often encouraged or even required for advancement. I suspect that this is a major contributing factor to the underemployment that all agree is endemic among the deaf population in the U.S." Williams and Sussman (1971) indicated that most deaf people have found ready employment because they have acquired important knowledge and skills in residential schools which have vocational training programs. These skills are very salable in the employment market. However, the jobs are usually semi-skilled in nature such as printing, woodworking, bookbinding, shoe repairing, and so forth. These authors state that "employed deaf people are very often seriously underemployed. The deaf college graduate linotype operator or pressman is quite common, for example. Everywhere we find deaf men and women of normal or above abilities operating automatic machines, performing simple assembly line operations, or otherwise occupied in unchallenging routines." Moreover, they add that it is very seldom that the ladder for advancement in responsibility and function is available. One further example should suffice to complete the picture. According to Schein and Delk (1974), "almost 43 percent of deaf adults who have completed 13 years or more of school (*i.e.* have one or more years of higher education) have principle occupations in the following categories: clerical, transit and nontransit operatives, farm and nonfarm laborers, and service and household workers." Although Schein and Delk would not describe all of these job placements as underemployment, they do feel that it is true in many cases.

At least a partial solution to the underemployment situation may be provision of special continuing education programs for the deaf adult. Hopefully, in the future more and more communities will be responsive to the needs and problems of deaf adults. "When classes for deaf adults are an integral part of adult basic education programs, then perhaps all deaf people will be able to enjoy the full benefits of community life and realize their personal goals" (Donnels, 1976).

In the previous section concerned with the general employment outlook of the deaf adult, Grant *et al.* (1980) cited that the Bureau of Labor Statistics of the U. S. Department of Labor has been unable to develop the methodology to accurately measure underemployment for the general population. In an attempt to provide such information as it concerns deaf RIT graduates, Grant *et al.* (1980) mentioned that three measures of underemployment were built into the Graduate Feedback Questionnaire (GFQ) distributed to all certified deaf graduates during 1977 (*n* = 644) and 1978 (*n* = 832). These three measures of underemployment were (1) determining earning adequacy by asking graduates if they have enough money to pay their bills; (2) determining if graduates are employed commensurate with training by checking exit degree level and program against job titles and responsibilities; and (3) determining

if those graduates who are employed part-time desire full-time employment. "The third question is much clearer since the other two require interpretations and judgment." Other measures which these authors used to examine possible underemployment were mobility of deaf RIT graduates, measures of independent action, and measures of accommodation and integration within employment and personal environments. Their conclusions from studying the data from each of the measures were that much evidence exists that NTID does make a difference in helping to eliminate initially and prevent future underemployment. Their data indicate that "Graduates are mobile in terms of employment, they exhibit a high degree of independence, and are in many ways integrated and accommodated into the greater personal and professional hearing world." In addition, the Employment Opportunities Department at NTID has ascertained, through the above and other methods, that of the 914 initially employed graduates, 93% (*n* = 850) were employed in jobs commensurate with their degree level and training.

It would seem that considerable progress has been made in breaking down the historical barriers of entry into a wide variety of professional and educational opportunities for deaf adults through advanced education such as that provided by NTID and through other continuing education programs located throughout the United States. Some of these other programs will be examined in a later subsection dealing specifically with educational opportunities for the adult deaf.

Educational Attainment and Employment

Job Satisfaction—Although not necessarily exemplary of the entire deaf civilian labor force, the returns from the Graduate Feedback Questionnaire (GFQ) distributed to 832 deaf RIT graduates over a 2-year period (1977–78) were examined by Welsh (1980) to solicit information concerning job satisfaction. The areas examined were satisfaction with (1) internal opportunities, (2) co-workers, (3) supervisor, (4) content of work, (5) safety conditions, (6) education and training by firm, and (7) way firm treats deaf people. Table 7.6 presents the data derived from the results of the GFQ administration.

Welsh stated his statistics demonstrated

Table 7.6
Percentage Figures Relative to Job Satisfaction of RIT Deaf Graduates by Age, Race, Sex, and
Marital Status (*n* = 832)

	Age		Sex		Race		Marital Status	
	25 and Under	26 and Over	Male	Female	White	Non-White	Single	Married
	%		%		%		%	
Money	75.8	78.5	76.4	78.9	78.0	55.5	77.6	76.2
Internal opportunities	93.5	83.5	82.1	83.9	87.6	66.7	83.6	80.2
Co-workers	94.4	91.8	91.3	95.3	92.9	90.0	91.7	94.4
Supervisor	86.5	90.4	87.9	88.7	88.2	88.8	87.3	89.3
Content of work	83.8	87.2	85.5	85.2	86.0	90.0	87.8	87.9
Safety conditions	92.5	98.2	94.6	96.9	95.3	100.0	95.3	95.5
Education and training by firm	83.3	83.3	80.2	87.4	83.3	77.7	84.1	81.9
Way firm treats deaf people	85.2	81.9	86.6	81.3	83.3	77.7	83.9	83.6

Note: The figures in this table were reproduced from Welsh (1980).

that generally there were 5.7% more older persons (CA 26 years and older), more males (5.2%), and more single persons (4.2%) in the deaf graduate population studied. According to Welsh "this is much the same as is the case with hearing persons. The data on race is really not interpretable because of the small number (*n* = 10) of minority persons who responded to the questionnaire."

In reviewing Table 7.6 there are few important differences based on age, race, sex, or marital status. It appears that older persons are slightly happier with their salaries, but seem a bit more unhappy with internal opportunities and the way their firm treats deaf people. "Apart from these things, however, there are few real differences and perhaps the main point, in any event, is that most RIT deaf graduates are well satisfied with most aspects of their jobs." This does not seem to be true of deaf adults in general. For example, as reflected in the information presented by Costello (1977), such items as (1) increased income through better jobs, (2) improved communication and interaction between deaf and hearing persons, and (3) reduction of unemployment were high on the list of needs and desires of those 574 deaf persons participating in needs assessments conducted in 15 cities throughout the United States. These deaf persons hoped to achieve their goals through continuing education.

Technical Education Suggestions—An unpublished study of a demographic nature carried out by NTID Career Opportunities and Professional Development in 1973 represented an initial attempt to ascertain from NTID graduates the types of technical education which would have made their educational experiences more applicable to their existing jobs. Alumni (*n* = 194) who had successfully completed educational programs at various levels from certificate through master's degree participated in the 3-month, postemployment survey. The resulting data indicated that 50–55% would (1) recommend training, and in more depth, on equipment with which they had not had previous experience, (2) modify the training to make it more like the "real" job environment, (3) increase the amount of training in technical vocabulary, and (4) provide additional cooperative work experiences (experience during the academic training period where the student spends time on a job(s) similar to that in which she/he intends to seek employment). The percentages from the 1-year employee questionnaire were essentially the same.

The above data were preliminary to a more in-depth review of technical training needs of employed NTID alumni, and although they may be accurate, they must be viewed with caution since they represent perceptions related to a short duration of employment. A subsequent study by Parker and Welsh (1980) demonstrated that many of these technical training needs were probably met through on-the-job training and other types of continuing education in which the employed NTID graduates were later involved. According to these authors, 85% of the employed graduates ($n = 455$) participating in the 1978 Graduate Feedback Questionnaire (GFQ) had had some form of post-graduate educational experience(s) including: (1) on-the-job training for orientation (32%), (2) on-the-job training for skills (37%), (3) college degree courses (21%), (4) college continuing education (5%), (5) apprenticeship training (4%), and (6) other educational training (29%). The largest single reason for participating in educational experiences was to "increase technical skills for their current job (42%) .... Acquiring new technical skills for a new job accounted for another 16%." Parker and Welsh feel that these graduates are a highly motivated group who recognize the need for continuing education and know how to get it.

Communication Skills Recommended for Job Success—In the same preliminary 3-month and 1-year survey of NTID graduates performed in 1973 by NTID Career Opportunities and Professional Development, the graduates were asked which, if any, communication skills were essential for successful employment. In order of priority, the respondents indicated that the following skills should be emphasized during the academic careers of all deaf students: (1) ability to lipread (78%), (2) ability to read and understand written instruction (71%), (3) ability to make their speech understood by others (71%), (4) ability to read and understand technical materials (63%), (5) ability to understand job-related vocabulary (61%), and (6) ability to make their writing understood by others (61%).

Although these suggestions are very important in supplying information for strengthening communication development programs for deaf clients, Welsh (1980) reported that pre-employment scores obtained on communication variables such as speech intelligibility, reading, writing, and simultaneous receptive ability are not necessarily useful predictors of future labor force involvement, employment status, and job satisfaction, at least for NTID graduates. However, it must be emphasized here that the most NTID graduates are significantly more adept at most of these communication skills than the average adult deaf client in many communities around the United States.

Educational Opportunities and Employment—Several types of extended educational

opportunities for the deaf adult are already in existence (Costello, 1977; Donnels, 1976; Johnson, 1976b; Kelly, 1975; LeBuffe, 1976; and others). However, it is essential that a thorough examination be made concerning the types and nature of that available education. This is necessary in order to ensure appropriate placement of clients into those programs which will both meet their needs adequately and provide the maximum opportunity for success. Those programs which will be examined within this section are (1) continuing education programs, and (2) post-secondary and technical/vocational education programs. A third program which embraces both of the aforementioned programs, "Regional Education Programs," will be included in the discussion for the primary purpose of making the reader aware of its existence. Finally, there will be some discussion of the new National Center on Employment of the Deaf and the implications of this program for employment for the adult deaf client.

Continuing Education Programs—These programs have already been defined by Costello (1977) as being synonymous with adult education and "refer to a process whereby persons who no longer attend school on a regular basis undertake sequential and organized activities with the conscious intention of bringing about changes in information, knowledge, understanding, skills, appreciation, and attitudes." They are exclusive of post-secondary and technical/vocational education which award certificates or degrees. This definition will be adhered to within this section.

The LeBuffe (1976) article provides an excellent resource not only as a historical review of the subject, but also as a listing of cities with existing programs. According to LeBuffe, the need for these types of programs was recognized as early as 1904. Sporadic attempts were made to rekindle interest in such programs for the deaf in 1932, during World War II, and occasionally during the 1950s and 1960s. "Yet, until recently it was still credible to speak of 'Adult Education for the Deaf—A Long Neglected Need.' ... We have, I believe, a reason to hope that the exclusion of the deaf from adult education will be a thing of the past all over the nation by 1980."

LeBuffe stated that currently there are large and permanent adult deaf education programs in several cities including San Diego, New York, various cities in North Carolina, and Washington, D. C. Additional programs were beginning in Atlanta, Newark, Delaware, the San Francisco Bay area, St. Louis, Florida, South Carolina, Richmond, Baltimore, Tulsa, and Denver; plans for organization of programs were underway in Iowa, Milwaukee, White Plains, New York, New Orleans, Minneapolis, and Kansas City. "Currently every county in the United States receives A.B.E. (Adult Basic Education) money from the Federal government under the 'Right to Read' act." Moreover, information presented earlier in this chapter indicates that lack of basic language skills (including English reading comprehension) is a major deterrent to occupational and vocational success and a major cause of underemployment for the deaf adult. These funds, according to LeBuffe, could rightfully be applied toward the establishment of ABE programs for the deaf which are ". . . the single most important part of continuing education for the deaf adult."

Most aspects of adult and deaf education, including personal and social counselling, communication instruction, basic information of importance to occupational and vocational success, and successful community involvement, apparently have been omitted or have not been made available through ABE programs to adult deaf clients. However, any program already in existence or in the planning stage must appropriately assess the "real" needs of the deaf client before initiating an instructional program.

Post-Secondary and Technical/Vocational Education Programs—A second very important educational source for deaf adults is the certificate and degree-granting program. These are programs for deaf adults who have demonstrated the desire, motivation, and wherewithal to compete successfully within such programs to enhance their career opportunities. These programs are not necessarily limited to young deaf adults. More recently, older deaf adults are beginning to take advantage of this type of educational experience which previously was not available. For many years only a liberal arts program (Gallaudet College in Washington, D. C.) existed. This program did not provide that type of academic exposure of interest to many deaf

persons, and some of these deaf persons did not possess the appropriate educational base for acceptance within that program.

An example of the CA range of deaf adults involved in full-time post-secondary level educational programs today is given by the NTID student population. Although the average entering student in 1980 was 19.5 years, the CA range extended from 16 through 45 years. This CA range is typical of other academic years as well.

Any counsellor, speech-language pathologist, audiologist, or other allied professional providing career guidance for deaf adults interested in technical/vocational or post-secondary education must be aware of certain criteria which must be inherent in the selected program if the desired outcome to be realized is successful program completion. Program selection is highly dependent upon career interest, expressive and receptive communication skills, math and science skill levels, motivation, and availability of special support services.

Two of the most important resources for program selection available to the career advisor are (1) *A Guide to College/Career Programs for Deaf Students: Revised 1981 Edition* (Rawlings et al., 1981), and (2) a summary of an earlier guide (Rawlings and Trybus, 1976).

Career selection is contingent upon many personal attributes such as personal aspiration, interest, aptitude, level of educational attainment, and even a physical disability such as vision. For example, although not impossible, it would not be advisable for a deaf person with color deficiency to seek a career in photo finishing where visual perception of color is an essential ingredient for success. Likewise, the selection of a career in deaf education would not be a wise choice for a person who had not mastered the basic syntax of the English language. The general outlook for career selection is, however, quite encouraging. Schein and Delk (1974) stated ". . . deafness need not hinder employability. Deaf persons are employed in all principal occupations from professional to domestic." This point has been further verified by Grant et al. (1980) and Parker and Welsh (1980).

Also of primary importance to career selection, among those attributes already mentioned, is the job market. It makes no sense for any individual, deaf or hearing, to train for a career in any area where there is no job market or where a surplus of trained individuals already exists.

Rawlings and Trybus (1976) stated that there were at least 43 post-secondary programs throughout the country and Canada which accept deaf students. These programs were located in 23 states, the District of Columbia, and two Canadian provinces. The size of enrollment in these programs ranged from 10 to over 800 full-time deaf students. The major emphasis in 5 of these programs was reported as liberal arts, while 29 reported emphasis in technical/vocational offerings and 9 reported emphasis in both liberal arts and technical/vocational offerings.

By 1981 the number of programs which met the criteria for inclusion within the *Guide* (Rawlings *et al.*, 1981) had expanded to 57. These criteria included (1) has either a full-time director specifically for the deaf program or a part-time director who devotes a minimum of 50% of his/her time to the deaf program; (2) has a minimum of 15 full-time students enrolled in the deaf program; (3) is part of an accredited post-secondary program; and (4) generally complies with the principles of the Conference of Executives of American Schools for the Deaf. Of the 57 programs listed within the main body of the *Guide*, 52 are located within the United States, and 5 are located in Canada.

As in the earlier versions of the *Guide*, there still remains a preponderance of programs which specialize in technical/vocational education (43). However, 27 of these programs also offer a degree in liberal arts, and 11 offer degrees in various aspects of rehabilitation. In addition, four programs offer degrees in liberal arts only, seven offer degrees in liberal arts at the graduate level only, and three offer degrees in rehabilitation only.

Table 7.7 shows twelve (12) different support services which are provided for deaf students in many of these post-secondary level programs. As can be seen in the table, most of the programs provide interpreting, tutoring, notetaking, vocational development, personal counselling, and vocational placement services. However, it is surprising to note that only 28 programs provide speech and hearing services. That this fact is true is somewhat disheartening since deficiencies in receptive and expressive communication skill

Table 7.7

Availability of Special Services in Post-Secondary Programs for the Deaf in 1981

Special Services Co-ordinated by Programs for the Deaf[a]	Number of Programs		
	Total[b]	Services Available	Services not Available
Special classes for deaf students	57	30	27
Interpreters in regular classes	57	56	1
Tutoring services	57	56	1
Notetaking services	57	56	1
Vocational development services	57	49	8
Personal counselling services	57	50	7
Social/cultural services	57	44	13
Vocational placement services	57	42	15
Speech and hearing services	57	28	29
Manual communication training for deaf students	57	47	10
Manual communication training for instructors	57	48	9
Supervised housing	57	24	33

[a] Update on post-secondary programs for hearing-impaired.
[b] Fifty-two of the 57 programs are located in the United States, and 5 programs are located in Canada. There are other known post-secondary programs which serve deaf students, but do not meet one or more of the criteria for inclusion within *A Guide to College/Career Programs for Deaf Students* (Rawlings *et al.*, 1981).

development have always been one of the primary problems of deaf students/clients and are often the cause for other academic/personal-social problems which they encounter.

That language and other communication skills are essential ingredients for certain post-secondary education and technical/vocational programs has already been established. For instance, acceptance at both NTID and Gallaudet College, the two national post-secondary programs for the deaf, requires that the student possess the equivalent of an overall 8th grade achievement level (including English reading comprehension). This is not true of some vocational programs. The absence of good speechreading, speech discrimination, and speech and English skills may be a hindrance to deaf students electing to enter college or technical/vocational programs which do not offer special classes or preparatory programs for deaf students. "Individual students must consider what special services they will or will not require to obtain their educational training" (Rawlings and Trybus, 1976). For this reason, it is highly recommended that students and counsellors consult the *Guide* (Rawlings *et al.*, 1981) for more explicit information concerning available support services.

Regional Education Programs—In August 1974, a new program, referred to as Regional Education Programs, was formally created by Congress to meet the needs of deaf individuals who, because of educational deficiencies, could not meet the requirements for entrance into either Gallaudet College or NTID. According to information recently obtained from the coordinator of Regional Education Programs, approximately 50% of the applicants for enrollment into these two institutions fail to meet their entrance criteria. Under the auspices of the newly created program, four institutions of higher education were awarded grants and contracts to accommodate these adult deaf individuals. They are (1) California State University in Northridge, CA (CSUN), (2) Delgado College in New Orleans, LA, (3) Seattle Community College in Seattle, WA, and (4) St. Paul Technical Vocational Institute in St. Paul, MN (TVI). More information concerning these four programs can be obtained by consulting *A Guide to College/Career Programs for Deaf Students* (Rawlings *et al.*, 1981).

In 1975, the law was appended to accommodate individuals with other handicapping conditions. According to the Office of Education (1976), now known as the U. S. Department of Education, the law now reads "to award grants and contracts to institutions of higher education, including junior and community colleges, vocational and technical institutions, and other appropriate non-profit educational agencies for the development and operation of specially designed or modified programs of vocational, technical, post-secondary, or adult education for the deaf or other handicapped persons." Funds from these grants or contracts cannot be used for payment of tuition or subsistence allowances.

The *Federal Register* (Office of Education, 1976) explains the final rules and regulations governing Regional Education Programs as they pertain to handicapped persons who are ". . . mentally retarded, hard of hearing, deaf, speech impaired, visually handicapped, emotionally disturbed, crippled, or in other ways health impaired and by reason thereof require special education programming and related services."

The process for filing initial application for Federal assistance through Regional Education Programs is an annual competition, and includes: (1) requesting and filling out the required application form (Note: application forms and a copy of the *Federal Register* containing provisions covering application requirements, criteria, priorities, and types of activities which will be supported may be obtained by writing directly to the Coordinator of Regional Education Programs, Office of Special Education, 3121 Donohoe Building, 400 Maryland Avenue S. W., Washington, D. C. 20202.), and (2) submitting an appropriate "Program Narrative" inclusive of such items as (a) description of the handicapped population to receive services, (b) objectives and need for assistance, (c) results or benefits expected, and (d) geographic location to be served.

The purpose of establishing Regional Education Programs was not to create a new type of program, since it inherently includes both continuing education and post-secondary and technical/vocational education programs. Rather it is an attempt to expand educational opportunities for handicapped persons at the post-secondary or adult education levels.

Since its inception, grants or contracts have been awarded to 15 already established colleges, universities, and other non-profit educational agencies throughout the country demonstrating a desire to provide educational opportunities for persons with the handicapping conditions cited above. In addition to their regular student enrollment, five of these post-secondary institutions now provide educational opportunities for the deaf exclusively, five for deaf and hard-of-hearing students and those with other handicapping conditions, and five for handicapping conditions other than deafness. The five programs serving the deaf exclusively are already listed in the *Guide* (Rawlings *et al.*, 1981). The other five programs now serving deaf students are:

(1) University of North Dakota, Grand Forks, ND; (2) Wright State University, Dayton, OH; (3) Southern Illinois University, Carbondale, IL; (4) Columbia Teacher's College, New York, NY, and (5) State University of New York, Buffalo, NY. Priority consideration in awarding grants or contracts is given to applicants who intend to serve a multi-state area or large population centers. Other priorities are cited in the *Federal Register* including demonstration of alternative financial and other types of commitment to program continuance following expiration of the initial Federal Funding period.

National Center on Employment of the Deaf—In 1979, a new program was created at NTID in Rochester, NY. This program, the National Center on Employment of the Deaf (NCED), is an expansion of placement and employer development services regarding deafness, and according to Martin (1980, p. 14) performs five major functions. (1) *Employer development*, which is "a systematic, targeted, marketing process which moves potential employers of deaf RIT students, graduates, and other qualified deaf persons from a stage of awareness to acceptance of the idea of hiring a qualified deaf person." (2) Provision of a *career matching system* for deaf persons in an effort to link their abilities with employers' needs. Within this system, NCED has compiled information on scores of employers interested in hiring deaf people. The next step, once the system is fully operational, "will be to include names and job qualifications of deaf people who are seeking employment opportunities." By using an information-processing system to match the needs of the deaf applicant and the employer, materials regarding the applicant will be sent to the employer giving the employer the option of contacting the candidates. (3) Provision of *professional and employer training* for professionals working with deaf persons in employment such as vocational rehabilitation counsellors and employers themselves. Professionals in employment will be trained to select, approach, and prepare employers for deaf employees. Employers will be given in-depth instruction on the implications of deafness in the work environment. (4) *Continuing education* for NTID Alumni to keep them competent and competitive. (5) Provision of *information services* as a means of upgrading and

expanding the literature and media to strengthen the entire field of deaf education and employment of deaf people.

Martin (1980), in explaining the NCED, stated that "Not only will its activities be of benefit to deaf RIT students and graduates, but also to other post-secondary program completers and ultimately to all deaf people."

NCED had its first national conference in Rochester, NY for vocational rehabilitation counselors and other professionals working to improve job opportunities for the hearing-impaired in November, 1980. Similar conferences are planned for the future. For additional information concerning the NCED, see NTID Public Information Office (1980), Ritter (1980), or contact the NCED directly through the Career Opportunities Office, NTID, One Lomb Memorial Drive, Rochester, NY 14623.

Comments—Underemployment, rather than unemployment, is among the major factors causing dissatisfaction within the deaf community. Lack of job mobility, career choice, and secondary employment within the civilian labor force creates part of this dissatisfaction that is often related to underachievement in the area of communication skills, according to many of those authorities cited. Surveys of deaf individuals enrolled in adult basic education courses have indicated that English language skills are high on the list of communication needs for successful primary employment. Other surveys have indicated that speech, speechreading, and other communication skills are also felt to be important, although not necessarily a predictor, for job success.

Although provision of educational opportunities may pose a partial solution to the problem of underemployment, especially in the area of communication skill development, Gochnour (1973) stated that "many deaf people have decidedly antagonistic feelings toward oralism, hearing aid use, and speech therapy. Often the client has come to see a pathologist (speech-language) only because his vocational counselor or welfare worker has sent him and not because he has a motivation to acquire oral-aural skills."

It thus appears that, although deaf clients are aware of their needs to develop better receptive and expressive communication patterns, many may not be highly motivated to take advantage of communication programs when they are made available.

Thus, professionals must be sensitive to the feelings as well as the needs of adult deaf clients if they are to work with them successfully. They must also be aware of educational opportunities which are available, and keeping in mind individual differences, be able to make an accurate assessment of the appropriateness of these programs for each deaf client.

COMMUNICATION AND THE ADULT DEAF CLIENT

Increasingly, speech and language pathologists (and audiologists) are coming in contact with adult deaf clients. Generally, these professionals are asked to act in consultative, evaluative, or therapeutic capacities. This trend has been developing in the past five or six years, and more interaction with this population can be expected (Gochnour, 1973).

Since speech and hearing therapists and other professionals and para-professionals are beginning to interact more frequently with the adult deaf client, it is important that these professionals understand and appreciate the various types of receptive and expressive communication modes which deaf clients utilize in their communication episodes. In the mid-seventies, authors such as Gochnour (1973), Johnson (1976a), and Walter (1976) expressed their concern for the difficulty involved in dealing appropriately with the communication needs of deaf clients because of the dearth of experimentally documented information.

However, increasingly, more information is becoming available concerning communication assessment techniques, program planning, and instructional strategies which can be employed with this clientele. For example, and in-depth review of the applicability of existing techniques and test instrumentation for assessing the language, English reading and writing, oral/aural, and manual/simultaneous receptive and expressive communication skills of deaf students CA 5–9, 10–14, and 15+ years has recently been made available for dissemination (Johnson et al. 1980b). In addition, an entire special issue of the *American Annals of the Deaf* (Caccamise, 1978) has recently been devoted specifically to the linguistic, psychologic, and instruc-

tional ramifications of the various sign symbol systems employed by adult deaf clients. This issue of *Annals* explores the most current research and makes recommendations concerning assessment and instructional strategies. A second special *Annals* issue (Crandall and Orlando, 1980) has been devoted entirely to research, assessment, and instructional strategies concerned with the spoken language (English and oral/aural) systems of adult deaf clients. The information contained within these three documents should greatly enhance our knowledge of adult deaf clients and facilitate the chance of more appropriate interaction.

It is often difficult for persons unfamiliar with the adult deaf client to determine what form of communication will be easiest for the deaf client to understand during the initial interview. Gochnour (1973) stated that "Easy communication in the client's language is of primary importance in establishing rapport." Related to this, Gochnour (1973) and Caccamise *et al.* (1978) emphasized the importance of professionals becoming proficient in various types of manual-simultaneous communication. However, some clients will not be proficient in manual, oral, or simultaneous communication, and it may be necessary to use pantomine, drawings, writing of key words, or combinations of these modes of expression.

The NTID Public Information Office (1977) has stressed the diversity in receptive and expressive communication skills among deaf individuals: "Communicating with a deaf person is not necessarily hard or easy. There are no standardized lists of words, phrases or sentences that can always be understood. Intelligence, personality, age of onset of deafness, language background, listening skills, lipreading, and speech abilities all vary with each deaf person. . . ." Deaf persons will often try every possible way to communicate or convey an idea. The hearing person, in return, must be willing to experiment with ways to communicate with the deaf client. The important thing is not how ideas or feelings are exchanged, but that they are communicated.

Gochnour (1973), Caccamise *et al.* (1978), and the NTID Public Information Office (1977) have offered some psychosocial and communication guidelines to facilitate communication with the deaf adult. These guide-lines are summarized in the following three paragraphs.

Psychosocial Considerations

(1) Idiomatic expressions and colloquial-isms are often misunderstood and should be avoided; (2) facial and body gestures should be used liberally, but should coincide with intended meaning; (3) the viewpoints of the deaf concerning communication should be treated as valid and adult; (4) age of onset can provide important information concern-ing speech and English skill levels; (5) etiol-ogy can provide clues to existing disorders secondary to deafness; (6) reception of rapid fingerspelling may be difficult for the post-lingually deaf person; (7) forcing the deaf person to use speech during the early part of the interview may have a negative effect; (8) many deaf persons will not readily admit when conversations or instructions have not been understood; and (9) all program rec-ommendations should be appropriate rather than ideal.

One-to-One Communication Considera-tions

(1) Be certain to secure attention before speaking; (2) speak slowly and clearly, but without exaggeration; (3) look directly at the person while speaking; (4) use a written mes-sage when necessary; (5) always maintain good eye contact; (6) rephrase rather than repeat statements; (7) use body language and facial expressions which facilitate meaning.

Group Communication Considerations

(1) In groups, seating should be advanta-geous to the deaf; (2) attempt to avoid light sources from behind the speaker; (3) brief outlines and print-outs can facilitate lectures, movies, and filmstrips; (4) provide lists of new vocabulary in advance; (5) use visual aids to support lectures and discussions; (6) avoid pacing the floor or facing the chalk-board while speaking; (7) slow the pace of communication; (8) special instructions and assignments should be written; and (9) repeat questions or statements made by persons seated behind the deaf. (The reader is advised to review the Gochnour (1973), Caccamise, *et al.* (1978), and NTID Public Information Of-fice (1977) articles for rationales and detailed information concerning the above commu-nication considerations.)

In addition, a film *Deafness and Commu-nication* has been prepared for dissemination by NTID. This film can be used as an aid in educating those who have little knowledge of deafness, and who have a high likelihood of associating with the deaf. It deals with the nature and severity of hearing loss and with the channels of communicating with the deaf. The film may be borrowed at no charge from the Media Services Department, NTID, One Lomb Memorial Drive, Rochester, NY 14623. Other instructional products and re-sources developed at NTID can be obtained by writing directly to the NTID Public Infor-mation Office and requesting a copy of the *NTID at RIT Deaf Education and Rehabili-tation Resource Catalog.*

The remainder of this chapter will be de-voted to (1) suggesting techniques for assess-ment of the communication skills of deaf clients, (2) demonstrating a systematic ap-proach to communication program planning, and (3) recommending some strategies for providing communication instruction or ther-apy.

Assessment of Communication Skills

Assessment, if undertaken in the appropri-ate manner, will quickly demonstrate that no two deaf clients have identical communica-tion skills (Johnson, *et al.*, 1980a; Johnson and Kadunc, 1980). Because of the great variation in communication performance and personality among clients, care must be taken to make certain that the client understands the purpose of the evaluation. Once the client understands the rationale behind the com-munication evaluation, he will feel more com-fortable and probably approach the test sit-uation with a more positive attitude (Goch-nour, 1973).

Communication assessments are under-taken for a variety of reasons: (1) rapid iden-tification of clients in need of communication skill(s) development; (2) explaining an indi-vidual client's communication strengths/ weaknesses not only to the client, but to other professionals and family members (upon con-sent of the client); (3) use in developing a communication individualized education program (CIEP)) for the client; (4) language and communication program management (defining personnel, equipment, and space needs); and (5) studying trends within client populations.

Relative to the second objective, surveys conducted on students entering NTID have shown that often these young deaf adults have not acquired sufficient knowledge of the extent and nature of their hearing loss and their various receptive and expressive communication skill levels. As a result, they are poor candidates for habitual use of amplification and the communication remediation process (Galloway, 1975; Gauger, 1978a and 1978b; Gauger and McPherson, 1978; Johnson, 1974; Moore, 1975a; Schmalz and Walter, 1980). To combat this problem, all entering students are required to participate in the course "Introduction to Communication" (Schmalz and Walter, 1980). In this course: (1) students are oriented to the NTID Communication Program; (2) communication performance assessments are conducted; (3) instruction is provided in interpreting communication profile assessment results; and (4) each student has an opportunity to discuss her/his communication skills and needs and begins her/his communication program planning together with a communication advisor. Thus, the students are prepared to interact with their advisor and other communication team members in development of their formal CIEP. Providing the adult deaf client with information of this nature can help eliminate some of the antagonistic feelings toward oralism, hearing aid use, and speech therapy which are often encountered by clinicians working with deaf adults who use primarily manual communication (Gochnour, 1973).

Definitions—Often, teminology concerning assessment and/or evaluation techniques, methodologies, instrumentation, and profiles is used interchangeably, or not having been properly defined, becomes a source of confusion to the reader. To prevent such confusion, the terms, performance, diagnostic profile, and communication individualized education program (CIEP) will be defined as they are meant to be interpreted within this chapter.

Performance versus Diagnostic—The word performance, as used in relation to communication, is used only in conjunction with the

Table 7.8
Difference between Performance Assessments (Screening) and Diagnostic Evaluations (Tests/Examinations)

	Performance	Diagnostic
Definition	Separation of those persons among a group who will need further examination from those who are not likely to need attention for the communication parameter in question	Determination of nature and cause(s) of problem(s) when screening has demonstrated the existence of the problem(s)
Methods	Use of special fast and relatively easy to administer assessment instruments usually resulting in raw scores which may be converted to simple ratings or pass/fail scores (such as in visual screening)	Use of all available clinical and laboratory diagnostic procedures
Personnel[a]	Persons especially trained in administration and limited interpretation of assessment results. Could include members of CIEP planning team	Professionals such as speech-language pathologists, audiologists, English language specialists, manual/simultaneous communication specialists
Examples	Administration of assessment instruments for screening speechreading, speech intelligibility, manual reception, etc.	Administration of tests of speech articulation competency, determination of auditory site-of-lesion, or ability to recognize speech sounds, etc.

[a] All personnel administering screening assessments or diagnostic examinations to deaf students should be experts in manual/simultaneous communication or have access to a certified interpreter to enhance communication during screening and diagnostic procedures.

Table 7.9

Six Receptive and Two Expressive Communication Parameters Included in the NTID Communication Profile and Their Corresponding Test Instruments

Profile Parameter	Test Instrument
Receptive tests	
1. Hearing (speech) discrimination	10 Selected Spondee Words (Johnson and Yust, 1976) and NTID audiocassette versions of CID Every day Speech Sentences
2. Speechreading without sound	NTID filmed or videocassette versions of CID Everyday Speech Sentences (Davis and Silverman, 1970)
3. Speechreading with sound	(Same as Item 2)
4. Manual reception	(Same as Item 2)
5. Simultaneous reception	(Same as Item 2)
6. English reading comprehension	California Reading Test: Junion High Level, WXYZ Series, 1963 Norms (Tiegs & Clark, 1967)[a]
Expressive tests	
1. English written language intelligibility	NTID videotaped versions of Mr. Koumal Film Series developed by SIM Corporation (Crandall, 1978)
2. Speech intelligibility	Audiotapes of students reading the rainbow passage (Fairbanks, 1960)

[a] For secondary-level deaf students, the Paragraph Meaning Subtest of the Stanford Achievement Test, Special Edition for Hearing Impaired Children (Madden and Gardner, 1973) should be used to derive skill levels for English reading comprehension.

terms assessment, screening, or gross identification procedures. Performance assessments provide *approximations* of general skill levels for the various receptive and expressive communication parameters being assessed. The instruments used for performance assessments (screening) should be relatively fast and easy to administer (although not necessarily always easy to interpret), inexpensive (in terms of equipment and personnel), valid, reliable, and productive (they should yield a worthwhile number of cases for referral).

Given the nature of the performance assessment instruments used at NTID to measure communication skills (see Table 7.9), persons with severe to profound hearing losses may show a rather large range (up to 15–16%) in their scores between initial assessment and reassessment for any single receptive communication parameter. Since assessment instruments are used to provide approximations of general skill levels, this amount of variability is acceptable although it would not be acceptable in the case of diagnostic test scores.

When the results of communication performance assessments suggest that a student/client has weak receptive and/or expressive communication parameter(s), an in-depth diagnostic evaluation/test/examination should be performed by a communication/language or medical specialist to discover the reason(s) for the existing problem(s). Diagnostic information is used for planning strategies for medical or non-medical remedial intervention while performance assessments are used only for the purpose of initial problem identification. The terms evaluation, test, and examination are used only in conjunction with in-depth diagnostic procedures, and the term examination is more properly employed in relation to physical examinations such as those administered by otolaryngologists and ophthalmologists. Table 7.8 shows the conceptual differences between performance (screening) assessments and diagnostic evaluations (tests)/examinations.

Profiles—The term profile as used herein refers to an assemblage of scores/ratings arranged in such a manner as to permit a review of an individual's skill levels for a particular type of performance such as communication. For example, based on the results of a series of receptive and expressive communcation performance assessments, a *profile* of communication skills (strengths and weaknesses) can be assembled, and this profile can be utilized to develop a communication individualized education program (CIEP) for each student/client. Table 7.9 shows the various components which currently make up the assessment battery which is used to develop a communication profile for individual NTID students. This battery of tests, referred to as the NTID Communication Performance Profile, has been described by Johnson (1975), Johnson (1976a), Johnson and Kadunc (1980), and Johnson *et al.* (1980a). In addition, other communication profiles have been described by Gochnour (1973) in relation to adult deaf clients and Moeller and Eccarius (1980) in relation to hearing-impaired children.

For every assessment instrument within a communication performance battery, there should be a corresponding series of diagnostic test instruments which, in turn, when administered, are used to make up a diagnostic profile. Such a profile has been described by Subtelny (1977) and Subtelny *et al.* (1981) in relation to the communication performance parameter of speech intelligibility. According to Subtelny, when a deaf student/client has unintelligible or semi-intelligible speech, an in-depth diagnostic evaluation is performed to determine which one(s) of a number of aberrant speech and/or voice characteristics is causing the problem. The diagnostic profile corresponding to the performance parameter of speech intelligibility includes ratings for articulation, pitch register, pitch control, loudness, rate, prosody, control of air expenditure during speech, and voice quality. Voice qualities are rated in terms of breathy, tense, harsh, or faulty nasal and/or pharyngeal resonance. Once the diagnostic profile has been developed, the language/communication specialist uses this information to determine the appropriate content and sequencing of instructional strategies to provide the deaf student/client with remedial intervention. (Note: Subtelny *et al.* (1981) have developed a special training package complete with audio cassettes and self-instruction manuals to train speech-language pathologists and students in speech-language pathology and deaf education to identify/diagnose the various deviant speech and voice characteristics of the deaf. This package, *The Speech and Voice Characteristics of the Deaf (A0235)*, or information concerning the package, may be obtained by writing directly to Publications and Sales, The Alexander Graham Bell Association for the Deaf, 3417 Volta Place, N. W., Washington, D. C. 20002.)

Communication Individualized Education Programs (CIEP)—According to the Education for All Handicapped Children Act, the term individualized education program means a written statement for each handicapped child developed in any meeting by representatives of the local educational agency or an intermediate educational unit who shall be qualified to provide, or supervise the provision of, specially designed instruction to meet the unique needs of a handicapped child. The written document shall include ". . . a statement of the present levels of educational performance of such child." (P.L. 94-142, The Education for All Handicapped Children Act, Sec. 4, Item a19). This is a direct charge by the United States Congress for educational programs to assess the instructional needs of handicapped students, and based on the results of these performance assessments, to develop appropriate "individualized education programs" (IEP). IEP planning should cover *all* aspects of each student's education including communication development. A "communication individualized education program" (CIEP), as it relates to a deaf student/client, is a written plan devised specifically to make certain that all aspects of the individual's receptive and/or expressive communication receive appropriate educational attention when the need has been established. In order to develop a CIEP, it is first necessary to administer a battery of receptive and expressive communcation performance assessments, and subsequently, generate a communication performance profile for the individual student/client. The profile should minimally include representative scores/ratings in the areas of: (1) English reading and writing, (2) oral/aural communication (speech, speechreading, and listening), (3) sign language (manual codes for English and American Sign Language), and (4) simultaneous communication (use of spoken and sign English together).

It is the intent within this chapter to discuss specific instrumentation and techniques for performing a complete communication performance assessment for adult deaf clients, and ultimately, to demonstrate techniques for developing CIEPs for these clients. However, appropriate CIEP planning is not an easy task. Because it involves a number of communication skills, the process requires a group of skilled professionals working together as a team. Professionals involved should minimally include a speech-language pathologist, audiologist, English language specialist, and manual/simultaneous communication specialist. Frisina and Williams (1976) have stressed that, "No single individual nor profession is capable of providing the full scope of services required by the special learner. A 'comprehensive approach' must include professionals, the parents, and the student in complementary efforts."

Communication Profiles—Concerning the first and third objectives, Gochnour (1973), Johnson (1975 and 1976a), Johnson and Kadunc (1980), Johnson et al. (1980a and 1980b), and Moeller and Eccarius (1980) have discussed the concept of obtaining a communication profile on each client for the purpose of CIEP planning. These profiles include information obtained from assessment of each client's auditory, English, speech, speechreading, and manual/simultaneous communication skills.

Johnson (1976a) has provided a full description of the NTID communication profile system including seven receptive and three expressive communication test instruments, methods for assessment, a rating system, functional descriptors, and information of a demographic nature obtained on more than 800 entering students over a 4-year period. "Utilization of these evaluation tools at NTID over a four-year period clearly demonstrates that a large segment of students, upon entrance at NTID, are lacking many communication skills essential for success in the academic environment and later on the job and in the community." Johnson's study clearly demonstrated the efficacy of utilizing a communication performance-type system as an adjunct to program planning in the development of the communication skills of the adult deaf client. Because research has demonstrated redundancy of information for one profile parameter and the information was not deemed to be pertinent for another, two of the parameters are no longer assessed. It is expected that further experience and research will lead to additional modifications that will refine the precision of these screening instruments. Thus, the current performance profile system includes six receptive and two expressive components (see Table 7.9 and Johnson and Kadunc, 1980). Additional components have been recommended for fu-

ture inclusion as soon as appropriate assessment instruments have been developed (Johnson et al., 1980b).

The materials, equipment, and scoring procedures for the current NTID Communication Performance Assessment Battery have been described by Crandall and Albertini (1980), Johnson (1976a), Johnson and Kadunc (1980), and Subtelny (1977). Validity and reliability data collected on NTID students have been reported by Caccamise (1979), Caccamise et al. (1979), and Sims (1975).

In addition, Johnson and Kadunc (1980) and Johnson et al. (1980a) reported on the usefulness of the NTID communication performance profile for assessment and program planning for deaf secondary-level students. These two reports were based on field tests conducted with 420 deaf students at two residential schools for the deaf and led to the following conclusions: (1) the NTID communication performance battery, excluding the California Reading Test: Junior High Level (Tiegs and Clark, 1967), is appropriate for use with deaf students at the secondary level (CA 13.6 + years); (2) the Paragraph Meaning Sub-test of the Stanford Achievement Test, Special Edition for Hearing Impaired Students (Madden and Gardner, 1973) should be used for secondary-level students in lieu of the California Reading Tests as a measure of English reading comprehension.

As mentioned above, the NTID system for assessment of performance in major communication skill areas include 8 components which are defined as follows.

A. Receptive.
1. Hearing (speech) discrimination. Under optimum conditions, how well the student receives information when audition is her/his only mode of information reception.
2. Speechreading without sound. Under optimum conditions, how well the student receives information when s/he has only speechreading (lipreading) as her/his mode of information reception.
3. Speechreading with sound. Under optimum conditions, how well the student receives information when speechreading and audition are combined.
4. Manual reception. Under optimum conditions, how well the student receives information when signs and fingerspelling are her/his only mode of information reception.
5. Simultaneous reception. Under opti-

mum conditions, how well the student receives information when s/he has a combination of listening, speechreading, and manual communication as her/his mode of information reception.

6. Reading comprehension. Under optimum conditions, how well the student reads and understands written English.

B. Expressive.

1. Writing intelligibility. Under optimum conditions, how well the student makes her/himself understood when written English is her/his only mode of communication.

2. Speech intelligibility. Under optimum conditions, how well the student makes her/himself understood when reading aloud from a preselected passage, and speech is her/his only mode of communication.

Scoring and interpretation of the six receptive parameters is relatively easy. The raw scores derived from administration of each instrument can be converted to a rating on a 5-point (1 to 5) rating scale. Each rating has a simple functional descriptor for ease of interpretation to students/clients. In CIEP planning, however, it is essential that the raw scores be examined. A 5-point rating scale is too gross a measure to be used by itself for student program planning. For example, the raw score range for persons with ratings of 3 for hearing (speech) discrimination extends from 0–48%. Thus, the rating scale does not truly reflect achieved student skill levels. It is more appropriate to refer to the actual raw scores for more accurate information. See Table 4 in Johnson and Kadunc (1980, p. 343) for raw score to profile rating scale conversions. Table 7.10 lists each of the 5 ratings and their matching functional descriptors.

Scoring of the two expressive parameters (speech intelligibility and English written language intelligibility) is somewhat more difficult and requires considerably more training. Moreover, although administration of the screening for both of these two parameters is simple to conduct, scoring and interpretation of the results requires background and knowledge in speech-language pathology for the former and in linguistics and written English for the latter. As in the case of the receptive parameters, the raw scores for speech intelligibility and English written language intelligibility can be converted to a 5-point rating scale.

Interpretation of Results of Performance

Table 7.10
Rating System and Corresponding Functional Descriptors Utilized by NTID for Defining Student Receptive and Expressive Communication Skills

Profile Rating	Functional Descriptor
5	Under optimum conditions, the complete content of the message is received or expressed with no difficulty.
4	Under optimum conditions, most, but not all of the content of the message is received or expressed with little difficulty.
3	Under optimum conditions, with great difficulty, only about half of the message is received or expressed appropriately.
2	Under optimum conditions, only an occasional word or phrase is received or expressed appropriately.
1	Under optimum conditions, the content of the message is neither received nor understood.

Note: The content for hearing discrimination, speechreading, and manual and simultaneous reception is derived from simple everyday social discourse and not the technical vocabulary utilized in academic and career environments.

Profile Administration—Table 7.11 shows the comunication scores of 299 students entering NTID during the Summer Session, 1980. These students were grouped on each of seven profile parameters according to severity of hearing loss. Group 1 had the least severe hearing loss (65–84 dB ANSI) with Groups 2 (85–98 dB ANSI) and 3 (99 dB+ ANSI) demonstrating successively greater losses throughout the speech range.

Of the total population of entering students, approximately 75% were suspected of having lost their hearing prior to or at birth, 85% by CA 1 year, 90% by CA 2 years, and 95% by CA 3 years. (Note: this type of descriptive information concerning age-of-onset of hearing loss has remained essentially the same over a 10-year period.) Depending upon the definition of prelingual deafness utilized, this information could be interpreted to mean that as many as 95% of entering NTID students could be considered to be prelingually deaf with subsequent implications for development of English language and other communication skills.

Hearing (Speech) Discrimination—Hearing discrimination is the ability of the client to listen to and understand the speech of others. At NTID, taped versions of CID Everyday Sentence lists (Davis and Silverman, 1970) and 10 selected spondaic words (Johnson and Yust, 1976) are utilized to determine hearing discrimination skill levels.

Of 299 students entering NTID during the Summer Session, 1980, 43 were classified (according to ODS classification for severity of hearing loss) as Group 1, 62 as Group 2, and

194 as Group 3. Approximately 65% of the students in Group 1, 40% of those in Group 2, and 15% in Group 3 showed some ability to discriminate speech (performance profile ratings of 3, 4, or 5). The remaining students had not attained skill levels essential to speech discrimination. Results of application of the Duncan Multiple Range Test (Duncan, 1955) indicated that, with respect to speech discrimination, there were three statistically different groups.

This information should not be interpreted

Table 7.11
Performance Profile Data Elicited from Administration of Tests of Skill Levels for Eight Communication Parameters for Students Entering NTID during the Summer Session, 1980 (*n* = 299)

Communication Parameter	Test Material	*n*	Mean Score	Score SD
Receptive skills				
Hearing (speech) discrimination	NTID audio-cassette versions of CID			
Group 1[a]	everyday sentences and 10 selected	43	3.1[b]	1.34
Group 2	spondees	62	2.7	0.66
Group 3		194	2.2	0.85
Speechreading (no sound)	NTID film version CID everyday			
Group 1	sentences	43	44%	12.33
Group 2		62	39%	16.61
Group 3		194	38%	16.38
Speechreading (sound)	NTID film version CID everyday			
Group 1	sentences	43	67%	28.41
Group 2		62	42%	24.41
Group 3		194	36%	22.94
Manual reception	NTID film version CID everyday			
Group 1	sentences	43	52%	30.50
Group 2		62	64%	25.16
Group 3		194	73%	22.14
Simultaneous reception	NTID film version CID everyday			
Group 1	sentences	43	81%	17.39
Group 2		62	72%	14.51
Group 3		194	72%	16.29
Reading comprehension	California Reading Test, Junior High			
Group 1	Level, Form W	43	8.4[c]	1.00
Group 2		62	7.8	0.98
Group 3		194	8.2	1.11
Expressive skills				
Speech intelligibility	Rainbow passage			
Group 1		43	4.2[d]	0.92
Group 2		62	3.1	1.05
Group 3		194	2.8	1.09
Writing intelligibility	NTID Test of Written Language,			
Group 1	Form A	43	7.5[e]	1.71
Group 2		62	7.0	1.33
Group 3		194	7.1	1.50

[a] Better ear pure tone average for Groups 1, 2, and 3 are 65 to 84 dB, 85 to 98 dB, and 99 dB+ (ANSI) respectively. The Office of Demographic Studies technique was applied to derive better ear averages; that is (1) always computing a three-frequency average for 500–1000–2000 Hz, and (2) substitution of 120 dB when there is no response at the limits of the audiometer for any of the frequencies 500, 1000, or 2000 Hz.
[b] Profile rating on a scale from 1 to 5.
[c] GLE, grade level equivalent.
[d] Intelligibility ratings on a scale from 1 to 5.
[e] Intelligibility points on a scale from 1 to 10.

to mean that students with hearing discrimination profile ratings of 1 or 2 are not candidates for amplification or auditory training. In fact, 17% of those students with profile ratings of 1 and 2 owned their own hearing aids and wore them 5 or more hours per day. Both Johnson (1974) and Moore (1975a) have stated that lack of auditory skill development may be related to retarded English language skills, inconsistency of hearing aid usage, site of lesion (location of damage within the auditory pathways), insufficient auditory training experience, and various other factors. Moore (1975a) found that as the range of available frequencies is narrowed (based on cut-off frequency), the number of students who use a hearing aid "all or most" of the time decreases. This is not surprising since the less hearing a person has, the less likely it is that s/he will receive tangible benefit from amplification. However, with proper training they (NTID students) often derive some benefit from amplification as an aid to speechreading. The implications seem to be for recommended use of amplification even where limited hearing is present. That this fact is true of the students in the population being discussed is evidenced by the large number of "all or most" of the time hearing aid users with very little hearing discrimination ability.

Speechreading with and without Sound— NTID-filmed versions of the CID Everyday Sentence Lists (Johnson, 1976a) were utilized to measure skill levels of the 1980 entering NTID student population. The data for speechreading without sound are shown in Table 7.11. These data are grouped according to increasing severity of hearing loss. The data show that the average student in Group 1 is able to speechread, with difficulty, about half of the information in everyday social-type sentences. The average student in Group 3, those with the most severe hearing losses, received a mean raw score rating of 38% which means that, under optimum conditions, s/he could speechread only occasional words in social sentences.

When the Duncan Multiple Range Test was used to determine whether the three groups were in fact distinct from one another, it showed Group 1 to be significantly different from Groups 2 and 3 for speechreading without sound and each group significantly

different from one another for speechreading with sound.

Group 1 experienced a great deal less difficulty when speechreading and sound were combined to receive social information. Group 1 increased its average communication reception by approximately 23%, while students in groups 2 and 3 did not demonstrate a significnant change in their speechreading skills when sound was available. The implications of these data are (1) that speechreading skill levels decrease with increased severity of hearing loss, and (2) that persons with greater hearing losses (86 dB and more) are evidently not utilizing hearing to much advantage during the speechreading process. Erber (1972) reported that typically, for profoundly hearing-impaired subjects, the addition of acoustic cues results in a mean improvement of 1 to 15% over speechreading alone. The above data for Groups 2 and 3 are in agreement with this finding.

*Manual Reception—*NTID-filmed versions of CID Everyday Sentence lists (Johnson, 1976a) were utilized to assess the manual receptive skills of those students entering NTID during Summer Session, 1980. These films contain no sound and no lip movements, only signs and fingerspelling.

The data in Table 7.11 show that skill in receiving signed and fingerspelled information increases as hearing loss increases. Caution should be used in interpreting this type of information in relation to the post-lingually adult deaf client. Gochnour (1973) stated that "adults who have learned sign language after childhood also often display difficulty in reading rapid fingerspelling."

When the Duncan Multiple Range Test was applied to the data for manual reception, Groups 1, 2, and 3 were each shown to be statistically different from each other. This information is interpreted to mean that, under optimum conditions, those students with less hearing loss are generally not as reliant upon manual communication, and, thus, have developed less skill in receiving information through this mode of information reception. Evidence for this statement is contained within the raw percentage scores for speechreading with sound in Table 7.11. Group 1 achieved a mean raw score of approximately 67% for the test of speechreading with sound under optimum conditions. However, under similar conditions for manual reception, they received only 52% of the information in everyday social sentences.

Simultaneous Reception—Simultaneous reception is the ability of the client to receive information through the combination of signs and fingerspelling, lipreading, and listening simultaneously. NTID film versions of the CID everyday Sentence lists (Johnson, 1976a) are utilized to assess performance skill levels for this communication parameter. Table 7.11 shows the average simultaneous receptive skills of 299 students entering NTID during Summer Session, 1980. The data in the table show that all three groups receive more information through this combined mode of information reception than when any single mode or combination of two receptive modes are utilized. Further evidence substantiating this finding has been provided by Caccamise and Blasdell (1977). These authors have shown that students can identify sentence-type materials under simultaneous test conditions better than interpreted conditions in which an interpreter is employed to sign and silently mouth the words of a speaker. This fact lends credence to the contention that teachers, clinicians, and counsellors should become facile with and use the simultaneous communication approach when attempting to communicate with their clients during classroom lectures and in one-to-one conversational situations.

When the Duncan Multiple Range Test was applied to the data for simultaneous reception, there were two unique groups—Group 1 and Groups 2 and 3—when arranged according to the ODS hearing loss categories. This is another indication that the ODS system for grouping clients according to severity of hearing loss is appropriate.

Reading Comprehension—The California Reading Test: Junior High Level (Tiegs and Clark, 1967) was utilized to assess the reading comprehension skills of the 1980 entering NTID student population. Table 7.11 shows that the average reading score of this population is at approximately the 8th grade level. All three groups would experience difficulty in reading college level materials. Approximately 25% of the entire population received profile ratings of 4 and 5 on this measure of reading comphrension. These ratings can be equated to fall within the grade level range

between 9.0 and 12.0+. Approximately 50% received ratings of 1 and 2 for reading comprehension. These ratings place this group of students at the −5.0–7.9 grade level for English reading skills. The Duncan Multiple Range Test demonstrated that for this measure of reading skill the three groups were not unique. Information in reading comprehension has profound implications for designing programs for communication skill building as will be demonstrated in the section on program design. There are also important implications for adult basic education classes, underemployment, and, ultimately, job dissatisfaction.

Writing Intelligibility—Form A of the Koumal film series developed by SIM Corporation and modified by NTID (the NTID Test of Written Language) to include pre- and post-film instructions (Johnson, 1976a) was utilized to elicit writing samples from this NTID population. The average writing intelligibility scores for all three groups are shown in Table 7.11. Possible scores range from 1 to 10, with a 10 indicating a composition free of linguistic anomalies and a 1 indicating no evidence of any word-combining attempts (Crandall, 1980b). Table 7.12 gives an overview of characteristics associated with each score. This score can be converted to a profile rating range from 1 to 5. The writing samples of the average student in this population include spelling and punctuation errors, article errors, inflectional and derivational morpheme errors, function word errors, and contentive word substitutions. These samples would be approximately 70% intelligible to the naive reader. There was not a significant difference between the three groups' written language skills as indicated by the Duncan Multiple Range Test.

Approximately 5% of this population received profile ratings of 2, which can be interpreted to mean that these students cannot use English syntax in simple sentences. Without knowledge of basic English syntax, the adult deaf client would be a poor candidate for courses in speechreading, auditory training, and spontaneous speech production, which place great reliance on the utilization of contextual clues to fill in missing information (closure). Furthermore, there is no assurance that communication will occur through utilization of manual and/or simul-

Table 7.12
Description of Score Categories Used with the NTID Test of Written Language

Score	Category	Description
10	Acceptable	Free of mechanical and linguistic anomalies.
9	Mechanical	Punctuation errors, spelling errors, word division errors, contiguous repetition of a word within a sentence.
8	Inflection	Bound inflectional morphemes, articles, phrase and clause series "and."
7	Derivation	Bound derivational morphemes within nouns, verbs, and modifiers.
6	Functor	Free functors including prepositions, verb particles, selected modifiers, conjunctions, infinitive "to," pronouns, auxiliaries, modals, determiners, and negatives.
5	Contentive	Contentive stem substitutions and additions.
4	Structural	Word order involving subject, verb stem, object, auxiliary, modal, verb particle, or modifier.
3	Multiple structural	Two or more 4-type anomalies within one t-unit.[a]
2	Unconnected	Listing of single words or naming of substantives.
1	Unrecognizable	Unrecognizable words in lists, letter lists, scribble, only pictures.

[a] Note: A t-unit is a structural unit that can stand alone: that is, an independent clause with all of its dependent clauses (Crandall, 1980b).

taneous communication if they are expressed in English syntactical format. Thus, it is no wonder that the adult deaf client places the development of written English and other English language skills high on her/his list of priorities when considering courses in adult basic education (Costello, 1977; Donnels, 1976).

Speech Intelligibility—Speech intelligibility is the ability of the client to make her/himself understood when speech is her/his primary mode of information expression. The procedures for establishing profile ratings for speech intelligibility have been described by Subtelny et al. (1981). According to Subtelny and Walter (1975), on the average (for profile rating levels of 2, 3, and 4), ratings of readings are 1 profile rank higher than ratings based on spontaneous speech production. Apparently the difference is related to the student's difficulty in generating appropriate English for conversational purposes.

Table 7.11 shows dramatic differences among the average speech intelligibility ratings of the three groups. The Duncan procedure, when applied to the ranges of the three groups, clearly demonstrates the important relationship between amount of hearing loss and ability to generate intelligible speech. Each group was statistically different from each other.

This information should not be interpreted to mean that students with profound hearing loss cannot develop intelligible speech. Although Subtelny and Walter (1975) have also indicated that " . . . speech status is commensurate with hearing," they also reported instances of students in their population with intelligible speech who had prelingual hearing loss onset with some residual hearing, but no ability to discriminate speech sounds.

Physical Examinations

A detailed quantitative account, along with a description of all hearing tests administered to all students entering NTID during the Summer Session, 1974, has been reported by Johnson (1977). This battery of audiologic tests includes an audiometric assessment (speech discrimination and pure tone tests), immittance tests (to determine the integrity of the tympanic membrane and middle ear and the possible presence of recruitment), hearing aid checks (acoustic and biologic), and otoscopic screening. The otoscopic screening and immittance tests are considered here to be physical in nature; that is, they are assessments/evaluations which help to determine the possible presence of ongoing outer and/or middle ear anomalies and consequently the need for referral for possible medical intervention. Of utmost importance to this entire procedure is the follow-up explanation between the student and audiologist to ensure complete understanding of the results and any necessary medical/non-medical remedial intervention.

In addition to physical tests for acute or chronic middle and other ear anomalies, assessments and/or examinations for visual functioning are administered routinely on all entering students, and in-depth laryngoscopic examinations are recommended in all cases of suspected laryngeal dysfunction.

Such a battery of physical tests is recommended for routine administration not only for adult deaf clients, but for all hearing-impaired persons. The supporting rationale is included in the following paragraphs.

Otoscopic and Immittance Assessments/Examinations—During the Summer Sessions of 1974 and 1975, a team of local Rochester otolaryngologists otoscopically examined the outer and middle ears of all entering NTID students (approximately 275 students per summer) for the presence of impacted wax and other outer and middle ear pathologies. In addition to finding a significant number of students with impacted wax, approximately 3% of these two populations were found to have clinically confirmed anomalies of the outer and/or middle ear and were in need of medical intervention.

During the summer Session of 1976, immittance tests were performed on all entering students ($n = 295$) using the Grason-Stadler 1701 Otoadmittance (immittance) Meter with a 1701 X-Y Recorder and 1701-9670 Recorder Adapter. Approximately 10% of these students demonstrated abnormal tympanograms and were subsequently referred for in-depth medical examinations. Although a significant number of this 10% demonstrated existing pathologic conditions which were not amenable or not in need of medical remediation, approximately 3% had confirmed anomalies which called for medical intervention.

Since 1976, the immittance equipment and otological procedures have changed. Otological examinations performed on entire populations of entering NTID students such as those conducted in 1974 and 1975 are no longer carried out routinely. However, otoscopic and immittance examinations/assessments are performed routinely by the audiologic staff before conducting audiometric assessments, making earmold impressions, performing hearing aid evaluations, and when

impacted wax is suspected if students complain of acoustic feedback. Under the new procedures, students with impacted wax, abnormal immittance, suspected anomalies of the ear canal or eardrum, complaints of pain, ear drainage, and severe tinnitus or dizziness are referred to the RIT Student Health Center for cursory otological examinations. When students are not responding to treatment, or if there is any question concerning diagnosis, etc., the students are seen for an in-depth diagnostic examination by RIT's consulting otolaryngologist.

Visual Assessments and Examinations—Vernon (1977) stated "The issue is that vision represents the key sense remaining in deaf people. Therefore, it must be assessed thoroughly." In another statement, Stuckless (1978) emphasizes not only the importance of the visual channel for deaf persons, but also stresses the need for professionals working with these individuals to pay more attention to that mode of information reception.

In my opinion, those of us who work with and on behalf of deaf children, have given altogether too little attention to what the eye does well and what the eye does poorly. I have difficulty understanding why our field has focused so much clinical and scientific attention on the deaf child's ears while virtually ignoring the principal sensory modality for receiving information, his eyes . . . . it is likewise curious that educators of the blind have been highly attentive to the blind child's eyes while largely ignoring his hearing.

In 1974, in response to reports from NTID professionals (and in some instances the students themselves) relative to students with suspected visual problems, a decision was made to initiate a visual screening program. The program was designed to identify already enrolled and entering NTID students with uncorrected visual problems in need of medical/non-medical remedial intervention and students with non-correctable functional visual problems (such as acuity, color, or binocular vision problems) who might be in need of special attention in order to be successful in the academic environment. Because of a variety of problems encountered with the initial visual screening techniques such as high incidence of over-referral (false positive condition) for ophthalmological examinations and lack of knowledge concerning appropriate follow-up procedures, in 1976 a Vision Task Force was formed at NTID to study the various problems and make recommendations based upon the results of research. The task force identified the following three objectives: (1) to determine the most appropriate means of identifying NTID students with visual impairments and make recommendations for medical and personal/social follow-up (Objective 1); (2) to determine the types and incidence of visual impairments among these students (Objective 2); and (3) conduct research that would assist in the provision of appropriate counseling relative to academic and career opportunities/experiences for persons with both auditory and visual impairments (Objective 3). The results of research conducted over a 3-year period (1977–79) to successfully complete these three objectives has been reported by Caccamise et al. (1980 and 1981), and Johnson et al. (1981). The results relative to Objectives 1 and 2 are of concern in this section and summarized in the following paragraphs.

Recommended Visual Screening Procedures for Adult Deaf Clients—In order to develop visual screening procedures which would identify all students with visual impairments and/or pathologies in need of immediate or periodic attention with a minimum of over-referrals (false-positive condition) or under-referrals (false-negative condition), both off-campus and on-campus procedures were studied. None of the off-campus procedures were found to be appropriate for the NTID population studied for a variety of reasons (Johnson et al., 1981). Thus, they will not be discussed here.

During the research phase of the project, on-campus visual screening procedures included assessments for near and far (distance) visual acuity, color vision, and binocular vision (muscle balance and depth perception). The equipment used for this screening included Bausch and Lomb Orthorater Vision Testers, the Ishihara Color Vision Test with a MacBeth Lamp for proper illumination, and Titmus Stereopsis Tests.

Table 7.13 demonstrates the visual assessment instruments, functions assessed, and referral criteria for the recommended NTID visual screening program. The rationales for selection of these parameters were based on research conducted at NTID during 1977–79 and are described in depth in Johnson et al. (1981).

As shown in Table 7.13, Orthorater far visual acuity and Isihara Color Vision assess-

Table 7.13
Visual Assessment Instruments, Functions Assessed, and Referral Criteria for the Recommended NTID Visual Screening Program

Visual Assessment Instruments and Functions Assessed	Recommended	Referral Criteria[a] for an On-Campus Ophthalmological Examination[b]
Orthorater		
Near acuity	Yes[c]	Jaeger 4 or worse in one or both eyes
Far acuity	Yes	20/40 or worse in one or both eyes
Color vision	No	
Phorias		
Near lateral	No	
Far lateral	No	
Near vertical	No	
Far vertical	No	
Stereopsis	No	
Ishihara color vision test	Yes	7 or more misses on first 13 plates
Titmus stereopsis tests	No	
Vision questionnaire (personal/family ocular history)	Yes	Any indication of visual problems

[a] Use of these recommended referral criteria with the 1980 entering NTID student population ($n = 306$) netted an ophthalmological referral rate of approximately 24% ($n = 73$ students).
[b] If the student is presently under the care of an ophthalmologist, and/or results indicate adequate remediation has been provided, then referral for an on-campus ophthalmological examination may be unnecessary.
[c] Recommended at NTID for all students 30 years and older only.

ments together with a personal/family ocular history are recommended as components for visual assessments conducted on all NTID students. In addition, the Orthorater assessment for near visual acuity is conducted on all students 30 years and older. Appendix C in Johnson *et al.* (1981) describes in detail the recommended visual screening procedures. The referral criteria shown in Table 7.13 for each of those visual parameters assessed during visual screening of NTID students have been shown to maintain false-positive and false-negative results at a minimum in each instance.

Examinations for binocular vision (Phorias) are conducted by the NTID consulting ophthalmologist in conjunction with history-taking procedures for all students referred for suspected far visual acuity problems. In addition, the ophthalmologist checks for near visual acuity problems during the course of the ophthalmological examination. Recommended minimal ophthalmological procedures are described in detail in Appendix E of Johnson *et al.* (1981).

The Orthorater is an expensive visual screening device, and only one or two of ten visual parameters which can be screened with this instrument are being recommended for use in the NTID visual screening program in the future. Thus, research is currently under way at NTID to determine whether a less expensive Snellen chart with rear illumination can be substituted for the Orthorater to screen students for far visual acuity problems and still attain the same results.

Incidence and Types of Visual Pathologies and Impairments—The National Society to Prevent Blindness (NSPB) has stated that "Statistical studies showhat 25% of children of school age may have some eye difficulty which may require professional care" (NSPB, 1979). Objective 2 for the NTID Vision Task Force was to study the incidence and types of visual impairments within entering NTID student populations in order to determine prevalence rates of various functional visual problems.

During the Summer Sessions of 1978 and 1979, 620 students entered NTID. Table 7.14 shows that, using the visual screening and ophthalmologic techniques described in Johnson *et al.* (1981), 363 students (58.4%) were identified as having a far visual acuity

Table 7.14

Incidence of Functional Visual Problems within the Student Population Entering NTID during the Summer Sessions of 1978 and 1979 (*n* = 620)

Visual Problem	Number	Percent
Far acuity	302	48.7
Color deficiency	25	4.0
Binocular vision	70	11.3
Two problems	33	5.2
Three problems	1	0.002

Note: The above figures do not reflect the actual overall incidence within the population since some students had more than one functional visual problem. The exact number of students with a functional visual impairment(s) was 363 (58.4%).

problem, a color deficiency problem, a binocular vision problem, or combinations thereof. Of this group, by far the greatest number 302 (48.7%) had far visual acuity problems. In addition, the data collected on 1979 entering NTID students (*n* = 311) demonstrated that at least 21 (6.7%) with ocular pathologies did not have functional visual problems involving far visual acuity, color, and/or binocular vision. This latter group would not have been identified through routine screening procedures although some were in need of medical attention because of the nature of the pathology. Thus, the estimated incidence of *all* visual problems among entering students, when functional visual problems and pathologies are considered, is approximately 65%.

Further study of the 1978 and 1979 entering student populations revealed that most, but not all, of the students entering NTID have had adequate professional care, at least for far visual acuity problems, by the time they reach the post-secondary school level (the average chronological age of students entering NTID is approximately 19.5 years). However, among those 302 students who were found to have far visual acuity problems, 20 (6.6%) did not own corrective lenses and 7 (2.3%) were found to have inadequate correction. These data point out why it is so important that programs serving deaf adults not assume that these clients will have received appropriate visual attention by the time they have reached adulthood. Furthermore, it is not known whether, for those who were inadequately corrected, the problem was due to progression of the visual impairment since they received their last prescription or because they received inappropriate correction because of inadequate communication during the visual examination. That this latter problem probably did occur in several instances can be demonstrated by the fact that several of the students had poorer vision with than without their corrective lenses. Thus, it is important to stress here the importance of having interpreters present, as necessary, during visual examinations and persons with good manual/simultaneous communication skills conducting all visual screening programs for hearing-impaired clients.

Table 7.15 presents the incidence of non-correctable functional visual problems among the 573 entering NTID students seen for on-campus ophthalmologic examinations during 1977, 1978, and 1979. The table shows that there were 111 (19.4%) students with far visual acuity which could not be corrected to 20/40 or better in one or both eyes and an additional 34 (5.9%) students with color deficiency problems. These results, especially in the case of those 25 students who could not be corrected to better than 20/40 far visual acuity in both eyes, have strong implications for both personal/social and academic/career

Table 7.15
Incidence of Ophthalmologically Confirmed, Non-Correctable, Functional Visual Problems for Students Entering NTID during the Summer Sessions of 1977, 1978, and 1979 ($n = 955$)

Type of Problem	Number	Percent(s)
1. Far visual acuity		
A. Both eyes 20/40 or poorer	25	2.6 (4.4)
B. One eye 20/40 or poorer	86	9.0 (15.0)
2. Color deficiency	34	3.6 (5.9)
Total(s)	145	15.2 25.3

Note: Caution must be advised in interpretation of the percentage figures since they were derived by two different methodologies. The figures outside of parentheses are based on the total entering student population ($n = 955$); those inside the parentheses are based only on those students who were referred for and received an on-campus ophthalmologic examination ($n = 573$). The referral screening procedures for the 321 students entering NTID in 1977 were quite different from those used in 1978 and 1979 and might be suspect.

counselling and possible environmental modification(s) if these students are to be successful in the academic and later in their employment environments. Also, similar consideration needs to be given to those students who have near visual acuity problems (which may impact on reading and other near visual acuity tasks) and color vision problems.

During 1977, 1978, and 1979, 179 (31.2%) of the entering NTID student population seen for on-campus ophthalmologic examinations ($n = 573$) were found to have 23 different ocular pathologies and/or conditions existing as a direct result of these pathologies. While only 109 of these students had related functional visual problems (such as far visual acuity, color deficiency, and binocular vision problems) there were 50 among this group who have those types of pathologic conditions for which they are in need of periodic ophthalmologic examinations because of the progressive nature or possible recurrence of the problem. Unfortunately, of these 50 students, 40 were not aware of the existence and/or significance of the problem before their on-campus ophthalmologic examinations took place.

Table 7.16 shows the most frequently occurring ocular pathologies and/or conditions directly related to such pathologies within this population. It must be emphasized again that not all of the students with pathologies or resulting conditions have associated functional visual problems. For example, 13 of the students with rubella retinopathy and 3 with chorioretinal scars have normal functional vision. (A detailed description of the full array and discussion and definition of these pathologies and/or conditions can be obtained from reviewing Johnson et al., 1981.)

It is extremely important that clients, clinicians, and career counsellors become aware of existing visual problems from the standpoint of career selection, involvement in adult basic education, and program planning for communication development. For example, Vernon (1976) states that " ... Usher's syndrome is the leading cause of deaf-blindness in most scientifically advanced countries. The disease involves primarily a profound congenital hearing loss and a progressive loss of vision due to retinitis pigmentosa. It is transmitted genetically by an autosomal recessive gene." Approximately 3–6% of those persons born deaf have Usher's syndrome. This syndrome is often associated with such symptomatology as night blindness, tunnel vision, and vertigo. According to Vernon, many cases of Usher's syndrome go undiagnosed because of lack of knowledge on the part of medical and other professionals associated with deaf persons. Since persons with Usher's syndrome eventually are legally blind (20/200 or poorer far visual acuity in both eyes with best correction and/or lateral and vertical peripheral fields reduced to 20° or less; these criteria vary somewhat by state) by their mid-30s or early 40s, there are obvious implications for career selection. (Note in Table 7.16 that during 1977, 1978, and 1979, the 13 NTID students identified as having retinitis pigmentosa were verified as having Usher's syndrome.)

Laryngeal Examinations.—Each entering NTID student receives an assessment of speech intelligibility and, as necessary, an in-depth speech and voice diagnostic evaluation (Subtelny 1981). During these evaluations the speech-language pathologists are alert for possible laryngeal problems referred to as "source function voice disorders." Such disorders may be related to anomalies at the level of the vocal folds such as vocal nodules and contact ulcers. The voice characteristics associated with the attending aberrant laryn-

Table 7.16
Most Frquent Pathologies and/or Resultant Pathological Conditions Found among all Entering NTID Students Receiving On-Campus Ophthalmologic Examinations during the Summer Sessions of 1977, 1978, and 1979 ($n = 573$)

Type	Number	Percent
1. Strabismus	51[a]	8.9
2. Rubella retinopathy	43[a]	7.5
3. Color deficiency	34	5.9
4. Retinitis pigmentosa (RP)	13	2.3
5. Retinopathy (other than rubella)	9	1.6
6. Conjunctivitis	7	1.2
7. Iritis	4	0.7
8. Maculopathy	4[b]	0.7
9. Chorioretinal scars	4	0.7

[a] One strabismus case and one rubella retinopathy case also have color deficiency.
[b] Two cases of ocular maculopathy also have strabismus.

geal function may involve excessive breathiness and vocal weakness, vocal tension, and/or hoarseness.

In one year, eight (approximately 3%) of the entering student population were referred to otolaryngologists for suspected laryngeal anomalies. Of this number, laryngeal pathology was confirmed in three students. In light of this evidence, it is important that clinicians working with adult deaf clients remain alert to the possible presence of laryngeal anomalies and make appropriate medical referrals when such procedures are warranted.

Comments

During the initial interview with the new adult deaf client, care should be taken to ascertain the most appropriate means of communication in order to develop rapport as rapidly as possible. Remember that most of these clients have been referred by other agencies and not because they have the motivation to acquire oral-aural skills. Gochnour (1973) stated: "It is not unusual for the deaf to approach communication evaluation with some hostility, for they may be expecting the examiner to force oralism on them."

Communication performance and corresponding diagnostic profiles are recommended. The former profile should be utilized to ascertain communication strengths and weaknesses. The latter profile is used to provide information for determining instructional strategies.

In addition to assessment of receptive and expressive communication skill levels, therapeutic plans involving the use of audition, vision, and speech or voice require the performance of immittance, otologic, visual, and possibly laryngeal examinations.

Communication Program Planning, Rationales, and General Instructional Strategies

The results of communication assessments carried out on two entering NTID students will be examined within this subsection. This information will be used to devise communication program designs, discuss rationales for those designs, and recommend general instructional strategies. Those assessment techniques and instructional strategies presented are currently in use at NTID and in various stages of design, development, and evaluation. Teacher handbooks and student workbooks together with related media and materials are packaged and made available for general distribution when development and evaluation are completed. Those materials that are currently available are referenced later in this chapter.

Evidence from research data accumulated on NTID students indicates that it is possible to effect a positive change in the various communication skills of that population utilizing those instructional techniques which will be examined here. For instance, Orlando (1975) has shown in a research project involving 89 students that it is possible to reduce vowel and consonant articulation errors by approximately 10% in 18 1-hour individual therapy sessions. Crandall (1980a) and Crandall and Albertini (1980) reported that NTID students are improving their English skills at a faster rate than evidenced in their past educational history. The data indicated that the average NTID student ($n = 265$) increased her/his reading comprehension skills by approximately one grade level equivalent in three 10-week quarters (5 to 7 1-hour group and individual sessions per week) as opposed to approximately one half grade level equivalent during each of the past 13 years of her/his educational history. The increases were related to such parameters as student career area, skill level at entry, instructional hours per week, quantity of utterances in the class, and instructional approach. Crandall states, however, that " . . . this improved rate of learning is not great enough to allow the average student to learn independently from college level reading materials during her/his second year of college experience. Continued effort must be exerted to further increase the NTID student's rate of learning English language skills." Moore (1975b) presented auditory training instructional strategies utilized with 55 NTID students. She reported an average improvement of 30% (the range was 13% to 83%) in discrimination of sentence materials practiced. In a follow-up study, Snell and Managan (1976) reported that retention of these sentence materials appears to be related to speech discrimination skill levels and is poorest for those students with low discrimination skills prior to initiating therapy. Once training ceases, discrimination of sentence materials drops but then stabilizes and remains consistent at 5, 10, 15, and 20 weeks.

Other NTID research indicates that (1) significant changes in pitch register and control can be brought about for students with profound hearing losses (Orlando, 1975), and (2) in 18 1-hour sessions, student speechreading skills can be increased by an average of 28% using videotaped materials for individualized practice (Jacobs, 1975). Subsequent unpublished data collected by Jacobs on 97 students enrolled in advanced speechreading at NTID in 1976 and 1977 have indicated that the average student increased her/his skills in recognizing sentence materials related to career area by approximately 54% (the range was 32% to 100%) in 18 practice sessions utilizing instructional strategies similar to those described in her 1975 report. Seven of these students who had an average 49% post-course gain in technical sentence recognition were retested 12 months after course completion. The resulting data demonstrated an average drop in speechreading of technical/vocational sentences of approximately 13%. However, this drop, although significant, is relatively small when one realizes that these students still retained an average increase of approximately 40% in pre- and post-course evaluations.

This information shows that it is possible for adult deaf clients to develop and/or strengthen their communication skills providing they are given appropriate instruction or therapy. However, the clinicians involved in designing communication programs must be realistic concerning the goals they set for their clients. Time and motivation are definite factors to be considered. The client may very well be motivated to develop her/his communication skills, but time may pose a definite constraint. For example, if an adult deaf client has 4th or 5th grade reading comprehension skills, usable residual hearing, but no hearing aid, completely unintelligible speech with both voice and articulation problems, and little or no ability to speechread, the time commitment would be considerable. As shown above, (1) it would take about 30 weeks, meeting for 5 to 7 hours per week to raise reading comprehension by one grade level equivalent; (2) it may take 30 weeks or more at 2 hours per week to select, fit, and orient the client to amplification and provide the essential auditory training preparation for impending voice and/or speech training; (3) it could take 36 1-hour sessions or more to help the client learn to coordinate respiration and phonation with additional time for work on pitch and other voice problems before proceeding with work in reduction of articulation errors; (4) at an average articulation error reduction rate of approximately 10% in 18 1-hour sessions, it may take as many or more than 72 1-hour individual sessions to bring a client with an 86% articulation-error rate to speech levels intelligible to the general public. Subtelny and Walter, 1975 have suggested that " . . . the speech of the deaf should be intelligible if a 75% score in articulation (25% error) can be achieved."

As already indicated (Costello, 1977; Donnels, 1976), adult deaf clients are particularly interested in developing and/or strengthening their English skills. Crandall (1980a) has been able to demonstrate that such development is within the realm of possibility for young deaf adults at NTID. The adult deaf client, however, may not be inclined to expend the time, effort, and practice necessary to upgrade these skills, especially if s/he is beginning at very basic English levels. Bochner (1977) has itemized some important concepts concerning English language drills.

1. Language is a set of habits. These habits are internalized via large amounts of practice.

2. Language is unconscious. Learning this unconscious behavior does not proceed by assimilating detailed explanations, but by imitating and repeating the actions of a model.

3. The goal of a drill is to give the student practice with a highly restricted set of structures or to teach one specific structure.

4. The material and the tasks presented to the student must be sequenced according to their level of difficulty. There is both a hierarchy of skills (structures) that the student must internalize and a hierarchy of drills that the teacher must present.

At NTID the instructional designs used in English language instruction vary according to individual needs. That is, amplified speech, manual communication, simultaneous communication, glossynography, or a combination of these modes may be used. Sargent and Malcolm (1979) and Sargent and Nyerges (1979) have described glossynography as a system which presents a pre-programmed written message on a television monitor; the written message is synchronized with an auditory message which is received by both students and instructor.

The presentation design used in English language instruction may be sequenced (grammatical structures and vocabulary are isolated and taught in a developmental sequence), controlled (structures and vocabulary are restricted but not presented in any particular order), or natural (structures and vocabulary are handled as they arise in materials not specifically adapted). The instruction takes place in small groups and in a monitored self-learning environment (Crandall and Albertini, 1980).

NTID students are placed into the English curriculum according to the test scores they receive on the reading comprehension and written language tests which have been described in the section on assessment within this chapter. An English score is obtained on each student by using a matrix to combine her/his scores on these two tests. This English score is then used to place students within one of the five levels of English curriculum offered by the Communication Program of NTID. Table 7.17 shows the English score

Table 7.17
English Score Ranges and Placement.

English Score Range	Typical Reading GLE	Typical Writing Score	English Level Placement	Communication Instructional Department (CID) Placement
32.0 and above	11.0	9.50	Proficient	IV
29.0–31.9	10.5	9.00	Level 5	IV
26.0–28.9	9.5	8.00	Level 4	III
23.0–25.9	8.5	7.00	Level 3	II
20.1–22.9	7.5	6.00	Level 2	I
20.0 and below	6.5	5.00	Level 1	I

ranges and the resultant English curriculum placement. All students entering NTID except those with English scores 32 or more are required to enroll in English instruction. Students functioning at or above this level may voluntarily enroll in English instruction.

Specific linguistic items are prescribed for each level within the curriculum. The vocabulary and reading materials used at each level relate to specific content areas. The content defined for each level provides students with experiential referents ranging from general to specifically related to technical majors.

All of the above must be considered before devising a communication program plan for an adult deaf client. Program plans should be based upon a complete assessment of existing communication skills as discussed above, and should be discussed and mutually agreed upon by both client and clinician. Gochnour (1973), speaking of adult deaf cleints, stated, "Experience has shown that most clients will not do what they do not want to do." She also emphasizes the point that programs for these clients must be realistic. "It is crucial to make realistic recommendations based on both the test results and the patient's lifestyle. The evaluator should keep in mind the possible rather than the ideal."

These concepts concerning realistic program planning are not presented to dissuade the clinician from undertaking a course of therapy with a motivated deaf client, nor are they meant to provide the clinician with a rationalization for precluding therapy when conditions are appropriate for such an undertaking. A statement by Nickerson (1975) is used here to emphasize this point.

Moreover, the lack of both hearing and speech is such a severe handicap in our society that the acquisition of speech competence is worth a very considerable effort. To take this position, it is not necessary to disparage manual communication nor to endorse the idea that speech should be taught to the exclusion of signing. What is asserted is the desirability of being able to communicate by speech if at all possible, regardless of whatever other means of communication one may have at one's command.

With these thoughts in mind concerning the adult deaf client and the communication development process, it is possible to proceed with development of CIEPs and discuss general instructional content and strategies with two distinctly different NTID student case studies.

Subject 1 (S1) Background Information—S1, a male, was born on June 12, 1955, a seemingly healthy, full-term baby. Pre-natal history was essentially negative with no reason to suspect hearing loss. The parents are middle-class high school graduates, and neither they, two older siblings, nor other relatives demonstrate any history of hearing deficit. Hearing loss was first suspected by the parents at CA 2 years because of both lack of response to sound and retarded speech development. Severe to profound hearing loss was confirmed shortly thereafter by a local otologist. Age of probable onset was listed as birth with unknown etiology.

The parents were referred to a local hearing and speech agency where they received counselling, and S1 was fitted with a body-worn hearing aid on the left ear. Parent-oriented therapy was initiated shortly thereafter. The client entered a hearing pre-school program at CA 4 years where he received intermittent auditory, speech, and language training for approximately 1 year before entering a residential school for the deaf at CA 5 years. Approximately 1 year thereafter, according to the parents, although he still owned a hearing aid, he was using it infrequently.

S1 remained in the residential school, completing the remainder of his elementary and secondary school career in June, 1976. He entered NTID in July of that year at CA 19.1 years. At the time of entrance at NTID he still owned a body-worn hearing aid which was 7 years old and in need of repair. He seldom, if ever, attempted to use the aid.

S1 and Physical and Communication Examinations/Assessments—An otologic examination, visual screening, and a complete communication assessment were performed shortly after entrance at NTID. The otologic examination and visual screening results were essentially negative. A laryngeal examination did not appear to be warranted and was not performed.

Table 7.18 shows the results of the communication assessments including the descriptive hearing information, receptive and expressive communication performance profile rating information, and speech diagnostic information. According to this information

Table 7.18
Descriptive Hearing, Receptive, and Expressive Performance Profile, and Speech Diagnostic Information for Two Students Entering NTID.

Descriptive Hearing Information

Subject No.	Age at onset	Pure Tone Average		Frequency Cut-Off		Hearing Aid Usage	
		Right Ear	Left Ear	Right Ear	Left Ear	Right Ear	Left Ear
S1	Birth	105 dB	95 dB	4000 Hz	4000 Hz	Never	Seldom
S2	CA 4 years	93 dB	100 dB	4000 Hz	500 Hz	5–8 hours per day	Never

Receptive Performance Profile Information

Subject No.	Speech Discrimination				Speechreading No Sound		Speechreading with Sound		Manual Reception		Simultaneous Reception		Reading Comprehension	
	Right Ear		Left Ear											
	Rating[a]	%	Rating	%	Rating	%	Rating	%	Rating	%	Rating	%	Rating	GLE[b]
S1	1	0	1	0	2	21	1	8	5	86	4	72	2	7.5
S2	4	53	1	0	4	72	5	100	2	28	5	100	5	10.6

Expressive Performance Profile Information

Subject No.	Speech Intelligibility		Writing Intelligibility Score
	Read Speech Rating	Spontaneous Speech Rating	
S1	1.2	2	6.5
S2	4.6	5	8.0

Speech Diagnostic Information

Subject No.	Motivation for Speech Therapy Rating	% Articulation Errors	Stimulable Consonants Initial Word Position	Pitch Ratings		Loudness Ratings		Speech Rate Rating	Rating Respiration Duration Speech	Breath Control	Prosody Rating[c]	Quality Ratings[d]
				Register	Control	Appropriateness	Control					
S1	2	70	3/15 (20%)	5	4	4	3	3	2	3 seconds	2 (all)	(T) 3, (PR) 1, (H) 3
S2	1	28	1/6 (17%)	5	5	4+	5	5	5	9 seconds	5 (all)	5 (all)

[a] Note: In all cases, ratings of 1 are poor and 5 good.
[b] GLE, grade level equivalent.
[c] Prosody ratings are blending (B), stress (S), and inflection (I).
[d] Quality ratings are normal (N), harsh (H), breathy (B), tense (T), hoarse (HO), excess nasal resonance (NR), and excess pharyngeal resonance (PR).

an "ideal" program for S1 would include (1) hearing aid evaluation and selection procedures, (2) individualized auditory training, (3) English language instruction including reading comprehension and writing intelligibility, (4) individualized voice and speech therapy, (5) speeachreading instruction, and (6) other courses for communication refinement—not necessarily in that order. Order of programming would be dependent upon student progress.

S1 Program Design and Rationale—Tentatively, S1's program might be sequenced as shown in Table 7.19 below. These and all other communication courses available at NTID are described in the RIT Official Bulletin (1980).

First Quarter—Introduction to Communication Skills. This course helps students un-

Table 7.19
Projected Quarterly Communication Individualized Education Program (CIEP) Designed for Subject 1 (S1).

Quarter	Communication Courses and Tentative Sequencing
1	Introduction to Communication Skills
2	English 2: Modern Life—ASL Complement
2	Orientation to Acoustic Hearing Aids
3	English 3: Famous Scientists
3	CID II Basic Speechreading I
4	English 3: The Earth and the Universe
4	CID II Intermediate Speechreading
4	Understanding English Through Sign Language
5	English 4: Careers
5	Communicating with Other People—Unintelligible Speech
6	English 4: Beginning Scientific English
6	CID III Speech Therapy I
7	CID III Speech Therapy II
7+	CID III Speech Therapy III
7+	Telecommunication Aids
7+	CID III Idioms and Slang
7+	Vocabulary Skills
7+	Technical Speechreading and Speech
7+	CID III Basic Communication for Group Presentation

Note: Program sequencing is tentative since it is highly dependent upon student progress or lack thereof.

derstand their own communication skills. Basic information about the communication process, English language, sign language, and hearing and speech is taught. Students learn about communication courses they can take at NTID and design a communication training program to improve their communication skills. This is a required course for all new NTID students. A student text has been developed for this course by Schmalz and Walter (1980) and is available through the RIT Bookstore, One Lomb Memorial Drive, Rochester, NY 14623.

Minimally, in a clinical situation with an adult deaf client, this course would be substituted with a series of counselling sessions. These sessions should include interpretation of the results of the communication assessment, a discussion of communication needs based upon the assessment results, and a joint (clinician/client) planning session to devise a "realistic" program plan.

Second Quarter—English 2: Modern Life-ASL Complement. This course helps students improve their skills in writing English and using English words. It provides instruction in two different areas: the structure of sentences with two clauses with some kind of connector between them, and analyzing vocabulary words independently. In addition, the course concentrates on improving writing and developing reading skills. Reading and Writing Labs to provide practice are required. The Reading Lab work is related to the classroom grammar units. The course is taught using both American Sign Language (ASL) and English. It is for students with English scores from 20.1 to 22.9 and with good ASL skills.

S1 received an English score of 22.3 which places him at English level 2 (see Table 7.17); thus, the content and instructional strategies would be structured accordingly. Noting that S1 has a writing intelligibility rating of 6.5, he would be expected to manifest some or all of the following errors in his compositions (see Table 7.12 and Crandall, 1980b): (1) spelling and punctuation errors, (2) inflectional and derivational morpheme errors, (3) article errors, (4) phrase and clause series "and" errors, (5) functor word errors, and (6) contentive word errors. Such being the case, instructional content would be utilized in a combined approach of vocabulary, reading, and writing development.

At NTID, English skill development takes place simultaneously with all other therapeutic endeavors. Thus, speech pathologists, audiologists, manual communication specialists and English specialists work together in each of the four communication instruction departments (CIDs) to develop communication instruction to meet individual student needs. This same approach could be utilized with any adult deaf client. However, it would be essential that the instructor/therapist be in close contact with appropriate persons within the client's current employment environment to obtain pertinent high-usage vocabulary and related sentence materials.

Concurrently with the above course, during S1's second quarter, he would also enroll in *Orientation to Acoustic Hearing Aids.* This course is for students who have not used a hearing aid in a long time. It helps students learn to use a hearing aid daily. Students learn how to take care of hearing aids, and about guarantees, earmolds, and repairs. They have the opportunity to borrow different aids and to use them daily while keeping accurate records about the advantages and disadvantages of each hearing aid for later discussion with the audiologist. These activities help students decide the best, most comfortable hearing aid for themselves. Students who have not used a hearing aid in the last three years may enroll in this course with the recommendation of an audiologist.

Student materials and an audiologist manual have been developed for this course by Gauger (1978a, 1978b). These materials are available from the Alexander Graham Bell Association for the Deaf. The student package contains seven short manuals covering the following general areas: (1) hearing aids and what they do, (2) earmolds and hearing aid batteries, (3) maintenance and care of hearing aids, (4) troubleshooting hearing aid problems, (5) consumer information about hearing aids, (6) a hearing aid record, and (7) a student manual (including course preparation and a hearing aid performance checklist). The course booklets are written in English levels appropriate to the congenitally deaf adult and can be used with individual clients or in small groups.

Third Quarter—If we assume that S1 is now a hearing aid user and has improved his reading and writing skills, he would enroll in the following courses during his third quarter

at NTID. At this time, S1 is majoring in electromechanical technology leading to the AAS degree. *English 3: Famous Scientists.* This course gives students a knowledge of vocabulary and structural forms that are common in social, academic, and professional situations. Students practice vocabulary and grammar used in engineering and science and every class includes writing practice. The reading and writing exercises center around the lives and accomplishments of famous scientists from ancient times to the Industrial Revolution. Reading and Writing Labs are required. The course is for students majoring in engineering or science with English scores from 23.0 to 25.9. Reading selections and practice exercises that form a part of this course are available through the RIT Bookstore (Malcolm, 1980). During this third quarter, S1 would be advised to register for *CID II Basic Speechreading I.* This course helps students use their visual skills to understand speakers. Students learn speechreading strategies. They practice these strategies in a variety of lighting and noise conditions. They learn how to understand facial expressions, eye glances, and gestures and body movements as people talk. Both individual words and everyday sentences are included in the practice. Students who have speechreading scores (with or without sound) from 10% to 34% may enroll in this course. Jacobs (1978) has prepared a booklet entitled "Speechreading Strategies" which covers factors that affect speechreading ability and contains suggestions for strategies to improve the student's ability to communicate with hearing people. This booklet can be purchased through the RIT Bookstore.

Fourth Quarter—It typically takes a student two quarters to raise his English skill levels from English 3 to English 4 (Malcolm and Augustin, 1979). Therefore, in S1's fourth quarter, he would probably need to enroll in another English 3 course, *English 3: The Earth and Universe.* As in the previous English course, this course covers vocabulary and structural forms that are common in social, academic, and professional situations. Vocabulary and grammar used in engineering and science are incorporated within the writing practice which takes place in every class. Reading and writing exercises are about astronomy and geology. Reading and Writing Labs are required. This course is for engineering and science majors with English scores from 23.0 to 25.9.

S1's best speechreading score at entry was 21%. According to Jacobs (1975), his score would now probably be about 35% if he has shown appropriate improvement in Basic Speechreading I. This would qualify him for *CID II Intermediate Speechreading* which is designed for students with speechreading scores from 35% to 54%. This course helps students speechread common sentences and incorporates strategies and practice concerned with job interviews and conversations at work. Students also practice these sentences in short conversations. Some students practice speechreading hearing people in an interview.

If S1 has the time and desire, it would be recommended that he also enroll in *Understanding English Through Sign Language* during this quarter. The purpose of this course (designed for students with manual reception scores of 77% or greater) is to improve students' knowledge of English through the use of sign language. Students learn English forms for signs they know and use daily. They practice changing ideas presented in sign language to written English. Signs for technical and other difficult English words are practiced using sign language to help understanding.

Fifth Quarter—At this point, S1 will most likely possess an English score that will place him in Communication Instruction Department III (see Table 7.17). It is recommended that he take two courses during this quarter. The first course, *English 4: Careers,* is an introductory level 4 English course which helps students continue to develop their reading and writing skills. Social issues like child abuse and drug abuse are discussed to help students better understand themselves and the people with whom they will interface in the future on the job and in the community. Reading and Writing Labs are required. The course is for students with English scores from 26.0 to 28.9. The second course is *Communicating with Other People—Unintelligible Speech.* The purpose of this course is to analyze communication with other people and to solve problems that cause communication to break down. The course helps students understand their own problems and the problems of others in communication situations.

Students explore different ways to solve communication problems in social, job, and other experiences. They discover their own strengths and weaknesses in everyday communication. Students with spontaneous speech intelligibility scores from 1.0 to 2.5 and manual reception scores greater than 74% may enroll in this course.

Sixth Quarter—During this quarter, S1 will take his last required English language course. If he continues to make the typical progress reported for NTID students, he will now need to enroll in *English 4: Beginning Scientific English.* This course helps students improve reading and writing skills used in scientific English. Various topics related to physics and engineering are discussed. General topics are also included in the course. Students practice writing short compositions and changing sentences from one syntactic pattern to another. Students also work on other grammar and vocabulary exercises. The course is most useful for engineering and science majors. Reading and Writing Labs are required. The course is designed for students with English scores from 26.0 to 28.9.

During the summer quarter between S1's fourth and fifth quarter, he was involved in a cooperative work experience. Upon his return, he indicated a strong desire to improve his speech skills. Thus, it was recommended that S1 begin a program of individualized speech therapy. He would, therefore, enroll in *CID III Speech Therapy I.* This course helps students improve their speech and voice. Special diagnostic tests help the teacher evaluate the student's individual needs. The student meets with a speech instructor 2 hours a week and practices outside class for 1 hour each week. Instruction may include training in voice, pitch control, articulation, or loudness control. Students practice words, phrases, sentences, and conversations. Students with spontaneous speech intelligibility scores less than 4.1 may enroll in this course.

The speech diagnostic information section in Table 7.18 indicates that, at the time of entrance to NTID, S1 was not highly motivated to undertake a prolonged program of voice and speech therapy. Subtelny (1976a) has described an attitudinal questionnaire developed at NTID which provides a motivation index for speech therapy. Based on a 5-point rating system, ratings below 3 are indicative of poor attitudes toward speech instruction. S1 had a motivation rating of 2. However, at this point S1 has completed *Orientation to Acoustic Hearing Aids* and has elected to use amplification consistently. His attitude toward speech improvement has been altered. Accordingly, he should be advised of his chances of attaining intelligible speech.

Additional voice and speech diagnostic information indicates that S1 needs at least 18 to 36 individual therapy sessions (1–2 10-week academic quarters with two 1-hour sessions per week) on voice before initiation of an intensive articulation program. That is, his rating of 2 for respiration during speech and his inability to sustain the vowel /a/ for more than 3 seconds both indicate a lack of coordination between respiration and phonation. Thus, the major thrust of voice therapy would be concerned with therapeutic efforts directed toward facilitation of this necessary coordination.

The percentage of articulation errors as measured by the "Fisher-Logemann Test of Articulation Competence" (Fisher and Logemann, 1971) indicates an approximate incidence of errors (omissions, Substitutions, and distortions) in initial, medial, and final word positions of 70%. Fifteen of these errors appeared in initial word positions and only 3 of them were stimulable (could be imitated satisfactorily after demonstration) within the allowed three trials.

Although the consistent use of amplification may help S1 progress more rapidly in articulation therapy, it may still take more than three 10-week academic quarters (54 individual therapy sessions) to reduce the total error rate to a desired level of intelligibility (at a 25% or less error rate a client's speech is normally intelligible to the general public, according to Subtelny and Walter, 1975). Data relative to the client's auditory function and functional usage of English can furnish the clinician with vital information concerning prognosis for speech improvement. For instance, Subtelny (1976a) stated, "If the speech therapist knows exactly which sounds can be perceived, this information can be compared with the accuracy of the student's speech sound production. Following this procedure, the therapist should be in a much better position to select reasonable pho-

neme targets for correction and achieve faster progress in therapy."

Orlando (1975) has also stressed the importance of selecting the appropriate speech practice materials. The results of his research demonstrated the importance of using a variety of vowel contexts in carefully structured speech practice materials. "If materials are designed for the purpose of sequentially varying the target within varied vowel contexts, and within relevant language units (functional word groupings), training will be more effective and successful carryover into conversational speech facilitated." Also, greater improvement in vowel articulation was identified with greater gain in word intelligibility.

Seventh and Following Quarters—During S1's seventh quarter at NTID and in quarters subsequent to that, he would be eligible for several recommended courses. In his sixth quarter, S1 began a program of individual speech therapy and completed his English language course requirements. If he has made average progress in reading and writing skill development, his English score would now be 28.3. Malcolm and Augustin (1979) reported that 8% of the students beginning at Level 2 reach Level 5 at the completion of their English requirement, while 38% reach Level 4. S1 would, therefore, remain a part of the student population for whom CID III are responsible.

If S1 had shown good motivation in *CID III Speech Therapy I*, he would register now for *CID III Speech Therapy II* and then for *CID III Speech Therapy III*. These courses are a continuation of the individual speech therapy program begun in S1's sixth quarter. In these courses, students work on their own individual speech needs. After completing this program, S1 will most likely demonstrate semi-intelligible speech in situations in which the content is familiar and highly redundant to the listener.

All NTID students, regardless of their communication skill levels, have access to individualized instruction in telecommunication devices for deaf (TDD) and hearing persons. Castle (1977, 1978) and Johnson (1976b) have described some instructional strategies and equipment that can be utilized to carry out this essential aspect of instruction for adult deaf clients. Students/clients who have not acquired aural/oral skills permitting them to use the acoustic telephone should still be afforded the opportunity for instruction with different telephone-connected equipment for use at home or at work: Magsat, MCM, TTY, and TV phone are examples of such equipment.

It is recommended that S1 enroll in *Telecommunication Aids*. This course helps students learn about different kinds of TDD equipment and also helps students experiment with their ability to use an acoustic telephone. Using a TDD, students learn how to make long distance calls, appointments, emergency calls, and what to do if they have a bad connection or if they get disconnected. Students make TDD calls after class to practice using the different equipment and practice using special codes for listening and speaking. Students with hearing discrimination scores less than 25% may enroll in this course. Student and teacher materials used in this course have been prepared and can be purchased through the RIT Bookstore (Castle, 1981).

If S1 is interested in receiving more instruction related to English language skills, there are two courses that would be recommended. The course *CID III Idioms and Slang* helps students understand and use common idiomatic and slang expressions that are spoken, written, or signed. In this course, the *Dictionary of Idioms* (Boatner and Gates, 1966) is used and student materials for each unit are used to help students practice using idioms and slang correctly. Simultaneous communication is used in the classroom. Students with manual reception scores greater than 77% may enroll in this course. The course *Vocabulary Skills* is also recommended for students wishing more English language instruction. This course helps students understand and use new and difficult vocabulary words. Students learn several methods to help them use vocabulary in reading and writing. Also, common word prefixes, suffixes, and roots are taught. Skills developed in this course can also help students develop vocabulary skills in speech, speechreading, listening, signing, and fingerspelling.

To assist students in incorporating new vocabulary in their speech, Webster's diacritical markings have been useful. This diacritical symbol system was selected rather than other existing systems because adult clients generally have access to a *Webster's New Collegiate Dictionary* in academic and employment environments. NTID has developed a package consisting of 7 videotapes, 6 response sheets, a student manual, and a teacher's manual designed to improve students' independent skills in word pronunciation (Subtelny, 1976b). A Hawaiian firm, Camwil, Inc., at the request of NTID, has produced a mold (Element #2489M) which has the capability of manufacturing on a standard type element (Letter Gothic, 12 pitch type face) 15 diacritical symbols and International Phonetic Alphabet characters. This standard type ball can be used on any IBM selectric typewriter with 12 pitch type face, thereby making it a relatively easy task to generate new practice materials for students learning the diacritical symbol system (Clymer, 1977).

If now S1's speechreading score is at least 55%, it would be recommended that he enroll in *Technical Speechreading and Speech*. This course helps students improve their speechreading of "on-the-job" sentences. Students practice speechreading sentences specifically related to their own majors. They work individually with videotapes and practice speechreading a variety of people. Students are also able to practice pronouncing the technical vocabulary in the Self-Instruction Lab (McQuay and Coscarelli, 1980). Students must have completed at least three quarters in their major before taking this course because understanding of the technical vocabulary used in the exercises is essential to success in this course (Jacobs, 1975).

Experience with young deaf adults at NTID has demonstrated that these clients have difficulty in organizing their thoughts for lucid presentation of information. However, if these individuals are to become leaders in their respective communities and on their jobs, they must possess these essential communication skills. It is recommended that before graduation S1 enroll in a course designed to provide skills in organizing and delivering presentations. The course *CID III Basic Communication for Group Presentation* prepares students to give short presentations to groups of people. Students learn how to search for information and how to present their ideas to an audience. They also learn how to observe other presenters and how to evaluate these presentations. Students with simultaneous reception scores greater than 53% may enroll in this course.

Comments—The program designed for S1 may appear to be highly idealistic in nature. However, this type of individualized program planning for communication development is carried out with each entering NTID student, and many highly motivated students reach their mutually agreed-upon program goals.

Time and progress are important factors in the consideration of overall program goals. The program designed for S1 would require that he be enrolled at NTID for 4 years and be registered in communication courses for 4 quarters in his first year and three academic quarters during each of the other years. The average student remains at NTID for eleven quarters and receives an associate degree upon graduation (DiLorenzo and Welsh, 1981). Programs must be designed realistically with time and other constraints in mind. The student must be a participant in the overall communication program planning and be constantly appraised of progress or lack thereof.

Realistic program planning would be more constrained for the adult deaf client enrolled in community programs. Generally these clients are employed in daytime jobs and have much less time available for special study programs outside of work. Because of these constraints, it may be possible to help these clients upgrade only one receptive and expressive skill. If this is true, the highest priority should be given to English skill development.

Subject 2 (S2) Background Information— The communication program for S2 is distinctly different from that described for S1. Whereas S1 was beginning his communication program at basic levels, S2 is working at the level of refinement. The reader will note, however, that some of the courses are the same because they contain information pertinent to all students/clients.

S2, a female, was born on May 22, 1956. She is the second and only girl of four children. Her oldest and youngest brother and parents have normal hearing. The third child was born deaf from unknown etiology. S2's hearing loss was discovered at CA 4 years by her mother and family physician shortly after a severe case of measles. The suspected etiology was measles with age of onset listed as

CA 4 years. However, considering the deafness of her younger brother, there remains some question as to actual etiology and age of onset of her hearing loss although, according to her mother, speech and language appeared to be developing normally.

S2 received her first hearing aid shortly after her hearing loss was discovered and has worn amplification consistently since that time. There has been no evidence of hearing loss progression since first discovered.

Although her entire educational career took place in hearing schools, there is no reason to assume that this environment was more conducive to her superior communication attainment relative to that of S1. None of her education took place within special classes, nor did she receive special tutoring or communication therapy within the school system. In this case, other factors to be considered concerning communication attainment are (1) possible age-of-onset of hearing loss after development of basic speech and language skills, (2) constancy of hearing aid usage, (3) the advantage of considerable speech and language therapy in a local hearing and speech center, and (4) 2 years of community college before enrolling at NTID.

S2 transferred to NTID in 1976 at CA 20.2 years after experiencing considerable difficulty in a local community college. Thus far, at NTID, she has been highly successful and plans to attempt to obtain a baccalaureate degree in Medical Laboratory Technology.

S2 Physical and Communication Examinations/Assessments—An otologic examination, visual screening, and a complete communication assessment was performed shortly after entrance to NTID. The otologic examination disclosed a large bolus of cerumen impacted against the right tympanic membrane; the cerumen was removed, and subsequently the otologic examination and visual screening results were essentially negative. A laryngeal examination did not appear warranted and was not performed.

A consideration with all new clients wearing hearing aids is the appropriateness of that amplification; that is, is the hearing aid in good repair and does it adequately meet the needs of the client? S2's hearing aid, a behind-the-ear model, was 2 years old. It was checked acoustically for gain, saturation output, frequency response, second and third harmonic distortion, and total harmonic distortion and found to meet factory specifications (Hearing Aid Check—Acoustic). Her performance was then evaluated under optimum conditions wearing her own hearing aid (Hearing Aid Check—Biologic). The results of this latter evaluation were positive; that is, she did at least as well in the aided as the unaided condition performed under headphones in a sound-treated environment. Her earmold was in good condition, fit snugly, and there was no apparent problem from acoustic feedback. (Note: Hearing aid and earmold checks should be performed periodically at 6-month or 1-year intervals or aperiodically whenever the client suspects that some change has occurred.)

The results of the communication assessments are shown in Table 7.18. Examination of these results demonstrates a need for instruction/therapy in the areas of (1) manual communication, (2) speech refinement and auditory discrimination, (3) advanced speechreading, and (4) advanced reading and writing, but not necessarily in that order.

S2 Program Design and Rationale—Tentatively, S2's program might be sequenced as shown in Table 7.20. The reader is again referred to the RIT Official Bulletin (1980) for communication course offerings and descriptions.

First Quarter—As indicated in the section concerning S1, all adult deaf clients are in need of either a course similar to *Introduction to Communication Skills* or several counselling sessions to acquaint them with the results of their communication assessments and to discuss a potential realistic program design. Thus, S2 would enroll in this course during her first quarter at NTID.

Although S2 has demonstrated some ability to receive information through manual communication (profile rating of 2) upon entrance to NTID, she understands only an occasional word or phrase. Even though she receives 100% of the information under optimum conditions when speechreading is combined with sound, it is probable that in less than optimum conditions, this communication level will not be achieved. She would benefit from additional skills in manual communication in the academic and social environments where conditions are not optimum. Her past history indicates that she has no

Table 7.20
Projected Quarterly Communication Individualized Education Program (CIEP) Designed for Subject 2 (S2).

Quarter	Communication Courses and Tentative Sequencing
1	Introduction to Communication Skills
1	CID IV Basic Simultaneous Communication
2	English 5: Mechanics of Grammar
2	CID IV Intermediate Simultaneous Communication
2	CID IV Intermediate Auditory Training I
3	English 5: Grammar, Reading, and Summarizing
3	CID IV Intermediate Auditory Training II
4	CID IV Speech Improvement Through Listening
5	Telephone Communication
5	Speech for Telephone Communication
6	CID IV Speechreading for the Technical Major
7	Prefixes, Suffixes, and Roots—Speech
8	CID IV Basic Communication for Group Presentation
9	Advanced Communication for Group Presentation

Note: Program sequencing is tentative since it is highly dependent upon student progress or lack thereof.

previous experience with sign language and has limited herself entirely to the hearing community. Given these circumstances, such clients may believe that the learning of sign language will cause a deterioration of speaking abilities. Conklin *et al.* (1980) studied 78 students who were evaluated over a 2-year interval of residency at NTID. Analysis of data revealed that these students made significant gains in manual communication with no associated deterioration in speech or speechreading skills.

We would recommend that S2 also enroll in *CID IV Basic Simultaneous Communication* during her first quarter at NTID. The CID IV section of this course is recommended because S2's reading and writing scores place her in CID IV (see Tables 7.17 and 7.18). This course introduces students to sign language and helps students develop a basic sign language vocabulary for social, classroom, and work situations. Basic principles of sign language are also covered. These principles include: (1) proper hand orientation, movement, shape, and position, (2) how to ask questions in manual/simultaneous communication, (3) how to use space for location of people and objects, (4) how to use space for distinguishing among time periods, (5) how to use reduplication for plurality, and (6) others (Caccamise *et al.*, 1977; Caccamise, 1978). The class also teaches students how to use speech and signs together. Students with manual reception scores less than 40% may enroll in this course.

Second Quarter—The reading and writing tests S2 took at entry to NTID yielded an English score of 30.5. This score requires that she enroll in a level 5 English language course. Her first English course would be *English 5: Mechanics of Grammar*. This course helps students improve their skills in writing and understanding materials using multiple clause sentences. Practice is provided on parts of speech, verb tense, and word endings used in clauses in addition to other rules of grammar. The course uses material selected from important events that have occurred during the past two decades. These readings help students improve their understanding of current world events and their relationship to the past. There is also a lab for small groups of students to help them understand and use the skills learned in class. The course is for students with English scores from 29.0 to 31.9.

It is expected that S2 would obtain a score above 40%, but below 80%, on the manual reception test after completing *CID IV Basic Simultaneous Communication*. If she is motivated to further develop her sign language skills and is finding this skill useful, it is recommended that she enroll in *CID IV Intermediate Simultaneous Communication* during her second quarter. This is a course for students who already know some signs and who want to improve their skills. Students work on sign fluency, fingerspelling, and the use of signs and speech together. They learn more advanced vocabulary and the multiple meanings of some signs. Students with manual reception scores from 41 to 78% may enroll in this course.

If S2 has time, it would also be advantageous for her to begin courses in auditory training during her second quarter. *CID IV Intermediate Auditory Training I* would be recommended. This course is designed to help students improve their ability to listen to and understand sentences. Students practice listening to sentence materials and can choose units on different topics such as history, getting an apartment, and restaurants. They listen to both male and female speakers and work individually using headphones or their own hearing aids in class. Students with hearing discrimination scores from 15 to 70% may enroll in this course. Another important prerequisite is that students must also use a hearing aid all or most of the time. Mapes and Moreau (1980) reported that students enrolled in this course demonstrated an average gain of 33% on sentences related to those practiced in the course. In a follow-up study, Moreau (1980) investigated variables related to gains in this course. The variables included in her study were English ability at the onset of the course, pure tone average, aided hearing discrimination, hearing discrimination under headphones, the difference in hearing discrimination under headphones and with hearing aids, improvement in English score during the training period, speechreading with sound, speechreading without sound, auditory training pre-test score, and high frequency cut-off for the better ear. She found the best predictor of gains in this course was the student's English ability at the onset of the course. Students with higher level English reading and writing skills made the greatest gains. This finding would indicate that S2 would be an excellent candidate for this course and has an excellent prognosis for making significant gains in auditory discrimination skills.

Third Quarter—It is projected that during this quarter, S2 would enroll in her last English language course before demonstrating proficiency (Malcolm and Augustin, 1979). Proficiency, an English score of 32 or more, was established by determining the level at which the average entering hearing student enrolled at RIT was functioning (Crandall and Malcolm, 1977). During this third quarter S2 would enroll in *English 5: Grammar, Reading and Summarizing*. The purpose of this course is to assist students in improving their skills using English grammar, doing critical reading, making inferences, and developing basic skills for summarizing paragraphs. The content of the course involves materials on current issues such as crime, the energy crisis, and foreign policy. There is also a lab that helps students analyze what they read. This course is for students with English scores from 29.0 to 31.9.

Since S2 has an excellent prognosis for improving her listening skills, it will be assumed that she did make progress in the auditory training course she enrolled in during the second quarter and her instructor has recommended that she enroll for more work in this area during her third quarter. Thus, she would register for *CID IV Intermediate Auditory Training II*. This course is a continuation of *Intermediate Auditory Training I* and further improves a student's ability to listen to and understand sentences. Students must complete *Intermediate Auditory Training I* and receive a recommendation from the instructor of that course to enroll.

Fourth Quarter—It is now appropriate for S2 to begin using her listening skills in speech refinement and in learning to pronounce new vocabulary. During her fourth quarter, it is recommended she enroll in *CID IV Speech Improvement Through Listening*. This speech class helps students improve their speaking and critical self-listening skills. They also learn meanings of new words. Students listen to pre-recorded material on tapes and use a workbook that accompanies the taped material. They record their voice, listen to their own speech, and learn how to correct their own speech errors. Students with speech intelligibility scores greater than 3.6 and hearing discrimination profiles of 3 or greater may enroll in this course. This course uses the speech lab described by Humphrey *et al.* (1979) and Johnson (1976b). This communication learning center is equipped with 10 individual student carrels for listening and speaking, and a teacher station which permits intermittent monitoring by the instructor. Students with some discrimination for speech are scheduled for work within the lab (1) to practice and maintain speech skill, (2) to develop the habit of critical self-listening, (3) to reinforce auditory discrimination, and (4) to increase functional vocabulary.

It is doubtful that these types of special equipment will be available to the adult deaf client in the average clinical environment. However, a creative clinician, utilizing those instructional strategies described by Humphrey *et al.* (1979), can probably provide the client with the environment and materials essential for this much-needed practice.

Fifth Quarter—S2 is an excellent candidate for the Telephone Communication course. Johnson (1976b), in a questionnaire administered to 161 potential candidates for this course, determined that 57% of these students were not using the phone regularly because " . . . based on past experiences, they were afraid of making mistakes." S2 possesses all those skills necessary for inclusion within such a course including (1) intelligible speech, (2) constant hearing aid usage, (3) adequate hearing discrimination skills, and (4) an appropriate knowledge of the English language. However, she has limited her telephone usage to close friends and/or relatives because of extreme anxiety concerning phone conversations with strangers. It is, therefore, recommended that she enroll in the *Telephone Communication* and the *Speech for Telephone Communication* courses during her fifth quarter at NTID. The *Telephone Communication* course helps students improve their ability and confidence in using the telephone to talk with strangers. Students learn the best way to use their hearing aid with the phone, how to make long distance calls, how to make appointments over the phone, how to get information, what to do if they have any problems, and what to do in an emergency. Students learn special strategies to improve their talking and listening over the phone. They also learn how to use business phones, pay phones, and TDDs. Students are required to make phone calls every week for practice. The instructor works individually with students during four special appointments. Students with hearing discrimination scores greater than 24%, speech intelligibility scores greater than 3.5, and written language scores greater than 7.4 may enroll in this course. Also, they must have a telephone in their room or apartment, use a hearing aid all or most of the time, and have completed at least 2 quarters at NTID. Instructor and student materials used for this course can be purchased through the RIT Bookstore (Castle, 1980).

The *Speech for Telephone Communication* course helps students improve their speech and their use of telephone strategies so that people can understand them better on the telephone. Students have individual meetings with a speech instructor and practice speech and telephone strategies with pre-recorded audio-cassette tape units. In the class, students review these tapes with the instructor, practice speech, and make telephone calls. Students must have completed or be registered for *Telephone Communication* to enroll in this course.

Sixth Quarter—Table 7.18 indicates that S2 attained a score of 72% for speechreading everyday social sentences without sound under optimum conditions. In addition, when sound was applied to the speechreading process, under these same conditions, she attained a score of 100%. Although S2 has the skills necessary to function in many social environments, Jacobs (1975) has pointed out that "most of the language associated with job-related materials is very technical and often difficult to speechread." Jacobs was able to demonstrate that after reviewing her videotaped job-related materials "all students became more aware of the need for improving their speechreading skills to levels necessary to be able to receive language associated with their academic work and future job careers. Clinicians working with adult deaf clients must be certain to assess the client's knowledge and understanding of vocabulary before beginning speechreading therapy. Part of Jacobs' strategy is to have the students read key vocabulary words, their definitions, and sentences on a randomized list before they begin practicum with a videotape, because " . . . the student must be familiar with the language before any work begins."

Thus, at this point in her academic program, after having attained some knowledge and understanding of her career-related vocabulary, S2 is a good candidate for *CID IV Speechreading for the Technical Major*. The purpose of this course is to improve students' ability to speechread messages in their technical majors. Students practice identifying key words, phrases, and sentences in specific technical and professional situations. Practice materials also include passages of connected sentences that are spoken by different speakers using different kinds of materials. Speech-

reading practice is conducted with videotapes. Students with speechreading scores from 55 to 100% and who have completed at least 3 quarters in their majors may enroll in this course.

Seventh and Following Quarters—There are three additional courses which would be recommended for S2. In her seventh quarter, she should register for *Prefixes, Suffixes, and Roots—Speech*. In this course students learn how to determine the meaning and pronunciation of new words independently. Instruction and practice is provided in recognizing and pronouncing common prefixes, suffixes, and word roots, determining word meaning from context, and achieving proper pronunciation of technical words within the student's special area of study. One hour of practice each week in the Self-Instruction Lab (McQuay and Coscarelli, 1980) is required. Students with English scores greater than 29.0, speech intelligibility scores greater than 3.5 and hearing discrimination profiles of 3 or more may register for this course.

During S2's eighth quarter, she would benefit from instruction offered in the *CID IV Basic Communication for Group Presentation* course. The content of this course has been described for S1. The difference in this course for S2 would be that she would enroll in a section with other students having English language skills similar to hers. The final communication course recommended for S2 is *Advanced Communication for Group Presentation*. This course is designed to refine and increase speaking ability by giving students more experience in researching and organizing information for presentation to different audiences and for interview situations. Students review and practice basic organizational public speaking skills required for successful presentations and interviews before hearing groups. Their presentations focus on topics learned in class related to hearing impairment and its effect on communication, psychosocial development, and habitation. Students serve as a speaker representing NTID. The course is highly recommended for students enrolled in Social Work and those aspiring to managerial positions. One hour per week critiquing and recording speeches in the Self-Instruction Lab is required as a supplement to classroom activities. Students with English scores of 29.0 or more and with simultaneous reception scores greater than 77% may enroll in this course. Gustafson (1980) has described the four major content areas (readings, assignments, speaking and interviewing activities, and grading) used in this course.

Comments—A program has been designed for a young deaf client who has a need for communication refinement. This type of profoundly hearing-impaired client might very well be accommodated by a communication program in any community hearing and speech agency or clinic. The program plan presented is not only ideal, but realistic as well, provided she is motivated and willing to expend both time and effort.

References

BENDERLY, B. L., Dancing without Music. Garden City, NY: Anchor Press/Doubleday (1980).

BERGER, K. W., *Speechreading: Principles and Methods.* Baltimore: National International Press, Inc. (1972).

BERGER, M. L., and BERGER, P. J., *Group Training Techniques.* New York: John Wiley and Sons (1972).

BERGER, D. G., HOLDT, T. J., and LaFORGE, R. A., *Effective Vocational Guidance of the Deaf Adult: The Oregon Vocational Research Project.* Washington, D. C.: Social Rehabilitation Services (1972).

BOATNER, M. T., and GATES, J. E. *A Dictionary of Idioms for the Deaf.* Washington, D. C.: National Association of the Deaf (NAD) (1966).

BOCHNER, J., An evaluation of a computerized verb drill program designed for deaf young adults. *Teach. Engl. Deaf,* 18–45 (1977).

CACCAMISE, F. C., Reliability of CID Sentence Lists for performance assessment of receptive English simultaneous and manual communication skills. *Am. Ann. Deaf,* 124, 726–730 (1979).

CACCAMISE, F. C., ed., Sign language and simultaneous communication: linguistic, psychological, and instructional ramifications. *Am. Ann. Deaf,* 123, 795–906 (1978).

CACCAMISE, F. C., and BLASDELL, R., Reception of sentences under oral-manual interpreted and simultaneous test conditions. *Am. Ann. Deaf,* 122, 414–421 (1977).

CACCAMISE, F. C., MEATH-LANG, B., and JOHNSON, D. D., Assessment and use of vision: critical needs of hearing-impaired students. *Am. Ann. Deaf,* 126, 361–369 (1981).

CACCAMISE, F. C., JOHNSON, D. D., HAMILTON, L. F., ROTHBLUM, A. M., and HOWARD, M., Visual assessment and the rehabilitation of hearing-impaired children and adults. *J. Acad. Rehab. Audiol.,* 13, 78–101 (1980).

CACCAMISE, F. C., FISCHER, S., and BLASDELL, R., *Validity of CID Everyday Sentence Lists for Performance Assessments of Receptive English Simultaneous and Manual Communication Skills.* National Technical Institute for the Deaf (NTID), Rochester, NY (1979).

CACCAMISE, F. C., HATFIELD, N., and BREWER L., Manual/simultaneous communication (M/SC) research:

results and implications. *Am. Ann. Deaf,* 123, 803–823 (1978).

CACCAMISE, F. C., BLASDELL, R., and MEATH-LANG, B., Hearing-impaired persons' simultaneous reception of information under live and two visual motion media conditions. *Am. Ann. Deaf,* 122, 339–343 (1977).

CARROLL, A. W., *Personalizing Education in the Classroom.* Denver: Love Publishing Company (1975).

CASTLE, D. L., *Telecommunication Training for the Deaf.* Rochester, NY: NTID Communication Program (1981).

CASTLE, D. L., *Telephone Training for the Deaf.* Rochester, NY: NTID Communication Program (1980).

CASTLE, D. L., Telephone communication for the hearing impaired: methods and equipment. *J. Acad. Rehab. Audiol.,* 11, 91–104 (1978).

CASTLE, D. L., Telephone training for the deaf. *Volta Rev,* 79, 373–378 (1977).

CLYMER, E. W., Webster's diacritical markings typewriter element. *Audiovisual Instruction,* 22, 21–22 (1977).

CONKLIN, J. M., SUBTELNY, J. D., and WALTER, G. G., Analysis of communication skills of young deaf adults over a two year interval of technical training. *Am. Ann. Deaf,* 125, 388–393 (1980).

COSTELLO, E., Continuing education for deaf adults: a national needs assessment. *Am. Ann. Deaf,* 122, 26–32 (1977).

CRANDALL, K. E., English proficiency and progress made by NTID students. *Am. Ann. Deaf,* 125, 417–426 (1980a).

CRANDALL, K. E., *Written Language Scoring Procedures for Grammatical Correctness According to Reader Intelligibility.* Rochester, NY: NTID Communication Program (1980b).

CRANDALL, K. E., Reading and writing skills and the deaf adolescent. *Volta Rev,* 80, 319–332 (1978).

CRANDALL, K. E., Assessment of reading and writing skills in an adult deaf population. *J. Acad. Rehab. Audiol.,* 8, 64–69 (1975).

CRANDALL, K. E., and ALBERTINI, J., An investigation of variables of instruction and their relation to rate of English language learning. *Am. Ann. Deaf,* 125, 427–434 (1980).

CRANDALL, K. E., and MALCOLM, A., *Writing Skills of College Transfer Students.* Paper presented at NTID Miniconvention, Rochester, NY (1977).

CRANDALL, K. E., and ORLANDO, N. A., eds., The use and learning of spoken language systems. *Am. Ann. Deaf,* 125, 333–448 (1980).

DAVIS, J., Report of the ARA committee on educational models and continuing education. *J. Acad. Rehab. Audiol.,* 9, 17–21 (1976).

DAVIS, H., and SILVERMAN, S., *Hearing and Deafness* (3rd ed.). New York: Holt, Rinehart & Winston, Inc. (1970).

DELGADO, G., *Survey of Graduates from 1959 to 1963.* Berkeley: California School for the Deaf (1963).

DENTON, D. M., *Educational Crises.* Maryland School for the Deaf paper presented at the Tripod Conference, Memphis, Tennessee (1971).

DiLORENZO, L. T., and WELSH, W. A., *Concept Paper-Follow-Up: Report I, How Long to Receive a Degree?* Working paper, National Technical Institute for the Deaf (NTID), Rochester, NY (1981).

DONNELS, L., Adult basic education programs for deaf

people. In R. R. Davila (Ed.), *Report of the Proceedings of the 47th Meeting of the Convention of American Instructors of the Deaf*, 480–483. Washington, D. C.: U. S. Government Printing Office (1976).

DUNCAN, D. B., Multiple range and multiple F tests. *Biometrics*, **11**, 1–42 (1955).

EMERTON, G. R., HURWITZ, T. A., and BISHOP, M. E., Development of social maturity in deaf adolescents and adults. In L. J. Bradford and W. G. Hardy (Eds.), *Hearing and Hearing Impairment*. New York: Grune & Stratton (1979).

ERBER, N. P., Auditory, visual, and auditory-visual recognition of consonants by children with normal and impaired hearing. *J. Speech Hear. Res.*, **15**, 413–422 (1972).

FAIRBANKS, G., *Voice and Articulation Drillbook*. New York: Harper & Row (1960).

FISHER, H. B., and LOGEMANN, J. A., *The Fisher-Logemann Test of Articulation Competence*. Boston: Houghton Mifflin Co. (1971).

FITTS, W. H., *Tennessee Self Concept Scale: Manual*. Nashville, TN: Counselor Recordings and Tests, Department of Mental Health (1965).

FRISINA, D. R., and WILLIAMS, W. H., Managing programs for the handicapped. In F. B. Withrow and C. J. Nygren (Eds.), *Language, Materials, and Curriculum Management for the Handicapped Learner*, 214–225. Columbus, OH: Charles E. Merrill Publishing Company (1976).

GALLOWAY, A., A review of hearing aid fittings on young adults with severe to profound hearing impairment. *J. Acad. Rehab. Audiol.*, **8**, 95–109 (1975).

GARRISON, W. M., and EMERTON, R. G., *Relationships of the California Psychological Inventory to Social Knowledge and Behavior in a Deaf Population (or Absence Thereof)*. Working paper, National Technical Institute for the Deaf (NTID), Rochester, NY (1978).

GARRISON, W. M., DeCARO, P., TESCH, S., and EMERTON, R. G., *Deafness and Self-Disclosure: Some Problems in Interpreting Self-Concept Measures, Paper Series No. 24*. Rochester, NY: Department of Educational Research and Development (1978a).

GARRISON, W. M., EMERTON, R. G., and LAYNE, C. A., *Self-Concept and Social Interaction in a Deaf Population*. Working paper, National Technical Institute for the Deaf (NTID), Rochester, New York (1978b).

GARSTECKI, D. C., Survey of school audiologists. *ASHA*, **20**, 291–296 (1978).

GAUGER, J. S., *Audiologist Manual: Orientation to Hearing Aids (N6575)*. Washington, D. C.: Alexander Graham Bell Association for the Deaf, Inc. (1978a).

GAUGER, J. S., *Orientation to Hearing Aids (N6362)*. Washington, D. C.: Alexander Graham Bell Association for the Deaf (1978b).

GAUGER, J. S., and McPHERSON, D. L., A support system for hearing aid evaluations at NTID. *J. Acad. Rehab. Audiol.*, **11**, 66–90 (1978).

GOCHNOUR, E. A., Evaluating the communication skills of the deaf adult. *ASHA*, **15**, 687–691 (1973).

GRANT, D. J., WELSH, W. A., and MARRON, M. J., *An Analysis of Selected Measures of Job Success of Graduates of the National Technical Institute for the Deaf at the Rochester Institute of Technology (Report No. 32)*. Rochester, NY: NTID Department of Institutional Planning and Research (1980).

GUSTAFSON, M. S., Advanced communication for group presentation: learning and speaking about hearing impairment. *Am. Ann. Deaf*, **125**, 413–416 (1980).

HARTBAUER, R. E., *Aural Habilitation: A Total Approach*. Springfield, IL: Charles C Thomas (1975).

HASPIEL, G. S., *A Synthetic Approach to Lipreading*. Magnolia, MA: Expression Company (1969).

HAZARD, E., *Lipreading for the Oral Deaf and Hard-of-Hearing Person*. Springfield, IL: Charles C Thomas (1971).

HUMPHREY, B. K., SUBTELNY, J. D., and WHITEHEAD, R. L., Description and evaluation of structured speaking and listening activities for hearing-impaired adults. *J. Commun. Disord.*, **12**, 253–262 (1979).

JACOBS, M. A., *Speechreading Strategies*. Rochester, NY: NTID Communication Program (1978).

JACOBS, M. A., Programmed self-instruction in speechreading. *J. Acad. Rehab. Audiol.*, **8**, 106–108 (1975).

JOHNSON, D. D., Rationale and design of a hearing aid service center and shop. *Hearing Aid J.*, **30**, pp. 13 and 48–52 (1977).

JOHNSON, D. D., Communication characteristics of a young deaf adult population: techniques for evaluating their communication skills. *Am. Ann. Deaf*, **121**, 409–424 (1976a).

JOHNSON, D. D., Communication learning centers at NTID. In D. D. Johnson and W. E. Castle (Eds.), *InfoSeries 2: Equipment Designed to Improve the Communication Skills of the Deaf (PB-292046)*, 55–76. Springfield, VA: National Technical Information Services (NTIS) (1976b).

JOHNSON, D. D., Communication characteristics of NTID students. *J. Acad. Rehab. Audiol.*, **8**, 7–32 (1975).

JOHNSON, D. D., The need for continual use of amplification and auditory training. *Maryland Bull.*, **94**, 81–85 (1974).

JOHNSON, D. D., and KADUNC, N. J., Usefulness of the NTID communication profile for evaluating deaf secondary-level students. *Am. Ann. Deaf*, **125**, 337–349 (1980).

JOHNSON, D. D., and YUST, V. R., Rationale and design for a student response system. In D. D. Johnson and W. E. Castle (Eds.), *InfoSeries 2 (PB-292046)*, 32–38. Springfield, VA: National Technical Information Services (NTIS) (1976).

JOHNSON, D. D., CACCAMISE, F. C., ROTHBLUM, A. M., HAMILTON, L. F., and HOWARD, M., Identification and follow-up of visual impairments in hearing-impaired populations. *Am. Ann. Deaf*, **126**, 321–360 (1981).

JOHNSON, D. D., CACCAMISE, F. C., and KADUNC, N. J., Development of communication individualized educational programs (CIEP) for deaf secondary-level students. *J. Acad. Rehab. Audiol.*, **13**, 32–50 (1980a).

JOHNSON, D. D., WALTER, G. G., CRANDALL, K. E., McPHERSON, D. L., SUBTELNY, J. D., LEVITT, H., CACCAMISE, F. C., and DAVIS M. S., EDS., *Communication Performance Evaluation with Deaf Students: A Review (PB80-101082)*. Springfield, VA: National Technical Information Services (NTIS) (1980b).

JOHNSON, D. D., TWYMAN, L., and PASSMORE, D., *Continuing education for adult deaf: the 1977 Rochester, New York needs assessment and questionnaire results*. Rochester, New York: NTID Public Information Office (1978).

KELLY, J. F., NTID training program in interpersonal

communication. *J. Acad. Rehab. Audiol.*, **8**, 131–133 (1975).

KELLY, J. F., and SUBTELNY, J. D., *Interpersonal Communication.* 3rd Ed. Rochester, NY: NTID Communication Program (1980).

KRONENBERG, H. H., and BLAKE, G. D., *Young Deaf Adults: An Occupational Survey.* Washington, D. C.: Vocational Rehabilitation Administration (1966).

LAYNE, C. A., *Cultural Aspects of Mental Health and Deafness.* Working paper, National Technical Institute for the Deaf (NTID), Rochester, NY (1980).

LEBUFFE, L., Adult education for deaf people: icing on the cake? In R. E. Davila (Ed.), *Report of the Proceedings of the 47th Meeting of the Convention of American Instructors of the Deaf,* 474–480. Washington, D. C.: U. S. Government Printing Office (1976).

LEVINE, E. S., Psycho-cultural determinants in personality development. *Volta Rev.,* **78**, 258–267 (1976).

LEVINE, E. S., Studies in the psychological evaluation of the deaf. *Volta Rev.,* **65**, 496–512 (1963).

LUNDE, A., and BIGMAN, S., *Occupational Condition Among the Deaf.* Washington, D. C.: Gallaudet College and National Association for the Deaf (1959).

MADDEN, R., and GARDNER, E., *Stanford Achievement Test, Special Edition for Hearing Impaired Children.* New York: Harcourt, Brace, Jovanovich, Co. (1973).

MALCOLM, A., ED., *Famous Scientists: Vol. I. Ancient Times to the Industrial Revolution.* Rochester, NY: NTID Communication Program (1980).

MALCOLM, A., and AUGUSTIN, M., *Progress of Students Through English Levels.* Paper presented at NTID Miniconvention, Rochester, NY (1979).

MAPES, F. E., and MOREAU, R., The use of decoy sentences to measure auditory training gains. *Am. Ann. Deaf,* **125**, 394–399 (1980).

MARTIN, K., National Center on Employment of the Deaf: helping to "make it happen." In *NTID Focus: Employment,* 14–15. Rochester, NY: NTID Public Information Office (1980).

McGOWAN, J. F., and VESCOVI, G. M., Counselor selection, education, and training. In A. E. Sussman and L. G. Stewart (Eds.), *Counseling with Deaf People,* 108–158. New York: Deafness Research and Training Center, New York University School of Education (1971).

McQUAY, K. C., and COSCARELLI, L. S., A self-instruction lab for developing communication skills of deaf post-secondary students at NTID. *Am. Ann. Deaf,* **125**, 406–416 (1980).

MEADOW, K. P., Personality and social development of deaf people. *J. Rehab. Deaf,* **9**, 1–12 (1976).

MOELLER, M., and ECCARIUS, M., Evaluation and intervention with hearing-impaired children: a multidisciplinary approach. *J. Acad. Rehab. Audiol.,* **13**, 13–31 (1980).

MOORE, E. M., Hearing characteristics: implications for auditory training and hearing aid use. *J. Acad. Rehab. Audiol.,* **8**, 81–89 (1975a).

MOORE, E. M., Programmed self-evaluation in auditory training. *J. Acad. Rehab. Audiol,* **8**, 90–94 (1975b).

MOREAU, R., Factors affecting auditory training gains. *Am. Ann. Deaf,* **125**, 439–441 (1980).

MYKLEBUST, H. R., *Your Deaf Child.* Springfield, IL: Thomas Bannerstone House (1950).

NICKERSON, R. S., *Speech Training and Speech Reception Aids for the Deaf, Report No. 12980.* Cambridge, MA: Bolt, Beranek and Newman, Inc. (1975). (Copyright 1975, Bolt, Beranek and Newman, Inc.)

NOAR, G., *Individualized Instruction: Every Child a Winner.* New York: John Wiley and Sons, Inc. (1972).

NSPB (NATIONAL SOCIETY TO PREVENT BLINDNESS), *Vision Screening of Children (P-257),* 1–12. New York: NSPB (1979).

NTID PUBLIC INFORMATION OFFICE, *NTID Focus: Employment.* Rochester, NY: NTID Public Information Office (1980).

NTID PUBLIC INFORMATION OFFICE, Communication tips. *NTID Focus,* 24 (winter, 1977).

OFFICE OF DEMOGRAPHIC STUDIES, *Characteristics of Hearing Impaired Students by Hearing Status: 1970–71, Series D, Number 19.* Washington, D. C.: Gallaudet College (1973).

OFFICE OF EDUCATION, *Federal Register,* **41**, 24101–24336. Washington, D. C.: The National Archives of the United States (1976).

ORLANDO, N. A., Evidence of success in speech and voice training. *J. Acad. Rehab. Audiol.,* **8**, 51–63 (1975).

PARKER, C. A., and WELSH, W. A., *A Report on the Comparative Status of NTID Graduates in 1977 and 1978 (Report No. 30).* Rochester, NY: NTID Department of Institutional Planning and Research (1980).

PATTERSON, C. H., and STEWART, L. G., Principles of counseling with deaf people. In A. E. Sussman and L. G. Stewart (Eds.), *Counseling with Deaf People,* 43–86. New York: Deafness Research and Training Center, New York University School of Education (1971).

QUIGLEY, S., The vocational rehabilitation of deaf persons. In S. Quigley (Ed.), *The Vocational Rehabilitation of Deaf People,* 1–4. Washington, D. C.: Rehabilitative Services, Administration (1966).

RAWLINGS, B. W., and TRYBUS, R. J., Update on post-secondary programs for hearing impaired students. *Am. Ann. Deaf,* **121**, 541–546 (1976).

RAWLINGS, B. W., TRYBUS, R. J., and BISER, J., *A Guide to College/Career Programs for Deaf Students.* 4th Ed. Washington, D. C.: Gallaudet College (1981).

RIT OFFICIAL BULLETIN, *The RIT Official Bulletin (USPS 715-400).* Vol. LXXX, No. 3, Rochester, NY: Rochester Institute of Technology (May 1980).

RITTER, A., *National Center on Employment of the Deaf: An Annotated Bibliography of Literature Related to Employment of Deaf Persons.* Rochester, NY: NTID Staff Resource Center (1980).

SANDERS, D. A., *Aural Rehabilitation.* Englewood Cliffs, NJ: Prentice-Hall, Inc. (1971).

SARGENT, D. C., and MALCOLM, A., *The Presentation of Continuous Speech with Synchronous Text.* Paper presented at IEEE International Conference on Acoustics, Speech, and Signal Processing, New York, NY (1979).

SARGENT, D., and NYERGES, L. D., A system for the synchronization of continuous speech with printed text. *Am. Ann. Deaf,* **124**, 530–535 (1979).

SCHEIN, J. D., *Economic Status of Deaf Adults: 1972–1977.* New York: Deafness Research and Training Center, New York University School of Education (1978).

SCHEIN, J. D., and DELK, M. T., JR., *The Deaf Population of the United States.* Silver Spring, MD: National Association of the Deaf (1974).

SCHMALZ, K., and WALTER, G. G., *Introduction to Communication.* 3rd Ed. Rochester, NY: NTID Communication Program (1980).

SIMS, D., The validation of the CID Everyday Sentence

Test for use with the severely hearing impaired. *J. Acad. Rehab. Audiol.*, **8**, 70–79 (1975).

SNELL, K. B., and MANAGAN, F. E., Effectiveness of an auditory training program at the National Technical Institute for the Deaf. NTID paper presented at the American Speech and Hearing Association Convention, Houston, TX (1976).

SNELL, K. B., MANAGAN, F. E., and CLYMER, W., Instructional technology principles applied to an auditory training program. *Audiol. Hear. Educ.*, **4**, 8–10 (1976).

STRENG, A., FITCH, W. J., HEDGECOCK, L. D., PHILLIPS, J. W., and CARRELL, J. A., *Hearing Therapy for Children*. New York: Grune & Stratton (1967).

STUCKLESS, E. R. *Deaf People as a Population*. Monograph under preparation, Rochester, NY: NTID Office of Integrative Research (1980).

STUCKLESS, E. R., Technology and the visual processing of verbal information by deaf people. *Am. Ann. Deaf*, **123**, 630–636 (1978).

SUBTELNY, J. D., Assessment of speech with implications for training. In F. H. Bess (Ed.), *Childhood Deafness*. New York: Grune & Stratton (1977).

SUBTELNY, J. D., The assessment of aural and oral skills program planning for NTID students. In R. R. Davila (Ed.), *Report of the Proceedings of the 47th Meeting of the Convention of American Instructors of the Deaf*, 603–615. Washington, D. C.: U. S. Government Printing Office (1976a).

SUBTELNY, J., Ed., *Webster's Diacritical Markings*. Bloomington, IN: Handicapped Learner Materials Distribution Center (HLMDC) (1976b).

SUBTELNY, J. D., Speech assessment of the deaf adult. *J. Acad. Rehab. Audiol.* **8**, 110–116 (1975).

SUBTELNY, J. D., and WALTER, G. G., An overview of the communication skills of NTID students with implications for planning of rehabilitation. *J. Acad. Rehab. Audiol.*, **8**, 33–50 (1975).

SUBTELNY, J. D., ORLANDO, N. A., and WHITEHEAD, R. L., *Speech and Voice Characteristics of the Deaf (A0235)*. Washington, D. C.: The Alexander Graham Bell Association for the Deaf (1981).

THORESON, R. W., and TULLY, N. L., Role and function of the counselor. In A. E. Sussman and L. G. Stewart (Eds.), *Counseling with Deaf People*, 87–107. New York: Deafness Research and Training Center, New York University School of Education (1971).

TIEGS, E. W., and CLARK, W. W., *California Reading Test: Junior High Level, WXYZ Series, 1963 Norms*. Monterey, CA: McGraw-Hill, Inc. (1967).

U. S. BUREAU OF CENSUS, *Census of Population, 1970: General Social and Economic Characteristics, Final Report, PC (1)-C1 U. S. Summary*. Washington, D. C.: U. S. Government Printing Office (1972).

U. S. BUREAU OF CENSUS, *General Population Characteristics, 1970: PC (1)-B1 U. S. Summary*. Washington, D. C.: U. S. Government Printing Office (1970).

U. S. BUREAU OF CENSUS, *Statistical Abstracts of the United States, 1977*. 98th Ed. Washington, D. C.: U. S. Government Printing Office (1977).

U. S. BUREAU OF EDUCATION FOR THE HANDICAPPED, Notice of proposed rule-making: November 11, 1975. *Federal Register*, 24101–24336. Washington, D. C.: U. S. Government Printing Office (1975).

U. S. BUREAU OF LABOR STATISTICS, Explanatory notes. In C. L. Green, G. P. Green, and J. A. McCall (Eds.), *Employment and Earnings: December 1976*, 145–163. Washington, D. C.: Bureau of Labor Statistics (1976).

U. S. BUREAU OF LABOR STATISTICS, Explanatory notes. In C. L. Green, G. P. Green, and J. A. McCall (Eds.), *Employment and Earnings: March 1974*, 129–144. Washington, D. C.: Bureau of Labor Statistics (1974).

VERNON, M., Editorial. *Am. Ann. Deaf*, **122**, 4 (1977).

VERNON, M., Usher's syndrome: problems and some solutions. *Hear. Speech Action*, **44**, 6–13 (1976).

WALTER, G. G., English skills assessment and program planning for NTID students. In R. R. Davila (Ed.), *Report of the Proceedings of the 47th Meeting of the Convention of American Instructors of the Deaf*, 592–602. Washington, D. C.: U. S. Government Printing Office (1976).

WELSH, W. A., *The Relationship of Selected Demographic, Achievement, and Communication Variables to Labor Force Activities of Graduates of Rochester Institute of Technology Through the National Technical Institute for the Deaf (Report No. 35)*. Rochester, NY: NTID Department of Institutional Planning and Research (1980).

WILLIAMS, B. R., and SUSSMAN, A. E., Social and psychological problems of deaf people. In A. E. Sussman and L. G. Stewart (Eds.), *Counseling with Deaf People*, 13–29. New York: Deafness Research and Training Center, New York University School of Education (1971).

WINAKUR, I., Results of the Winakur survey. Gallaudet Alumni Newsletter, **9**, 6 (1975).

8

The Adult Deaf-Blind Client and Rehabilitation

Linda M. Hirsch, M.S.

In his poem, "Shared Beauty," Robert Smithdas describes sensations conveyed to him despite the absence of vision and hearing.

I cannot see a rainbow's glory spread
across a rain-washed sky when storm is over;
nor can I see or hear the birds that cry
their songs among the clouds, or through
    bright clover.
You tell me that the night is full of stars,
and how the winds and waters sing and
    flow;
and in my heart I wish that I could share
with you this beauty that I cannot know.
I only know that when I touch a flower,
or feel the sun and wind upon my face,
or hold your hand in mine, there is a bright-
    ness
within my soul that words can never trace.
I call it Life, and laugh with its delight,
though life itself be out of sound and sight.

Robert J. Smithdas, with permission

The senses of smell, of taste, and of touch provide the primary pathways through which the world around him may be explored. In communication, in travel, and in daily living, he must function with life literally at his fingertips.

The focus of this chapter is to explore the dual handicapping condition of deaf-blindness. Since the onset and degree of each disability plays a major role in one's overall functioning, the effects of early *versus* late onset, as well as partial *versus* total impairment will be discussed. Some common etiologies of deaf-blindness, including Usher's Syndrome and Congenital Rubella Syndrome, will be presented.

The loss of hearing and vision strongly affects one's ability to communicate. Special methods of communication used with deaf-blind persons will be discussed in depth, in an effort to provide the reader with practical knowledge of such communication techniques. The audiologic, speech, and language evaluation of the deaf-blind individual possesses some unique aspects because of the client's dual impairment, as does the communicative (re)habilitation of such an individual. Some common speech and language problems seen in the deaf and in the blind will be discussed including the unique aspects of the communicative (audiologic, speech, and language) evaluation and rehabilitation process. It is important to keep in mind that each deaf-blind person is an individual first, with needs and aspirations that set him apart from others, deaf-blind or not. It is our responsibility to help him to achieve these goals.

"We can say this about deaf-blind people: They are human beings who serve to exercise their curiosity and who have the courage to live if they are given the opportunity and the assistance they need to reach their goals." (Smithdas, 1976.)

STATISTICS AND PREVALENCE OF DEAF-BLINDNESS; AVAILABILITY OF SERVICES

Deaf-Blind Youths and Adults

Identification of deaf-blind adults is a difficult task. Unfortunately, despite recent attempts to mainstream handicapped individuals into the general population, it is thought that many deaf-blind adults presently reside in custodial institutions where access to specialized rehabilitation services for them are, at best, limited. The Helen Keller National Center for Deaf-Blind Youths and Adults, a rehabilitation facility operating under authorization contained in Section 305 of Title III of the Rehabilitation Act of 1973, maintains a National Register of deaf-blind youths and adults. Through the efforts of their regional representatives, located in nine offices throughout the country (see Appendix 8A), as well as affiliates of the Center, approximately 5100 deaf-blind youths and adults have been identified to date and are listed on the register. Despite continued efforts to update and expand the register, it is thought that there are still many deaf-blind adults not yet identified. Individuals interested in reporting suspected cases of deaf-blind individuals for addition to the Register should contact the Center (see Appendix 8C).

Many deaf-blind youths and adults receive services through the Helen Keller National Center for Deaf-Blind Youths and Adults, headquartered in Sands Point, NY. The Center is operated by the Industrial Home for the Blind under an agreement signed in 1969 with the U. S. Department of Health, Education, and Welfare. At present, it operates under the general supervision of the Rehabilitation Services Administration, Department of Education. Funds for it's operation are appropriated annually by Congress.

According to the Helen Keller National Center Annual Report, covering the period March 1, 1979 through Feb 29, 1980, 798 deaf-blind clients received services. Approximately 75% of these services were provided by regional representatives (see Appendix 8A) or affiliated agencies. Here, isolated services may be provided, such as training in mobility, training in communications, or a refresher training program to upgrade skills and enhance employability. Clients who require in-depth comprehensive evaluation and rehabilitation training in multiple rehabilitation areas (*i.e.* communication, mobility, daily living, work ability skills, psycho-social development, etc.) are served at the Helen Keller National Center headquarters facility. The objectives of the Helen Keller National Center are listed in Table 8.1.

As stated in *Introducing the Helen Keller National Center* (1980), ". . .to be eligible for the evaluation at the Helen Keller National Center, an individual must have substantial visual and auditory losses such that the combination of the two causes extreme difficulty in learning. Such losses constitute the basic condition of eligibility for any of the services of the Center. This includes eligibility for services of the regional representatives and affiliated agencies. Eligibility for enrollment in the evaluation and rehabilitation training program conducted at the Center's headquarters is limited to persons who are deaf-blind within the following definitions. *Deafness*, a physiological chronic hearing impairment so severe that most speech cannot be understood through the ear with optimum amplification. A speech discrimination score of 40% or less in the better ear would generally indicate a hearing impairment within the Center's criteria for enrollment in the evaluation and rehabilitation training program. *Blindness*, visual acuity not exceeding 20/200 in the better eye with correcting lenses, or visual acuity greater than 20/200 if the visual field is constricted to 20° or less. Exceptions to this basic definition may be made for a deaf-blind individual with an auditory or visual condition that shows poor prognosis, or one whose ability to use his hearing and/or vision is so limited as a result of protracted inadequate use of either or both of these senses that he functions as a deaf-blind person. Some individuals with substantial visual and auditory deficits requiring a period of careful training and practice to make optimum use of newly acquired hearing aids and/or special corrective lenses, may also be eligible."

Agencies for the deaf, as well as for the blind, are beginning to provide services to deaf-blind individuals. A nationwide survey has recently been conducted by the Helen Keller National Center in conjunction with

Table 8.1
Objectives of the Helen Keller National Center for Deaf-Blind Youths and Adults[a]

1. To provide initial assessment of physical and psycho-social functioning of deaf-blind individuals to determine feasibility for admission to the Helen Keller National Center, or referral to other agencies with services appropriate to their individual needs.
2. To provide multidisciplinary evaluation to those deaf-blind individuals for whom rehabilitation is feasible, and to determine their rehabilitation needs, interests, and potentialities.
3. To then provide comprehensive individualized rehabilitation training to achieve in each case (a) meaningful contact with the environment and effective means of communication, (b) constructive participation in the home and community, (c) initial or enhanced employability, and (d) any other development important to the optimum rehabilitation of the deaf-blind individual.
4. To act as a resource center for the deaf-blind, the families and friends of deaf-blind individuals, and professionals in the field who work with the deaf-blind.
5. To identify and locate youths and adults who are deaf-blind in order to develop a national register of those individuals which will provide information as to the composition and distribution of the deaf-blind population that will aid in the planning of services appropriate to the needs of this population.
6. To encourage and develop research regarding the implications of deaf-blindness and the impact this disability has for the deaf-blind in terms of personal adjustment, employment, education, and technical/accessibility requirements.
7. To innovate and/or improve techniques of rehabilitation that will best serve the deaf-blind.
8. To design and/or improve sensory aids to help reduce the handicapping effects of deaf-blindness.
9. To provide training for workers in service for deaf-blind persons.
10. To provide community education programs designed to sensitize both the lay and professional communities to the special needs and aspirations of deaf-blind individuals.
11. To encourage, assist, and educate public and private agencies to develop and increase services for deaf-blind individuals.

[a]Reprinted by permission from *Introducing the Helen Keller National Center* (brochure). Sands Point, NY: Helen Keller National Center (1980).

the American Deafness and Rehabilitation Association (ADARA) in an effort to locate rehabilitation agencies serving deaf-blind individuals and to determine the nature of their services. A directory of agencies reporting to serve deaf-blind persons has been compiled as a result of this survey. (See Appendix 8C, Abordo and Thomas (1980) for information regarding publication and availability).

Deaf-Blind Children

The rubella epidemic of 1963–65 increased the number of deaf-blind children in the United States to more than 5000 (Lowell, 1975). According to Dantona (1974), "surveys conducted by the Regional Centers for Deaf-Blind Children have located... 5,064 deaf-blind children." Hicks and Pfau (1979) report that "...during the 1977–78 program year the regional centers identified 5,614 deaf-blind children (under 21 years of age).... During the 1978–79 program year, 5,872 deaf-blind children are projected to be served.... This represents the total number of deaf-blind children identified in the U. S."

Services to deaf-blind children are provided by Regional Centers for Services to Deaf-Blind Children, which operates ten regional centers across the country (see Appendix 8B). Their services are offered to "children who have both auditory and visual impairments, the combination of which causes such severe communication and other developmental and educational problems that they can not be properly accommodated in special education programs for the hearing-handicapped child or for the visually handicapped child." (Dantona and Salmon, 1972).

DEFINITION AND DISCUSSION OF DEAFNESS AND BLINDNESS: EFFECTS OF THE DUAL HANDICAP

As workers with the hearing-impaired are well aware, the term "deafness" does not necessarily connote total absence of hearing. The "deaf" range from those who function as hard-of-hearing individuals to others who have little or no hearing. Similarly, "blindness" does not necessarily connote total absence of vision. Although there is no legal or generally accepted definition of deafness among agencies serving the hearing-impaired, there is a legal definition of blindness. Blindness is defined along two parameters, one which pertains to limited visual acuity, and the other which deals with the restriction on peripheral vision (visual fields). The definition of blindness most commonly accepted in the U. S. is central visual acuity not exceeding 20/200 in the better eye with correcting lenses or a visual field that is constricted to 20° or less regardless of visual acuity (Carroll, 1961). An individual who falls within the first definition may experience difficulty reading small print and identifying details visually; however, he still retains significant useful vision and generally functions as a "visually impaired" individual. An individual who retains good acuity but has restricted visual fields, or "tunnel vision," may appear to the casual observer to have normal vision. Such an individual may be capable of reading small print, and performing daily activities visually. However, difficulties may be encountered in crossing streets, or in group communication where peripheral vision is as vital as central vision.

Just as the degree of hearing and vision loss affects functioning, so does age at onset of each disability. It is well known that congenital hearing loss causes significant difficulties not found in the adventitiously hearing-impaired individual, particularly in language development. Similarly, congenital vision loss tends to cause difficulties with development of such visual concepts as color, size, and position in space. Individuals who are adventitiously blinded still retain visual memory based on past experience with such concepts, just as those who lose their hearing later in life retain auditory recall of sounds and sound sources.

Individuals who are totally congenitally deaf-blind are a rarity; in fact, whether or not such individuals exist is an issue of question among some educators of the deaf-blind. Rather, "most deaf-blind people tend to fall into one of two groups: either deafened *blind* people or blinded *deaf* people. The distinction rests on the relative functioning of the two senses and the age at onsets of their impairment. Deaf persons who became blind, as in Usher's Syndrome, tend to react as deaf persons. Similarly, blind persons who lose their hearing continue to resemble blind persons more than deaf persons in their daily functioning." (Kates and Schein, 1980). This distinction plays an important role in one's ori-

entation to communication, mobility, and daily living skills, as well as to the approach a clinician takes in improving skills in these areas.

For the purposes of clarification, an operational definition of terms has been adapted from Kramer *et al.*, 1979. "A *total* impairment of hearing or vision is one in which the magnitude of dysfunction precludes a significant contribution to the reception or development of language through the particular sensory modality. Total impairment is not necessarily synonymous with the total absence of hearing or vision. Thus, a partial impairment becomes one that significantly hinders, but does not rule out the reception or development of language. These definitions have been made for convenience and are not meant to discount the value of minimal sensory function. Light perception and gross auditory awareness can affect significantly an individual's conceptualization, ultimately contributing to his ability to function. In like manner, a congenital impairment, in either sensory modality, is defined as one whose onset is so early as to rule out a contribution to the reception or development of language. Alternatively, a subsequently acquired disability is labeled adventitious."

Etiologies of Deaf-Blindness

There are many causes of deaf-blindness. Some causes are genetically linked syndromes which cause loss of both hearing and vision, and perhaps other coincident impairments as well. Other individuals become deaf-blind due to auditory and visual defects, each of which may be caused by genetic factors, trauma, or illness/disease.

Usher's Syndrome—According to Vernon (1974), "the leading cause of deaf-blindness in most scientifically advanced countries" is Usher's Syndrome. Nance *et al.* (1976) define Usher's Syndrome as "a genetic disorder characterized by severe neural hearing loss and Retinitis Pigmentosa." Retinitis Pigmentosa (R. P) is "a slowly progressive degeneration of the retina and pigment epithelium (a layer of pigmented cells next to the neural retina) characterized by loss of side vision, loss of night vision, pigmentary clumping, and loss of electrical response on the electroretinogram." (Bergsma, 1976). Electroretin-ography (ERG) is an objective measurement of "electrical potential produced in the retinal and pigment epithelium in response to light. This electrical potential is diminished or absent in R. P." (Bergsma, 1976). ERG permits the diagnosis of Retinitis Pigmentosa before its obvious symptoms are evident. In R. P., the vision loss progresses to at least legal blindness due to restricted visual fields, with a gradual loss of central visual acuity (Bergsma, 1973). According to McLeod et al. (1971), R. P. "frequently does not become symptomatic until late childhood or adolescence. The earliest visual symptom is usually night blindness, followed by progressive restriction of the visual fields, leading to almost complete loss of useful vision by the fourth or fifth decade of life. Defects in color vision and the development of cataracts may also be observed as the disease process progresses." R. P. can appear without hearing loss as well.

McLeod et al. (1971) note that "among congenitally deaf persons, the incidence of R. P. has been variously reported to range from 3.0 to 10.4%," making the deaf a high risk group for this disease. Further, "hearing loss has been found in 3.4 to 6.3% of patients with pigment degeneration of the retina" (McLeod et al., 1971). The 1980 Annual Report of the Helen Keller National Center for Deaf-Blind Youths and Adults states that approximately 45% of all clients served were diagnosed as having Usher's Syndrome.

It is generally agreed that those having a congenital severe to profound sensorineural hearing loss, in addition to R. P., fall within the definition of Usher's Syndrome. However, there are cases of individuals having R. P. in combination with normal or mildly impaired hearing at birth. The hearing loss may be stable or progress in later life, concurrent with the visual loss. The classification of such individuals as being affected by Usher's Syndrome is still a topic of debate among providers of service to the deaf, blind, and deaf-blind. Presently, however, many investigators believe the definition should be broader, including those individuals demonstrating less severe hearing loss. McLeod et al (1971) have documented cases of siblings affected with the combination of R. P. and hearing loss, displaying sigificant variation in the degree of hearing loss present among siblings. This evidence supports the need for inclusion of a broader range of hearing loss in the definition of Usher's Syndrome.

At present, there is no cure for Usher's Syndrome. However, early detection and intervention can make a significant difference in affecting a positive change for the individual's future. The concept of early detectiion and intervention of hearing impairment is well accepted among audiologists, speech-language pathologists, teachers of the deaf, and other workers with the hearing-impaired. The value in early detection of concurrent visual impairment, achieved through visual screenings, can be realized when one considers the importance of the visual mode in the deaf population. As noted by Barrett (1979), "for persons who are deaf, good vision becomes paramount for learning communication, mobility, recreation, social interaction, and vocational pursuit." In view of the importance of good vision among the deaf, Barrett (1979) cites several justifications regarding implementation of vision assessment programs: "(a) to identify these persons with vision problems who may require further treatment, (b) to make the appropriate referral for treatment, and (c) to initiate appropriate counselling services when visual conditions are diagnosed which cannot be treated medically." In proposing a theoretical model to assess vision in a school for the deaf, Barrett (1979) includes "evaluation of possible refractive error, eye muscle coordination, intraocular pressure (tonometry), eye pathology, and overall visual functioning." Levin and Erber (1976) suggest that a comprehensive visual screening among deaf children include: (1) tests of visual acuity, (2) tests of binocular vision, (3) tests of color vision, and (4) tests of peripheral vision. Such tests would detect not only the presence of R. P., but other visual disorders as well.

In recognition of the importance of visual assessment and follow-up on the habilitation of the hearing-impaired, the National Technical Institute for the Deaf has initiated a comprehensive project on identification of visual impairments among deaf college students (Caccamise et al., 1980). Visual parameters assessed include near and far (distance) acuity (the ability of the eyes to resolve or differentiate detail), color vision (the ability to discriminate colors), and binocular vision (muscle balance and depth perception) (Caccamise et al., 1980).

Following detection of R. P., genetic counselling for patients and their families is indicated. Effective genetic counselling would, hopefully, cause a significant reduction in the occurrence of Usher's Syndrome. However, it should be noted that Usher's Syndrome can not be completely eliminated even through the combination of visual screening and genetic counselling because, as Vernon (1976) notes, "it is transmitted by an autosomal recessive gene. This means men and women may be carriers even though they do not have Usher's Syndrome." In addition to genetic counselling for individual's having Usher's Syndrome, appropriate recommendations for vocational and personal/social follow-up are indicated.

Public and professional education is an important component in any program of detection and intervention. In promoting detection of Usher's Syndrome, individuals who work with the deaf are the prime audience for such information, as they deal with this group which is high risk for the disease. It is interesting to note that in schools and colleges for the deaf, individuals who have been diagnosed as having Usher's Syndrome often make the identification of another individual who unknowingly also has the disease. Thus, in its middle or advanced stages, it is not difficult to detect by one who is familiar with the symptoms.

There are numerous other genetic syndromes which include symptoms of congenital hearing loss and R. P. Some of these, as cited by McLeod *et al.* (1971) are Hallgren's Syndrome (retinitis pigmentosa, cerebellar ataxia, and deafness); the Laurence-Moon-Biedl Syndrome (Retinitis Pigmentosa, retardation, obesity, polydactyly hypogonadism, and deafness); Alstrom's Syndrome (Retinitis Pigmentosa, obesity, diabetes, and deafness); and Refsum's Syndrome (Retinitis Pigmentosa, ichthyosis, polyneuritis, and deafness). However, statistics reveal that Usher's Syndrome is seen in greater numbers than any of these more distinct syndromes.

Rubella—Congenital Rubella Syndrome, also known as German measles, is one of the leading causes of congenital deafness. Among children enrolled in programs for the hearing-impaired who were not born during the 1963–65 epidemic years, approximately 8–10% are deaf due to rubella. However, this figure increases to 41–44% of those born in 1964 and

34–37% for those born in 1965. (Jensema, 1974; Trybus *et al.*, 1980). According to Castle (1980), "this dramatic increase, sometimes described as the 'rubella bulge' was due directly to the calamitous rubella epidemic which swept this country in 1963, 1964, and 1965, resulting in 8000 or more children being born deaf and 4000 or more other children being born deaf and blind."

There are several characteristics that comprise the Congenital Rubella Syndrome.

Hearing Loss—Hearing loss is the most common defect associated with rubella babies (Jensema, 1974), with incidence placed at approximately 73% of the cases (Chess *et al.*, 1978). Ziring (1975) notes that deafness may be the only defect present in the child whose mother contracted rubella after the eighth week of pregnancy. The hearing loss is sensorineural and is generally bilateral, although unilateral losses may be seen.

Some investigators have suggested that rubella-deafened children have more severe hearing losses as a group than those whose deafness was due to other causes. Jensema (1974) notes that "49% of those in the rubella group with known better ear averages had a profound hearing loss and 83% had a loss of over 70 dB. In contrast, only 69% of the other-causes group had a better ear average of 70 dB." Others suggest that the loss is not as severe. Myklebust (1964) states that rubella results in a degree of deafness which is moderately severe but not total. Vernon and Hicks (1980) note that the hearing losses range over the full spectrum, but in general tend to be flat or cup shape in audiometric configuration. They suggest that rubella-deafened youth have better functional use of their hearing than would be expected by determining a pure-tone average in the better ear. E. R. Stuckless (reported by Trybus *et al.*, 1980) reports slightly better hearing in the speech range among rubella than non-rubella students at NTID and significantly better auditory discrimination and speech intelligibility among rubella students. In most cases, the hearing loss is stable; however, Smith (1974) notes that 30% may experience further deterioration in auditory functioning at age five or six due to cochlear degeneration.

Cardiac Defects—Cardiac defects may be found in 32–76% of rubella youth (Vernon *et al.*, 1980; Chess *et al.*, 1978). The most common cardiac defect noted in rubella children is patent ductus arteriosus (Ziring, 1975). Vernon *et al.* (1980) describe this as "failure of the opening between the aorta and pulmonary artery to close after birth." Surgical repair is possible. Ziring (1975) notes that other cardiac disorders, particularly defects of the aortic arch, may also be seen, but less commonly than patent ductus arteriosus. Some of these are aortic stenosis, coarctation, and ventricular septal defect (Ziring, 1975).

Visual Defects—Visual problems are found in approximately 33% of rubella children (Chess *et al.*, 1978). The most common ocular defect in children with congenital rubella is retinopathy. The rubella virus causes clumping of the retinal pigments to give it a "salt and pepper" appearance when viewed with an ophthalmoscope. This condition does not interfere with vision; however, evidence of pigmentary clumping in combination with deafness suggests the etiology of deafness as due to congenital rubella. This information is helpful in cases where the etiology of deafness was previously unknown, and may be confirmed by laboratory tests (Cooper, 1969; Ziring, 1975).

Cataracts are "the most characteristic, although not the most common, ocular manifestation of congenital rubella. . . . The cataracts result from direct virus infection of the lens of the developing eye. After birth, the virus may persist in the lens for an indefinite period of time after it can no longer be detected elsewhere in the body" (Ziring, 1975). Cataracts may be bilateral or unilateral. They may be present at birth, but often are undetectable due to their small size. In addition, eyes of rubella children are frequently microphthalmic (very small). Surgical removal of cataracts is possible; however, the optimal time for removal of cataracts is still a subject of some debate. Some ophthalmologists prefer to wait until the eye has grown to sufficient size to increase surgical facility and chances of successful vision restoration; others feel that earlier intervention is preferable, particularly in consideration of critical periods of sensory development.

Congenital glaucoma is present in approximately 4–10% of rubella infants (Menser *et al.*, 1967; Cooper, 1969). Glaucoma is a condition in which pressure in the eye builds resultant of improper drainage of fluid, causing damage to the retina (Vernon *et al.*, 1980). The condition requires prompt treatment, generally through surgery, since delay in diagnosis or treatment often leads to blindness.

Neurological Damage—Neurological damage is not uncommon among rubella children. Chess and Fernandez (1980) found a low incidence of neurologic damage (10%) among rubella deaf children who had normal intelligence. However, among the rubella deaf-mentally retarded, and deaf-blind-mentally retarded, the incidence of neurologic damage was much higher (70 and 51%, respectively).

Behavior problems frequently accompany neurologic damage. Chess and Fernandez (1980) make a distinction between behavioral problems caused directly by damage to the brain (Chronic Brain Syndrome) and those behavioral problems which are resultant of coping with motor and perceptual difficulties (Reactive Behavior Disorder). Behavioral symptoms commonly noted are "perseveration, difficulty in shifting from one task to another, sudden shifts of mood or overreaction to minor stimuli, motility disturbances which may consist of hyper- or hypomotility (great movement or great inertia), and high distractibility" (Chess and Fernandez, 1980). Impulsivity is also commonly found among rubella youth (Vernon *et al.*, 1980). Aphasia and other learning disabilities may be found in rubella children as well (Vernon *et al.*, 1980). Chess (1977) reports a 7.4% rate of autism among rubella children. This represents a significant increase over the incidence of autism among the general population.

In summary, hearing loss, cardiac defects, visual defects, and psychoneurologic and behavioral factors comprise the most prevalent characteristics found among rubella children. Additionally, urogenital disorders and endocrine disturbances may be found, as well as a failure to thrive during infancy (Vernon *et al.*, 1980).

Usher's Syndrome and Congenital Rubella Syndrome are the two most common causes of deaf-blindness. However, deaf-blindness can also occur as a result of unrelated hearing and visual losses. Some of the visual defects found among blind and deaf-blind individuals, described by the National Eye Institute, can be found in Table 8.2.

COMMUNICATION TECHNIQUES USED WITH THE DEAF-BLIND CLIENT

There are many methods of communication that can be used by deaf-blind individ-

Table 8.2
Visual Disorders Found among Blind and Deaf-Blind Individuals [a]

Retinitis Pigmentosa	an inherited condition that gradually impairs the retina's ability to respond to light, causing night blindness and progressive loss of peripheral vision.
Myopia	also known as nearsightedness; a common condition in which the image is focused in front of instead of on the retina. Can be corrected with eyeglasses or contact lenses.
Astigmatism	the refractive, or light bending, power of the cornea is not equal in all directions. Only part of the image is sharply focused on the retina. Can be corrected with eyeglasses or contact lenses.
Retinal detachment	separation of the light sensitive layer of the retina from underlying tissue causes impaired vision. Can be treated with surgery if diagnosed early.
Strabismus	the muscles of the two eyes do not work together properly and one or both eyes may turn inward or outward. The brain is unable to fuse the input from each eye into a single image. Is often treated successfully with bifocals, eye exercises, or surgery.
Cataract	a cloudiness in the lens of the eye which interferes with vision. Surgery is the only effective treatment.
Glaucoma	gradually impairs peripheral vision when increased pressure in the eye damages the optic nerve causing "tunnel vision." It can be usually controlled by medication or surgery.
Macular degeneration	progressive loss of central vision usually associated with aging. There is no effective treatment for most cases.

[a] Reprinted by permission from *How Eye Problems Affect Our Vision.* Bethesda, MD: National Eye Institute, National Institutes of Health (1977).

uals. Some of these methods are primarily visual and can be used by the deaf-visually impaired adult who retains significant residual vision. Other methods which are primarily auditory are more suitable for the individual who retains significant residual hearing. Many methods of communication used by deaf-blind persons, however, rely on the sense of touch alone in conveying messages to those individuals who possess little or no residual sight or hearing.

The following section will discuss close range methods of communicating: (1) with those deaf-blind individuals having residual hearing, (2) with those deaf-blind individuals having residual vision, and (3) with those deaf-blind individuals having neither residual hearing nor residual vision (see also Table 8.3). Subsequently, long range methods of communication with these groups will be discussed.

Close Range Methods of Communication Used with Deaf-Blind Individuals Having Residual Hearing or Vision

Amplified Speech—For the deaf-blind individual who retains significant residual hearing, every effort should be made to maximize use of audition in reception of communication. To this end, competing background noise should be avoided and a favorable acoustical environment employed to enhance message reception. The intensity level of the speaker's voice, as well as distance and orientation of the speaker to the hearing- and visually-impaired listener should be modified in accordance with the listener's needs. These factors are particularly important in the absence of any residual vision. In such a case, the individual must rely entirely on his impaired residual hearing for message reception, having no access to speechreading cues.

The individual who has significent residual hearing and uses audition as a primary mode of receptive communication will most likely use amplification. If appropriate amplifiction is not possessed, a speech audiometer or auditory trainer may be helpful in determining the contribution of amplified residual hearing to message reception in establishing effective communication.

The individual who relies on audition for message reception most likely uses speech as an expressive means of communication. Although this client's speech may be defective, it is generally intelligible enough to be understood even by an individual unfamiliar with the speech patterns of the deaf.

In communicating with the deaf-blind individual who has significant residual vision, it is important to be aware of the type of visual condition that the client possesses; that is, whether his visual disability is due to poor visual acuity or to restricted visual fields. "In the case of reduced visual acuity, as in myopia, there is a need for the message sent to be in close visual range. Additionally, appro-

Table 8.3
Methods of Communication Used with Deaf-Blind Persons, Based on Onset and Severity of Hearing and Visual Losses.[a,b]

Vision	Hearing							
	Adventitious				Congenital			
	Partial		Total		Partial		Total	
	RECEPTIVE	EXPRESSIVE	RECEPTIVE	EXPRESSIVE	RECEPTIVE	EXPRESSIVE	RECEPTIVE	EXPRESSIVE
Adventitious — Partial	1. Amplified speech with speechreading 2. Block print or script writing	1. Speech 2. Block print or script writing	1. Block print or script writing 2. Print-on-palm 3. Speechreading 4. American one-hand manual alphabet	1. Speech 2. Block print or script writing	1. Amplified speech with speechreading 2. Block print or script writing 3. Sign language with interpreter for the deaf, if necessary 4. American one-hand manual alphabet	1. Speech 2. Block print or script writing 3. Sign language, with interpreter for the deaf, if necessary 4. American one-hand manual alphabet	1. Sign language, with interpreter for the deaf, if necessary 2. American one-hand manual alphabet 3. Block print or script writing 4. Speech reading	1. Sign language, with interpreter for the deaf, if necessary 2. American one-hand manual alphabet 3. Block print or script writing 4. Speech
Adventitious — Total	1. Amplified speech 2. Print-on-palm 3. Alphabet plate 4. American one hand manual alphabet (tactual) 5. Braille	1. Speech 2. Block print or script writing 3. American one-hand manual alphabet 4. Braille	1. Print-on-palm 2. Alphabet plate 3. American one-hand manual alphabet (tactual) 4. Braille	1. Speech 2. Block print or script writing	1. Amplified speech 2. American one-hand manual alphabet (tactual) 3. Sign language (received tactually), with interpreter for the deaf, if necessary 4. Print-on-palm 5. Alphabet plate 6. Braille	1. Speech 2. Sign language, with interpreter for the deaf, if necessary 3. American one-hand manual alphabet 4. Block print or script writing 5. Braille	1. Sign language (tactual), with interpreter for the deaf, if necessary 2. American one-hand manual alphabet (tactual) 3. Print-on-palm	1. Sign language, with interpreter for the deaf, if necessary 2. American one-hand manual alphabet 3. Speech 4. Block print or script writing 5. Braille 6. Gestures and demonstration

Congenital Vision	RECEPTIVE	EXPRESSIVE	RECEPTIVE	EXPRESSIVE	RECEPTIVE	EXPRESSIVE	RECEPTIVE	EXPRESSIVE
Partial	1. Amplified speech with speechreading 2. Block print or script writing	1. Speech 2. Block print or script writing	1. Block print or script writing 2. Speechreading 3. Print-on-palm 4. American one-hand manual alphabet (visually or tactually)	1. Speech 2. Block print or script writing	1. Amplified speech with speechreading 2. Block print or script writing 3. Gestures and demonstration 4. Sign language, with interpreter for the deaf, if necessary 5. American one-hand manual alphabet	1. Speech 2. Block print or script writing 3. Gestures and demonstration 4. Sign language, with interpreter for the deaf, if necessary 5. American one-hand manual alphabet	1. Sign language, with interpreter for the deaf, if necessary 2. Gestures and demonstration 3. Block print and script writing 4. American one-hand manual alphabet	1. Sign language, with interpreter for the deaf, if necessary 2. Gestures and demonstration 3. Block print and script writing 4. American one-hand manual alphabet
Total	1. Amplified speech 2. Braille 3. Tellatouch 4. Braille card	1. Speech 2. Braille	1. Tellatouch 2. Braille card 3. Braille 4. Gestures and demonstration (tactual)	1. Speech 2. Braille	1. Amplified speech 2. Gestures and demonstration 3. Braille 4. Tellatouch 5. Sign language (tactual), with interpreter for the deaf, if necessary 6. American one-hand manual alphabet (tactual)	1. Speech 2. Gestures and demonstration 3. Braille 4. Sign language, with interpreter for the deaf, if necessary 5. American one-hand manual alphabet	1. Gestures and demonstration (tactual) 2. Sign language (tactual), with interpreter for the deaf, if necessary	1. Gestures and demonstration 2. Sign language, with interpreter for the deaf, if necessary

[a] Adapted from Kramer, L. C., Sullivan, R. F., and Hirsch, L. M., *Audiological Evaluation and Aural Rehabilitation of the Deaf-Blind Adult*, Sands Point, NY: Helen Keller National Center (1979), by permission from Helen Keller National Center.

[b] Numbering indicates order of preference within each category.

priate lighting is very important in eliminating excessive glare or shadows on the speaker's face, hands, or printed material, depending on the mode of communication. The client may be questioned as to his optimal communicating distance based on his past experience. In the case of an individual having retricted visual fields or "tunnel vision," as in Retinitis Pigmentosa, the distance consideration is generally reversed. The message sent must be farther from the deaf-blind person so that the entire message fits within his restricted visual field. Since light and dark adaptation difficulties, also known as night blindness, generally occur in the individual having reduced visual fields, as in Retinitis Pigmentosa, consideration should be given to appropriate lighting" (Hirsch and Morton, 1981).

Print Writing—As seen in Fig. 8.1, print writing is highly successful in receptive and expressive communication with some deaf-blind individuals who retain significant vision. It can be used in two way communication with some deaf-blind peers, as well as with the general public. In writing messages to deaf-blind persons, the type and severity of visual impairment will determine which format and print size will be most effective. (Kates and Schein, 1980). DiPietro (1978) notes that letter styles, letter size, writing implements, types of paper, and sentence modification are all variables in sending written communications to the deaf-blind individual having residual vision and must be chosen appropriately. Hirsch and Morton (1981) state that "in the case of reduced visual acuity, large print, using upper case letters printed on white or yellow unlined paper with a black felt tipped pen has met with best reception. In the case of restricted visual fields, small or regular sized print may be more acceptable so as not to exceed the limits of the visual field with excessively large printed letters." In addition, use of print writing as an effective means of communication requires that the client knows the English print alphabet and has linguistic competence to read and write simple messages. Systematic exploration is usually required to find the person's optimal print size and language level. (Kramer *et al.*, 1979).

Speechreading—Speechreading can be an effective method of receptive communication with the partially sighted individual, particularly when supplemented with aided residual hearing. Use of speechreading is most successful among deaf-blind individuals having residual vision who (1) are congenitally deaf and have been educated aurally/orally, or (2) are adventitiously deaf. Congenitally deaf manually oriented adults can often speechread common phrases and sentences; however, extended conversation with such an individual is generally not possible.

As with print writing, knowledge of the type of visual impairment will aid in determining the appropriate environmental conditions for optimal speechreading capabilities. Lighting plays an important role. Direct lighting on the speaker's face is preferable, as lighting from the sides or from behind may cause shadows on the face. Avoidance of shadows on the face is of particular importance when the speechreader has a visual condition, such as Retinitis Pigmentosa, in which difficulties with light and dark adaptation are found. The distance of the speaker from the speechreader is another critical factor which can determine success or failure at speechreading. In the case of reduced visual acuity, the speaker should be close enough so that his face can be clearly seen by the speechreader. This may be as close as 1 or 2 feet. In the case of reduced visual fields, a distance of 6 feet or more is generally indicated, depend-

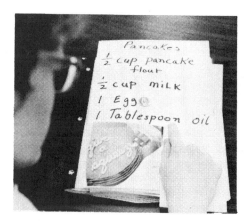

Figure 8.1. Print Writing. Reprinted with permission of publisher from Kramer, L. C., Sullivan, R. F., and Hirsch, L. M., Audiological Education and Aural Rehabilitation of the Deaf-Blind Adult. Sands Point, NY: Helen Keller National Center for Deaf-Blind Youths and Adults, copyright, 1979.

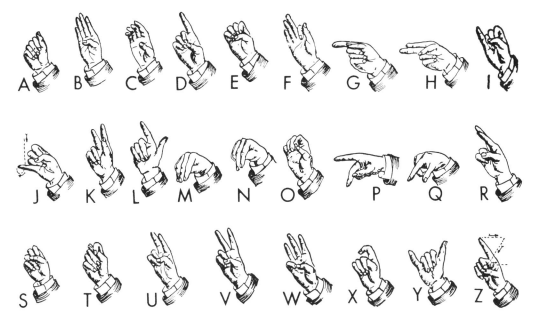

Figure 8.2. American One-Hand Manual Alphabet (Visual). Reprinted with permission of publisher from Kramer, L. C., Sullivan, R. F., and Hirsch, L. M., Audiological Evaluation and Aural Rehabilitation of the Deaf-Blind Adult. Sands Point, NY: Helen Keller National Center for Deaf-Blind Youths and Adults, copyright, 1979.

ing primarily on the degree of constriction of the visual fields. In addition to these guidelines, it is usually best to seek advice from the speechreader regarding lighting and distance requirements, based on his own experience.

The language skills possessed by the deaf-blind speechreader contribute significantly to his ability to receive a message accurately since "verbal content, the natural redundancy of conversational speech, and an intuitive knowledge of the probability of words spoken can all contribute to speechreading success" (Kates and Schein, 1980). Further, "perceptual efficiency (visual acuity, attention span, speed of focusing or receptive speed)" (Kates and Schein, 1980) may be a contributing factor in achieving success in speechreading.

American One-Hand Manual Alphabet— The American One-Hand Manual Alphabet, also known as fingerspelling, is a widely used form of communication with and among the deaf-blind in the United States. Each of the distinctive one-hand configurations, displayed in Fig. 8.2, represents a letter or number. Messages are spelled out letter by letter. Fingerspelling is most commonly used in conjunction with sign language in receptive and expressive communication among the deaf-

normally sighted. Therefore, its use is well suited for the congenitally deaf individual having a partial visual loss, as he may be already familiar with this method of communication. Kramer *et al.* (1979) note, however, that one must keep in mind possible language limitations of this client.

The American One-Hand Manual Alphabet is also an excellent method of communication to be taught to the adventitiously deaf-partially sighted individual. It is easy to learn and can be sent and received accurately at fairly rapid rates.

As with any method of communication used with the partially sighted, consideration must be given to proper lighting and distance. The same general guidelines may be followed as those used in communicating through speechreading or print writing. Communicating with individuals having poor visual acuity will require the hand configuration to be close enough so that the presented handshape can be distinguished from other similar handshapes. Of course, adequate lighting on the hand, with a minimum of glare, should be present. Communicating with the individual having restricted visual fields may require the deaf-blind individual to position the sender's hand so that it can be seen within his limited visual field. In such a case, it is particularly important to maintain all handshapes in that limited area, with an effort not to "drift" out of his visual field. The most generally used hand placement is adjacent to the speaker's face. In this way, if the visual field is wide enough, the deaf-blind person may be able to take advantage of simultaneous speechreading cues. The American One-Hand Manual Alphabet may also be used with the totally deaf-blind individual. This is discussed under "Tactual Methods of Communication."

Sign Language—Sign language is a complex system of communication in which a one- or two-handed movement represents a word, phrase or concept. (Hirsch and Morton, 1981). There are many forms of sign language presently in use. Recently, linguists have begun to place these forms into classifications which describe their grammatical structure and relationship to English. The three most common classifications in use at present are American Sign Language (ASL), Pidgin Sign English (PSE), and Manually Coded English (MCE).

Woodward (1974) and Wilbur (1979) present the concept of sign language as a continuum, with ASL found at one end and MCE systems at the other. PSE lies somewhere in between.

According to Wilbur (1979) "American Sign Language (ASL or Ameslan) is, in the United States, the native language of many deaf people who have deaf parents and is the language used by many deaf adults among themselves." Kates and Schein (1980) note that "the signs in ASL are word-like units which have stable meanings, both concrete (MOTHER, SPOON, CLOTHES) and abstract (DECIDE, HAPPY, RULE, IDEA). Signs are made by either one or both hands assuming distinctive shapes in particular locations and executing specific movements. ASL grammar uses spatial relations visually displayed within the signing frequency, direction, and orientation of the hands' movement articulation space to indicate grammatical relations (subject *versus* object; singular or action *versus* plural or continuous action, etc.). Facial expression and body shift may be employed in the grammar also."

Manually Coded English includes those sign language systems that correspond to spoken and written English. These systems have been created in order to permit concurrent signing and speaking using English syntax (Wilbur, 1979), as well as to facilitate teaching written English. Therefore, use of these systems is generally found within educational settings and not among the deaf signing community. Such systems do not simply reorganize ASL signs into English grammatical structure; rather they drastically alter the morphologic and phonologic processes that users of ASL are accustomed to producing and perceiving (Wilbur, 1979). Manually Coded English systems include Seeing Essential English (SEE₁), Signing Exact English (SEE₂), and Manual English.

Pidgin Sign English (PSE), also known as Amelish, Siglish, and Signed English (Kates and Schein, 1980), "uses ASL signs strung together in English word order by the use of fingerspelling and some conjunction words" (Wilbur, 1979). Kates and Schein (1980) note that "PSE has some ASL elements, *e.g.* vocabulary and much of the formational structure. It also employs some of the English modeling techniques used comprehensively in MCE, such as use of one form of the verb TO BE and some tense marking." Whereas ASL is transmitted among the deaf community, and MCE is overtly taught in the schools, PSE is often "looked upon as broken English signs by educators, and in contrast regarded as imperfect ASL signs by the deaf signing community" (Kates and Schein, 1980). Wilbur, (1979) notes that in some instances, PSE may employ more aspects of English than of ASL; in other, less formal situations, ASL may predominate. She parallels this variation in signed expression to that found in spoken langues, whereby the speaker chooses the appropriate style according to the formality of the situation and individual with whom they are communicating (Wilbur, 1979).

Since sign language systems are widely used among the congenitally deaf-normally sighted, their use is well suited to the congenitally deaf individual having a partial loss of vision. Every effort should be made to communicate using the sign language system preferred by the deaf-blind client. ASL or PSE tends to be preferred by most deaf adults. MCE forms may be found among some young adults or children who have encountered these systems in their schooling. Since knowledge of MCE requires use of English grammatical devices, it is likely that the individual who prefers MCE has good mastery of English language structure. This may be an individual who has partial loss of hearing or who is adventitiously deaf.

If sign language is the only mode of communication used by a deaf-blind individual and the clinician is not proficient in sign language use, an interpreter for the deaf should be employed. A list of the local chapters of interpreters for the deaf may be obtained from the National Association of the Deaf, 814 Thayer Ave., Silver Spring, MD 20910, or from the Registry of Interpreters for the Deaf, P.O. Box 1339, Washington, D.C. 20013.

Sign language, seen in Fig. 8.3, involves not only hand movements, but also facial expression and body movement in conveying semantic, syntactic, and phonologic information. Therefore, every effort should be made to maximize the deaf-blind person's visual reception of all these cues. It is preferable that the sender's face and hands be seen clearly, and if possible, the upper half of the body as well. If vision is so limited that only one or both hands may be seen, effective communication may still be possible. However, loss of each visual cue contributes to a possible communication breakdown. The client having severely restricted visual fields will require a distance of 6 or more feet between speaker and listener. He should direct the clinician as to the best distance for maximal sign language reception. Signs should be smaller than usual to accommodate the limited signing space. If the visual loss is one of acuity, the clinician should be at fairly close range so that the signs may be clearly seen. If the sender is using an MCE form of sign language, which permits simultaneous use of speech, it is important that the signs do not block the view of the mouth so that speechreading cues are accessible to the deaf-blind individual.

Sign language may also be used with the totally deaf-blind individual. This is discussed under "Tactual Methods of Communication."

Gestures and Demonstration—In dealing with the individual who possesses significant residual vision but who is unable to communicate through any of the formal communication methods already described, gestures and demonstration may be the only effective method in bridging the communication gap.

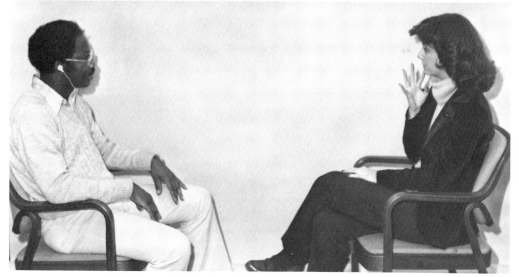

Figure 8.3.   Sign language (visual). Note the distance between the sender and the receiver of the message due to the receiver's restricted visual fields. Reprinted with permission of publisher from Kramer, L. C., Sullivan, R. F., and Hirsch, L. M., Audiological Evaluation and Aural Rehabilitation of the Deaf-Blind Adult. Sands Point, NY: Helen Keller National Center for Deaf-Blind Youths and Adults, copyright, 1979.

An individual such as this has either not had exposure to an appropriate education, or more likely has been unable to comprehend and assimilate communication methods which have been taught to him. Additional disabilities such as mental retardation and neurologic impairment are not uncommon among adults having hearing and vision impairments who have not learned one or more formal methods of communication.

It is likely, however, that this individual's residual vision has permitted him to observe the world, allowing him to become familiar with the functions of common objects. Therefore, use of gestures and demonstration simulating familiar items and actions may be more successful than initially anticipated.

Tactual Methods of Communication

There are several methods of close range communication which can be used with the deaf-blind adult who has no residual sight or hearing. These methods rely on tactual reception of information which may be spoken, printed-Brailled, or manually conveyed.

As mentioned earlier, the vast majority of deaf-blind adults were not born with a total loss of both hearing and vision. It is likely that one disability was present at birth and the second disability subsequently acquired. As children, such individuals were deaf-sighted or blind-hearing. The following discussion will describe tactual methods of communication used with the totally deaf-blind adult falling into one of three categories: (1) those who are congenitally totally deaf and adventitiously totally blind, (2) those who are congenitally totally blind and adventitiously totally deaf, and (3) those who are congenitally totally deaf-blind.

Congenitally Totally Deaf-Adventitiously Totally Blind Individual—An individual having congenital total deafness and adventitious total blindness is likely to have been educated in a school for the deaf. Experience has shown that the largest proportion of totally deaf-blind adults is in this category, having total congenital deafness and total adventitious blindness due to Usher's Syndrome. In this case, the visual condition of Retinitis Pigmentosa has advanced to a state of total blindness with little or no central residual vision remaining. These individuals tend to be in their late 30's or older at this stage.

Having been educated as deaf-normally sighted, these individuals are generally most familiar with printed and manual forms of communication. Therefore, the modification of printed and manual forms into a tactile medium is desirable for message reception.

Two commonly used methods of tactile communication, based upon the print alphabet, are print-on-palm and the alphabet plate.

Print-on-Palm—Print-on-palm requires the sender to use his fingertip in printing upper case letters in the deaf-blind person's palm. As seen in Fig. 8.4, dotted lines, arrows, and numbers indicate the proper direction, sequence, and number of strokes. Each letter or number is made individually in the center of the palm. The letters are not connected. A pause is inserted between words. Although this method is rather slow, it is effective and highly useful with the general public (Kramer et al., 1979; Kates and Schein, 1980).

Alphabet Plate—The alphabet plate, seen in Fig. 8.5, is a pocket-sized plastic card displaying the upper case print alphabet, as well as numbers zero through nine, in raised figures which can be identified tactually. "Words can be spelled out by having the 'speaker' use the deaf-blind person's index finger as a pointer and pressing it on the appropriate letter. The sighted speaker, with no training, can easily use these cards to communicate a message to the deaf-blind individual." (Kramer et al., 1979). If the deaf-blind individual does not have intelligible speech, expression may be achieved by his pointing to each letter and spelling out the words (Kates and Schein, 1980).

Since individuals in this category are congenitally deaf, language limitations may be present. Therefore, simple language should be used to shorten the length and complexity of the message sent. It is often helpful for the deaf-blind person to fingerspell or speak each letter as it is received by him as a safeguard against incorrect tactile reception of each letter. These methods may be applicable to a congenitally blind individual. However, having never seen print, additional time will be required to familiarize this individual with the characteristic shapes of each letter of the alphabet.

American One-Hand Manual Alphabet—The American One-Hand Alphabet, described earlier, is "the most widely used and

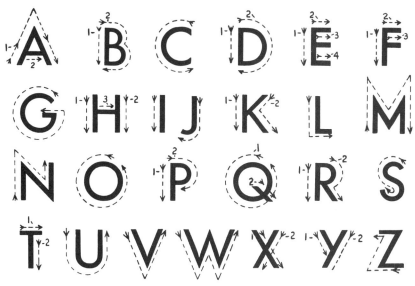

Figure 8.4. Print-on-palm. Reprinted with permission of publisher from Kramer, L. C., Sullivan, R. F., and Hirsch, L. M., Audiological Evaluation and Aural Rehabilitation of the Deaf-Blind Adult. Sands Point, NY: Helen Keller National Center for Deaf-Blind Youths and Adults, copyright, 1979.

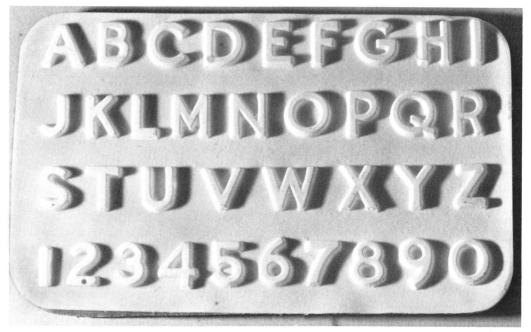

Figure 8.5. Alphabet plate. Reprinted with permission of publisher from Kramer, L. C., Sullivan, R. F., and Hirsch, L. M., Audiological Evaluation and Aural Rehabilitation of the Deaf-Blind Adult. Sands Point, NY: Helen Keller National Center for Deaf-Blind Youths and Adults, copyright, 1979.

best known form of tactual communication with deaf-blind people" (Kates and Schein, 1980). To receive a message tactually, the deaf-blind person lightly covers the sender's hand with his own slightly cupped hand. The "in-the-hand" method and the "over-the-hand" method, illustrated in Fig. 8.6, are common hand-to-hand positions used in tac-

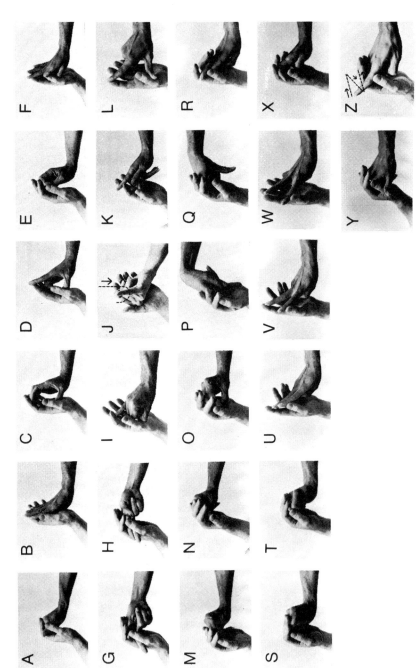

Figure 8.6A. American One-Hand Manual Alphabet (tactual), in-the-hand method. The letters are formed within the deaf-blind person's slightly cupped hand. Reprinted with permission of publisher from Kramer, L. C., Sullivan, R. F., and Hirsch, L. M., Audiological Evaluation and Aural Rehabilitation of the Deaf-Blind Adult. Sands Point, NY: Helen Keller National Center for Deaf-Blind Youths and Adults, copyright, 1979.

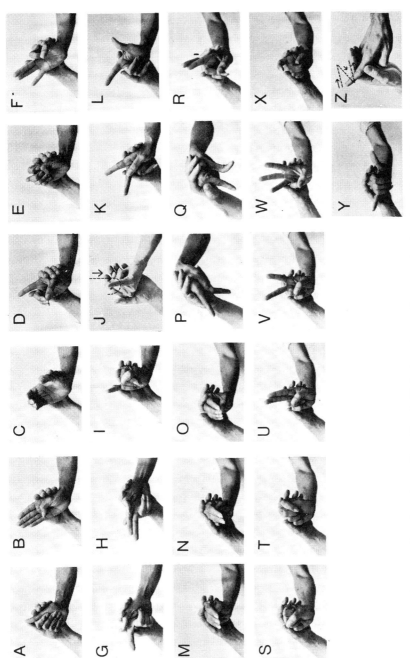

Figure 8.6B. American One-Hand Alphabet (tactual), over-the-hand method. The deaf-blind person lightly cups his hand over the sender's letter formations. Some deaf-blind persons prefer this method to the in-the-hand method. Reprinted with permission of publisher from Kramer, L. C., Sullivan, R. F., and Hirsch, L. M., Audiological Evaluation and Aural Rehabilitation of the Deaf-Blind Adult. Sands Point, NY: Helen Keller National Center for Deaf-Blind Youths and Adults, copyright, 1979.

tual reception of the American One-Hand Manual Alphabet. Since this alphabet is used among congenitally deaf-normally sighted individuals, its tactile adaptation to the congenitally deaf-adventitiously blind is well suited. Language limitations tend to be the presiding difficulty among this group.

Surprisingly, adventitiously totally deaf-totally blind individuals also use this system with great facility. Since individuals in this group have developed language normally, through previously intact auditory channels, the speed of transmission and uniformity of the manual alphabet make it an attractive method of communication. In addition, it is rather easy to learn and universal in its use with other deaf-blind individuals.

Sign Language—Sign language, discussed earlier, can be received tactually by a totally deaf-blind individual. The cogenitally totally deaf-adventitiously totally blind individual often prefers tactual sign language to other methods of tactile communication which are slower and require the deaf-blind individual to have the ability to receive spelled words. Despite the absence of visual cues such as facial expression and speechreading cues, effective message reception can be achieved, especially by the individual whose first language is sign language.

As illustrated in Fig. 8.7, the deaf-blind client and sender face each other, with the deaf-blind individual's hands resting lightly on the sender's. As the sender performs the

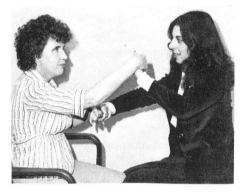

Figure 8.7. Sign language (tactual). Reprinted with permission of publisher from Kramer, L. C., Sullivan, R. F., and Hirsch, L. M., Audiological Evaluation and Aural Rehabilitation of the Deaf-Blind Adult. Sands Point, NY: Helen Keller National Center for Deaf-Blind Youths and Adults, copyright, 1979.

signs naturally, the client follows the motions of the signs tactually (DiPietro, 1978; Kramer *et al.*, 1979).

Congenitally Totally Blind-Adventitiously Totally Deaf Individual—An individual having congenital total blindness and adventitious total deafness is likely to have been educated in a school for the blind. These individuals often have hearing and visual disorders due to unrelated etiologies, to illness, or to trauma. Genetic factors are not as common in causing both deafness and blindness in this category as is found in the prior category.

Having been educated as blind-normally hearing children, these individuals have generally learned Braille as a method of communication. Therefore, Braille and methods that incorporate the Braille alphabet are highly effective among this group.

Braille—Braille is a system of touch-reading employing a maximum of six raised dots arranged in cells consisting of two vertical columns having three dots each. Each Braille character is formed by one or more of these dots (Kramer *et al.*, 1979; Kates and Schein, 1980). The Grade 1 Braille alphabet, as well as numbers zero through nine, is shown in Fig. 8.8.

The two most common forms of Braille are Grade 1 and Grade 2. "In Grade 1 Braille, each word is spelled out letter by letter. It consists of the letters of the alphabet, punctuation, numbers and composition signs. Grade 2 Braille uses all the Grade 1 signs plus 189 contractions and short-form words." (Kates and Schein, 1980).

Braille may be produced either with a Brailler or with a slate and stylus. A Brailler may be thought of as a Braille typewriter. It has six keys that correspond to each dot in a Braille cell, a space bar, a back spacer, right and left margin stops, and a key to move the paper upward one or more lines (Kates and Schein, 1980). A slate and stylus may be used to write Braille manually, without the aid of a Brailler. After the paper is secured in the plate, the deaf-blind individual presses the stylus against the plate, leaving rounded embossed dots on the paper (Kates and Schein, 1980).

Other methods of communication used with this group employ the Braille alphabet in a device that more easily allows one-to-one communication. A Tellatouch, seen in Fig.

1	2	3	4	5	6	7	8	9	0
a	b	c	d	e	f	g	h	i	j

k	l	m	n	o	p	q	r	s	t

u	v	w	x	y	z

Figure 8.8. Braille Grade I alphabet. Reprinted with permission of publisher from Kramer, L. C., Sullivan, R. F., and Hirsch, L. M., Audiological Evaluation and Aural Rehabilitation of the Deaf-Blind Adult. Sands Point, NY: Helen Keller National Center for Deaf-Blind Youths and Adults, copyright, 1979.

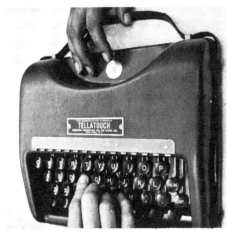

Figure 8.9. Tellatouch. Reprinted with permission of publisher from Kramer, L. C., Sullivan, R. F., and Hirsch, L. M., Audiological Evaluation and Aural Rehabilitation of the Deaf-Blind Adult. Sands Point, NY: Helen Keller National Center for Deaf-Blind Youths and Adults, copyright, 1979.

8.9, is a portable device having a standard typewriter keyboard. There are also six keys similar to those on a Brailler (Kates and Schein, 1980). "As each key for a letter of the alphabet is depressed, the corresponding Braille symbol is raised on a plate on the back of the device. The sender types out his message, pausing between words or using the space bar" (Kramer et al., 1979). Only Grade I may be transmitted using a Tellatouch. Use of the Tellatouch is highly effective in communicating with the general public.

Braille Card—The Braille card, seen in Fig.

8.10, is a pocket-sized card that is similar to the alphabet plate, except that it displays the Braille alphabet with corresponding printed letters, rather than the raised print alphabet found on the alphabet plate. Following the same procedure as with the alphabet plate, words can be spelled out by having the 'speaker' use the deaf-blind person's index finger as a pointer and pressing it on the appropriate letter (Kramer *et al.*, 1979). Use of the Braille card may be effective in communicating with the general public. If necessary, the Braille card may be used to achieve expressive communication as well (Kramer et al., 1979; Kates and Schein, 1980).

Congenitally Totally Deaf-Congenitally Totally Blind Individuals—Few deaf-blind adults are born totally deaf and blind. In reporting cases seen at the Helen Keller National Center for Deaf-Blind Youths and Adults, Kramer *et al.* (1979) note that "although several individuals have been seen . . . who fall within the limits of total hearing and visual losses . . . we have not yet seen any documented evidence that these individuals were actually totally deaf and totally blind at birth."

Tadoma Method—In the past, one method of communication used with deaf-blind children was the Tadoma Method, also known as the Vibration or Hofgaard Method. Often referred to as "tactile speechreading," its purpose is to teach speech and speechreading based solely on vibrotactile information (Norton *et al.*, 1977). The deaf-blind individual's hand is placed on the face and neck of the speaker. As illustrated in Fig. 8.11, in an

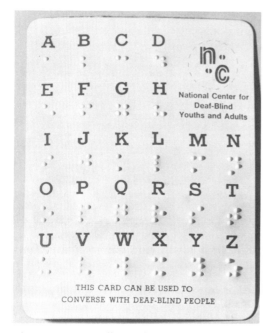

Figure 8.10. Braille card. Reprinted with permission of publisher from Kramer, L. C., Sullivan, R. F., and Hirsch, L. M., Audiological Evaluation and Aural Rehabilitation of the Deaf-Blind Adult. Sands Point, NY: Helen Keller National Center for Deaf-Blind Youths and Adults, copyright, 1979.

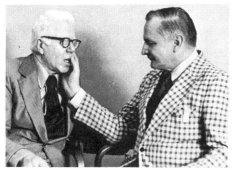

Figure 8.11. Tadoma method. Tactile speech-reading as demonstrated by Dr. Robert J. Smithdas (*right*) and Mr. Louis J. Bettica. Reprinted with permission of publisher from Kramer, L. C., Sullivan, R. F., and Hirsch, L. M., Audiological Evaluation and Aural Rehabilitation of the Deaf-Blind Adult. Sands Point, NY: Helen Keller National Center for Deaf-Blind Youths and Adults, copyright, 1979.

effort to tactually speechread the message, ". . . the fingertips, placed on the throat, provide information regarding voicing; the thumb on the lips provides information re-

garding lip formation and movement, as well as air pressure and air flow from the mouth and nose. The fingers on the jaw and cheek give information regarding jaw movement" (Hirsch and Morton, 1981). Using this method, some deaf-blind persons can receive connected speech through tactile means. Kirman (1973) notes that Tadoma is "the only tactile display which permits comprehension of spoken language." This is so despite numerous unsuccessful attempts to build a device which would allow tactile reception of connected speech. For a comprehensive review of such attempts, the reader is referred to Kirman, 1973.

Although Tadoma has been in use for several decades, it has received little attention in the literature or in clinical, educational, and research investigations (Norton *et al.*, 1977). However, a group of investigators (Norton *et al.*, 1977; Reed *et al.*, 1978) have recently begun a systematic study of the Tadoma method in order to (1) "demonstrate that the method makes it possible to perceive speech and language skills through the tactile and kinesthetic sense" (Norton *et al.*, 1977); (2) "provide insight into the perceptual cues used by Tadoma readers, to provide important background knowledge for the development of artificial tactile speechreading displays" (Norton *et al.*, 1977); and (3) "to contribute to the improvement of Tadoma" (Norton *et al.*, 1977).

Present use of Tadoma in educational programs for the deaf-blind is seldom found. It had once been "the exclusive method of instruction for deaf-blind students in some schools (for example, the Perkins School for the Blind in Watertown, MA) from the 1930's until the 1960's. Tadoma fell from favor and use due to the changing population of the deaf-blind—specifically, with decreases in infant mortality, there has been a significant increase in the multiply-handicapped and the intellectually impaired deaf-blind population. For many of these children, the development of oral comunication is an unrealistic goal" (Norton *et al.*, 1977).

The Tadoma method may have applicability to individuals who have residual hearing and/or vision as a supplement to auditory or visual speech reception (Norton *et al.*, 1977; Kates and Schein, 1980). Its use as an aid to speech production, particularly with the hearing-impaired, is more commonly accepted than its use as an aid to speech reception. For information regarding use of Tadoma (tactile) cues in speech production of the deaf, the reader is referred to Ling (1976) and Calvert and Silverman (1975). The use of Tadoma cues in aiding speech production of the deaf-blind is discussed in the section on "Communication Rehabilitation" found later in this chapter.

Tactile Gestures and Demonstration— Among the congenitally deaf-blind, use of tactile gestures and demonstration tends to be the most effective means of communication. They may employ some concrete formal signs which signify the actual object or motion being described. Tactual gestures may be made by holding both hands of the deaf-blind individual in the same manner as tactual sign language. These gestures must be gross, simple, and repeated many times to be sure they are understood (Kramer *et al.*, 1979).

Braille may be familiar to the congenitally deaf-blind individual who has benefitted from an appropriate education. Ability to read Braille may be limited to recognition of a few important words, such as one's name. In some cases, congenitally deaf-blind individuals may be able to follow a continuous spelled message conveyed by Braille. It is likely that such an individual can communicate through more formal methods than gross gestures such as the American One-Hand Alphabet (received tactually) or use of the Tellatouch. A congenitally deaf-blind individual who has these capabilities is likely not to have severe intellectual limitations.

The most important element in achieving successful communication is, above all, a desire to communicate. Kramer *et al.* (1979) note that "the clinician should not be embarrassed at his apparent ineptitude or lack of success in expressing ideas to and receiving ideas from some clients. As so few individuals in the limited social sphere of many of the clients attempt any form of communication, generally, the client's patience, attempts at understanding, and willingness to meet the clinician much more than half-way make the communicative task far less awesome than it would appear at initial assessment . . . . In the authors' experiences, the greatest barriers to communication have been more in the psychological dimension than in the physiological impairment."

Long Distance Methods of Communication Utilizing Residual Hearing or Vision

As is found among the general population, deaf-blind individuals have a need to communicate over distances. This is important not only for social interaction, but for expanding employment opportunities as well.

The ability to use long distance communication depends, in large part, on the deaf-blind individual's language skills. Those deaf-blind individuals who have well developed language skills through spoken or printed/Brailled modes may be able to communicate with strangers by long distance communication. Those having semi-developed skills may be limited to family and friends in distance communication. Individuals who are severely limited in close range receptive and expressive language abilities may be unable to communicate effectively through methods of distance communication, since these methods generally require comprehension and production of spoken or printed/Brailled messages.

In addition to linguistic abilities, the appropriate devices and methods used in distance communication are determined by residual sensory function. Those having significant residual hearing may be successful in using amplified speech with the aid of appropriate devices, while those having significant residual vision may have success in using printed materials. For the totally deaf-blind, Braille and other tactile methods may be used in communication over distances. Methods of communication among each of these groups will be discussed.

Amplified Speech via Telephone—Telephone communication may be facilitated by a telephone amplifier, or by use of a telephone switch on a hearing aid, or a combination of these. A successful program of telephone training includes appropriate use of such devices, as well as strategies for obtaining desired information in telephone communication.

According to Castle (1977a), individuals who attempt to use the telephone with persons unfamiliar with deaf speakers should possess "(a) ability to understand most words and sentences through hearing only, (b) speech that is understood by most people, and (c) good language skills." She suggests helpful strategies to aid in accurate reception of information. Some of these strategies are: (1) ask the individual to repeat the message, (2) ask the speaker to rephrase the message, (3) ask the speaker to spell the message, (4) use of code words (using a familiar word which starts with the letter spelled, (5) use of digits, (6) use of the alphabet, (7) use of counting, and (8) use of key words (spelling the important word in the sentence) (Castle, 1977a).

An individual having more limited auditory and/or speech abilities may use the telephone in distance communication which is limited to family, friends, and other familiar persons. With the use of a telephone amplifier or telephone switch on a hearing aid, the individual having a profound loss of hearing can often detect and discriminate among rhythmic patterns conveyed on the telephone. Such phone signals as a dial tone, ring signal, and busy signal may be discriminated, as well as recognition of interruption of signals when the phone is answered by "Hello?" at the receiving end. (Castle, 1977a; Kramer et al., 1979). Since the conversation is with a familiar person, a pre-arranged code may be used, such as Morse code, which is received auditorily by the hearing-impaired listener. Expression may be achieved by speech, if it is intelligible, or by sending the code by tapping or blowing on the telephone mouthpiece. If the hearing-impaired individual has fairly intelligible speech, he may use a system whereby he verbally asks questions and seeks a response of either (1) No, (2) Yes-Yes, or (3) Please repeat. He can determine which of the three responses was conveyed by the distinctive syllable pattern of each response (one, two, or three syllables respectively). This method is also useful in tactile message reception via telephone, discussed under "Long Distance Tactile Methods of Communication" (see discussion of the Tactile Speech Indicator).

For use of amplified speech via telephone with the totally blind individual, consideration should be given to tactile orientation to the telephone and appropriate devices. Castle (1977b) notes the availability of portable telephone amplifiers, modified telephone bells that may vary pitch and loudness of the ring, and a flashing light which signals that the telephone is ringing.

Telephone Devices for the Deaf (TDD)/Teletypewriters (TTY)—The invention of microelectronics has promoted development of Telephone Devices for the Deaf (TDD), which are portable, battery-operated electronic devices having either an alpha-numeric readout or printer (Ryan, 1981). TDDs are essentially modern electronic versions of the older stationary teletypewriters (TTYs) used in telephone communication by deaf-normally sighted individuals. The caller places the telephone handset into an acoustic coupler on the unit. Dial tone, busy, and ring signals are indicated by a flashing light. Once contact has been made with another individual having a TDD or TTY, messages are typed back and forth and may be displayed in fluorescent (on TDD) or hard copy display. Therefore, both individuals communicating must have residual vision that is sufficient to read the printed signal. (See Appendix 8C for availability).

A large type TTY attachment is available which is compatible with the Model 28 TTY. This attachment enables individuals who can read only large print to use a TTY (see Appendix C for availability).

Long Distance Tactile Methods of Communication for the Totally Deaf-Blind

In recognition of the need for distance communication by totally deaf-blind individuals, several devices have been developed for this purpose. An individual who is proficient at reading Braille may be able to use the Telebraille. The Telebraille is a device which enables the deaf-blind person to communicate over the telephone using Braille. It may be used in two-way communication; however, both individuals must be able to read Braille tactually (most likely this will be a conversation between two deaf-blind individuals or a deaf-blind and blind-normally hearing individual). The sender types out his message either on a typewriter keyboard or on six keys resembling the design of a Perkins Brailler. The signal is sent through a telephone handset which is acoustically coupled to the Telebraille, much like a TTY. The message is received by tactually reading the Braille characters which appear in a single cell, much like a Tellatouch.

The totally blind individual familiar with Braille may also use the Model A Braille Phone-TTY, which is fully compatible with existing telecommunications for the deaf. This unit consists of a teleprinter having a Grade 1 Braille embosser that prints Braille on a paper tape readout. The totally deaf-blind individual may receive the message through Braille and may maintain a permanent Brailled record of the telephone conversation. Also available are signal lamps or fan attachments which will alert the deaf-blind individual that the phone is ringing (Telephone Devices in Review, 1981) (see Appendix 8C for information regarding availability of these items.)

The Tactile Speech Indicator (TSI), seen in Fig. 8.12, is "a device used in conjunction with the telephone to enable the deaf or deaf-blind person having intelligible speech to receive telephone communication through vibrational patterns" (Kramer et al., 1979). Using this device, which converts auditory signals to vibrations, the individual "can be taught the basic vibration patterns in telephone signals, including a dial tone, ring signal, busy signal, and voice communication" (Kramer et al., 1979). Once it is determined that the phone has been answered, the deaf-blind person having intelligible speech can then state, "My name is _____. I am a deaf-blind person and cannot hear what you say. I have a device that will indicate to me when you say "No," "Yes-Yes," or "Please repeat." Please answer my questions accordingly." The three responses can be felt as one, two, or three beats respectively. (Kramer et al., 1979). This method is most successful with normally hearing family and friends who are already familiar with the system. However, it can be used with the general public to a limited degree and is a method that can be used effectively in emergency situations.

In addition to this procedure, the Morse code may be conveyed vibrotactually using a TSI. If a TSI is not accessible, a bone conduction vibrator attached to a hearing aid with telecoil may effectively receive auditory signals and convert them to vibration for the individual having little or no residual hearing (Kramer et al., 1979). As mentioned earlier, individuals having some residual hearing, although limited, may be able to receive these signals auditorily.

The methods of distance communication discussed so far all involve use of the telephone. However, written communications are also effective in achieving distance communication. The individual having residual vision may receive small or large printed communications. The totally blind individual may receive Braille. Unfortunately, totally blind individuals often receive letters and documents which are in print rather than Braille. In the past, the printed matter had to be transcribed from print to Braille by a third party. A device known as the Optacon has served to decrease that need to some degree.

The Optacon (OPtical-to-TActile CONverter) is "a reading aid which converts the image of a printed letter into a vibrating form that the blind or deaf-blind person can feel." (Kates and Schein, 1980). As each letter is scanned with a camera, a tactile array of the visual (printed) image is presented and felt by the fingertip. It is a time-consuming method but it allows the blind or deaf-blind individual to read printed material independently, without dependence on others for transcription.

UNIQUE PROBLEMS IN AUDIOLOGICAL ASSESSMENT OF THE DEAF-BLIND ADULT

The purpose of audiologically evaluating the deaf-blind adult is not only to determine the site of auditory impairment and amount of residual hearing possessed by the deaf-blind individual, but also to determine the

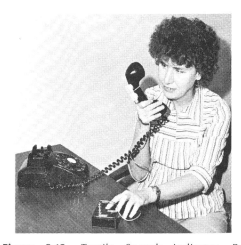

Figure 8.12. Tactile Speech Indicator. Reprinted with permission of publisher from Kramer, L. C., Sullivan, R. F., and Hirsch, L. M., Audiological Evaluation and Aural Rehabilitation of the Deaf-Blind Adult. Sands Point, NY: Helen Keller National Center for Deaf-Blind Youths and Adults, copyright, 1979.

client's functional use of receptive sensory capabilities at present and their potential for improvement. Receptive sensory capabilities refer not only to auditory reception, but to visual and tactual reception of signals as well. Assessment of receptive abilities in multiple sensory modalities is critical, in view of the presence of sensory impairments in the two primary sense receptors, vision and hearing. This information is then applied to a rehabilitation program which may include auditory, visual and/or vibrotactile training to enhance reception of speech and environmental information.

Pure-Tone Audiometry

As in a standard audiologic evaluation, pure-tone and speech audiometry are assessed first. In selecting appropriate conditioning procedures, consideration should be given to the client's sensory (auditory and visual) and linguistic functioning as well as experiential base. A deaf-blind adult who possesses basic communication skills should be able to respond to standard stimulus-response procedures such as a hand raise or push button response. The key is to simplify instructions and communicate them to the client through his preferred mode. Most clients having long standing hearing losses will be familiar with the test procedure, having had a history of prior audiologic evaluations. This client can usually demonstrate response modes used in the past (*i.e.* hand raise) simply upon recognition of the audiometric instrumentation.

Evaluation of a more limited deaf-blind client, particularly one who is totally blind, requires special consideration in conditioning and testing. Having no visual reception to provide cues regarding his environment, it is advisable to tactually orient the client to his surroundings (Kramer *et al.*, 1979). This includes tactual exploration of the audiometer, earphones, and test suite, which will not only promote the client's comfort with these unfamiliar surroundings but also facilitate the evaluation process.

Experience has shown that a combination of Behavioral Observation Audiometry (BOA) and tactual demonstration yields a high degree of success in conditioning the severely limited deaf-blind individual. If previous audiometric data is available, conditioning is initiated at a point well above

threshold, if there is one that is measureable. If previous data is not available, 500 Hz is the first frequency used in presentation of pure-tone stimuli, followed by 250 and 125 Hz. Intensity is increased gradually and the client is observed for a change in facial expression or behavior. If no change is noted by the time maximum audiometric limits are reached, conditioning is initiated by pointing the client's index finger to the earphone and physically raising his hand in a tactual demonstration of the desired response. Repetition and a great deal of reinforcement is needed for the client to raise his hand independently in response to the perceived stimulus. If no consistent response is noted to 500 Hz or lower frequencies, speech stimuli is presented instead. At approximately 90 dB SPL and above, a substantial vibrotactile artifact accompanying the high intensity sound is evident. If no consistent response is obtained to high intensity speech stimuli, the individual is considered not conditioned, as he is not responding to the overt vibrotactile artifacts at the earphones that should be perceived, regardless of auditory sensitivity. We have found that by using this conditioning procedure, about 90% of deaf-blind clients can be successfully conditioned quickly and easily.

Calibrated noisemakers and other selected stimuli may also be effective in eliciting a response. Franklin (1978) reports behavioral changes to such stimuli as a trumpet, music, calibrated sound toys, and speech when evaluating deaf-blind children who were untestable with conventional audiometric procedures.

Those who are not conditioned by the procedures described above are generally highly limited clients, often having little or no functional hearing or vision. Among this group, paired auditory and vibrotactile stimuli are presented. Intense speech stimuli, using the stimulus "buh-buh-buh" is presented simultaneously through earphones and a hand-held bone conduction vibrator. A traditional hand raise or block-in-the-box is used as the response mode. After the client has been conditioned to respond to the paired auditory and vibrotactile stimulus, the vibrotactile component is eliminated, and testing of auditory function continues (Hirsch and Morton, 1981). If no consistent response is noted, it is likely that auditory function is beyond audiometric limits. Objective test results, to be discussed shortly, may support this finding.

Occasionally, the false positive rate for a client will be high; however, experience has demonstrated that among the congenitally deaf, these responses are usually in addition to reliable responses rather than in their place. In such a case, repeat testing on a daily basis, often in combination with other means of auditory training, yields more reliable results. Among the adventitiously deaf, however, different problems are encountered. Although the adventitiously deaf can understand the most complex of instructions, they tend to be highly erratic in their responses. Most often, the adventitiously deaf complain of tinnitus and tend to confuse their internal head noises with external stimuli.

Once the client is finally conditioned, pure-tone testing may proceed. "One must be sure to note if responses are in the range of vibrotactile stimulation at the earphones, an artifact of the high intensity auditory stimulus, and be sure not to interpret all responses as auditory in nature. Because many deaf-blind clients have profound losses of hearing, bone conduction testing is usually of negligible value. Impedance measurements, to be discussed shortly, are far more valuable as a predictor of middle ear pathology in the profoundly deaf" (Hirsch and Morton, 1981).

When testing at frequencies and intensities where vibrotactile artifacts accompany high intensity sound, an attempt may be made to have the client distinguish whether the stimulus to which he responded was heard or felt. Some higher functioning clients may attempt to make a distinction, but more often than not, the profoundly congenitally deaf who have never used amplification are unable to make such a distinction. Sound and vibration are one and the same to them. The adventitiously deaf, however, are more capable of making such a distinction.

Speech Audiometry

Numerous investigators (Franklin, 1977; Ewing and Ewing, 1944; Eisenberg, 1976; Condon and Sander, 1974) have demonstrated that speech is a more effective elicitor of response than pure-tone and other stimuli in assessing hearing of newborns, young infants, children, and other difficult-to-test populations. Therefore, it is possible that individuals who do not respond to pure-tone or other stimuli may be more responsive to speech. Clinical experience in audiologic assessment of difficult-to-test deaf-blind adults supports this finding.

"In performing speech audiometry, the first measures attempted are Speech Detection Threshold (SDT) and Threshold of Discomfort (TD). For SDT, the same response procedure is used as for pure-tone testing. In assessing threshold of discomfort, if the client has sufficient communication skills, it is important for the clinician to provide an explanation of what is to happen next so as not to shock the client upon reaching the threshold of discomfort" (Hirsch and Morton, 1981). For the client having more limited communication skills, clinical observation of the client's behavior at intense sound pressure levels must suffice in determining threshold of discomfort. In the deaf-blind client having little or no speech discrimination ability, SDT and TD are often the only speech audiometric measures that can be obtained and are available for determining choice of appropriate amplification. The individual having more developed communication skills will most likely be capable of judging his most comfortable listening level (MCL), in addition to SDT and TD.

Standard speech reception threshold (SRT) testing is attempted; however, "often minimal residual hearing as well as limited language skills precludes obtaining a conventional SRT in response to an open set of spondees. Therefore, a modified SRT may be obtained, using a closed set of five known spondees first conveyed to the client through his preferred mode of communication" (Hirsch and Morton, 1981). This procedure may be carried out during a hearing aid evaluation as well, whereby aided results may be compared with unaided results in determining the effects of amplification.

"Measures of auditory discrimination ability are directed at finding the client's present level of auditory functioning and determining prognosis for improvement of discrimination abilities in a program of auditory training" (Hirsch and Morton, 1981). Prognosis for improvement of auditory discrimination abilities is determined by including a brief training period within the audiologic evaluation, in order to determine the effects of training. "Detection and training of minimal sensory function is of greater importance in the individual having both auditory and visual deficits than in the individual having only one impaired sensory modality. Therefore, evaluation procedures are modified to evaluate discrimination among monosyllabic words, discrimination among sentences, and discrimination among gross environmental sounds" (Hirsch and Morton, 1981).

In assessing speech discrimination for monosyllabic words, every attempt should be made to use standardized CID W-22 or PB word lists. Since many clients who have the linguistic and auditory abilities to respond to these tests also have semi-intelligible speech, it is important that the client's response mode be one which will not cause the clinician to misinterpret the client's responses. Writing the responses may serve as an appropriate substitute; however, fingerspelling or Brailling the words are more likely modes in view of the visual impairment.

In the case of an individual who does not have sufficient language skills to respond to CID or PB words, the Word Intelligibility by Picture Identification test (WIPI) (Ross and Lerman, 1970) may be employed. This test has wide applicability among those clients who retain sufficient vision to recognize the items represented in the pictures; however, it is not appropriate for use with the totally blind. It is also useful in comparing reception through audition alone, audition plus vision (speechreading and/or manual receptive abilities), and vision alone.

Unfortunately, there is a large population of deaf-blind clients who retain auditory discrimination abilities to discriminate among selected monosyllabic words, but do not possess the linguistic competence to respond to the words employed in the CID, PB, or WIPI tests. This is often due to experiential limitations and/or intellectual barriers. In such a case, discrimination among monosyllabic words that are *known to be* in this client's vocabulary is helpful in determining differences in left *versus* right ear, aided *versus* unaided function, and auditory only *versus* auditory plus speechreading and/or manual receptive abilities. Often, tactual identification of common objects and pointing to body parts and articles of clothing serves to provide this information. If the client is accompanied by a friend, family member, or professional worker, this individual can serve as a valuable resource in providing information regarding words in the client's vocabulary.

If a deaf-blind client does demonstrate some ability to discriminate among monosyllabic words, where possible, the CID Everyday Sentences Test (Davis and Silverman, 1970) should be administered in addition to previous auditory discrimination tests. In planning a comprehensive program of aural rehabilitation, it is helpful for the clinician to know how well the client can synthesize the partial auditory information he receives into a meaningful sentence by utilizing contextual cues. This is particularly important with the totally blind-hearing impaired individual who has no access to speechreading cues to supplement the auditory signal. In the case of the partially sighted individual, this test may also be administered with the addition of speechreading and/or manual cues to determine auditory plus visual reception of spoken sentences.

Frequently, one may encounter a deaf-blind individual who demonstrates no ability to auditorily discriminate among speech, even among a closed set of spondees. In such a case, an assessment of his gross auditory discrimination abilities is performed in order to determine the potential application of these discrimination abilities in communication training, as well as in mobility (travel) training. Those parameters assessed are: (1) presence *versus* absence of sound, (2) discrimination among gross environmental sounds, (3) discrimination among number of stimuli, (4) discrimination among duration of stimuli (long *versus* short), (5) discrimination among intensity of stimuli (loud *versus* soft), and (6) discrimination among pitch of stimuli (high *versus* low) (see Appendix 8D). Securing information regarding these discrimination abilities aids in determining potential for their improvement and application in a program of auditory training (discussed under "Aural Rehabilitation"). In a case where no speech discrimination abilities exist, this information, in conjunction with SDT and TD, is the only information upon which to judge an appropriate hearing aid selection.

Site-of-Lesion Tests

Administration of behavioral site-of-lesion tests is often not feasible in the audiologic evaluation of the deaf-blind adult. The most limiting factors are the small amount of remaining residual hearing as well as difficulty in conveying instructions for appropriate responses to these more complex tasks. Objective measurements such as acoustic impedance measurements and evoked response audiometry are generally more informative in providing site-of-lesion data.

Objective Clinical Measurements

The importance of acoustic impedance testing to determine the presence of middle ear pathology in the deaf-blind individual cannot be overemphasized. Frequently, the inability to secure bone conduction data due to the severity of the client's hearing loss leaves impedance testing as virtually the only audiometric tool by which a conductive loss may be detected. Additionally, acoustic reflex testing can provide gross information regarding the presence and degree of residual hearing to confirm behavioral results. Differential diagnostic tests in the impedance batter may also be helpful in determining the site of auditory impairment.

Evoked response audiometry (ERA) has gained wide applicability among the difficult-to-test in recent years. ERA can be a helpful tool in assessing residual auditory function and site-of-impairment in the deaf-blind individual in the event that behavioral results cannot be obtained. However, it should not be viewed as a substitute for conditioning and attempts to obtain behavioral thresholds. Experience with the deaf-blind has shown that, given sufficient time, it is a rare case that cannot be conditioned through the methods described earlier. Further, since behavioral procedures require an appropriate response by the client to the presence of a stimulus, the testing process can be viewed as a first step in the process of initiating an effective comprehensive program of communicative rehabilitation. Therefore, in evaluating the deaf-blind, ERA should be employed only as a last resort in the absence of any reliable behavioral responses, despite the clinician's most creative efforts. In such a case, the fact that ERA must be used indicates that the deaf-blind individual is functionally not using residual hearing that may be physiologically present. Such cases tend to be the most difficult in training functional use of residual hearing.

ENT Exam

Prior to initiation of a hearing aid evaluation, an ear, nose, and throat exam should be carried out routinely. Deaf-blind clients, particularly the profoundly congenitally deaf, traditionally view ENT exams as unimportant and the ears tend to be neglected. Among this population, there is a high incidence of impacted cerumen. "Audiologic results should be reviewed by the ENT physician, and, in the absence of any contraindications, the client should be cleared for use of amplification. The use of an interpreter during the ENT exam is important in keeping the client in touch with what is happening" (Hirsch and Morton, 1981).

UNIQUE PROBLEMS OF AURAL REHABILITATION WITH THE DEAF-BLIND CLIENT

"The deaf-blind individual experiences severe sensory isolation due to his impairments in two primary sense receptors. This sensory isolation is compounded by experiential and linguistic limitations which serve to further isolate the deaf-blind individual in communication with people and in contact with the environment. Therefore, maximum use of residual auditory and visual capabilities in establishing contact with the environment, as well as in developing communication is of prime importance in a program of aural rehabilitation." (Hirsch and Morton, 1981). Additionally, optimal reception of tactile and vibrotactile stimulation is important as an adjunct to residual sight and hearing, or as a primary receptor of sensory information in the totally deaf-blind individual.

Motivation

In initiation of an aural rehabilitation program, the first step is assessment of the client's motivation for improvement of communication skills. Although prognosis for development of communication skills may appear to be good based on the audiometric results, clinicians will agree that no program of communicative rehabilitation will be successful without the client's interest and active participation.

Assessment scales, such as the Denver Scale of Communicative Function (Alpiner et al., 1971) may be helpful in subjectively assessing the client's attitude toward his hearing impairment. However, the presence of the visual impairment is cause for some unique considerations in assessing the client's attitude toward his present status and future rehabilitation goals. "Specific motivational problems are often linked to the individual's onset and degree of hearing and visual losses. The deaf-blind adult having a congenital hearing impairment may demonstrate a lack of interest in amplification use due to negative experiences with hearing aids during childhood. In the case of the individual who has a progressive visual impairment, in addition to hearing loss, as in Usher's Syndrome, acceptance of amplification has a high correlation with acceptance of impending blindness. Those individuals who have accepted their prognosis as deaf-blind, rather than deaf-normally sighted, are generally anxious to help prepare themselves through use of aids and techniques that may facilitate living with the dual handicap. Rejection of amplification, particularly body type amplification, on a cosmetic basis is not uncommon, especially among the adventitiously blind. Motivation among lower functioning clients is often difficult to assess; however, amplification should be tried to see if it is even slightly successful. Because of the importance of contact with the environment, no matter how minimal, all deaf-blind individuals should be candidates for hearing aid evaluations" (Hirsch and Morton, 1981). If motivational problems are so severe as to preclude initiation of a hearing aid evaluation, assistance from counselling personnel should be sought in an attempt to overcome the client's negative attitudes toward use of amplification. Clients having a negative attitude toward use of amplification are likely to have negative attitudes toward other aspects of rehabilitative training as well.

Hearing Aid Evaluation

The procedures used in performance of a hearing aid evaluation, determined by an individual's sensory, linguistic, and experiential functioning, are similar to those to which the individual responded in the unaided condition. A deaf-blind individual demonstrating significant speech discrimination ability in the unaided condition should be able to respond to standard hearing aid evaluation procedures assessing aided discrimination at representative levels of conversational speech. The influence of speech-reading and/or manual (*i.e.* sign language) cues on aided speech reception should be assessed in the individual retaining useful vision in order to determine the client's optimal communicative ability and the role that the auditory channel plays.

In the case of a more limited deaf-blind individual, every attempt should be made to assess the benefits of amplification, no matter how small. This is necessary even if the client has demonstrated no ability to discriminate speech during the unaided assessment. Aided thresholds to warbled pure tones or narrow band noise should be compared to unaided thresholds. In addition, speech detection thresholds (SDT), thresholds of discomfort (TD), and speech reception thresholds (SRT), if possible, using an open or closed set of spondees can provide helpful information on which to base a hearing aid selection. In clients having no speech discrimination ability, an assessment of gross auditory discrimination abilities is particularly important. The gross auditory parameters to be evaluated were detailed under "Audiological Evaluation," and may also be found in Appendix 8D. Just as aided speech discrimination scores attempt to achieve an unaided PB Max, aided gross discrimination abilities should replicate the client's ability to perform these discriminations made in the unaided condition. This may give the clinician some additional information regarding the quality of aided sound received by the deaf-blind individual in choosing optimum amplification. In addition, the client's gross auditory discrimination abilities may be improved, in a program of auditory training, and applied to use in various aspects of an aural rehabilitation program (see "Auditory Training").

In selecting aids to be assessed in a hearing aid evaluation, consideration should be given not only to optimizing auditory discrimination abilities, but also to optimizing auditory localization abilities. "Because of the presence of the visual impairment, enhancement of auditory localization and its use in travel by the blind individual takes on equal importance to enhancement of auditory discrimination abilities. The importance of auditory localization in such a case must be considered in making decisions regarding directional *versus* non-directional aids, body *versus* ear level aids, and monaural *versus* binaural fittings" (Hirsch and Morton, 1981).

The monaural-binaural controversy in choosing appropriate amplification for the hearing impaired has not yet been completely resolved. Despite anticipated gains in aided function through binaural hearing, particularly in the area of speech intelligibility, "most of the evidence showing a binaural advantage for hearing-impaired listeners has been observed under controlled laboratory conditions, and even then there is some variability between studies in terms of the magnitude of this binaural improvement. Objective data on the superiority of the binaural hearing aid under conditions of actual use are sparse" (Levitt *et al.*, 1980). For a critical review of monaural-binaural hearing and hearing aids, the reader should refer to Levitt *et al.* (1980), Ross (1977), and Ross and Giolas (1978).

One parameter that is definitively enhanced by binaural hearing, however, is auditory localization. To a limited degree, auditory localization can be performed monaurally; this is achieved primarily through the use of scanning head movements, effectively simulating the binaural condition (Stevens and Davis, 1938) and may be improved with training (Altman, 1978). As demonstrated by Markides (1977) in hearing-impaired subjects, significant improvement in their ability to localize was noted using binaural amplification. For this reason, it is important that binaural amplification be used in the aural rehabilitation of the hearing- and visually-impaired individual whenever possible.

The problems involved in choosing ear-level *versus* body type amplification are not as severe today as they were years ago. Because of improved hearing aid technology, high powered ear level aids are now available. Since ear level amplification reduces the body baffle effect, and enhances auditory localization due to microphone placement at the ears rather than at the chest, it is preferable to body type amplification in the deaf-blind individual. There are some clients, however, demonstrating profound hearing loss who seem to make more substantial gains in sound reception with body type amplification than with ear level amplification. In these individuals, localization cues are generally not accessible; therefore, the benefits to be derived from binaural amplification are minimized in comparison to the need for hearing aid conditions which will permit sound reception at lower sound pressure levels.

Some visually-impaired individuals may find directional hearing aids beneficial in enhancing auditory localization. Directional hearing aids may be particularly applicable in cases of asymmetric hearing loss, where balanced binaural amplification cannot be achieved, but optimum auditory localization remains an important consideration. "In other cases, however, the 'tunnel hearing' characteristic of aided listening with directional microphones may prove to be subjectively unsatisfactory. The client may complain about an unduly restricted field of auditory input. Rear approaching acoustic stimuli may be missed or misinterpreted. Consequently, a well supervised trial period of directional *versus* non-directional ear level aids is essential to accommodate individual differences" (Kramer *et al.*, 1979). Recently, a few commercial hearing aid manufacturers have developed aids which are available with a directional/non-directional switch. This may be helpful to some clients in accommodating listening needs according to the environment.

Where hearing is asymmetric, with a significant disparity in discrimination between ears, "the binaurally aided intelligibility scores may actually be inferior to a best monaurally aided score. A critical decision must then be made as to whether auditory localization is to be sacrificed in the interest of intelligibility. A compromise may be achieved in instructing the client to alternate between monaural and binaural fittings. He should wear two hearing aids when traveling independently. Use of a single instrument in the better ear should be reserved for specific auditory communicative situations. When using binaural instruments, a set procedure, using a broad band noise source, should be established for balancing gain controls on the aids" (Kramer *et al.*, 1979) (see also Appendix 8E).

In addition to the above considerations, the hearing aid selected should be one which is easy to manipulate solely through tactile means. If possible, the aid should have a setting for "off," rather than moving the battery casing in and out. The battery holder should be hinged to the case rather than totally removable. In addition, it should be possible for battery insertion to be performed tactually so that the deaf-blind client can become an independent hearing aid wearer. Most hearing aids are designed so that battery insertion can be performed solely through tactual means; however, the clinician should assess this for any aid chosen for a trial period of hearing aid use.

The hearing aid evaluation should be seen as a primary evaluation of aided auditory function. The choice of amplification, using clinic loaners, should be continually re-evaluated during an extended trial period of amplification use. During this period, auditory, speech, and language training should help to determine the benefits of amplification to the client, as well as to provide a comparison among aids while further developing communication abilities. This is of particular importance with a severely limited deaf-blind client, where results of a single evaluation may be unreliable (Hirsch and Morton, 1981).

Hearing Aid Orientation

Following selection of appropriate amplification to be used for a trial period, a thorough program of hearing aid orientation should follow. The goal of a hearing aid orientation program is for the client to become an independent hearing aid wearer. "Independent manipulation of on-off and volume controls, as well as ability to change batteries, clean the mold, and perform simple repairs serves as an excellent motivator for development of further interest in using amplification. These tasks can be performed through tactual means alone in the case of the totally blind. Severely limited deaf-blind individuals may be unable to perform independent hearing aid operation on a constant basis; however, it is likely that such an individual will live in a supervised group home or semi-independent living situation where assistance will be available for such tasks. With this individual, the goal of a hearing aid orientation program is for the client to function as independently as possible. With training, these clients are often able to independently insert the mold and consistently operate the on-off and volume controls; however,

hearing aid repairs and maintenance require assistance" (Hirsch and Morton, 1981). For a detailed program outlining tactual cues and methods of teaching hearing aid orientation to severely limited deaf-blind clients, please refer to Kramer et al. (1979).

Individuals having more developed language abilities, as well as significant residual vision may obtain significant benefits from the Orientation to Hearing Aids Program, designed by Gauger (1978). These materials, developed for use with deaf college students at NTID, have been found very useful in teaching some deaf-blind individuals about their aids, as well as in encouraging their active participation in the process of evaluating their performance with various loaner aids.

Auditory Training

The importance of providing some amount of sensory input, no matter how small, to the deaf-blind individual, requires that auditory training play a major role in the communicative rehabilitation of the deaf-blind individual. Auditory training may proceed in any of three major areas: (1) training to improve speech discrimination abilities; (2) auditory localization training; and (3) training to promote recognition and discrimination of gross environmental sounds.

"For the individual having enough speech discrimination ability to discriminate from among an open set, training fine auditory discrimination among speech sounds, suprasegmental patterns, and use of contextual cues takes on extra importance, particularly in the totally blind individual who has no access to speechreading cues" (Hirsch and Morton, 1981).

Some clients who demonstrate poor auditory discrimination of connected speech will be able to discriminate from among a closed set of common phrases. These individuals generally can achieve SRT scores to a closed set of known spondees, but not to an open set. Individuals such as these are often highly successful in a program of auditory training with emphasis on "survival" phrases and sentences that the client may encounter in work, travel, and daily living. Such stimuli may range from everyday sentences encountered in social situations to specific phrases encountered in vocational situations. The client should be able to suggest numerous phrases and sentences which he feels are important for him to recognize auditorily (Hirsch and Morton, 1981).

Clients displaying the ability to discriminate speech, either in an open or an expanded closed set, will probably benefit from auditory localization training. "Training may begin in a clinical environment, such as a sound-treated room, and progress to real life situations such as quiet streets and later, busy intersections. Emphasis should be on localization of stationary, as well as moving sound sources. Aid from a mobility specialist may be of great value here" (Hirsch and Morton, 1981). Suggested instrumentation and procedures used in auditory localization training with the deaf-blind individual can be found in Appendix 8E.

Individuals having a profound loss of hearing may demonstrate aided sound reception and some discrimination among intensities, frequencies, and duration of stimuli, but be unable to discriminate among speech stimuli. Such individuals are excellent candidates for a program of auditory training for reception and discrimination among gross environmental sounds. Included in such a program should be information regarding sources of sound one would find in specific environments (i.e. indoor versus outdoor) and their unique sound patterns, as well as appropriate behavioral responses to these sounds. "Emphasis should be placed on survival sounds, such as the client's name, door knocking, alarms and sirens, and car motors. Training should be performed in natural environments where these sounds may be found, as many deaf-blind individuals having limited language, experience, and sensory awareness may have difficulty relating tape-recorded stimuli to actual settings in which such sounds may be found" (Hirsch and Morton, 1981). A program that has been found helpful in training discrimination of parameters which will aid gross sound discrimination may be found in Appendix 8D.

Speechreading

Consideration of speechreading training with the deaf-blind individual should be approached cautiously, as many deaf-blind individuals have progressive visual losses (i.e. Usher's Syndrome). In view of this, consultation with the client's eye specialist, preferably an ophthalmologist, should be sought prior to initiation of speechreading training. In addition to securing information regarding the etiology and projected course of visual loss, the eye specialist may impart valuable information regarding the nature of the client's visual impairment, as well as possible benefit to be derived from visual aids (i.e. glasses, magnifiers, etc.) While it is difficult to determine the future course of one's visual impairment, knowing the etiology and past history (onset, course) of the impairment may be helpful in determining the possibility and rate of future progression. Some general guidelines may be followed with respect to the appropriateness of speechreading training. In the individual who retains stable vision, and can discriminate among gross lip movements, speechreading training should be attempted. The individual having a slowly progressive loss of vision may have many useful years ahead as a partially sighted, rather than totally blind individual. While preparation for impending total blindness is an important part of the client's rehabilitation, one must ensure that the client is not treated as totally blind until visual function is severely decreased. An individual such as this may benefit from speechreading training and incorporate it in receptive communication during the years that he retains significant residual vision.

Alternatively, an individual having a rapidly progressive loss of vision should not be encouraged to depend on rapidly decreasing residual vision for receptive communication. Rather, every effort should be made to prepare him for impending total blindness in the near future. This includes teaching tactual methods of communication, discussed under "Communication." An individual such as this is most likely receiving rehabilitative training in other areas (i.e. mobility, daily living skills, vocational preparation) where tactual cues will be stressed. Obviously, dependence on speechreading should not be encouraged in such a case.

In cases where speechreading training is indicated, emphasis should be placed on the functional needs of the client. Some clients may require only refinement of skills or a refresher course, while other clients, particularly those who are adventitiously deaf, may require a complete speechreading program. Other clients, particularly congenitally deaf manually oriented adults may be more suited to a program of speechreading "survival" sentences that they may encounter in work, travel, or daily living. As with any hearing-impaired individual, residual hearing should be optimized as a supplement to speechreading. In the deaf-blind individual, reduced auditory and visual function increases the need for maximizing residual sensory capabilities.

The most significant difference between speechreading training in the deaf-normally sighted and in the deaf-blind individual is the need for strategies to facilitate effective speechreading. As discussed under "Communication," proper lighting and distance require special attention in accordance with the speechreader's visual requirements. In a program of speechreading training, interpersonal strategies, such as having the deaf-blind individual inform the speaker of his visual limitations as well as his lighting and distance requirements, should be stressed.

Vibrotactile Amplification

Despite diligent efforts to evaluate and train aided auditory function, some clients may appear to obtain minimal benefit from conventional air conduction amplification. Yet, there remains a great need for sensory input to provide a form of gross environmental input to the deaf-blind individual who has made minimal progress with air conduction amplification. In such a case, vibrotactile amplification may be considered. The instrumentation required generally includes a body aid, 36-inch cord, bone conduction vibrator, and wristband, as described in Appendix 8F. Using this arrangement, auditory stimulation is received, vibrotactually, at the wrist. Using such a device, discriminations such as presence *versus* absence of sound, number of stimuli, duration, intensity, and discrimination among gross environmental sounds may be achieved with training of reception of the vibratory information. This may be helpful not only in reception of gross environmental input with the totally deaf-blind, but also in speech training, in telephone communication, and, as demonstrated by Decker and Folsom (1978), as an adjunct to speechreading in the deaf individual retaining residual vision. For

detailed information regarding the advantages and limitations of such a device, as well as specific application with deaf-blind individuals, please refer to Appendix 8F.

By maximizing the client's reception of information, we are achieving part of our goal of improving communicative abilities. Emphasis on strengthening expressive modes is of equal importance in the aural rehabilitation of the deaf-blind adult. Since the onset of hearing and vision losses plays a major role in contributing to speech and language difficulties, the following section will present an overview of some common speech and language problems of the prelingually deaf and of the congenitally blind. Given this information, a discussion of unique aspects of the speech and language evaluation and rehabilitation with the deaf-blind adult will follow.

SPEECH AND LANGUAGE PROBLEMS OF THE DEAF

Speech Problems

"The fact that profound prelingual deafness prevents the normal acquisition of speech is well known" (Nickerson, 1975). A classic study by Hudgins and Numbers (1942), supported by the more recent findings of Smith (1975), Nickerson (1975), and others describes various classes of segmental and suprasegmental errors which are commonly found in the speech of congenitally deaf individuals. A brief review of these will be presented here; however, the reader is advised to refer to original sources for a thorough discussion of this topic.

For convenience, errors in the speech of the deaf are generally placed in two classes; segmental errors and suprasegmental errors. It should be noted, however, that the segmental and suprasegmental errors in the speech of the deaf are not necessarily independent of each other. Rather, these segmental and suprasegmental errors are often very much interrelated.

Segmental Errors—The segmental structure of speech refers to "the features and characteristics of individual phonemes" (Levitt and Nye, 1971). Segmental errors in speech of the deaf include consonant errors and vowel errors.

Consonant Errors—Hudgins and Numbers

(1942) noted seven categories of consonant errors in deaf speakers.

CONFUSION OF VOICED (SONANT)-VOICELESS (SURD) DISTINCTION—This is the largest category of error in the speech of subjects in the Hudgins and Numbers study. Intended voiced plosives are perceived as voiceless (devoiced) plosives or vice versa (Nickerson, 1975). Examples of this are substitution of /p/ for /b/ or /t/ for /d/. Smith (1975) found that "among voiced-voiceless cognates, substitution toward the voiced member of the pair was more common than substitution toward the voiceless." Calvert and Silverman (1975) suggest that the causes of distortion in voiced-voiceless consonants are "(a) inadequate coordination of voicing and articulation . . . , (b) inappropriate force of articulation causing duration distortion of the consonant and (c) distortion of the duration of vowels preceding consonants."

MIXED SUBSTITUTIONS—Substitution of one consonant for another ranked sixth in frequency of errors in the Hudgins and Numbers study. Several investigators have identified /s/ as a particular problem and Hudgins and Numbers note high rates of substitution between /s/ and /ʃ/. Calvert and Silverman (1975) note that the substituted sound often provides more oral sensory (tactile) feedback to the speaker than the intended sound.

NASALITY—These are errors involving inappropriate substitution of nasal consonants for others, most notably, stops; or, the lack of nasality where it should be produced in /m/, /n/, or /ŋ/. Calvert and Silverman (1975) note that "nasal-oral substitution rests primarily on improper coordination . . . of the nasopharyngeal closure."

COMPOUND CONSONANTS—Errors of this type may take one of two forms: (a) dropping one member of the compound (i.e. st ɪŋ for strɪŋ); (b) the compound is spoken too slowly, therefore additional syllables are added to the word (i.e. su nɪk for snɪk) (Hudgins and Numbers, 1942).

ABUTTING CONSONANTS—In words or phrases where the final or arresting syllable abuts with the releasing consonant of the next, the deaf speaker often fails to "observe the arresting function of the one consonant and disjoin the articulatory organs before closure of following consonant occurs" (Hudgins and Numbers, 1942). The result is

the addition of an intrusive syllable (i.e. flæg ə poul for flæg poul) (Hudgins and Numbers, 1942).

The last two categories involve errors of omission. Smith (1975) found "the single most frequent error for nearly all consonants was omission."

DROPPING ARRESTING (FINAL) CONSONANT—The consonant movement is completely lost, is incomplete, or is too slow to have a dynamic effect on the preceding vowel. As a result, the syllable is not arrested and the vowel trails off slowly (i.e. Pau' for Paul) (Hudgins and Numbers, 1942).

DROPPING RELEASING (INITIAL) CONSONANT—The consonant movement is too slow or incomplete resulting in failure to close or make the proper juncture with the opposing surface. This prevents a sufficient constriction for air pressure to produce the consonantal effect upon the syllable (ɔr for your) (Hudgins and Numbers, 1942).

Vowel Errors—Hudgins and Numbers (1942) identified five vowel error categories.

SUBSTITUTION OF ONE VOWEL FOR ANOTHER—Typically, there is "a tendency for vowels to drop to a more neutral position" (Smith, 1975).

DIPTHONGS—Errors involving dipthongs take one of the following two forms. (a) "The dipthong is split, making two distinct vowels instead of a fusion of the two components. This is caused by the slowly executed movements of articulation which allows too much time for the vowel and improper coordination of breathing muscles." (Hudgins and Numbers, 1942). "(b) One of the components of the dipthong, usually the final member, is dropped. This is caused by a failure to make the complete articulatory movement" (Hudgins and Numbers, 1942).

DIPTHONIZATION OF PURE VOWELS—Due to poor coordination of articulatory movements and breath pulses, deaf speakers make slow transitory movements during articulation of a vowel. The continuation of voice during these transitions causes the vowel to be produced as a dipthong (Hudgins and Numbers, 1942).

NEUTRALIZATION OF PURE VOWELS—Oral movements required for producing the pure vowel are not precise enough and causes the vowel to become more like the neutral vowel /ə/ (Hudgins and Numbers, 1942).

NASALIZATION OF PURE VOWELS—Poor velum control can cause nasalization of pure vowels. "It is often difficult to determine whether the consonant movement or the vowel is at fault for the nasality present in both" (Hudgins and Numbers, 1942).

Suprasegmental Errors— The suprasegmental features are "those features and characteristics that relate to entire phrases and sentences" (Levitt and Nye, 1971). Suprasegmental characteristics may be divided into two classes. (1) Prosodic characteristics are those which affect the meaning of what is said. The key suprasegmental characteristics which affect meaning directly are intonation, the modulation of voice pitch; stress, whereby the syllable is spoken so as to make it more perceptually prominent; rhythm, the pattern in which certain syllables are stressed and others are left unstressed; and phrasing, whereby words are grouped together according to the linguistic structure of the utterance (Levitt and Nye, 1971). (2) Voice quality characteristics "have little effect on meaning but ... convey a good deal of information as to who is speaking, the physical or mental state of the speaker, and other intangibles, such as emotion and feeling" (Levitt and Nye, 1971). "Factors that affect voice quality are loudness, average pitch, stridency, breathiness, hoarseness, and nasality, to mention a few" (Levitt and Nye, 1971).

Errors of Prosody—Deaf speakers often fail to make the differentiation between stressed and unstressed syllables. Rather, all syllables tend to be produced as though they are stressed, leading to flat and monotonous intonation (Nickerson, 1975; Levitt and Nye, 1971). Pauses are inserted more frequently and "of longer duration than is found in running speech of normal hearing speakers. Additionally, these pauses are often inserted at inappropriate places" (Nickerson, 1975). Poor use of appropriate rhythmic and intonational patterns is found. This is often related to problems in proper production of stress and proper use of pauses. Related to these is the problem of poor breath control, usually resultant of excessive air expenditure during speech (Hudgins and Numbers, 1942; Smith, 1975; Nickerson, 1975; Levitt and Nye, 1971).

Voice Problems—One of the most common voice problems among deaf speakers is improper fundamental frequency for the speaker's age and sex. "Both young male and female deaf talkers tend to speak with a higher fundamental pitch than hearing persons ... " (Calvert and Silverman, 1975). Further, poor pitch control is often present, resulting either in a monotone voice or erratic pitch variation. Improper control of the velum may cause hypernasality. Inappropriate vocal intensity is common in the speech of the deaf. Voicing may be too soft, too loud, or may vary erratically (Nickerson, 1975). This may be due to lack of awareness regarding appropriate vocal intensity as dictated by distance, social, and environmental requirements, or due to inability to physically control vocal intensity. Inability to speak loud enough may be due to inefficient use of the air stream at the glottis. This may result in breathiness as well. Regarding rate, Nickerson (1975) notes that "deaf persons tend to speak at a much slower rate than do hearing persons."

Language Problems

"It has been repeatedly demonstrated by researchers that language abilities of many hearing-impaired children are quite delayed ... (however) it is still not clear whether deaf children generally learn language like normal hearing children, albeit at a slower rate, or whether they are different or even deviant in their developmental patterns" (Streng *et al.*, 1978).

Kretschmer and Kretschmer (1978) present several considerations in regard to the delay *versus* deviance dilemma. They suggest that linguistic capabilities in deaf children may be viewed "(a) [as] delayed in nature because of a lack of linguistic/cognitive experience but shown to progress with age; (b) as deviant in nature because of the effects of hearing impairment on cognitive development as well as influences from an alternative symbol system (ASL); (c) as dialectical in nature because English is a second language, or more probably; (d) as showing language proficiency that is the result of some or all of the foregoing influences" (Kretschmer and Kretschmer, 1978).

In a review of studies regarding language development in older deaf children, Kretschmer and Kretschmer summarize five points regarding the relative abilities of deaf and normally hearing children to "generate spontaneous compositions, and to understand and/or produce meaningful English sentences through reading, writing, drawing, or pointing" (Kretschmer and Kretschmer, 1978).

"First, deaf subjects' written language ... is consistently immature when compared to normally hearing subjects.... Second, although deaf children's linguistic efforts are generally less accurate than those of normally hearing children, both in production of base structures and of more complex forms, their restricted forms or pattern deviations generally parallel those of subjects without hearing loss.... Third, deaf children depend highly upon surface structure organization in both comprehension and production of English written sentences.... Fourth, it seems to be time now ... to try to understand the semantic/pragmatic knowledge acquired by deaf children so that semantic field differentiation and other aspects of meaning may be brought into congruence with the majority of English language users. Fifth, the paucity of English deep structure intuitions of most deaf children can be clearly seen in tasks that test grammatical sensitivity ... " (Kretschmer and Kretschmer, 1978).

Streng *et al.* (1978) review studies dealing with language comprehension and production of deaf children in three basic areas: phrase structure rule acquisition; transformational rule acquisition; and pragmatic rule acquisition.

According to Streng *et al.* (1978), "research into phrase structure rules of spoken English indicates that deaf children do acquire many of the phrase structure rules of English much in the same way as do normally hearing children, but in a delayed fashion with some exceptions of deviant rule acquisition." They note that studies of phrase structure knowledge of written language seem to suggest that "the base structure of hearing-impaired children is deviant from that of normal hearing writers. . . ." Transformational growth in deaf children "seems to parallel that of normally hearing children, with some exceptions noted ... " (Streng *et al.*, 1978). Studies of pragmatic growth in deaf children, although limited, seem to demonstrate that "deaf children often lack an understanding of how to communicate information to others" (Streng *et al.*, 1978).

Clinical observation of the language abilities of congenitally deaf manually oriented adults often reveals good linguistic competence through use of Ameslan, with fair to poor mastery of English. In such a case, English may be thought of as a second language (Kretschmer and Kretschmer, 1978). Since ASL generally uses one signed concept (*i.e.* a congregation of people) to represent English words (*i.e.* team, society, class, group), the signed concept may be understood; however, the specific English word meant may not be recognized when printed. This causes semantic difficulties for ASL users. Additionally, since the syntactic structure of ASL is different than English, comprehension of printed English sentences (*i.e.* "I am finished working.") tends to be more limited than ASL ("Me work finish.") comprehension.

SPEECH AND LANGUAGE PROBLEMS OF THE BLIND

The congenitally blind-normally hearing population has not traditionally been thought of as displaying characteristic speech and language disorders. This may be, in part, due to the fact that experimental data assessing the communication skills of congenitally blind individuals has been sparse. However, a recent study by Bernstein (1978), assessed how congenital blindness affects "comprehension of dimensional adjectives (big-little, long-short, and thick-thin); relational terms (same-different); and locatives (front-back, side, in, on, under)." Bernstein's study revealed that, "on all tasks, blind children's performance was significantly delayed when compared to that of normal children. There were no indications of deviant development on the part of blind subjects" (Bernstein, 1978).

The speech patterns of the blind has received little, if any, attention. Bernstein (1978) cites a paper delivered by Fay (1975) which describes the evaluation of speech in 53 blind children entering nursery school. "Of those children studied, 25% of the children had normal speech, 25% of the children had no speech, and 50% of the children had delayed or defective speech" (Bernstein, 1978). The speech and language abilities of the congenitally blind remains an area in need of much further study.

UNIQUE ASPECTS OF THE SPEECH AND LANGUAGE EVALUATION OF THE DEAF-BLIND ADULT

In evaluation and rehabilitation of speech and language abilities of the deaf-blind individual, any and all of the aforementioned speech and language problems may be found. However, these problems are generally linked to the onset and severity of hearing and visual losses. Individuals who are congenitally severely impaired (auditorily and/or visually) demonstrate the most severe and most numerous speech and language problems, while adventitiously and/or partially impaired individuals may demonstrate few or no speech and language difficulties. Of course, the possible presence of additional disabilities, such as intellectual limitations or emotional disorders may compound speech and language problems to a greater extent than that seen in a deaf-blind individual who has no additional compounding disabilities.

To date, there are no speech and/or language tests standardized on a deaf-blind population which would allow the performance of the individual at hand to be compared with others through use of norms. However, careful selection and appropriate adaptation of available speech and language tests can be helpful in eliciting information to determine current functioning in various skill areas, as well as to determine specific communicative areas in need of rehabilitation. The clinician's choice of appropriate test instruments should be guided by knowledge regarding the onset and severity of hearing and visual losses; this history information should be secured by the clinician prior to meeting with the client. In this way, speech and language evaluation tools may be selected according to anticipated speech and language problems demonstrated by the deaf-blind client, as described in the previous section. Additionally, "all test materials that require reading should be prepared in large print, Grade One, or Grade Two Braille according to the client's visual functioning" (Hirsch and Morton, 1981). The clinician performing the evaluation should be competent in the deaf-blind client's preferred mode of communication so that the evaluation can proceed smoothly and results may be valid and reliable. If this is not possible, the services of an interpreter (see Appendix 8C) should be arranged prior to the evaluation.

Upon meeting the client, specific history information should be obtained to aid in determining current status and prognosis for rehabilitation. "In gathering a speech and language history, special attention should be given to the amount of residual hearing, hearing aid usage, level of language functioning, and prior and present use of speech as an expressive mode of communication" (Hirsch and Morton, 1981).

A standard oral peripheral examination of the speech mechanism (Johnson et al., 1963) which assesses various aspects of the respiratory, phonatory, and articulatory systems should be performed. In performing an oral peripheral examination on a deaf-blind individual possessing the linguistic abilities to understand directions, all instructions should be conveyed to the client through his preferred mode. Clients with more limited language may require tactual cueing in support of auditory and/or visual reception to produce the desired articulatory, respiratory, or phonatory responses. The Tadoma hand position (discussed under "Communication Methods") placed on the clinician's articulators can provide the client with a tactual model of the desired behavior (Morton, 1980).

The articulation evaluation should not only assess production of phonemes in isolated words, but also in connected speech. Since most deaf-blind clients one will encounter are congenitally deaf, as discussed under "Statistics and Prevalence," the articulatory errors of many deaf-blind clients will represent many segmental and suprasegmental errors characteristic of the speech of the deaf discussed in the previous section. In view of the prevalence of articulatory errors involving confusion of voiced and voiceless cognates, a distinctive feature analysis is desirable in order to determine if multiple errors are linked to confusion regarding manner and place of articulation (Morton, 1980). At the Helen Keller National Center, the Fisher-Logemann Test of Articulation Competence, (1971) which employs a distinctive feature analysis, is used for assessment of errors made in production of isolated words as well as sentences. The protocol and test sheets should be prepared in large print and/or Braille as appropriate (Morton, 1980). In addition to assessment of production in isolated words and sentences, stimulability for improvement of articulatory errors should be assessd as an aid in determining prognosis for improvement. Tactual models may be provided by the clinician, with the client receiving the information through use of the Tadoma hand position on the clinician's articulators.

The suprasegmental aspects of speech are assessed to determine the effects of suprasegmental errors on speech intelligibility. At the Helen Keller National Center, the Speech and Voice Diagnostic Form, designed by Subtelny (1975) has been found highly useful in evaluating these suprasegmental features. Since it was designed for use with a deaf population, it is particularly useful in pinpointing those suprasegmental errors and voice qualities that are characteristic of the speech of the deaf, discussed in the previous section.

Where possible, "standardized language tests are adapted for use with this population. The results are used to measure growth within the individual and to compare his performance with other deaf-blind individuals rather than by using the norms" (Hirsch and Morton, 1981). Standardized language tests which have been found applicable for use with some deaf-blind individuals are the Peabody Picture Vocabulary Test, aspects of the Illinois Test of Psycholinguistic Abilities, and the Test of Syntactic Abilities (Hirsch and Morton, 1981). Of course, decreased auditory and visual capabilities of the client limit the application of these tests to a narrow range of the deaf-blind population. Where significant residual auditory and/or visual capabilities exist, these standardized tests are generally appropriate for use with the client having at least fair to good language skills. In addition, a written or Brailled language sample should be obtained and compared to language conveyed through the client's preferred (*i.e.* manual, aural/oral) mode.

The congenitally deaf adult whose first language is Ameslan may demonstrate poor understanding of English semantic, syntactic, and phonologic structure, and yet demonstrate good mastery of language through ASL. In such a case, the language evaluation should attempt to assess communication abilities through the client's preferred mode, ASL, as well as through English, which may be thought of as a second language for such a client.

For a client demonstrating severely limited language abilities, an assessment of functional communication abilities is generally indicated (Morton, 1980). These should include linguistic concepts that the client needs to comprehend and/or express in his daily living. A client's family member or friend, as well as other professionals working with this client can be of invaluable assistance in providing the clinician with a list of words and commands that the deaf-blind client can comprehend and/or express. Where possible, the clinician should observe the client in various settings, such as vocational and social situations so that a true picture of the client's functional communication abilities may be assessed (Morton, 1980).

UNIQUE ASPECTS OF THE SPEECH AND LANGUAGE REHABILITATION PROCESS WITH THE DEAF-BLIND INDIVIDUAL

The results of a speech and language evaluation are not the only factors to consider in determining an individual's candidacy for speech and language training. "Motivation is of paramount importance. A well-motivated deaf-blind individual may succeed far more than may be expected" when simply viewing test results (Hirsch and Morton, 1981). "Motivation for improvement of communication ability tends to be linked to positive attitude toward other areas of rehabilitation as a deaf-blind person" (Hirsch and Morton, 1981). Some other factors to be considered are the client's functional use of aided residual hearing and willingness to use sensory (auditory, visual, and vibrotactile) aids, educational background, experience with and attitude toward aural/oral training, and willingness to use semi-intelligible speech with the hearing world (Hirsch and Morton, 1981).

Speech training programs with the deaf-blind individual who is congenitally deaf may be initiated on any of several levels. "The goals may range from a short term program of survival speech, emphasizing intelligible production of one's name, address, and such words as 'help' and 'hello,' to a goal of intelligible connected speech as a primary mode of communication. With the adventitiously deaf, the goal is generally to maintain the existing intelligible speech" (Hirsch and Morton, 1981).

"One of the major distinctions between speech training with hearing-impaired sighted individuals and hearing- and visually-impaired individuals is the need for special attention to use of tactile and kinesthetic cues in the speech rehabilitation process. These cues should be used as an adjunct to existing residual hearing and/or vision; however, in cases of total hearing and/or vision loss, reliance on tactile and kinesthetic cues becomes of paramount importance" (Kramer et al., 1979). Tactual and kinesthetic cues used in teaching speech to the deaf-blind are discussed in detail in Appendix 8G. These cues are used in conjunction with any existing residual hearing and/or vision in teaching correct speech production in the congenitally deaf, and for maintaining intelligible speech in the adventitiously deaf.

All speech rehabilitation materials used should be prepared in a mode (print, large print, Braille) that the client prefers. Additionally, the use of supportive speech instrumentation may be helpful in visualizing those aspects of speech which can not be received auditorily. Existing commercial speech instrumentation which uses a light to signal correct production (Risberg, 1968) may be used in a darkened room with the visually impaired individual in order to enhance illumination (Morton, 1980). Vibrotactile adaptors have been found highly effective in transferring output from a visual to tactile output useable with the totally blind. For more detail regarding these vibrotactile adaptations, please refer to Kramer et al., 1979.

In a program of speech rehabilitation, multiple target articulation therapy has been found highly effective wit deaf-blind individuals who are congenitally deaf. Because of the difficulty in production of voiced-voiceless distinctions among the congenitally deaf, teaching the overall concept with application to specific groups of phonemes (/p/-/b/, /t/-/d/, /k/-/g/, etc.) has been successful with this population (Morton, 1980). The clinician should take advantage of any auditory and visual cues available to the client; however, tactile cues serve as a strong support to auditory and visual information and may be used as the primary mode in conveying models of correct speech production in the totally deaf-blind individual.

Approaches to remediation of suprasegmental features and improvement of voice quality are similar to those traditionally used with the deaf-normally sighted; however, special attention should be given to the use of tactile and kinesthetic cues (see Appendix 8G) in support of aided residual vision and/or hearing. Additionally, vibrotactile devices such as a bone conduction vibrator (discussed under "Aural Rehabilitation") can be helpful in training correct production of suprasegmental features. For more detail regarding speech training in the deaf normally sighted adult, please refer to Chapter 7.

Pronunciation training is "designed to improve the student's independent skills in word production by teaching Webster's diacritical symbols and some general rules of pronunciation. Practice in using the dictionary and diacritical markings is also provided" (Johnson, 1978). The deaf-blind client having limited vision may use a large type dictionary, such as the Websters-New World Dictionary, (Second College Edition) (1970) while the totally blind individual may use the American Vest Pocket Dictionary, Braille Edition (1961). (Morton, 1981) (see Appendix 8C).

As stated by Levitt, (1980), ". . . it is generally believed that the earlier speech and language training is provided to a deaf child, the more effective are the results." The importance of early identification and intervention with the deaf is well accepted and has been supported by our knowledge regarding critical periods of development during the early years (for more information regarding critical periods of development, refer to Lenneberg, 1967). Our aim is not to dispute the value of early intervention, however, we must consider the case of the congenitally deaf adult who may not have developed a functional language system. Do we view this individual as a "hopeless case" in language acquisition?

Little emphasis has been placed on language development in the deaf adult; however, a few studies reveal that some gain in functional language acquisition can be achieved with careful training. Spidal and Pfau (1972) found that deaf adults who were termed "illiterate" prior to training were later able to "communicate with others at the simple sentence level in speech, writing, and the language of signs, . . . engaged each other in enjoyable and successful dialogue, . . . [and] progressed from the recognition of a small number of nouns to the reading and comprehending of simple connected language. . . . " In addition, they desired more contact with reading materials at their ability levels and significantly increased attention span related to learning activities as a result of training (Spidal and Pfau, 1972).

Rees *et al.* (1974) report a case study of first language acquisition in a deaf-blind adult. Their study demonstrated that, resultant of an extensive training program, their subject progressed "from a passive unreacting, noncommunicative organism" to a "young man with severe and limiting handicaps who could nonetheless relate meaningfully to others, use a limited linguistic system to communicate with those around him, and learn selected cognitive, linguistic, and academic skills" (Rees *et al.*, 1974).

The functional needs of the deaf or deaf-blind adult must be considered in designing a program of communicative development. Language training may be initiated on any of several levels. Deaf-blind clients who are severely limited in linguistic abilities may begin a "survival" language program, with emphasis on social, vocational, and other concepts that will facilitate daily living (Morton, 1980). It is likely that such a client will use manual (signed or gestural) methods of communication as his primary mode, with secondary support of print and/or Braille modes for word recognition and limited expression. Individuals interested in details of a program of first language acquisition in a deaf-blind adult should refer to Rees *et al.* (1974).

The congenitally deaf individual whose first language is ASL may require instruction in application of ASL into English semantic, syntactic, and phonologic structure, facilitating written and/or aural/oral communication. One approach that has been found effective at the Helen Keller National Center is the teaching of English as a second language, whereby knowledge of semantic, syntactic, and phonologic structure of a first language (*i.e.* ASL) is applied to learning new structures in a second language (*i.e.* English). This facilitates reception and production of English-based communication methods, such as reading/writing, aural/oral communication and use of Manually Coded English systems. Such individuals generally have some experience in use of speech as a means of expression; however, it is often unused. If motivated, such individuals may be candidates for a program of "survival speech."

Deaf-blind adults having more advanced language abilities may require refinement of conversational skills, including training in comprehension and use of idiomatic expressions and improvement of interpersonal skills. Programs such as these can develop pragmatic communication abilities, an area in need of improvement in the congenitally deaf, as noted by Streng *et al.*, (1978). These and other programs are described more fully in Chapter 7, "The Adult Deaf Client and Rehabilitation." The key to application of these programs with deaf-blind individuals is to be sure the materials and instructions account for the presence of the client's visual loss, in addition to his hearing loss. Clients such as these, having rather well-developed language skills, are often more apt than clients having limited language to use speech as a means of communication with the hearing public. This client's writing/Braille skills are generally sufficient to use print writing or Braille communication devices (*i.e.* Tellatouch, etc.) with the general public as well.

References

ABORDO, E. J., and THOMAS, L. J. (Eds.), *Directory of Agencies Serving the Deaf-Blind.* Sands Point, NY: Helen Keller National Center (1980).

ALTMAN, J., *Sound Localization, Neurophysiological Mechanisms: Translations of the Beltone Institute for Hearing Research.* Chicago: Beltone Institute for Hearing Research (1978).

ALPINER, J. G., CHEVRETTE, W., GLASCOE, G., METZ, M., and OLSEN, B., *The Denver Scale of Communicative Function.* Unpublished study. University of Denver (1971).

AMERICAN FOUNDATION FOR THE BLIND, *Directory of Agencies Serving the Visually Handicapped in the United States.* New York: American Foundation for the Blind, (1981).

American Vest Pocket Dictionary (Braille Edition) 7 vols. Louisville, KY: American Printing House (1961).

Annual Report, Helen Keller National Center for Deaf-Blind Youths and Adults, 3/1/79–2/29/80 Period. Sands Point, NY (1980).

BARRETT, S. S., Assessment of vision in the program for the deaf. *Am. Ann. Deaf,* **124,** 745–752 (1979).

BERGSMA, D., The Usher's Syndrome: clinical definition and related research. In N. Tully (Ed.), *Papers Presented at Workshop on Usher's Syndrome, Deceber 2–3, 1976,* pp. 8–14. Sands Point, NY: Helen Keller National Center (1976).

BERGSMA, D. R., Ophthalmologic aspects of Usher's Syndrome. *Symposium on Ushers Syndrome,* p. 22. Washington, D. C.: Gallaudet College (1973).

BERNSTEIN, D., *Semantic Development in Congenitally Blind Children.* Unpublished Ph.D. dissertation, The Graduate School of the City University of New York (1978).

BOOTHROYD, A., Sensory Aids Research Project—Clarke School for the Deaf. In G. Fant (Ed.), International

Symposium on Speech Communication Ability and Profound Deafness, pp. 375–377. Stockholm, Sweden (August, 1970).

CACCAMISE, F., JOHNSON, D. D., HAMILTON, L. F., ROTHBLUM, A. M., and HOWARD, M., Visual assessment and the rehabilitation of hearing impaired children and adults. *J. Acad. Rehab. Audiol.*, **8**, 78–101 (1980).

CALVERT, D. R., and SILVERMAN, S. R., *Speech and Deafness.* Washington, D. C.: Alexander Graham Bell Association for the Deaf (1975).

CARROLL, T. J., *Blindness: What It is, What It Does, and How To Live with It.* Boston: Little, Brown, and Co (1961).

CASTLE, D., Telephone training for the deaf, *Volta Rev.*, **79**, 373–378 (1977a).

CASTLE, D., Telephone and distance communication devices for the hearing impaired. *Deaf Am.*, **29(10)**, 15–16 (1977b).

CASTLE, W., Introduction, *Am. Ann. Deaf* **125**, 961–962 (1980).

CHESS, S., Follow-up report on autism in congenital rubella. *J. Autism Child. Schizophr.*, **7**, 69–81 (1977).

CHESS, S., and FERNANDEZ, P., Neurologic damage and behavior disorder in rubella children. *Am. Ann. Deaf,* **125**, 998–1001 (1980).

CHESS, S., FERNANDEZ, P., and KORN, S., Behavioral consequences of congential rubella. *J. Pediatr.*, **93**, 699–703 (1978).

CONDON, W. S., and SANDER, L. W., Neonate movement is synchronized with adult speech: interactional participation and language acquisition. *Science*, **183**, 99–101 (1974).

COOPER, L., The child with Rubella Syndrome. *New Outlook Blind*, **63 (10)**, 290–298 (December, 1969).

DANTONA, R., The deaf-blind population: implications for rehabilitation. *J. Rehab. Deaf*, **8**, 65–68 (1974).

DANTONA, R., and SALMON, P. J., The current status of services for deaf-blind persons. *New Outlook Blind*, **66 (3)**, 65–70 (March, 1972).

DAVIS, H., and SILVERMAN, S. R., *Hearing and Deafness*, pp. 492–495. 3rd Ed. New York: Holt, Rinehart, and Winston (1970).

DECKER, T. N., and FOLSOM, R. C., A tactile method for increasing speechreading abilities: two case studies. *Audio. Hear. Educ.*, **4**, 14–18 (1978).

DiPIETRO, L. J., Ed., *Guidelines on Interpreting for Deaf-Blind Persons.* Washington, D. C.: Gallaudet College (1978).

EISENBERG, R. B., *Auditory Competence in Early Life.* Baltimore: University Park Press (1976).

EWING, I. R., and EWING, A. W. G., The Ascertainment of Deafness in Infancy. *J. Laryngol. Otol.*, **59**, 309–333 (1944).

FAY, W., *The Triple Trauma of Blindness to Language Development.* Paper presented at the American Speech and Hearing Association Annual Convention, Washington, D. C. November, 1975 (1975).

FISHER, H. B., and LOGEMANN, J. A., The Fisher-Logemann Test of Articulation Competence. Boston: Houghton Mifflin Co (1971).

FRANKLIN, B., New techniques for the auditory evaluation of deaf-blind children. In *The Psychologist, Audiologist and Speech Pathologist and the Deaf-Blind Child*, pp. 94–96. Sacramento: California State Department of Education (1978).

FRANKLIN, B., Split-band amplification and speech band audiometry. *Hear. Instruments*, **28(11)**, 18–20, 47 (1977).

GAUGER, J., *Orientation to Hearing Aids.* Washington, D. C.: Alexander Graham Bell Association for the Deaf (1978).

HICKS, W. M., and PFAU, G. S., Deaf-visually impaired persons: incidence and services. *Am. Ann. Deaf*, **124**, 76–92 (1979).

HIRSCH, L. M., and MORTON, D., Deaf-Blindness. In L. J. Bradford and F. N. Martin (Eds.), Audiology: *An Audio Journal for Continuing Education.* New York: Grune & Stratton (1981).

HUDGINS, C. V., and NUMBERS, F. C., An investigation of speech of the deaf. *Gen. Psychol. Monograph*, **25**, 289–292 (1942).

Introducing the Helen Keller National Center (brochure). Sands Point, NY: Helen Keller National Center (1980).

JENSEMA, C., Post rubella children in special educational programs for the hearing impaired. *Volta Rev.*, **76**, 466–473 (1974).

JOHNSON, D. J. The Adult Deaf Client and Rehabilitation. In J. Alpiner (Ed.), *Handbook of Adult Rehabilitative Audiology.* Baltimore: The Williams & Wilkins Co. (1978).

JOHNSON, W., DARLEY, F., and SPRIESTERBACH, D. *Diagnostic Methods in Speech Pathology.* New York: Harper and Row (1963).

KATES, L., and SCHEIN, J., *A Complete Guide to Communication with Deaf-Blind Persons.* Silver Spring, MD: National Association of the Deaf (1980).

KIRMAN, J., Tactile communication of speech: a review and an analysis. *Psych. Bull*, **80**, 54–74 (1973).

KRAMER, L. C., SULLIVAN, R. F., and HIRSCH, L. M. *Audiological Evaluation and Aural Rehabilitation of the Deaf-Blind Adult.* Sands Point, NY: Helen Keller National Center (1979).

KRETSCHMER, R. R., JR., and KRETSCHMER, L. W., Language Development with the Hearing Impaired. Baltimore: University Park Press (1978).

LENNEBERG, E. H. *Biological Foundations of Language.* New York: John Wiley & Sons (1967).

LEVIN, S., and ERBER, N. P., A vision screening program for deaf children. *Volta Rev.*, **78**, 90–99 (1976).

LEVITT, H., Hearing aids: special problems. In H. Levitt, J. M. Pickett, and R. A. Houde (Eds.), *Sensory Aids for the Hearing Impaired.* New York: IEEE Press (1980).

LEVITT, H., and NYE, P., eds., *Sensory Training Aids for the Hearing Impaired.* Washington, D. C.: National Academy of Engineering (1971).

LING, D., *Speech and the Hearing Impaired Child: Theory and Practice.* Washington, D. C.: Alexander Graham Bell Association (1976).

LOWELL, E. L., A correspondence and direct service program for parents of deaf-blind children. Proceedings of the Forty-Seventh Meeting of the Convention of American Instructors of the Deaf, Greensboro, NC, June 22–27, 1975, pp. 260–263.

MARKIDES, A., *Binaural Hearing Aids.* New York: Academic Press (1977).

McLEOD, A. C., McCONNELL, F. E., SWEENEY, A., COOPER, M. C., and NANCE, W. E., Clinical variation in Usher's Syndrome. *Arch. Otolaryngol.*, **94**, 321–334 (1971).

MENSER, M. A., DODS, L., and HARLEY, J. D., A twenty five year follow-up of congential rubella. *Lancet*, **2**, 1347-1349 (1967).

MORTON, D., Speech Services: Vibrotactile Instrumentation as an Aid to Speech Rehabilitation. Paper presented at Seminar on Deaf-Blindness. Helen Keller National Center, July 14-18, 1980.

MYKLEBUST, H. R., *The Psychology of Deafness*. 2nd Ed. New York: Grune & Stratton (1964).

NANCE, W. E., CAMPBELL, J. B., and BEIBER, F. R., The Usher's Syndrome: a long neglected genetic disease. In N. Tully (Ed.), *Papers Presented at Workshop on Usher's Syndrome, December 2-3, 1976*, pp. 4-7. Sands Point, NY: Helen Keller National Center (1976).

NATIONAL EYE INSTITUTE, *How Eye Problems Affect Our Vision*. Bethesda, MD: National Institutes of Health (1977).

NICKERSON, R. S., Characteristics of the speech of deaf persons. *Volta Rev.*, **77**, 342-362 (1975).

NORTON, S. J., SCHULTZ, M. C., REED, C. M., BRAIDA, L. D., DURLACH, N. I., RABINOWITZ, W. M., and CHOMSKY, C., Analytic study of the Tadoma Method: background and preliminary results. *J. Speech Hear. Res.*, **20**, 574-595 (1977).

REED, C. M., RUBIN, S. I., BRAIDA, L. D., and DURLACH, N. I., Analytic study of the Tadoma Method: discrimination ability of untrained observers. *J. Speech Hear. Res.*, **21**, 635-637 (1978).

REES, N. S., KRUGER, F., BERNSTEIN, D., KRAMER, L., and BEZAS, M., The acquisition of a first language in a blind-deaf adult: a case study of a language development in an adult with a history of deaf-blindness. *J. Rehab. Deaf*, **8**, 11-23 (1974).

RISBERG, A., Visual aids for speech correction. *Am. Ann. Deaf*, **113**, 178-194 (1968).

ROSS, M., Binaural versus monaural hearing aid amplification for hearing impaired individuals. In F. Bess (Ed.), *Childhood Deafness, Causation, Assessment, and Management*. New York: Grune & Stratton (1977).

ROSS, M., and GIOLAS, T. G., Issues and exposition. T. G. Giolas and M. Ross (Eds.), *In Auditory Management of Hearing Impaired Children*, Chap. 9. Baltimore: University Park Press (1978).

ROSS, M., and LERMAN, J., A picture identification test for hearing impaired children. *J. Speech Hear. Res.*, **13**, 44-53 (1970).

RYAN, J. F., TDD's—the second invention of the telephone. *Hear. Instruments*, **32**, 18-19 (1981).

SMITH, B. J., Potentials of rubella deaf-blind children. In C. E. Sherrick (Ed.), *1989 is Now*. Los Angeles: John Tracy Clinic (1974).

SMITH, C., Residual hearing and speech production in deaf children. *J. Speech Hear. Res.*, **18**, 795-811 (1975).

SMITHDAS, R. J., Vocational education and the future of the deaf blind. In C. Rouin, (Ed.), The deaf-blind child and the vocational rehabilitation counselor. Sacramento: California State Department of Education, 1976, pp. 2-4.

SPIDAL, D. A., and PFAU, G. S. The potential for language acquisition of illiterate deaf adolescents and adults. *J. Rehab. Deaf*, **6**, 27-41 (1972).

STEVENS, S. S., and DAVIS, H., *Hearing*. New York: John Wiley and Sons, Inc. (1938).

STRENG, A. H., KRETCHMER, R. R., JR., AND KRETCHMER, L. W., *Language Learning and Deafness, Theory Application and Management*. New York: Grune & Stratton (1978).

SUBTELNY, J. D., Speech assessment of the deaf adult. *J. Acad. Rehab. Audiol.* **8**, 110-116 (1975).

Telephone Devices in Review, *Hear. Instruments*, **32**, 20-24 (1981).

TRYBUS, R. J., KARCHMER, M. A., KERSTETTER, P. P., and HICKS, W., The demographics of deafness resulting from maternal rubella. *Am. Ann. Deaf*, **125**, 977-984 (1980).

VERNON, M., Usher's Syndrome: problems and some solutions. *Hear. Speech Action*, **44**, 6-13 (1976).

VERNON, M., Overview of Usher's Syndrome—congenital deafness and progressive loss of vision. *Volta Rev.*, **76**, 100-105 (1974).

VERNON, M., and HICKS, D., Overview of rubella, herpes simplex, cytomegalovirus, and other viral diseases: their relationship to deafness. *Am. Ann. Deaf*, **125**, 529-534 (1980).

VERNON, M., GRIEVE, B. J., and SHAVER, K., Handicapping conditions associated with the Congential Rubella Syndrome. *Am. Ann. Deaf*, **125**, 993-997 (1980).

Webster's New World Dictionary (Second College Edition) (Large Type). 24 vol. Louisville, KY: American Printing House (1970).

WILBUR, R. B., *American Sign Language and Sign Systems*. Baltimore, MD: University Park Press (1979).

WOODWARD, J. C., Implication variation in American Sign Language: negative incorporation. *Sign Language Studies*, **5**, 20-30 (1974).

ZIRING, P., Current status of the rubella problem. Sharing deaf-blind methods—1975. In M. Collins (Ed.), *Proceedings of Two Regional Workshops for Professionals and Paraprofessionals Serving Deaf-Blind Children in Illinois-Indiana-Michigan-Minnesota-Ohio-Wisconsin*. Lansing, Michigan: Midwest Regional Center for Services to Deaf-Blind Children (1975).

8A

Service Regions of the Helen Keller National Center for Deaf-Blind Youths and Adults

New England region
89 State St., Suite 1130, Boston, MA 02109
(617) 523-7015
Connecticut, Maine, Massachusetts, New Hampshire, Rhode Island, Vermont

Mid Atlantic region
111 Middle Neck Road, Sands Point, NY 11050
(516) 944-8900 (TTY and voice)
New Jersey, New York, Puerto Rico, Virgin Islands

East Central region
Scott Plaza II, Suite 301, Philadelphia, Pa 19113
(215) 521-1370
Delaware, District of Columbia, Maryland, Ohio, Pennsylvania, Virginia, West Virginia

Southeastern region
1581 Phoenix Boulevard, Suite 14, Atlanta, GA 30349
(404) 996-2802 (TTY and voice)
Alabama, Florida, Georgia, Kentucky, Mississippi, North Carolina, South Carolina, Tennessee

North Central region
35 E. Wacker Drive, Suite 1268, Chicago, IL 60601
(312) 726-2090
Illinois, Indiana, Iowa, Michigan, Minnesota, Missouri, Wisconsin

South Central region
1111 W. Mockingbird Lane, Suite 1540, Dallas, TX 75247
(214) 630-4936 (TTY and voice)
Arkansas, Louisiana, New Mexico, Oklahoma, Texas

Mountain-Plains region

12075 E. 45th Avenue, Suite 222, Denver, CO 80239

(303) 373-1204 (TTY and voice)

Colorado, Kansas, Nebraska, North Dakota, South Dakota, Utah, Wyoming

Northwestern region

649 Strandler Boulevard, Suite C., Seattle WA 98188

(206) 575-1491

Alaska, Idaho, Montana, Oregon, Washington

Southwestern region

870 Market Street, Suite 885, San Francisco, CA 94102

(415) 956-4562 (TTY and voice)

Arizona, California, Guam, Samoa, and the Trust Territories, Hawaii, Nevada

8B

Federally Funded Programs for the Deaf-Blind*

Center and Services for Deaf-Blind Children, Bureau of Education for the Handicapped, U. S. Office of Education, Department of Health, Education, and Welfare, Donohoe Building, Room 4046, 400 Maryland Avenue, Washington, D. C. 20202
Robert Dantona, Project Coordinator

A. Multi-State Centers

1. Mid-Atlantic Regional Center for Deaf-Blind Children
%New York Institute for Education of the Blind, 999 Pelham Parkway, Bronx, NY 10469
(212) 547-1234
Khogendra Das, Coordinator
Serves deaf-blind children from Delaware, New Jersey, New York, Puerto Rico, and the Virgin Islands.

2. Midwest Regional Center for Deaf-Blind Children
% Michigan Department of Education, 5th Floor, Davenport Building, Ottawa and Capitol Streets, Lansing, MI 48933
(517) 373-0108
George Mouk, Coordinator
Serves deaf-blind children from Indiana, Michigan, Minnesota, and Wisconsin.

3. Mountain Plains Regional Center for Deaf-Blind Children
165 Cook Street, Denver, CO 80203
(303) 399-3070
John Ogden, Coordinator
Serves deaf-blind children from Idaho, Kansas, Montana, Nebraska, New Mexico, North Dakota, South Dakota, Utah, and Wyoming.

4. New England Regional Center for Deaf-Blind Children
% Perkins School for the Blind, 175 North Beacon Street, Watertown, MA 02172
(617) 924-3434
John B. Sinclair, Coordinator
Serves deaf-blind children from Connecticut, Maine, Massachusetts, New Hampshire, Rhode Island, and Vermont.

5. South Atlantic Regional Center for Deaf-Blind Children
% North Carolina Department of Public Instruction, 327 Hillsboro Street, Bunn-Hatch Building,

---

* Reprinted from American Foundation for the Blind, *Directory of Agencies Serving the Visually Handicapped in the United States*. New York: American Foundation for the Blind (1981). Reprinted with permission of publisher.

Raleigh, NC 27611

(919) 733-3619

Jeff Garrett, Coordinator

Serves deaf-blind children from District of Columbia, Maryland, North Carolina, South Carolina, Virginia, and West Virginia.

6. South Central Regional Center for Deaf-Blind Children

2930 Turtle Creek Plaza, Dallas, TX 75204

(214) 522-4540

7. Southeast Regional Center for Deaf-Blind Children

% Alabama Institute for the Deaf-Blind, Box 698, Talladega, AL 35160

Jack English, Coordinator

Serves deaf-blind children from Arkansas, Iowa, Louisiana, Missouri, and Oklahoma.

(205) 362-8460

John W. Crosby, Coordinator

Serves deaf-blind children from Alabama, Florida, Georgia, Kentucky, Mississippi, and Tennessee.

8. Southwest Regional Center for Deaf-Blind Children

% California Department of Education, 721 Capitol Mall, Sacramento, CA 95814

(916) 322-2173

William Blea, Coordinator

Serves deaf-blind children from Arizona, California, Guam, Hawaii, Nevada, and the Trust Territories.

B. Single State Centers

1. Alaska State Center for Deaf-Blind Children

650 International Airport Road, Anchorage, AK 99502

(907) 274-9591

Kenneth Crow, Coordinator

2. Colorado State Center for Deaf-Blind Children

% Colorado Department of Education, State Office Building, 201 E. Colfax, Denver, CO 80203

(303) 839-2219

Carlee Fundenberger, Coordinator

3. Illinois State Center for Deaf-Blind Children

% Illinois Office of Education, 100 North First Street, Springfield, IL 62777

(217) 782-6601

Kenneth Stonecipher, Coordinator

4. Ohio State Center for Deaf-Blind Children

% Ohio Department of Education, Division of Special Education, 933 High Street, Worthington, OH 43085

(614) 466-1470

Mark Guhardstein, Coordinator

5. Oregon State Center for Deaf-Blind Children

% University of Oregon, Health, Science and Child Development Center, 707 Gaines Road, Room 1250, Portland, OR 97210

(503) 225-8109

Maureen Otos, Coordinator

6. Pennsylvania State Center for Deaf-Blind Children

% Pennxylvania Department of Education, P.O. Box 911, Harrisburg, PA 17125

(717) 783-3238

Eleanor Long, Coordinator

7. Texas State Center for Deaf-Blind Children

   % Texas Education Agency, 201 E. 11th Street, Austin, TX 78701

   (512) 475-3501

   Kenneth Crow, Coordinator

8. Washington State Center for Deaf-Blind Children

   % Washington State Office, Old Capitol Building, Olympia, WA 98504

   (206) 242-9400

   Marie Thompson, Coordinator

8C

Resource List

Communication Aids and Devices

Alphabet Plate	Helen Keller National Center for Deaf-Blind Youths and Adults 111 Middle Neck Road Sands Point, NY 11050
Brailler	Howe Press Perkins School for the Blind 175 North Beacon St. Watertown, MA 02172
Slate and stylus	American Foundation for the Blind 15 West 16 St. New York, NY 10011
Tellatouch	American Foundation for the Blind (see above)
Braille Card	Helen Keller National Center (see above)
Telephone amplifier	your local telephone office
TTY or TTD	Teletypewriters for the Deaf P.O. Box 28332 Washington, D. C. 20005
Large Letter Type for TTY	Sales and Product Services Teletype Corp. 555 Touhy Ave. Skokie, IL 60076
Telebraille	Helen Keller National Center (see above)
Braille Phone-TTY	Phone TTY, Inc. 14–25 Plaza Rd. Fair Lawn, NJ 07410
Tactile speech indicator	Helen Keller National Center (see above)
Optacon	Telesensory Systems, Inc. 3408 Hillview Ave. P.O. Box 10099 Palo Alto, CA 94304

Services

Interpreter services	National Association for the Deaf 814 Thayer Ave. Silver Spring, MD 20910
	Registry of Interpreters for the Deaf 814 Thayer Ave. Silver Spring, MD 20910
National Register of Deaf-Blind Persons	Helen Keller National Center (see above)

Dictionaries

| Braille | American Vest Pocket Dictionary (7 vols.)
American Printing House
1839 Frankfort Ave.
Box 6085
Louisville, KY 40206 |
| Large type | Webster's New World Dictionary, 2nd College
Edition (24 vols.)
American Printing House (see above) |

Publications

Available from National Association for the Deaf:

Kates, L., and Schein, J., *A Complete Guide to Communication With Deaf-Blind Persons (1980)*

Available from the Helen Keller National Center for Deaf-Blind Youths and Adults:

Kramer, L., Sullivan, R., and Hirsch, L. *Audiological Evaluation and Aural Rehabilitation of the Deaf-Blind Adult (1979)*

Abordo, E. and Thomas, L. (eds) Directory of Agencies Serving the Deaf-Blind (1980)

Papers Presented at Workshop on Usher's Syndrome (1976).

Other publications may be available from:

Howe Press, Perkins School for the Blind, Watertown, MA 02172

American Foundation for the Blind, 15 West 16 St., New York, NY 10011

Alexander Graham Bell Association for the Deaf, 3417 Volta Place, NW, Washington, D. C. 20007

Gallaudet College Press, Kendall Green, Washington, D. C. 20002

8D

Auditory Training Sequence*

The following is the sequence of evaluation and training of auditory skills used with profoundly hearing-impaired adult clients at the Helen Keller National Center. Each of the skills described below is assessed during the audiologic evaluation. Based on the client's performance during this assessment, an auditory training program is initiated at the skill level at which the client had his last success, proceeding to more difficult skills when the earlier ones have been mastered. If bone conduction amplification (for vibrotactile stimulation) is used in lieu of air conduction amplification, each item of this sequence is followed for vibratory training.

PRESENCE OR ABSENCE OF SOUND IN PERIOD OF EXPECTATION

Evaluation—This is assessed through reliability of response to pure tone testing.

Training—The first step in developing auditory sensitivity is to get the client to respond to sound when he is expecting it. Let him know that you will call his name from behind him, and that he is expected to turn around at the sound of his name. (This can be achieved by demonstrating to him what must be done, using another individual in place of him and allowing him to watch the procedure.) Try this a few times.

Start with a very limited time frame. Have the client turn away, and within five seconds present the stimulus. Be sure to reinforce correct responses. Once a consistent response has been established, lengthen the time frame to ten seconds. It is likely that now he will respond with more false positives; that is, responding when no stimulus was presented. Initially, reinforce only correct responses to stimuli and ignore false positives. It is possible that they will extinguish with practice. If not, start again with a shorter time frame and establish a consistent response once again.

Extend this procedure so that the client is involved in another activity; however, he is aware that a stimulus will be presented in a particular time frame. In that way, hopefully, the "listening" channels will remain open even though he is involved in other activities. Once he has met with success, carry this procedure over to a situation where sound is not expected. Practical experience has demonstrated, however, that awareness of spontaneous sound will usually not be detected until the client demonstrates significant auditory discrimination abilities (approximately the fourth or fifth on this sequence). Even then, consistency of response to spontaneous sound may be erratic.

---

* Reprinted from Kramer L. C., Sullivan, R. F., and Hirsch, L. M., *Audiological Evaluation and Aural Rehabilitation of the Deaf-Blind Adult.* Sands Point, NY: Helen Keller National Center (1979). Reprinted with permission of publisher.

DISCRIMINATION BETWEEN ENVIRONMENTAL SOUNDS THAT ARE GROSSLY DIFFERENT

Evaluation—Tell the client that a sound is coming. Let him know what the choice will be (*i.e.* voice *versus* clap is a good start, as the clinician can present the stimuli without special equipment). Condition him to respond through a method appropriate to his level of communication (imitation, sign, fingerspelling, etc.).

Training—In training, gradually increase the variety of stimuli presented. Be sure to teach various contexts in which particular sounds are likely to occur, as well as appropriate responses to those sounds. Emphasize sounds that are necessary for survival (voice, particularly the client's name; siren; knocking on door; etc.)

DISCRIMINATION OF NUMBER OF STIMULI

Evaluation—Present one, two, or three claps, or white noise bursts. Have the client either imitate the pattern or communicate the number of stimuli perceived.

Training—This can be incorporated into training of environmental sounds, as various sounds have distinct rhythmic patterns. Training of number of stimuli is then carried over to number of syllables perceived (as in ba,ba-ba, ba-ba-ba).

DISCRIMINATION OF SOUND PATTERNS AND RHYTHMS

Evaluation—Using voice, horns, or drum beats, present a simple pattern. Allow client to get vibrotactile cues as well as auditory until conditioning is achieved. Client response can be an imitation of what is heard. Present stimuli groups of varying duration, number, intensity, pitch in variation of sound patterns and rhythms.

Training—Start with presentation of a single stimulus, either long or short (duration). When this is auditorily perceived correctly, present stimuli having two beats of varying duration of rhythmic patterns. Following learned auditory perception of these stimuli, present any of the one- or two-beat stimuli learned. Follow this procedure, gradually increasing the total number of stimuli presented by varying the duration of beat and number of beats. Follow the same procedure with stimuli of loud-soft (intensity); then high-low (pitch).

DISCRIMINATION OF KNOWN WORDS HAVING DIFFERENT NUMBERS OF SYLLABLES

Evaluation—Present a one-, two-, and three-syllable word to the client through his preferred mode of communication, making sure that the words chosen are in his vocabulary. Establish a response pattern, either through imitation; indication of one, two, or three; or by fingerspelling.

Training—Extend the procedure described above with various sets of three known words. Use of recorded stimuli are helpful in facilitating this auditory discrimination task. Choose three known words of varying syllable length (*e.g.* Hi; Bye-Bye; How are you?), taking care to choose "survival stimuli" (words, phrases or sentences that are most important for the client to be able to hear and understand). Suggestions as to the stimuli used should be sought from the client. Record these stimuli and allow the client to use the recorded stimuli to train auditory discrimination abilities. This technique is especially useful in allowing the client to work independently. When the client is successful in discriminating within a closed set, present words from an open set (words that are in his vocabulary, but do not let him know the choice of words). Assess his ability to discriminate the number of syllables in these words.

8E

Auditory Localization*

The extent to which an adult deaf-blind client is capable of using auditory cues for spatial orientation is largely contingent upon the extent of residual auditory sensitivity and early life exposure to environmental sounds, either aided or unaided. There is also a complex interaction between the time of onset of vision loss and hearing loss. One who loses hearing, subsequent to vision loss, should have a more firmly entrenched auditory-spatial cognitive mapping ability than one who has simultaneously lost both hearing and vision, either early or later in life.

Without residual hearing or vision, only tactile cues may serve to spatially orient the deaf-blind individual. Where residual hearing is present, there are prerequisites to be met prior to the consideration of formal training of auditory localization skills. First, is there sufficient aided dynamic range to permit the use of amplification? Is some form of output limitation necessary? Does the loss fall within the range of headborne amplification? Can a binaural fitting be used? Should directional microphones be considered?

In the normally hearing sighted individual and in the hearing blind individual, interaural comparisons serve as a primary means of auditory localization. Small interaural differences in time, intensity and spectrum provide the basis for auditory spatial orientation. These cues may be considered "static" or "passive" as the individual does not have to actively range about through head movements. Where hearing and vision are impaired or where hearing is asymmetrical, the interposition of dynamic head movements becomes the most important feature in auditory localization.

In the deaf-blind population, "dynamic" localization through head movements and, with body aids, bodily movements is the major method of auditory localization. In testing for and training auditory localization potential, the test setting should permit, rather than restrict, the use of dynamic localization cues. One may wish to test and train the client both in seated and unrestricted standing positions.

Initially, training should take place in an acoustically isolated environment, free of extraneous sounds. A sound room with multiple speaker array is used at the Helen Keller National Center. Initial stimuli include broadband noise, filtered noise, music, and speech. Pure tones are both difficult to localize and unrepresentative of the temporal and frequency response characteristics of environmental stimuli and should not be used. Stimuli should be both continuous and intermittent in order to allow for dynamic ranging to the sound source.

---

* Reprinted from Kramer L. C., Sullivan, R. F., and Hirsch, L. M., *Audiological Evaluation and Aural Rehabilitation of the Deaf-Blind Adult.* Sands Point, NY: Helen Keller National Center (1979). Reprinted with permission of publisher.

In the audiometric test room, the traditional two sound field speakers, located at 315 and 45 degrees, are supplemented with a set of four, high output miniature speakers, located at each 90-degree quadrant. Most clinical audiometers may be modified to provide calibrated stimuli through these additional speakers. The Bozak model 209B 6" speaker (or equivalent model) will provide up to 110 dB SPL at 2 feet through a standard audiometer sound field output. Small bookshelf type speaker enclosures may be used to conserve premium space in the sound room. Relatively inexpensive remote speaker selectors, such as those made by Switchcraft Corporation, may be used to accomodate as many as six additional output transducers.

At the outset, simple manually indicated localizations of sound stimuli are practiced. The test room is divided into quadrants with miniature speakers centered in each. The client is seated centrally in a chair with fixed base that allows easy 360 degree rotation. A head rest is not used as it tends to interfere with head movement. Initially, a response is reinforced positively if it occurs in the appropriate 90-degree quadrant. Each quadrant is further divided into 30-degree segments, with miniature speakers centered in the middle of each of four central thirty degree segments at 0, 90, 180, and 270 degrees, respectively. As training progresses, responses are deemed accurate if they occur in the appropriate twelfth-part division.

Starting the client in different chair positions allows for a variety of auditory angles to identify. Accuracy of side-to-side localization, as well as front-to-back localization should be assessed. Analysis of consistent aided localization errors provides significant information concerning the need for balance between binaural instruments, relocation of a body worn aid, possibly using shoulder mounted microphone(s), or attention to the directional microphone for head-borne instruments. Reinforcement of correct responses may be necessary, depending upon whether the session is one of hearing aid selection or of post-fitting auditory therapy. If reinforcement is provided during a comparative hearing aid evaluation, it is difficult to isolate performance factors from those attributable to differences in hearing aid quality.

As localization training progresses, background noise, first steady, then intermittent, should be introduced. Environmental sound recordings of both indoor and outdoor sounds, may be used in decreasing signal to noise ratios. In the later stages of localization training, both environmental stimuli and background noise may be used. Finally, the audiologist may accompany the client and mobility instructor in and out of doors, continuing localization training in a variety of environmental settings to promote the use of auditory localization for overall mobility in actual traveling situations.

8F

Use of Bone Conduction Amplification in Providing Vibrotactile Stimulation*

Among the trainees seen at the Helen Keller National Center, approximately 80 percent present audiometric contours that indicate no response to any stimuli at intensity levels other than those that are in the range of vibrotactile stimulation. Of these trainees, most are congenitally deaf individuals who have never used or have long ago rejected use of conventional amplification. In such cases a trial period of loaned amplification and a program of auditory training are generally tried. However, due to the profundity of the hearing loss and/or protracted disuse of the auditory mode, amplification is sometimes rejected or found to be of negligible value. Yet there remains a need for these individuals to obtain sensory input, at least in order to maintain contact with the environment. In consideration of this, we have begun to investigate the benefits of providing the much-needed sensory input through use of bone-conducted vibrotactile stimulation, and the possible benefits derived from this form of amplification.

Prior investigators have indicated that the ear is not a good receptor of vibrotactile stimulation. Therefore, if stimuli presented at high intensity levels is received vibrotactually rather than auditorily, reception of that information is not maximally received at the ear. Additionally, an air conduction receiver is not an efficient transducer of vibrotactile stimulation. (Boothroyd, 1970.)

Commercially available instrumentation has been adapted to provide sensory input through vibrotactile stimulation for use at the Helen Keller National Center. The instrumentation used includes a body aid, 30-inch cord, a bone conduction receiver, and a wrist band. The body aids used employ variable tone and output controls. Of major concern is the frequency response between 100 and 500 Hz. The literature on tactile perception (Kirman, 1973) indicates that the skin receives sensations maximally below 500 Hz.; however, below 100 Hz, nonauditory sensations may be transmitted. Therefore, it is helpful to try to eliminate frequencies below 100 Hz to minimize confusion.

The receiver chosen, which is also commercially available, is one that will enhance this same frequency range. It is important to try to match the impedances of the aid and receiver so that the transmission of sound is achieved more efficiently. The receiver is generally placed on an area of the body which the individual judges practical and most sensitive to vibration. At the Helen Keller National Center, the most common site of placement is at the wrist, either at the pulse or on the protrusion

---

* Reprinted from Kramer L. C., Sullivan, R. F., and Hirsch, L. M. *Audiological Evaluation and Aural Rehabilitation of the Deaf-Blind Adult.* Sands Point, NY: Helen Keller National Center (1979). Reprinted with permission of publisher.

of wrist bone. The mastoid process of the temporal lobe is not used as it is not an area especially sensitive to vibration. The receiver is held in place by a wrist band, usually either a Velcro strip or a tennis wrist band. As the sound enters the microphone, it is amplified and conveyed to the receiver as in a conventional air conduction arrangement. However, at the receiver the sound is converted into vibration rather than amplified sound.

Our preliminary observations have indicated that such properties as presence or absence of sound, duration, intensity, and number of stimuli can be discriminated. Reception of these stimuli can be trained and put to practical use in sound reception and environmental cueing, as well as in speech training.

In environmental cueing the client is taught about sound and various sounds that are likely to occur in different contexts. While he may initially have no means of determining the sources of sound around him, he can be made aware of the presence of sound. With training, the individual may learn to identify and make use of certain patterns, such as a voice, knocking on a door, traffic noise, etc., perceived through a combination of vibratory and contextual cues. This phase of training is frequently completed more rapidly by the adventitiously deaf individual who can associate the vibrotactile stimuli received with auditory memory. Where possible, vibrotactile amplification is fitted in conjunction with air conduction amplification. In this condition, the client obtains simultaneous sound reception through dual modes rather than through a single mode. New high powered air conduction/bone conduction aids with separate gain controls for each show promise for this application.

This form of amplification may also be helpful in speech training, both with the congenitally and the adventitiously deaf individual. Use of this device in detecting presence or absence of sound can be applied to teaching correct use of voice, particularly in correct production of voiced and voiceless cognates (*i.e.* /p/ *versus* /b/; /k/ *versus* /g/; /t/ *versus* /d/, a significant problem in the speech of those having congenital or long-standing hearing loss. Making use of duration cues can be applied to monitoring duration of phonemes, words, or more lengthy utterances. Utilization of intensity cues can be applied to teaching correct use of stress in words and sentences, as well as the rhythm of speech. Additionally, overall vocal intensity can be monitored, particularly in relation to background noise. Maximizing the ability to detect number of stimuli can be applied to detecting the number of syllables produced in words and sentences, both in the clinician's model and in the client's own speech.

The totally deafened individual having intelligible speech can, in addition, utilize the ability to detect a number of stimuli in telephone communication, using the same system as with a Tactile Speech Indicator. (See "Long Distance Communication Methods.") The aid must have a telecoil for this.

The research on tactual perception of speech has centered primarily on reception of elements that would facilitate speech understanding; thus far none of them has been highly successful. The device mentioned above is easily obtainable; it is commercially available, comparatively inexpensive, and wearable. Although it is a far cry from devices meant to convey phonetic elements of speech, it has numerous advantages for the deaf-blind, both for communication and for mobility. The use of bone-conducted vibrotactile stimulation as discussed here may have applicability to other populations, and this is an area that should be pursued. Likewise, use of this device as an adjunct to other means of receptive communication (*e.g.* speechreading, hearing) should be more thoroughly investigated.

8G

Tactile and Kinesthetic Cues for Speech Production*

One of the major distinctions between speech training with hearing-impaired sighted individuals and hearing- and visually-impaired individuals is the need for special attention to use of tactile and kinesthetic cues in the speech rehabilitation process. These cues should be used as an adjunct to existing residual hearing and/or vision; however, in cases of total hearing and/or vision loss, reliance on tactile and kinesthetic cues becomes of paramount importance.

In teaching correct production of articulatory features of speech, emphasis is placed on providing information regarding the distinctive features of speech, based on manner of formation and place of articulation in production of speech sounds. This can be done by having the clinician model correct production, and then allow the client tactually to perceive the production.

In modeling correct production, placement of the client's hand on the clinician's neck will give information regarding voicing characteristics. Placement of the tip of the thumb or other fingers at the lips gives information regarding place of production, as well as air flow from the mouth and nose. Placing the index finger along the side of the nose provides information regarding presence or absence of nasality.

Reception of this information can often be maximized by placing the client's hand on the clinician's articulators in the standard Tadoma position (see "Tactual Methods of Communication"), thereby receiving manner and place cues simultaneously. A modification of this position, particularly effective for speech training (rather than in use as a receptive means of communication) is to place the index finger along the side of the nose, with the tip of the thumb on the lips and remaining fingertips spread fanlike on the neck. A further modification of this method is to use the standard position, with thumb tip on lips, index finger on jaw and remaining three fingers on the neck, and placing the index fingertip of the opposite hand on the nose for cues of nasality. One must be sure that reception of information in this manner does not confuse, rather than aid the client in modeling correct speech production. Occasionally, the client may be more confused than aided by reception of three simultaneous channels of information (manner, voicing, nasality).

In utilizing this method, the clinician can teach the distinctive features that characterize each sound. By emphasizing the unique combinations of manner and placement of each speech sound, much of which can be perceived tactually, a tactual "roadmap" can be developed in facilitating correct production of speech sounds based on tactual demonstration. A sample is shown below.

* Reprinted from Kramer L. C., Sullivan, R. F., and Hirsch, L. M. *Audiological Evaluation and Aural Rehabilitation of the Deaf-Blind Adult.* Sands Point, NY: Helen Keller National Center (1979). Reprinted with permission of publisher.

phoneme	lips	throat	nose
/p/	Lips close (same as /b/ and /m/). Big air explosion from mouth upon opening.	no voice	No air escape or vibrations at nose.
/b/	Lips close (same as in /p/ and /m/). Small air explosion from mouth upon opening.	voice	No air escape or vibrations at nose
/m/	Lips close (same as in /p/ and /b/). No air escapes from mouth.	voice	Air escape through nose. Vibrations at nose.

Use of residual hearing and vision can be maximized in combination with these cues in description and demonstration of how the sound looks and what it sounds like. Additionally, kinesthetic awareness of how the articulators are operating in relation to each other can provide significant benefit. Such factors as pressure between articulators (*i.e.* lip closure; tongue tip-alveolar ridge), tension of the tongue, amount of air expenditure, and duration of vocalization should be stressed so that the client can use these self-monitoring cues in promoting speech intelligibility.

In addition to correct production of articulatory features, tactile and kinesthetic cues can be used in teaching use of suprasegmental features (stress, phrasing, rhythm, intonation) that have a major contribution to speech intelligibility.

Stress may be produced by raising the vocal pitch, by increasing duration or loudness of the syllable, or some combination of these. In teaching correct use of stress, a technique that has been found helpful is modeling the stress pattern through tactile demonstration (*i.e.* giving taps of varying stress on the arm to connote varying degrees of stress). In incorporating this concept with speech production, the client may be able to gain stress cues of the clinician's model by utilizing the Tadoma hand position and detecting the differences in pitch, loudness and/or duration among the syllables. Once this difference is discriminated, it can then be incorporated into the client's own speech, with him tactually monitoring his speech mechanism. It may also be helpful to point out the kinesthetic cues of breath and muscle control in producing stress.

Difficulties in phrasing may also be found. This difficulty may be based on incorrect use of breath groups or incorrect use of sense groups. If it appears to be attributable primarily to incorrect use of breath groups, tactile and kinesthetic cues to monitor breath control can be used. By having the client place one hand on his chest, and the other on his abdomen, he can receive tactile cues regarding inspiration and expiration. Additionally, he can concentrate on kinesthetic cues to respiration, to phonation, and to articulation. In this way he can use these cues to monitor his breath control and its relationship to phrasing.

Phrasing difficulties that are due to incorrect use of sense groups require language training to enable the client to form his expressions into organized groups.

Rhythm is generally referred to as the pattern in which certain syllables are stressed and others are left unstressed. In the hearing-impaired, frequently the syllables are given equal rather than varied stress, resulting in monotone speech. Since rhythm refers to stress patterns in connected speech, the tactile and kinesthetic cues for teaching correct use of stress can be applied to teaching rhythm as well.

Difficulties in intonation, the modulation of vocal pitch, is another characteristic found among hearing-impaired speakers. By having the client place his index finger and midfinger in a "V" position horizontally across the neck, the client can feel the larynx elevate as he produces rising intonation. Conversely, the lowering of the larynx can be felt with falling intonation. Emphasis can also be placed on kinesthetic awareness of changes in the speech musculature as intonation varies.

9

The Role of Ancillary Personnel in Rehabilitation

Dean C. Garstecki, Ph.D.

Some hearing-impaired adults are able to function with minimal hearing handicap. Medical or surgical care and/or successful use of a hearing aid may obviate their need for rehabilitative services. For others, hearing impairment of any degree, type, or duration may create a handicapping condition. These people may seek professional assistance when their hearing impairment prevents them from successfully participating in everyday conversation. They may experience communication problems in their job and with family members. Their hearing loss may influence all aspects of their life, how they feel about themselves and how they feel others perceive them. When problems relating to hearing impairment extend beyond the usual role and responsibilities of the audiologist, the cooperation of ancillary personnel should be enlisted in providing a comprehensive, individualized program of aural rehabilitation. Physicians, hearing aid dispensers, vocational rehabilitation counselors, psychologists, social workers, and family members may play an integral role in helping the hearing-impaired adult function optimally in social, vocational, and family communication (Alpiner, 1978).

The overall effectiveness of such a rehabilitation program, as with any other public service program, will be measured by how well it is able to recognize and meet its client's needs (Williams, 1961). With the cooperation of a group of resources, the services most relevant to an individual's particular needs, concerns, and lifestyle can be identified, evaluated and rehabilitated by professionals with specialized areas of expertise and family members with unique insight into the client's everyday communication problems. The relevance of this multiple-input approach to rehabilitation will become apparent to the client as he understands the multi-faceted nature of his particular problems. These may involve the need to be understood and treated as an individual, to gain social maturity, and to achieve educationally, vocationally, and socially (Alpiner, 1978). This chapter discusses the roles and responsibilities of ancillary personnel who may be involved in a comprehensive adult aural rehabilitation program.

A variety of people may constitute an adult aural rehabilitation team. Although not all of the resources covered in this chapter will be appropriate or necessary for comprehensive hearing health care for every hearing-handicapped adult, team members should know when and how to use these and other resources. It is important that one team member assumes primary case management responsibilities. The case manager should see that all appropriate evaluative and remediative services are provided. Although it is probably incidental who actually assumes the responsibility in practice, it may be the hearing-impaired person's first contact in the treatment of his hearing problem. For example, the physician may serve as the entry point in the treatment program and coordinate services that may be provided by others. All treatment decisions may be channeled through this person. A second approach is to assign case management responsibilities to the person or place providing the primary treatment need. The hearing-impaired adult who is unemployed may find it most appropriate and advantageous, for example to have the vocational rehabilitation agency coordinate and manage all appropriate services. A third approach is to alternate responsibility among hearing health care specialists. At one point in time, the physician may be the primary care provider. Beyond medical or surgical treatment, a psychologist may serve as the primary manager. When there are communication problems relating to hearing loss, the audiologist will assume major responsibility for managing the problems of the hearing-impaired adult. In all instances, benefit for medical evaluation should precede consideration of participation in a rehabilitation program. Medical treatment actually may obviate the need for rehabilitation in some cases. In every case, the individual diagnostic and rehabilitative needs of the hearing-handicapped adult should be held paramount.

THE PHYSICIAN

The hearing-handicapped adult generally finds help for his problem through self-referral to a family physician, otologist, hearing-aid dealer, or speech and hearing center (Marge, 1977). The physician, then, is likely to serve either as the entry point to other professional services or as the sole provider of hearing health care. The physician's examination and medical treatment often precedes consideration of enrollment in an aural rehabilitation program. Of all medical specialty areas, the otologist, by training and experience, knows most about evaluation and treatment of diseases of the ear and hearing. The otologist is able to provide case history, evaluation, and medical follow-up information which is important not only for determining the need for aural rehabilitation, but also for developing a prognosis for benefits to be accrued from participation in such a program.

Every member of the aural rehabilitation team should understand the importance of comprehensive medical care. The federal Food and Drug Administration (Food and Drug Administration, 1977) published a list of warning signs that can be used by hearing health care specialists to identify conditions which warrant prompt medical attention (see Table 9.1).

When medically irreversible hearing impairment remains, aural rehabilitation services may be appropriate and necessary. Physicians must understand that aural rehabilitation can serve to alleviate the handicapping effects of hearing impairment (Harless and Rupp, 1972). They should also understand why, therefore, responsibility for management of treatment and rehabilitation programs may alternate between the otologist and the audiologist depending on the hearing-impaired adult's changing needs. General medical education deals little with the role and responsibilities of the audiologist on the hearing health team. Unfortunately, physicians may cast the audiologist in a technician's role especially in those instances where the audiologist's primary job function is to provide objective measurement data rather than interpretation of data for consideration of alternatives in medical management and/or aural rehabilitation (Smith, 1975).

The audiologist, by training and experience, should be best equipped to manage the evaluation and treatment of communication problems resulting from hearing impairment. The roles and responsibilities of the audiologist and speech pathologist may interweave in this aspect of a comprehensive rehabilitative service program. However, the audiolo-

Table 9.1
Warning Signs of Potential Aural Pathology[a]

1. Visible congenital or traumatic deformity of the ear.
2. History of active drainage from the ear within the previous 90 days.
3. History of sudden or rapidly progressing hearing loss within the previous 90 days.
4. Acute or chronic dizziness.
5. Unilateral hearing loss of sudden or recent onset within the previous 90 days.
6. Audiometric air-bone gap equal to or greater than 15 dB at 500 Hz, 1000 Hz, and 2000 Hz.
7. Visible evidence of significant cerumen accumulation or a foreign body in the ear canal.
8. Pain or discomfort in the ear.

[a] Food and Drug Administration, 1977.

gist as a professional advocate for the hearing-handicapped person, should assume responsibility for the planning, coordination, and implementation of all hearing loss related services. The audiologist emphasizing work with hearing-handicapped adults has special knowledge and skill in the following.

1. Identification and measurement of aural pathology and hearing handicap found among an adult population such as those problems relating to noise trauma, otosclerosis, Meniere's disease, presbycusis, and others.

2. Evaluation and use of amplification systems with attention to orientation to hearing aid use and troubleshooting problems related to hearing aid operation.

3. Evaluation and remediation of communicative skills and the impact of hearing loss on the adult's personal, family, social, and vocational communication interests.

4. Conservation of residual hearing through periodic audiologic monitoring and referral as well as knowledge of the effects that environmental noise, improper use of a hearing aid, and certain physical agents may have on hearing ability.

5. Presentation of inservice and public information programs for allied health professionals and others concerned with identification, prevention and management of problems related to hearing loss.

6. Coordination and management of the evaluative and rehabilitative services provided by ancillary personnel on the aural rehabilitation team.

For the audiologist and physician to work together effectively, Smith (1975) offers the following suggestions. First, the audiologist should become familiar and comfortable with the medical treatment and management procedures used by the physician. In return, the physician should understand the range of concerns the audiologist has in designing an aural rehabilitation program. The physician should be generally informed of the types of rehabilitative procedures that might be warranted and employed and the rationale for such procedures. Second, hearing aid evaluation and fitting by an audiologist should be preceded by medical clearance. Otologists may dispense hearing aids, but they are encouraged not to retail hearing aids in their offices when adequate community facilities exist (Catlin, 1978). Physicians understand that a medical evaluation is required before a hearing aid may be sold and that fully informed adults over age 18 may request a waiver of this requirement for religious or personal beliefs. However, it is not always reasonable to assume that the physician will be conversant with such basic concepts as 1) types of hearing aids and electroacoustic modifications of basic hearing aid functions, 2) ear coupling methods and earmold acoustics, 3) types of hearing aid fittings with their advantages and limitations, 4) measurement of hearing aid electroacoustic characteristics, and 5) problems in hearing aid fitting (Schiff and Cohen, 1978). Third, every effort should be made to keep all professionals informed of evaluation results and progress made in rehabilitation. Reports exchanged among team members should be comprehensive yet brief, timely, and pertinent to the needs and interest of their intended reader.

Cooper (1971), a physician, notes that although each member of the hearing health care team has responsibilities for the welfare of the client, delays and inadequate services are sometimes experienced at all levels. Some of these problems may relate to a reluctance on the part of professionals to consider factors outside their specific discipline or field of practice. Obviously, it is not possible for one individual to function effectively as physician, audiologist, psychologist, social worker, and vocational counselor. The multi-faceted needs of the hearing-impaired adult are likely to be best served when a team of specialists addresses the adult's problems. One example of the physician's role in aural rehabilitation concerns a 21-year-old victim of von Recklinghausen's Disease. Audiologic test results confirmed the presence of bilateral meningiomas. Neither the client nor the family could accept the need for surgical intervention or the inevitability of a total loss of hearing. The physician, in preparing the client and her family for medical-surgical treatment, enlisted the cooperation of a psychiatrist and audiologist. The psychiatrist assisted the client and family in accepting the need for treatment and probable outcome. The audiologist designed and implemented an educational program considering the structures of the auditory mechanism and their function pre- and post-operatively. Attention was given to ways to cope with everyday living and communication problems resulting from deafness. Roleplaying activities were incorporated into the instructional program and alternate communication skills were developed. As the client progressed in her understanding of ways to communicate without hearing, psychiatric care for the client's and family's acceptance of the overall medical condition was increased. The physician, in this example, effectively managed and coordinated the scope and timing of the team's interrelated service program. He readily provided pertinent medical data, and also requested input from other team members. A cooperative working relationship existed and served to maximize the benefit to the client.

THE HEARING AID DEALER AND DISPENSING AUDIOLOGIST

At the present time, the hearing-impaired adult is most likely to visit a hearing aid dealer when he is interested in purchasing a hearing aid. About 70% of the nation's hearing aid users acquire their aids in this way. Over the past few years an increasing number of audiologists have begun to dispense hearing aids. The hearing aid consumer now has the option to choose whether to purchase the aid from a salesman or an audiologist. With this option, there is a need to clarify the similarities and differences in service provided by each of these individuals. Carhart (1975) noted that there are philosophical differences between these individuals which relate not to motivation toward serving the hearing-impaired, but to differences in focus in health care delivery.

The hearing aid dealer is a businessman who is concerned with product delivery from manufacturer to consumer. He is concerned with consumer satisfaction and, thus, may be involved in long-term technical maintainence and adjustment to enhance the wearer's use of the aid. He may assist the user in the care and minor repair of an aid and provide services and supplies to keep the aid in satisfactory working order, in addition to providing hearing aid fitting services. His training may range from a few hours of instruction from a hearing aid manufacturer to years of attendance at workshops, short courses, correspondence courses, and field training.

The early practice of hearing aid dispensing in a dealer-dominated delivery system led to sales abuses where consumers complained about the dealer's conflict of interest in that he charged a fee for the hearing evaluation and another fee for the aid itself. Complaints were registered which questioned dealer training and hearing aid costs. The U. S. Food and Drug Administration (1977) issued regulations and the Federal Trade Commission (1978) proposed rules to protect against hearing aid sales abuses. However, at this time there remain unresolved issues concerning provisions for clearance for hearing aid use, compatibility of federal regulations with state laws, and third party coverage of the cost of evaluations for hearing aid use and purchase of the aid (Wood and Marlin, 1980).

Despite efforts to control the practices of unscrupulous hearing aid dealers, sales abuses continue. Two recent incidents illustrate the seriousness of these abuses. The first example concerns a 65-year-old woman who contacted our Hearing Clinic requesting a second opinion before purchasing a hearing aid. She visited a local hearing aid dealer without first obtaining medical or audiologic consultation. The dealer evaluated her and recommended that she purchase two behind-the-ear aids for a total of $1100. Our hearing aid evaluation results suggested that she would not be considered a viable candidate for binaural amplification. Both ears were severely impaired, however considerable disparity in speech discrimination ability was demonstrated between ears. She was unable to demonstrate benefit from or interest in an aid worn on her poorer ear. Our recommendation was for a monaural system which ultimately cost less than one-third the price of the aids recommended by the dealer.

In a second situation, an 87-year-old widow who had been a successful hearing aid user for many years broke the plastic earhook portion of her behind-the-ear aid. She took her problem to a nearby hearing aid dealer who informed her that repair of her aid would be costly and it might be to her long-term benefit to consider purchasing a new aid. She indicated that she wanted to have an evaluation by an audiologist. In the interim, the dealer provided her with a loaner aid for a rental fee of $100. After one day of loaner aid use, she complained about the limited benefit she derived from the aid. She informed the dealer of her dissatisfaction and he delivered a second loaner aid to her home. She wore the second loaner aid to her evaluation in our clinic. She liked this aid so it was incorporated in our evaluation. Ultimately, she preferred the loaner aid over all others evaluated. When recording identification information from the preferred aid, it was noted that the serial number on the loaner aid was the same as the serial number of the aid that she wore during a previous visit to our clinic several years earlier. The dealer had replaced her broken earhook and had rented this woman's own aid to her as a "used" aid. When confronted with this information, the dealer regarded this as a simple mix-up among his office staff!

The dispensing audiologist is a hearing health professional who is concerned with provision of evaluative and remediative service to the hearing-impaired person. This service includes the selecting and dispensing of a hearing aid as part of a comprehensive program of audiologic care. The audiologist is concerned with the benefits that a hearing aid may have on a person's communicative skills.

As important, the audiologist is able to assist those who derive minimal benefit from an aid and those for whom an aid is not indicated. According to Hardick (1977) 10 to 20% of the hearing handicapped elderly adults seeking help through a hearing clinic may find little value in hearing aid use. The audiologist may provide a program of aural rehabilitation to these people which may consist of instruction in how to improve auditory and auditory-visual communication skills. They may be taught how to stage-manage difficult listening situations, thereby improving their self-confidence in social communication. They may be counselled in regard to changes in self-concept which may accompany hearing impairment and/or use of a hearing aid. In these and other ways, the audiologist is able to assist the hearing-impaired adult in self-management of problems related to hearing loss. These services typically are not provided by the hearing aid dealer (Libby, 1974).

Audiologists are trained to meet the standards for clinical certification by the American Speech-Hearing-Language Association. At minimum, this training includes academic coursework and clinical practice at the undergraduate and/or graduate degree level. A master's degree or its equivalent, 60 semester hours of academic coursework, 300 hours of clinical practice, 1 year of supervised professional experience, and successful completion of a national examination constitute the minimal requirements for a Certificate of Clinical Competence in Audiology (CCC-A). In addition, audiologists are encouraged to participate in continuing education programs available to all hearing health professionals.

Although such organizations as the Retired Professional Action Group (1973) and others (U. S. Department of Health, Education, and Welfare, 1975; American Speech-Hearing-Language Association, 1977) have been concerned about the sales of hearing aids when professionals from medicine and audiology are not involved, only 20% of all hearing aids fitted are the result of referral from professionals (Stutz, 1969). Whether a hearing aid is dispensed by a dealer or an audiologist, the best interests of the hearing-impaired person should be held paramount. Every effort should be made to prevent practices which may interfere with provision of proper hearing health care. Potentially harmful practices include those which may result in the following:

(a) Conflict of interest. When one person stands to profit from the evaluation of a person's hearing aid candidacy as well as from the sale of the aid, a potentially conflicting role is created. In the past, this practice has led to millions of dollars worth of hearing aids being sold to people who did not benefit from them or need them (Federal Trade Commission, 1978; Wood and Marlin, 1981). This danger may be reduced by requiring the hearing aid candidate to consult with a physician and/or audiologist prior to purchasing an aid. Statutes in the District of Columbia, Hawaii, New York, Vermont, and West Virginia currently call for medical and/or audiologic clearance for hearing aid purchase for all except those who object on the basis of religious beliefs. Six other states require a medical evaluation when certain otologic symptoms occur. These symptoms include the presence of a sudden hearing loss, rapidly progressing hearing loss, dizziness, or active drainage from the ear. Eleven other states advise hearing aid purchasers to consult a physician or sign a medical waiver prior to buying an aid. This option only serves to further weaken an already poor protection plan. In addition to the above, hearing aid dispensers are required to disclose to the hearing-impaired person that they are sellers of hearing aids. This is required under the FTC's 1975 "Hearing Aid Industry Proposed Trade Regulation" (Wood and Marlin, 1981).

(b) Poor quality of service. Assessment and remediation of aural pathology and its associated disorders is a complex series of events. Otologists and other medical specialists concerned with hearing loss spend years in academic instruction and practice to provide medical care to the hearing-impaired. Audiologists spend 1 or more years in graduate level coursework and clinical practice and 1 year of supervised experience in assessment and rehabilitation of hearing loss and its related problems in order to provide comprehensive hearing health care. Hearing aid dealers may have little formal training before selling aids as independent businessmen, but they may take advantage of workshops and short courses to increase their knowledge and skills in delivering health care service to the consumer. Each one of these individuals should be considered an integral member of the hearing health care team. It behooves each of these people to recognize the complementary roles they play in providing comprehensive health care and to educate the hearing-impaired person to the need for and desirability of taking advantage of the services that each of these people is prepared to provide.

(c) Exorbitant costs. Hearing health care expenses should be explained to the hearing-impaired person in a way in which he can understand the process involved in determining overall health care needs. It would be unwise, for example, to avoid obtaining an audiologic assessment in preparation for hearing aid use, when such test findings may alert one to the presence of a medically remediable condition or to the need for a different amplification system than originally planned. Fees for rehabilitative services should be explained to the client at the time of an audiologic evaluation. Since the costs for hearing aid component parts, construction of the aid, advertising, and sales promotion of the aid fall below the costs of the aid to the consumer, efforts should be directed toward minimizing the costs of the aid to the consumer. One approach would be for third party payers, such as Medicare and/or Medicaid, to cover the cost of hearing tests as well as the cost of the aid itself.

(d) Sales abuses. Consumer studies (Retired Professional Action Group, 1973; Public Interest Research Group in Michigan, 1973; Minnesota Public Interest Research Group, 1972; National Council of Senior Citizens, 1975), congressional studies (U. S. Subcommittee on Investigations of the Senate Committee on Government Operations, 1975), the Federal Interdepartmental Task Force on Hearing Aids (1975), and the Federal Trade Commission (1975), have revealed serious problems relating to the misevaluation and misfit-

ting of hearing aids, misrepresentations by hearing aid businessmen, and high-pressure sales tactics. Hearing aid consumers must be protected by laws restricting solicitation of hearing aid sales in their homes, by their right to a trial use period and right to cancel the purchase of an aid, and by penalties (fines, license suspension) for those dispensers who do not identify themselves as such, advertisers that claim an aid will restore hearing, provide significant benefits, or allow a person to understand speech in noise, and home-visiting dispensers who do not obtain written consent to visit the potential buyer prior to the actual visit. These considerations and others are important for the hearing-impaired person's well-being. Attention to these considerations should minimize the time, money, and effort wasted in hearing health care.

THE VOCATIONAL REHABILITATION COUNSELOR

When hearing impairment or other handicapping conditions such as visual impairment, orthopedic deformity or functional impairment, major extremity amputation, mental disorders, personality disorders, and other serious conditions create an employment problem, referral to a vocational rehabilitation counsellor is indicated. Vocational rehabilitation services are available through state and federally supported agencies and are usually known as the Division of Vocational Rehabilitation, Bureau of Vocational Rehabilitation, or some similarly titled office. In Illinois, this agency is the Department of Rehabilitation Services. The primary purposes of such agencies include the following.

(1) To arrange for quality treatment and rehabilitation services for all clients.
(2) To arrange for quality job development services and training to facilitate opportunities for gainful employment of all clients.
(3) To arrange for optimal use of available local and state resources by all clients (Illinois Department of Rehabilitation Services, 1981).

In some states, rehabilitation agencies employ counsellors specializing in service to clients with particular types of disorders. In lesser populated states, agencies have counsellors serving clients with a wide range of problems which restrict their opportunities for employment.

Classification of Disabling Conditions

Vocational rehabilitation services are provided first to those adults demonstrating the greatest need and potential for improvement. To assist the counsellor in categorizing population needs, various classification systems have been devised. Myklebust, *et al.* (1962) classified deaf adults as follows.

(1) Those with no problems or handicaps other than a lack of functional hearing ability.
(2) The superior.
(3) The emotionally disturbed.
(4) The academically limited.
(5) The retarded.
(6) Those with other handicaps.
(7) Those with other problems.

Hurwitz (1968) categorized vocational rehabilitation service differences according to those demonstrating the following.

(1) Vocational problems due to crises.
(2) Atrophied or non-competitive work attitudes.
(3) Disoriented work aptitudes.
(4) Underdeveloped work aptitudes.
(5) Underdeveloped personalities.

Sanderson (1973) classified hearing-impaired individuals in terms of degree of hearing loss and education categories and needs according to the following categories.

(1) Deaf—pre-lingual—manually oriented—special education.
(2) Deaf—pre-lingual—no special education.
(3) Deaf—post-lingual—manually oriented—special education.
(4) Deaf—post-lingual—no special education.
(5) Deaf—pre-lingual—orally oriented—special education.
(6) Deaf—post-lingual—orally oriented—special education.
(7) Deaf—multiple disabilities—special education.
(8) Hard of hearing—pre-lingual—orally oriented—special education.
(9) Hard of hearing—pre-lingual—manually oriented—special education.
(10) Hard of hearing—post-lingual—manually oriented—special education.
(11) Hard of hearing—post-lingual—orally oriented—special education.
(12) Hard of hearing—pre-lingual—no special education.
(13) Hard of hearing—post-lingual—no special education.
(14) Hard of hearing—multiple disabilities—special education.

(15) Deaf, hard-of-hearing, multiple disabilities, illiterate, non-verbal, no education—not otherwise classified.

In order to apply this information in determining eligibility for vocational rehabilitation services, agencies established their own coding system. Quigley (1966) described three levels of classification assigned to hearing-impaired individuals.

(1) Those who are termed deaf, unable to talk readily, with hearing too defective to interpret normal or amplified conversation through the ear.
(2) Those who are termed deaf, able to talk readily, with hearing too defective to interpret normal or amplified conversation through the ear.
(3) Hard-of-hearing who have defective hearing for communication, but understand loud or amplified speech.

At the present time, the Illinois Department of Rehabilitation Services classifies disabling hearing impairment into essentially the same categories as described by Quigley, however separate sub-divisions are now defined as follows:

(1) Deafness and inability to talk, due to
  (a) Degenerative and other non-infectious and specified diseases of the ear.
  (b) Upper respiratory infections and other infectious diseases.
  (c) Congenital malformation.
  (d) Accident, poisoning, exposure, or injury.
  (e) Ill-defined and unspecified causes.
(2) Deafness and ability to talk, due to
  (a) Degenerative and other non-infectious and specified diseases of the ear.
  (b) Upper respiratory infections and other infectious diseases.
  (c) Congenital malformation.
  (d) Accident, poisoning, exposure, or injury.
  (e) Ill-defined and unspecified causes.
(3) Other hearing impairments, due to
  (a) Degenerative and other non-infectious and specified diseases of the ear.
  (b) Upper respiratory infections and other infectious diseases.
  (c) Congenital malformation.
  (d) Accident, poisoning, exposure, or injury.
  (e) Ill-defined and unspecified causes.

According to this system, hearing-impaired adults in the first and second categories are classified as severely disabled. Those in the third category are classified as severely disabled only when two of the following conditions apply.

(1) Better ear pure-tone average exceeding 65 dB HTL with correction (hearing aid).
(2) Speech discrimination ability of 50% or poorer in the better ear with correction.
(3) Reliance on visual communication (speech-reading).

If only one or none of the above conditions is present, the hearing disability is not classified as severe.

As indicated by Alpiner (1978), the greatest problems in vocational rehabilitation are found among the deaf adult population, especially those who are impaired pre-lingually. The problems encountered relate primarily to delayed or disordered development, and limited communication skills. Co-existing handicapping conditions, such as mental retardation, visual impairment, emotional disorders, and others may compound the handicap created by hearing impairment.

Eligibility for Vocational Rehabilitation Services

At present, there are two conditions of eligibility for services in Illinois.

(1) Presence of a physical or mental disability which for the individual constitutes or results in a substantial handicap to employment.
(2) Reasonable expectation that vocational rehabilitation services will benefit the client in terms of employability (Illinois Department of Rehabilitation Services, 1978).

Eligibility is determined without regard to sex, race, age, creed, color, national origin, or type of disability. Clients served by one state cannot receive duplicate services in another state. Economic need is not a criterion of eligibility for services. Final decisions regarding an individual's eligibility are the counsellor's responsibility. For example, services are available to a secretary with impaired speech discrimination ability due to a progressive hearing loss, to a construction worker whose diabetes requires him to leave his present job, or to a stationery store clerk whose arthritis causes him to function from a wheelchair. Services are available to the hearing-handicapped, mentally retarded adult who needs job training and to the homemaker whose slipped disk prevents her from carrying out her normal duties.

Scope of Services

The following services are currently available through the Illinois Department of Rehabilitation Services.

(1) Evaluation of rehabilitation potential. This includes coverage for all diagnostic and related services necessary to determine eligibility for rehabilitation services and the nature and scope of services to be provided.
(2) Counselling and guidance. This includes coverage for personal adjustment counselling as well as maintenance of a counselling relationship throughout the client's program of service. It also includes the cost of referral for other services as needed.
(3) Physical and mental restoration services.
(4) Vocational training. Included is personal and vocational adjustment and books and materials.
(5) Maintenance of current or acquired vocational skills.
(6) Transportation.
(7) Services to families of handicapped clients.
(8) Interpreter services for the deaf.
(9) Reader, mobility, and related services for the blind.
(10) Telecommunication, sensory, and other technological aids and devices.
(11) Recruitment and training for new employment opportunities in the fields of rehabilitation, health, welfare, public safety, law enforcement, and other appropriate public service employment.
(12) Job placement.
(13) Maintenance of suitable employment.
(14) Occupational licenses, tools, equipment, and initial stocks and supplies.
(15) Other goods and services which can reasonably be expected to benefit a handicapped person's employability.

When individual prescriptions and fittings are required, they must be provided by appropriately licensed and certified individuals operating in accordance with state licensure laws. When a hearing aid is recommended, a hearing aid evaluation must be conducted. Referrals for a hearing aid evaluation must include the results of an audiologic assessment. Audiologists providing assessment and hearing aid evaluation services must hold the Certificate of Clinical Competence in Audiology (CCC-A) issued by the American Speech-Language-Hearing Association. In order for the vocational rehabilitation agency to cover the cost of a hearing aid, the reha-

Table 9.2.
Eight Service Tracks for All Stages of the Case Flow Sequence[a]

Case Flow Stage	Service Track							
	1	2	3	4	5	6	7	8
Referral	x	x	x	x	x	x	x	x
Application		x	x	x	x	x	x	x
Extended evaluation			x	x	x	↓	↓	x
Program development				x	x	x	x	x
Delivery of services	↓	↓	↓	↓	x	x	x	x
Closure	x	x	x	x	x	x	x	x
Post-employment services							x	x

[a] Adapted by permission from the Care Services Manual, West Virginia Division of Vocational Rehabilitation as reported in the Case Service Manual, Illinois Department of Rehabilitation Services, 1981.

bilitation counsellor must be able to justify its purchase on a vocational basis. Aids will usually only be purchased at an established state contract price. Except in instances of severe financial need, it is expected that the client will provide for the cost of any necessary parts, repairs, or hearing aid reconditioning services.

Case Flow

The case flow sequence consists of seven stages: referral, application, extended evaluation, program development, delivery of services, closure, and post-employment service. The entire process may be divided into eight tracks as illustrated in Table 9.2. The process begins with written referral to a vocational rehabilitation agency (see Appendix 9A). Receipt of a referral form and a physical condition survey form (see Appendix 9B) alerts the counsellor to a request for service. The counsellor follows with a referral contact (see Appendix 9C). At this time an interview is held with the potential client (see Appendix 9D). The counsellor provides the client with an outline of individual rights and responsibilities and the responsibilities of the Illinois Department of Rehabilitation Services (see Appendix 9E). This outline contains a listing of available services and a place to note the client's eligibility for service. The referral stage terminates with the potential client either applying for service or electing not to apply. If he chooses not to apply, the case is closed.

Those that apply for service complete an application and information release form (see Appendix 9F). Eligible clients move to the program development stage. Cases of ineli-gible clients are closed. In instances where the counsellor cannot determine if the client is eligible for services extended evaluation is required. For the hearing-impaired adult, this may mean a need to obtain test results, medical records, employment records, and other such information (see Appendix 9G). It may require reports of otologic, audiologic, and hearing aid evaluations (see Appendices 9H, 9I, and 9J). The extended evaluation stage ends when sufficient information has been obtained to determine that the client should either proceed to the program development stage or move to closure. When the client moves to program development, he jointly develops an individualized written rehabilitation program with the counsellor (see Appendices 9K and 9L). When this plan is formulated and approved, the client usually begins to receive services. The core of the rehabilitation process occurs during this time. From this stage, the client moves to closure, either being rehabilitated or non-rehabilitated. Of course it is desirable that the case be closed only when the client is fully rehabilitated and employed in a job suited to his aptitudes and abilities. However, closure may occur at any step along the way, depending on the particular individual and events occurring during client management. When certain routine services are necessary to continue satisfactory employment, post-employment services are provided. These services may be added at any time.

Young Adults

A small number of vocational rehabilitation projects are available for young deaf adults. Projects conducted at the Hot Springs

Rehabilitation Center (Blake, 1970; Bolton, 1974), St. Louis Jewish Vocational Service (Hurwitz, 1971), and Chicago Jewish Vocational Service (Chicago Jewish Vocational Service, 1974) are examples of rehabilitation research and demonstration programs conducted in existing rehabilitation facilities. A residential program at Northern Illinois University and a comprehensive vocational program at the National Technical Institute for the Deaf are examples of rehabilitation programs which are affiliated with universities.

The types of opportunities available in a residential program are exemplified in the Northern Illinois University program which offers diagnostic evaluation of communication, academic, vocational, and social skills and abilities. Counselling is provided to assist each student in the selection and development of vocational career goals. The program has two components, a 6-week summer diagnostic program and a 9-month work-study program. To be admitted to the summer program, the following standards must be met.

(1) Age: 16–24 years.
(2) I.Q.: Minimum score of 80 on the Performance Scale of the Wechsler Adult Intelligence Scale.
(3) Marital Status: Single.
(4) Disability: Hearing impairment sufficiently severe to affect academic, vocational, or social achievements.

Vocational rehabilitation counsellors usually initiate referrals to this program. Once admitted, the student participates in a summer program of evaluation of his vocational aspirations and abilities. They may be employed in a dormitory cafeteria where the staff evaluates their work performance and habits. The student's business and clerical skills are assessed. Reading and comprehension levels are determined. Finally, their communication skills are evaluated.

Students live in a dormitory with one roommate. They are provided with a complete program of recreational and social activities, many of which are planned by the students themselves. During the 9-month program, the student spends half his time in academic coursework and half his time in a work experience. Classes are offered in Language Arts, Business Education, Vocational Education, Mathematics, and Social Issues.

Remedial help, individualized instruction, and tutoring are also available, if needed. Each student is provided with a community or university work experience in business or industry. This gives him an opportunity to understand the world of work and to be exposed to various vocations. It provides each student with a worthwhile pre-vocational/vocational experience which gives him a better understanding of his interests and abilities, while demonstrating the work capabilities of hearing-impaired individuals to their employers. Money earned is deposited in a personal checking and/or savings account.

Throughout the 9-month program, students are assisted in forming realistic decisions about future employment. They are provided with aural rehabilitation services. A driver's education program is available. They also have access to all of the social and recreational facilities that are normally available to other university students. The 9-month program is staffed as follows. A Program Director is responsible for the administration and financial arrangements of the program. The Program Coordinator supervises other staff members, coordinates rehabilitative services and activities, selects students for the program and provides counsel and advice. The Program Counsellor develops and maintains student work opportunities, provides vocational counsel and guidance, and assists in future training or placement of each student, along with the referring counsellor, at the end of the program. The program also provides academic and remedial training, dormitory counsellors to assist in organizing social and recreational activities and graduate students to assist in academic and communication skill building areas. It is a superior model of services and activities that may be provided for young deaf adults in a university affiliated program. Evaluation of rehabilitation programs of this type suggest that they are highly successful. Hurwitz (1971) reported the outcome of a 5-year project to serve young deaf adults at the St. Louis Jewish Vocational Service. Of the 256 students served, one-half were placed in competitive employment. The 5-year project at the Chicago Jewish Vocational Service (1974) resulted in gainful employment for 49% of the 710 deaf adults served. Similar findings are reported for other projects.

Counselling Considerations

The goal of counselling hearing-impaired clients in a vocational rehabilitation program is to help them become independent, mature decision makers, able to deal competently with everyday problems. Both Stewart (1971) and Schein (1973) offer some suggestions for counselling the deaf which may also apply to hard-of-hearing adults. According to Stewart, it is not the nature of the counselling relationship, but the implementation of the counselling program that differs for normally hearing and deaf adults. Language problems of the more severely hearing-impaired adult may reduce his overall communicative effectiveness. Counsellors may need to structure their interaction with the hearing-impaired adult to include fewer opportunities for confusion. For example, he or she might ask briefer, more specific questions or perhaps a hearing-impaired person communicates most efficiently using sign language. The counsellor may need to prepare a variety of written and/or visual aid materials to facilitate a counselling session with a severely hearing-impaired adult. Finally, the counsellor may have to extend his normal counselling relationship with the hearing-impaired client to provide information and advice to assist the client in knowing how to relate to and interact with other people (Bolton, 1976).

Schein (1973) lists the necessary qualifications of a counsellor of hearing-impaired people.

(1) Knowledge of hearing impairment and all of its ramifications.
(2) Ability to communicate with the hearing-impaired.
(3) Ability to help determine an individual's employment potential.
(4) Ability to guide the client to his maximal achievement level.

Armed with appropriate knowledge of hearing impairment and the qualifications of an effective counsellor, the vocational rehabilitation counsellor is prepared to help individuals overcome personal obstacles and achieve optimal development of his personal resources (Martin, 1968).

Job Placement

The ultimate goal of vocational service is to prepare the client for gainful employment. This preparation may involve learning the role of a worker in addition to the skills entailed in a job. For the severely hearing-impaired, vocational maturity evolves through four stages.

(1) Vocational evaluation. This involves evaluation of work behavior to develop a "work personality" profile. It also involves assessment of training potential in various work areas.
(2) Vocational adjustment. This is a process in which actual working conditions are simulated, including use of incentives to modify behavior and close supervision.
(3) Skill training. Vocational possibilities are explored through review of the client's training profile, psychologic test results and expressed interests.
(4) Job placement. This may involve having to educate potential employers regarding hearing impairment, preparing the client to present himself positively, job orientation, and consideration of long-term adjustment matters (Bolton, 1976).

These matters will require less attention for those clients who are less seriously handicapped by their hearing impairment. For all clients to be successfully placed, certain conditions should be met.

(1) The job placement should be satisfactory to the worker.
(2) The job placement should not impose a medical risk.
(3) Job placement should be economically adequate.
(4) Job placement should be suitable to the interests of the employer.

Taking these considerations into account, job placement for the hearing-impaired adult should be a personally rewarding experience for the client as well as for the vocational rehabilitation counsellor.

THE PSYCHOLOGIST

At times it may be important to involve a psychologist in the rehabilitation program. When it is determined that the emotional or personal problems of the hearing-impaired person extend beyond those related directly to the improvement of communicative function, referral to a psychologist should be considered. The tools of psychology (interviews, tests, and therapy) provide us with deeper insight into the problems the hearing-impaired person may be encountering (Helfand,

1964). The psychologist can ferret out the complex and frustrating problems of the hearing-impaired adult.

Reports on the psychology of hearing impairment suggest that the same range of emotions and abilities to cope with everyday demands of employment, social, and family situations existing in normally hearing people are also present in the hearing-impaired. However, the frustrations caused by unsuccessful attempts at everyday interpersonal communication coupled with possible feelings of inferiority, fear, and stress may result in the need for professional counselling. Studies by Levine (1960), Knapp (1960) and others suggest that considerable variation in the behavior of hearing-impaired individuals can be observed which makes it difficult, if not impossible, to be able to predict the effect of hearing impairment on an individual. In this author's experience, adults with acquired hearing impairment of gradual onset generally tend to adjust to being less dependent on use of their residual hearing and more dependent on ways to compensate for hearing loss. The congenitally hearing-impaired adult with a severe-to-profound loss often is able to satisfactorily communicate and find a comfortable, active lifestyle. Adults with the greatest likelihood of need for psychological care seem to be those who experience either a sudden severe loss or further progression of a severe loss. In the first instance, the adult has had insufficient time to develop compensatory strategies. He or she suddenly is faced with having to depend on other input modalities for information needed in everyday conversation. They have not had time to explore ways in which they might optimize the use of their residual hearing, stage-manage difficult listening situations, maximize the use of their hearing aid, and associate knowledge of a conversation topic or situation with acoustic and visual (speechreading) cues to speech perception. They are frustrated by communication experiences and withdraw from them.

The adult who suffers a progression in loss after having had a long-standing severe hearing loss is often frightened at the possibility of having to cope with a world without sound. As Ramsdell (1970) indicates, they are fearful of losing their "relationship with the world." They may no longer be able to monitor the auditory events inherent in daily living. Fur-ther loss of hearing may result in severe depression. The services of a psychologist or psychiatrist are often the treatment method of choice in these cases.

Rousey (1971) suggests that a hearing-impaired adult under stress may react by accusing others of mumbling, not including him in conversations, or by blaming his communication difficulty on poor room acoustics. Once these projections are no longer valid, he may begin to withdraw from social communication situations. His self-esteem and self-image are lowered. He may fear being criticized, ostracized, or otherwise punished. The psychologist's role is to assist the client in adjusting to the emotional and personality changes brought about by hearing impairment in a manner which does not lower the client's lifestyle and self-image. The psychologist, as a counsellor, must create an emotional climate conducive to such growth and acceptance by a hearing-impaired person (Sanders, 1975). The need for psychologic services may be infrequent in many adult aural rehabilitation programs. When this need arises, however, one of the major problems is where to find a psychologist who is able to work effectively with hearing-impaired people. In a survey conducted in 1978, only 16 psychologists, 29 social workers, 27 psychiatric nurses, and 20 psychiatrists across the nation were able to be identified as emphasizing work with the hearing-impaired (Tucker, 1981). Therefore, it might be assumed that many mental health personnel in the United States are unaware of the specific needs of hearing-impaired adults. Most hearing-impaired adults are unable to receive outpatient assistance for mental health problems from someone who understands their unique communication difficulties and other problems associated with hearing loss. They are unable to benefit from mental health services available to the public at large.

Tucker's survey suggests that at least half of the states have made initial attempts to provide mental health services for their hearing-impaired citizens. In 1979, Arkansas hired a Program Specialist for the Deaf to generate mental health services for deaf patients, Connecticut hired a Director of Mental Health Services for the Deaf and Hearing-Impaired. Similar steps have been taken in Georgia, Hawaii, Maine, Maryland, Michigan, Oklahoma, Oregon, Rhode Island, Virginia, and Wisconsin. The major concern at this time is that there does not appear to be a uniform set of guidelines for states to follow to define the quality of mental health care due the hearing-impaired population. Myklebust (1964) noted some general characteristics of hearing-impaired people that may serve as a guide to psychologic needs.

(1) A loss of 30–40 dB. This is a moderate loss affecting mainly the scanning and background functions of hearing. It is also the point at which conversation becomes difficult without amplification. Psychologically, however, it is the impaired awareness and the environmental detachment which are most important. At this level, the restriction imposed on communication can be alleviated by getting closer to the speaker and by use of amplification. Thus, it is not socialization but basic awareness and monitoring that suffer most.

(2) A loss of 45–65 dB. With this degree of hearing loss, social intercourse is clearly affected and the background-foreground use of audition is essentially precluded. Because the scanning function of hearing is largely eliminated, the individual responds only in a foreground manner; whenever he hears, he scans, treating all sound as it first reaches his threshold as a sound requiring direct attention. The use of amplification makes conversation readily possible, but because he must give all sound equal attention, conversation is essentially limited to one person or to a small group. The individual experiences considerable detachment and seeks social relationships with others having a similar degree of deafness.

(3) A loss of 65–80 dB. The use of amplification, while effective for maintaining social inter-relationships, is less satisfactory than for those in Group 2. Both personal-social and general environmental contact is difficult. There is need for considerable reliance on other systems for monitoring, particularly on vision and taction. Feelings of identification are impeded and personal-social relationships are most satisfying when they are with others having deafness, usually to a similar extent.

(4) A loss of 80–100 dB. This is a profound hearing loss. The use of amplification is effective mainly in maintaining intelligible speech and focusing attention on loud environmental sounds. The use of vision and taction is mandatory for maintaining homeostatic equilibrium. Personal-social relationships are with others having profound deafness.

The audiologist and client eventually must decide whether or not it is in the client's best interests to seek psychologic service. When such service is indicated, the psychologist is an invaluable member of the rehabilitation team.

THE SOCIAL WORKER

The social worker is concerned with social interactions between people and with their environment (Pincus and Minihan, 1973). The social worker may be trained to focus on casework, group work, or community work. Those trained as caseworkers are concerned with the individual's ability to accomplish his or her life tasks, cope with distress, and realize aspirations. They may deal directly with hearing-impaired adults and their families by helping them decide how to manage some of their hearing loss related problems. The social worker can identify support services within a community which may benefit the hearing-impaired. They can explore and establish appropriate linkages between impaired individuals or their families and appropriate community agencies. Their information gaining skills are a valuable asset to the aural rehabilitation team.

Jablonski (1964) states that the social worker may play an important role in shaping an adult's attitude toward accepting his or her handicap. They may bring the hearing-impaired person to accept professional assistance in dealing with psychologic, social, educational-vocational and economic problems sometimes associated with their handicap.

To carry out his or her responsibilities most efficiently and effectively, the social worker must acquire some basic knowledge of hearing impairment and its ramifications. This is not usually part of the social worker's formal training. While serving the hearing-impaired, the social worker may be asked questions concerning the evaluation and treatment of various types of auditory disorders. They may be asked for their advice in regard to the services provided by hearing health professionals in the community or they may be asked for recommendations regarding the purchase of a hearing aid or enrollment in a "lipreading" class. At minimum, the social worker should be equipped with a basic knowledge of the simple classifications of aural pathology by anatomical site, degree of loss, and type of loss. With this, they should know that certain types of impairment are medically and/or surgically irreversible and might be further compensated for through use of a hearing aid and/or training to maintain or improve auditory communication skills. They should know the roles of the physician, audiologist, and hearing aid salesperson in the evaluation and treatment of auditory disorders and their related problems. The social worker must understand the complementary nature of the responsibilities assumed by each of these people.

Related to the provision of hearing health service is the possible need for financial assistance not only to pay for this service, but also to purchase a hearing aid. Medicare, under "Part A: Hospital Insurance," covers the costs of diagnostic and rehabilitative audiology services requested by a physician when provided to a hospital inpatient by an audiologist employee of that hospital. Under "Part B: Medical Insurance," audiologic assessment services are covered when this information is needed for purposes of medical or surgical treatment. A needed improvement is to expand Part B coverage to aural rehabilitation services that are provided in professional service settings that are not physician-directed. Medicaid programs may also cover some of the expenses incurred in hearing health care. Because of the state-to-state variations in benefits provided, the surest way of determining which service fees are reimbursable is to contact the specific government agency that administers the program in each state (Dowling, 1981).

Although financial assistance may be obtained to cover the costs of audiologic assessment and rehabilitation, costs involved in the evaluation, selection, and fitting of a hearing aid are not covered for most adults through third party payers. One exception is the veteran who may obtain hearing aids at no cost through the Veterans Administration for service-connected hearing loss. For others, the social worker can explore the possibility of acquiring re-built or re-conditioned hearing aids from community hearing societies or through local chapters of the Lion's Club or other such groups concerned with helping needy hearing-impaired people. The social worker may be able to assist the hearing-impaired adult in deciding which option to explore in the event of possible financial constraints, although these matters also may be addressed and resolved by the hearing aid dispenser.

Since social workers may be confronted with questions relating to the purchase of hearing aids and hearing health services, they should be informed of the nature of these products and services as they may vary not only in price, but in quality. As an extreme example, they must understand the differences between obtaining a hearing aid from a dispensing audiologist and buying an aid through the classified ads in a newspaper. Similarly, the social worker serving on an adult aural rehabilitation team should be aware of the availability and cost of other services and products that may be of interest to the hearing-impaired. They should know about public buildings, theaters, and churches that have group amplification systems to benefit the hearing handicapped. Social groups, clubs for the deaf, and community hearing societies provide opportunities for social interaction. Also, there are many hearing-impaired adults who would appreciate knowing the costs and availability of telephone warning devices and receiver-amplifiers, television captioning units, hearing-ear dogs, and other aids.

The hearing-impaired adult's rehabilitation program will be most successful when it provides practical solutions to everyday problems. Therefore, when designing a client-centered program it is necessary to consider cultural and economic factors that may influence the program format and/or client prognosis for success. The social worker is usually trained to determine where an adult lies on a socio-economic scale. The social worker's intervention in obtaining this information and providing it to the other members of the rehabilitation team may be invaluable when these factors are suspected to interfere with their self-management of hearing loss related problems. Cultural factors may inhibit an adult's acceptance of a hearing aid which may be regarded as a sign of weakness, age, or infirmity by his family or friends. Economic factors may dictate against the adult's ability to participate in a rehabilitation program, the acquisition of a hearing aid or other services and aids.

One example of the role the social worker may play on the rehabilitation team is demonstrated in the case of a 40-year-old severe-to-profoundly hearing-impaired woman who had experienced some hearing impairment due to meningitis at age 6. In her mid-thirties, she was diagnosed as having Meniere's disease and, shortly after childbirth, experienced a progression in hearing loss. She quit her job just prior to childbirth and was financially dependent upon her husband. He lost his job and all three family members were dependent upon her social security checks. When she enrolled in the rehabilitation program, it was obvious that the communication problems created by the progression in hearing loss were compounded by the family's financial crisis. Both she and her husband were under considerable strain and tension. They were referred to a family service agency and the social worker helped them organize a plan for financial and emotional recovery. With these matters on their way toward resolution, the client could better concentrate on rehabilitation of her communication skills.

The social worker served to strengthen the family relationship through use of community resources to help them regain financial solvency. This, in turn, served to bring the client to a receptive state for aural rehabilitation. The social worker provided emotional support for the client and her family. She helped the family adjust to their social problems and to deal with them in a constructive manner. The audiologist, then, concentrated on resolving family communication problems stemming from the client's hearing loss.

THE FAMILY

The family may serve as the hearing-impaired adult's primary communication outlet. Since each family member fills a role in the family unit which complements the roles of other members (Satir, 1967), changes in the communication skills of one member will impact on the others. In a constructive way, the family may provide the support needed for the hearing-impaired member to learn to self-manage his problems. Unfortunately, in other instances, they may regard the hearing-impaired member as the family scapegoat. All of the family's failures, real or imagined, are blamed on the impaired member (Haspiel et al., 1972) or the communication problems of one member may create high levels of anxiety among other family members (Webster and Newhoff, 1981). Because the role of the adult in his family unit cannot always be predicted, it is important for the rehabilitator to determine the status of the hearing-impaired member in his family structure before attempting to enlist their cooperation in the

rehabilitation program. Role changes naturally occur as the abilities of individual members to carry out their roles change and as there are changes in family composition. Members move away, divorce, or die. New members enter the family unit through marriage. Also, at one point a household may be dominated by younger people and at other times by older people. In order for family members to serve as ancillary personnel in rehabilitation, it is important to determine individual member roles, family dynamics, and family communication patterns. To determine family constellation, usual opportunities for family interaction and topics of family conversation, family members can be interviewed and/or asked to complete hearing handicap scales such as the Denver Scale of Communication Function (Alpiner et al., 1971) or the Denver Scale of Communication Function for Senior Citizens Living in Retirement Centers (Zarnoch and Alpiner, 1977) which assesses one's self-perceived competence in communicating with family members, the Hearing Performance Inventory (Giolas et al., 1979) which contains items referring to success in personal communication situations, and the McCarthy-Alpiner Scale of Hearing Handicap (McCarthy and Alpiner, 1980) which assesses family member attitudes and compares them to the attitudes of the hearing-impaired member, a process which defines the family member's role in the rehabilitation process. Once problems relating to hearing loss are understood by family members and they are incorporated in the rehabilitation program, the success of the program will depend largely on the participant's motivation toward involvement in and acceptance of rehabilitation program procedures. Harris (1977) classified hearing-impaired adults as "You-Fix-It," "Staller," or "Problem-Solver" types. The "You-Fix-It" type seeks information and advice, but might expect his family and/or the professional to assume major responsibility for management of his problems. The "Staller" also is collecting information for others or himself for use at some future time. The "Problem-Solver" type is most motivated toward improving his communication skills. This individual readily seeks, accepts, and applies information to help himself, as well as to assist others (family members) in understanding the problems they may be experiencing. Their success may depend on their ability to accept their loss, cope with feelings of anger, and deal with fealings of frustration, embarrassment, depression, and self-pity relating to their hearing loss. Once they are motivated toward making positive changes such as pursuing medical treatment, acquiring a hearing aid, seeking counsel, or whatever steps are appropriate, positive reinforcement by family members will foster greater self-motivation toward learning how to effectively deal with their problems. With help, they can gain confidence in assuming self-responsibility for increasing the likelihood of successful communication. The importance of family understanding of the problem and support for rehabilitation is illustrated in two recent clinical cases.

The first was a 35-year-old woman who had experienced an exceptionally difficult onset of Meniere's disease. Prior to this time, she was an active member of social organizations and volunteer groups. She enjoyed working as a newspaper reporter, housewife, and mother of two pre-teenage children. The changes in her personal and social life resulting from her hearing problem resulted in an eventual need for psychologic counselling. Her eventual adjustment to a bilateral moderate sensorineural hearing loss, constant tinnitus, recruitment, and hearing aid use was not easy. However, her family, with minimal understanding of her hearing problem, was able to provide emotional support and accommodate her personal needs through this difficult period. Family members assumed responsibility for helping her adjust to changes in her lifestyle by helping her develop interests in new activities. The family was drawn together by their genuine concern for her well-being and empathy for what she was experiencing in her personal and social life. Her family motivated her to accept her condition and to succeed at the challenges it presented.

In the second example, the family's influence was the reverse. When the family of the 21-year-old victim of von Recklinghausen's disease mentioned earlier in this chapter was presented with information concerning necessary medical, psychiatric, and audiologic treatment needs and procedures, they were not willing to accept the situation and its ramifications. They reacted by outwardly minimizing their concern for appropriate treatment. They viewed the educational/counselling information they were provided with as being interesting "especially for someone who might want to teach the deaf." Neither the client nor her family was about to admit to the possibility of sudden deafness, having successfully survived other potentially debilitating surgery for related problems. The family agreed to cooperate by arranging for her to receive professional care as long as her problems were addressed in a matter-of-fact general manner, rather than being personalized to the affected family member. The family essentially denied the presence of the problem the client occasionally expressed fear over. She found no emotional support from other family members.

When family members are involved in the rehabilitation process, they should be afforded opportunities for learning about hearing impairment and its effects. They should be able to find emotional support, if needed. Finally, they should have an opportunity to experiment with applying newly learned information in the security of the clinic environment. Family members must be given the opportunity to have their personal questions and concerns addressed by qualified professionals. They need to have their understanding of the family member's hearing impairment clarified. They should be allowed the opportunity to discuss their attitudes toward the family member and/or changes in family communication brought about by hearing loss. They should know the benefits and limitations of hearing aids and the expected communication capabilities of their hearing-impaired family member with and without an aid. Too often, family members may expect the hearing aid to restore hearing to normal. It is helpful for family members to listen to sound-field presentation of everyday conversation at the level of the impaired member's aided speech reception threshold and filtered to represent the hearing-impaired member's audiometric configuration and the speech distortion which results. This "live" demonstration helps them appreciate the sensitivity gap left by the hearing aid as well as the limited influence of an increase of signal intensity on speech discrimination. Family members should be provided with all the information necessary for them to understand the influence of aural pathology on everyday speech perception, otologic and audiologic care of hearing impairment, how to read and interpret an audiogram, how to acquire a hearing aid, and where to go for appropriate hearing health care. They may benefit from being provided with information concerning other aids for the hearing-impaired such as telephone warning devices, telephone receiver-amplifiers, hearing-ear dogs, cochlear implants, television captioning devices, infrared room amplification systems, TTYs, and literature pertaining to other problems associated with hearing loss.

Family members also may improve their capability in serving as ancillary personnel by having the opportunity to interact with other families whose members are hearing-impaired. Family members find much needed support in being able to interact with others who have learned to deal with some of the problems they are just beginning to encounter. They may have a continuiing or recurring need to maintain some contact with other families. The importance of this opportunity for family members was recently illustrated by a woman who called the Hearing Clinic asking if she could join a class where she could meet other hearing-impaired adults. She did not know of anyone who might be experiencing the types of problems she encountered daily. Finally, it is often beneficial for the family to have the opportunity to develop and practice ways to improve their communication through roleplaying. Some of the following "Communication Hints" may be incorporated in roleplaying and discussion activities in the rehabilitation program.

Communication Hints

I. General
  A. Be informed about national events and world affairs. Know what is going on in your community, neighborhood and social circle.
  B. Be informed about the interests of your family and friends.
  C. Be interested in encouraging a two-way conversation rather than monopolizing a conversation.
  D. Concentrate on understanding main ideas and concepts, rather than isolated words.
  E. Understand that everyone hears and understands less when they are tired or ill.
  F. Concentrate on being a good listener.
  G. Relax!
II. When speaking with hearing-impaired people
  A. Speak at a natural rate and rhythm. Don't shout or speak with exaggerated mouth movements.
  B. Simplify complex or lengthy messages.
  C. Rephrase misunderstood messages.
  D. Keep the hearing-impaired individual informed of the topic of conversation.
III. For hearing-impaired people speaking with others
  A. Wear recommended hearing aids (and glasses).
  B. Let the audible aspects of speech supplement visible speech movements.
  C. Position yourself so that the sun or light is on the speakers face, not in your eyes.
  D. Face the speaker directly and on the same level whenever possible. Sit across from and close to the speaker with your better ear toward the speaker.
  E. Watch facial expressions and body gestures while listening to the speaker.
  F. Become familiar with the way different people express themselves: facial expression, vocabulary, sentence structure, accent or dialect, etc.
  G. Learn to anticipate and understand the topic of conversation by using situational cues, contextual cues and understanding of the logical sequence of events. Also use the rhythm of a spoken message to help understand a conversation.
  H. If in another room, go to the speaker or have him come to you.
  I. In your home, reduce competing noises by turning off or lowering the volume of televisions, radios, stereo equipment, turning off running water, etc., for improved speech reception.
  J. Lessen room echoes by using sound-absorbing carpeting, ceiling tile, drapes, and overstuffed furniture in your home.
  K. Educate others to the fact that quiet, natural speech is easiest for you to understand.
  L. Be realistic! Don't blame your hearing loss for every communication problem. No one hears everything all the time.

References

ALPINER, J. G., *Handbook of Adult Rehabilitative Audiology*. Baltimore: Williams & Wilkins, Co. (1978).

ALPINER, J. G., CHEVRETTE, W., GLASCOE, G., METZ, M., OLSEN, B., The Denver Scale of Communication Function. Unpublished study (1971).

AMERICAN SPEECH-HEARING-LANGUAGE ASSOCIATION (ASHA), ASHA challenges new FDA hearing aid regulation. *ASHA* **19**, 261, 264–265 (1977).

BLAKE, G., *An Experiment in Serving Deaf Adults in a Comprehensive Rehabilitation Center, Final Report, SRS Grant No. RD-1932-S.* Little Rock, AR: Arkansas Rehabilitation Service (1970).

BOLTON, B., *Psychology of Deafness for Rehabilitation Counselors,* Baltimore: University Park Press (1976).

BOLTON, B., A behavior-oriented treatment program for deaf clients in a comprehensive rehabilitation center. *Am. J. Orthopsychiatry,* **44**, 376–385 (1974).

CARHART, R., Introduction. In M. C. Pollack (Ed.), *Amplification for the Hearing-Impaired.* New York, NY: Grune & Stratton (1975).

CATLIN, F. I., The otolaryngologist and the hearing aid delivery system: current federal regulations. *Otorhinolarngol.,* **86**, 559–562 (1978).

CHICAGO JEWISH VOCATIONAL SERVICE, *The Chicago Project for the Deaf, Final Report, SRS Grant No. RD-1576.* Chicago, IL: Chicago Jewish Vocational Service (1974).

COOPER, L. Z., Deafness: one physician's view. In D. Hicks (Ed.), *Medical Aspects of Deafness.* Atlantic City, NJ: Council of Organizations Serving the Deaf (1971).

DOWLING, R. J.. Federal health insurance for the elderly. In D. S. Beasley and G. A. Davis (Eds.), *Aging: Communication Processes and Disorders.* New York: Grune & Stratton (1981).

FEDERAL TRADE COMMISSION, *Hearing Aid Industry Report.* Washington, D. C.: Bureau of Consumer Protection (September, 1978).

FEDERAL TRADE COMMISSION, Hearing aid industry proposed trade regulation. *Code of Federal Regulations,* **16**, (1975).

FOOD AND DRUG ADMINISTRATION, Hearing aid devices: professional patient labeling and conditions for sale. *Federal Register,* **42(31)**, 9286–9296 (1977).

GIOLAS, T., OWEN, E., LAMB, S., AND SCHUBERT, E., Hearing performance inventory. *J. Speech Hear. Disord.,* **44**, 169–195 (1979).

HARDICK, E., Aural rehabilitation programs for the aged can be successful. *J. Acad. Rehab. Audiol.,* **10**, 51–66 (1977).

HARLESS, E. L., AND RUPP, R. R., Aural rehabilitation of the elderly. *J. Speech Hear. Disord.,* **37**, 267–273 (1972).

HARRIS, J., Adult aural rehabilitation: from the geriatric twenty's toward maturity. Paper presented at the California Speech and Hearing Association Conference, San Francisco (1977).

HASPIEL, M., CLEMENT, J. R., AND HASPIEL, G., Aural rehabilitation for hard of hearing adults. Unpublished paper, San Francisco Veterans Administration Hospital (1972).

HELFAND, I., The clinical psychologist. In *Auditory Rehabilitation in Adults, Proceedings of a Seminar.* Cleveland, OH: Cleveland Hearing and Speech Center and Case Western Reserve University (1964).

HURWITZ, S., *Habilitation of Deaf Young Adults, Final Report, SRS Grant No. RD-1804-S,* St. Louis, MO: Jewish Employment and Vocational Service (1971).

HURWITZ, S., A treatment nosology for vocational counseling of the deaf. *J. Rehab. Deaf,* **2**, 42–53 (1968).

ILLINOIS DEPARTMENT OF REHABILITATION SERVICES. *Case Services Manual.* Springfield, IL (1981).

ILLINOIS DEPARTMENT OF REHABILITATION SERVICES. *Case Services Manual.* Springfield, IL (1978).

JABLONSKI, M., The medical social worker. In *Auditory Rehabilitation in Adults, Proceedings of a Seminar.* Cleveland, OH: Cleveland Hearing and Speech Center and Case Western Reserve University (1964).

KNAPP, P. H., Emotional aspects of hearing loss. In D. A. Barbara (Ed.), *Psychological and Psychiatric Aspects of Speech and Hearing.* Springfield, IL: Charles C Thomas (1960).

LEVINE, E., *The Psychology of Deafness.* New York: Columbia University Press (1960).

LIBBY, E. R., Aural rehabilitation, 1974. *Hear. Instruments,* **25 (9)**, 11 (1974).

MARGE, M., The current status of service delivery systems for the hearing impaired. *ASHA,* **19**, 403–409 (1977).

MARTIN, D. G., Directions for rehabilitation counseling with deaf persons. *J. Rehab. Deaf,* **2**, 42–53 (1968).

MCCARTHY, P. A., AND ALPINER, J. G., The McCarthy-Alpiner scale of hearing handicap. Paper presented at the American Speech-Language-Hearing Association annual convention, Detroit (1980).

MINNESOTA PUBLIC INTEREST RESEARCH GROUP, *Hearing Aids and the Hearing Aid Industry in Minnesota.* Minneapolis, MN: MPIRG (November 13, 1972).

MYKLEBUST, H. R., *The Psychology of Deafness.* New York: Grune & Stratton (1964).

MYKLEBUST, H. R., NEYHUS, A., AND MULHOLLAND, A. M., Guidance and counseling for the deaf. *Am. Ann. Deaf,* **107**, 370–415 (1962).

NATIONAL COUNCIL OF SENIOR CITIZENS, *Survey of Hearing Aid Dealers in the District of Columbia* (October, 1975).

PINCUS, A., AND MINIHAN, A., *Social Work Practice: Model and Method.* Itasco, IL: F. E. Peacock (1973).

PUBLIC INTEREST RESEARCH GROUP IN MICHIGAN, *You Know I Can't Hear You When the Cash Register is Running: The Hearing Aid Industry in Michigan.* East Lansing, MI: PIRGIM (December 3, 1973).

QUIGLEY, S. P., The vocational rehabilitation of deaf people. In *A Report of a Workshop on Rehabilitation Casework Standards for the Deaf,* pp. 1–4. Washington, D. C.: U. S. Department of Health, Education, and Welfare (1966).

RANSDELL, D. A., The psychology of the hard-of-hearing and the deafened adult. In H. Davis and S. R. Silverman (Eds.), *Hearing and Deafness.* New York, NY: Holt, Rinehart and Winston (1970).

RETIRED PROFESSIONAL ACTION GROUP (RPAG), *Paying Through the Ear: a Report on Hearing Health Care Problems.* Philadelphia, PA: Public Citizen, Inc. (1973).

ROUSEY, C. L., Psychological reactions to hearing loss. *J. Speech Hear. Disord.,* **36**, 382–389 (1971).

SANDERS, D., Hearing aid orientation and counseling. In M. C. Pollack (Ed.), *Amplification for the Hearing-Impaired.* New York, NY: Grune & Stratton (1975).

SANDERSON, R. G., Preparation of hearing-impaired for adult vocational life. *J. Rehab. Deaf,* **5**, 12–18 (1973).

SATIR V., *Conjoint Family Therapy.* Palo Alto: Science

and Behavior Books (1967).

SCHEIN, J. D., Model for a state plan for vocational rehabilitation of deaf clients. *J. Rehab. Deaf*, **3,** 13 (1973).

SCHIFF, M., AND COHEN, I. J., What every otolaryngologist should know about hearing aids. *Laryngoscope*, **88,** 932–945 (1978).

SMITH, K. E., Professional relationships. In M. C. Pollack (Ed.), *Amplification for the Hearing Impaired*. New York: Grune & Stratton (1975).

STEWART, L., The nature of counseling with deaf people. In A. Sussman and L. Stewart (Eds.), *Counseling with Deaf People*, New York: Deafness Research and Training Center (1971).

STUTZ, R., The American hearing aid user—1968. *ASHA*, **11,** 459–461, (1969).

TUCKER, B. P., Mental health services for hearing-impaired persons. *Volta Rev.*, **83,** 223–235 (1981).

U. S. DEPARTMENT OF HEALTH, EDUCATION, AND WELFARE, *Final Report to the Secretary on Hearing Aid Health Care*. Washington, D. C.: U. S. Department of Commerce (1975).

U. S. FOOD AND DRUG ADMINISTRATION. *Code of Federal Regulations*, **801,** 420–421 (1977).

U. S. PERMANENT SUBCOMMITTEE ON INVESTIGATIONS OF THE SENATE COMMITTEE ON GOVERNMENT OPERATIONS, *Staff Study of the State Licensing Laws and Training Requirements for Hearing Aid Dealers*. 58–59 (October, 1975).

WEBSTER, E. J., AND NEWHOFF, M., Intervention with families of communicatively impaired adults. In D. S. Beasley and G. A. Davis (Eds.), *Aging: Communication Processes and Disorders*. New York, NY: Grune & Stratton (1981).

WILLIAMS, B. R., Basic needs of persons with impaired hearing. In *Proceedings of the Rehabilitation of the Deaf and Hard-of-Hearing*. Stowe, VT: University of Vermont College of Medicine (1961).

WOOD, E. F., AND MARLIN, D. H., A consumer prospective: the hearing aid delivery system. In D. S. Beasley and G. A. Davis (Eds.), *Aging: Communication Processes and Disorders*. New York, NY: Grune & Stratton (1981).

ZARNOCH, J. M., AND ALPINER, J. G., The Denver Scale of Communication Function for Senior Citizens Living in Retirement Centers. Unpublished study (1977).

APPENDIX

9A

Referral Form*

STATE OF ILLINOIS

DIVISION OF VOCATIONAL REHABILITATION

623 East Adams Street
Springfield, Illinois

REFERRAL

Date:

To:

From:_____   _____
                    Counselor   Office Address

Re:_____   _____
                                                          Street   City   County

Reason for Referral:

Parents:

Birth date:

Nature and diagnosis of disability:

Summary of treatment:

Summary of training:

Summary of work experience:

Comments: (Should include statement of preparation of client for referral).

_____

* Appendices 9A to 9L are reprinted by permission from the Department of Rehabilitation Services of the State of Illinois .

APPENDIX

9B

Physical Condition Survey

STATE OF ILLINOIS
DIVISION OF VOCATIONAL REHABILITATION

PHYSICAL CONDITION SURVEY

Name (please print)			Birthdate	Grade	Date
Address			County of residence		Phone
School			Vocational plan or goal		

This is a survey — <u>entirely voluntary on your part</u> — to indicate what disabling physical conditions you have, other than minor ones, which may substantially interfere with your efforts to find suitable employment when you are ready. Please be assured this Agency will treat all information confidentially.

Your Doctor's name and address: _____

Your Parent's or Guardian's name: _____

If you give permission for the DVR Counselor to get
information from your Doctor, please sign here: _____

Please answer each of the following questions and describe the condition if you check "Yes"

CONDITION	YES	NO	DESCRIBE (use back of form if needed)
Do you have any heart or lung abnormality?			
Do you have any deformities of bones, joints or muscles?			
Do you wear leg braces, orthopedic shoes or artificial appliances?			
Do you have poor hearing?			
Do you have blackouts or fainting spells?			
Do you require special dietary precautions or medications?			
Do you have severe scars or disfigurations?			
Do you have difficulty speaking smoothly or clearly?			
Do you have any other physical handicap?			
Are you under a doctor's care regularly? If so, why?			
Do you have very poor vision?			
Does your vision cause much difficulty in reading?			
Are you excused from regular physical education classes? If so, why?			
Additional comments:			

APPENDIX

9C

Referral Contact

REFERRAL CONTACT

Office Closed Case Card File Checked: Yes _____ No _____   Area Control Cards Checked: Yes _____ No _____

METHOD OF CONTACT:	Other	Representative	Telephone
Personal contact with Client _____	Individual _____	of Agency _____	

* Mr. Mrs. Miss Last Name	First	Middle	Date

* Number & Street	City	Zip Code	Telephone

* Referral Source	Address	Telephone

Other person or means to contact

BIRTHDATE			* Age	* Sex		
Month Day Year					Highest Grade Completed:	
					University Degree: Yes _____ No _____	

Social Security No.	SSDI Beneficiary:	SSI Recipient:	Race:
	Appl. for ____ Receiving ____	Appl. for ____ Receiving ____	White ____ Negro ____ A. Ind. ____ Other ____

* REPORTED DISABILITY	Primary (Describe in medical terms or how person is handicapped for work)
	Secondary

REASON FOR REFERRAL	

EMPLOYMENT STATUS	Salaried:		Unemployed _____	Never Employed _____
				Self Employed _____
	Employed Full-time _____	Employed Part-time _____		Student _____

APPOINTMENT	Month Day	Hour AM	Location:	
Call Client _____		PM	DVR Office _____ Client's Home _____ Other _____	
Call Referral Source _____	Other Location & Address			

Comments

_____

_____

_____

_____

_____

_____

_____

_____

_____

_____

_____

_____

_____

Person taking referral information	Referred to following Counselor:	District Number

DISTRIBUTION: File in Case Folder

* MINIMUM INFORMATION REQUIRED   REFERRAL CONTACT

APPENDIX

9D

Information Form

INTERVIEW INFORMATION

1. Last Name	First	Middle	2. Date of Application	3. District

4. Address	5. City	6. Zip	7. County

8. Telephone	9. Social Security No.	10. Date of Birth	11. Age	12. Sex M ___ F ___

13. Race
___ 1. White   ___ 2. Black   ___ 3. Indian   ___ 4. Asian
___ 5. Hispanic   ___ 6. N. African—Mid-Eastern

14. Disability   Code

15. Referral Source	16. Institution at Referral

17. Marital Status
___ 1. Married   ___ 3. Divorced
___ 2. Widowed   ___ 4. Separated
___ 5. Never Married

18. Living Arrangements
___ 0. Alone
___ 1. With Parent or Guardian
___ 2. With Own Children
3. With Siblings
4. With Spouse
5. With Friends
6. With Other

19. No. in Family _____

20. No. of Dependents _____

21. Members of Family Living At Home

Name	Age	Relationship	Employer	Job Title	Weekly Earnings

22. Primary Source of Income

00 - Current earnings, interest, dividends, rent
01 - Family and friends
02 - Private relief agency
03 - Public Assistance (at least partly with Federal funds)
04 - Public Assistance without Federal funds (G.A. only)
05 - Public Institution - tax supported
06 - Worker's compensation
07 - Social Security Disability Insurance benefits
08 - Other disability, sickness, survivors or age retirement benefits
09 - Annuity or other disability insurance benefits (private insurance)
10 - Benefits from other sources (Private insurance, savings)

23. Worker's Compensation
a. Is the disability the result of a job related accident or illness?
   Yes ___ No ___
b. If yes, is the client presently receiving any benefits or services under Worker's Comp?
   Yes ___ No ___

24. Public Aid
___ 0 - None
___ 1 - SSI: Aged
___ 2 - SSI: Blind
___ 3 - SSI: Disabled
___ 4 - AFDC
___ 5 - General Asst.
___ 6 - AFDC & SSI
___ 7 - MANG only
___ 9 - Food Stamp only

MONTHLY AMOUNT
$ _____

TIME ON AID
Years   Months

25.

SSDI Status	SSI	SSDI Claim Type	SSI Claim Type
___ 0 - No application	- 0 ___	___ 0 - None	___ 0 - None
___ 1- Allowed	- 1 ___	___ 1 - DIB	___ 1 - (DI) Disabled Ind.
___ 2 - Denied	- 2 ___	___ 2 - CDB-OA	___ 2 - (BI) Blind Individual
___ 3 - App. Pending	- 3 ___	___ 3 - CDB-DI	___ 3 - (DC) Disabled Child
___ 5 - Discontinued or terminated	- 5 ___	___ 4 - DWB	___ 4 - (BC) Blind Child
			___ 5 - (DS) Disabled spouse
			___ 6 - (BS) Blind spouse

WAGE EARNER NAME _____

WAGE EARNER SOCIAL SECURITY NUMBER _____

26. Highest Grade (G.E.D.=12) _____

27. Veteran
Yes ___
No ___

28. Work History
___ 0 - None
___ 1 - Current
___ 2 - Previous

29. Work Status
___ 1 - Competitive labor market
___ 2 - Sheltered workshop
___ 3 - Self-employed (except BEP)
___ 4 - State agency managed business (BEP)
___ 5 - Homemaker
___ 6 - Unpaid family worker
___ 7 - Not working-student
___ 8 - Not working-other
___ 9 - Trainees or workers (non-competitive)

30. Individual Weekly Earnings $ _____

31. Monthly Family Income $ _____

32. Hospital/Medical Insurance Yes ___ No ___

INSURANCE COMPANY   DD   POLICY NUMBER

33. PHYSICIANS PREFERRED (Names and Addresses)

General Medical _____
Specialist _____
Specialist _____

348

Appendix 9D *continued*

34. Work History

EMPLOYER	JOB DESCRIPTION	WEEKLY EARNINGS	DATES	REASON FOR LEAVING

35. Client's expressed needs _____

36. Services presently being received _____

37. Vocational plans & interests _____

38. Availability of transportation to meet client's needs _____

39. List two people outside the home through whom client can be contacted:

NAME _____ ADDRESS _____ PHONE _____

NAME _____ ADDRESS _____ PHONE _____

40. Directions to client's home

A summary of the interview on these items should be placed as an initial entry on the DORS: 58 Case Memorandum

1. Appearance and manner	3. Military service data	5. Social data	7. Source of information (GATB, school records, medical information)
2. Educational history & interests	4. Medical history	6. Accessibility of home, if ILR client	8. Describe disability

NOTES: _____

APPENDIX

9E

Individualized Program

ILLINOIS DEPARTMENT OF REHABILITATION SERVICES
Individualized Program
Part I

Client _____   Planning date _____
        (Last)   (First)   (Initial)

Social Security number_____   Date of birth _____

Program

  ☐ Individualized Educational   ☐ Individualized Written   ☐ Individualized Comprehensive
     Program   Rehabilitation Program   Rehabilitation Program

The statements in this document are the beginning of your individualized written program. Your rights and responsibilities and the responsibilities of the Illinois Department of Rehabilitation Services are outlined. This Program contains a list of objectives and services to be provided which you and/or your representative and staff of DORS will jointly prepare to meet your personal rehabilitation or educational goals. Your goals, objectives, and the provision of services may need to be revised from time to time because of changed circumstances and new information. Sometimes, a person's program cannot be carried out as originally planned.

Before any changes in the program plan take place, the entire situation will be disucssed with you and/or your representative.

A. Your responsibilities as a client

After you begin your program, your cooperation in carrying it out will affect its success. You must keep appointments and attend scheduled activities. You are responsible for carrying out medical and other professional instructions.

B. Evaluation and review of your program

This program will be reviewed and recorded at least once every 12 months to study your progress toward your goal.

C. Your rights and remedies

1. You and/or your representative have a right to discuss any problem or complaint you may have about your program with a DORS representative or his supervisor. If still dissatisfied with the results of the meeting, you are entitled to an Administrative Review, which allows your case and decisions to be reviewed by supervisory personnel.

2. If you are not satisfied with the Administrative Review or its results, you are entitled to a Fair/Due Process Hearing. The Director of the Department will make the final decision in such hearings. The Administrative Officer who conducted the Administrative Review will give you the information and any help you need to request a Fair/Due Process Hearing.

3. Additional appeals beyond a Fair/Due Process Hearing are available outside the Department. These include appeals to the courts or the Department of Education.

4. In addition to the DORS staff involved in your case, information and assistance are also available from the Client—Counselor Assistance Project (C-CAP), Illinois Department of Rehabilitation Services, P. O. Box 1587, Springfield, IL 62705. You may contact C-CAP directly at your expense at (217) 782-5374. If you prefer, you may telephone the Disabled Individual's Assistance Line (DIAL) by dialing "O" for Operator and placing a collect call to (312) 793-5000. DIAL will then contact C-CAP on your behalf and have them call you.

For all programs except Illinois School for the Deaf, Illinois Children's Hospital-School and the Illinois School for the Visually Impaired.

5. You have the right to discuss your case with DORS staff before any action is taken to change your status from eligible to ineligible. If you are found ineligible after this consultation, a written record of your views and the reason for the decision made by DORS will be placed in your file. You will receive a letter stating the reasons for ineligibility, if that occurs. Every person determined ineligible due to the impairment's being too severe is given an opportunity to participate in an annual review of that decision.

D. Notification of compliance

DORS will not discriminate in admission or access to, or treatment or employment in Department programs or services in compliance with the Illinois Human Rights Act, the Illinois Constitution, the U. S. Civil Rights Act, Section 504 of the Rehabilitation Act of 1973 45 CFR 104, and the U. S. Constitution. The Director of the Illinois Department of Rehabilitation Services is responsible for compliance.

E. Payment for services

DORS cannot pay for services without prior written authorization.

350

Appendix 9E *continued*

F. Services available

The groups of services listed as part of your program are available as needed. You must meet certain eligibility and financial requirements before some services can be provided.

Group 1 - Home Services

Types of services available in the Home Services Program include:

Health Support Service

Assistance to enable individuals to access services necessary to obtain and maintain a favorable condition of health by helping them identify and understand their health needs and obtain and utilize necessary medical treatment. Health services provided in the home by medically trained personnel (RN, LPN, P.T., Home Health Aide) such as injections, irrigations (catheter, colostomies, etc.) special diets, medical care training.

Chore and Housekeeping

Assistance with household tasks or personal care of the client in his or her home by a household employee under the supervision of the client or other responsible person.

Homemaker

Teaching of, and assistance in, household management and personal care. General support by trained and professional supervised homemakers to maintain and strengthen the functioning of individuals or families in their own homes where no responsible and capable person may be available for this purpose.

Group 2 - Community Services

Services available in the Community Services Program include:

Braille	Leisure-time activities
Homemaking skills	Mobility
Individualized instruction in personal care	Non-vocational counseling
techniques	Written communication skills

Group 3 - Illinois Visually Handicapped Institute (IVHI)

Services from IVHI include:

Assistance in preparing for the GED test	Limited medical services including specialized self-help instruction
Braille	for the blind diabetic and those undergoing renal dialysis
Classroom instruction in mobility	Oral communications
Counseling and testing with a special battery of	Personal management skills
tests for the visually impaired	Physical education
Help in preparing to attend college	Special activity program for senior citizens in the Chicago area
Hobby skills	Typewriting
Home management	Visual aid evaluation and training in the use of a visual aid
Industrial arts	

Group 4 - Residential Education Programs

Adaptive Physical Education	Mathematics
Communication Skills	Physical Education & Recreation
Extracurricular Activities	Reading
General Medical Services	Science & Health
Guidance & Counseling	Social Studies
Independent Living Skills	Vocational Education/Skill Training

Illinois School for the Deaf (ISD)	Illinois Children's Hospital-School (ICHS)
Total Communication Skills	Occupational Therapy
Daily Living Skills	Driver Evaluation & Education Program
Interscholastic Sports Program	Physical Therapy
	Special Medical Services

Illinois School for the Visually Impaired (ISVI)

Orientation & Mobility Training

Optacon Training

Deaf-Blind Program

Low Vision Clinic & Evaluation

Physical Therapy

Appendix 9E *continued*

☐ Group 5 - Vocational Rehabilitation (VR)
Services available in the VR program include:

Artificial Limbs & Training in their use	Occupational Licenses
Assistance in establishing a small business	Physical & Occupational Therapy
Braces & Orthopedic Devices	Placement Services
Clinical Evaluations	Psychiatric Examination
Dental Services	Psychotherapy
Eyeglasses	Reader Service
Guidance & Counseling	Speech Therapy
Hearing Aids	Transportation
Hospitalization	Vocational Testing
Interpreter Services	Vocational Training
Maintenance	Wheelchairs
Medical & Surgical Treatment	Work Evaluation
Medical Diagnosis & Evaluation	Other goods, services essential to rehabilitation

Eligibility requirements:

For Vocational Rehabilitation Services

A. Documentation of the existence of a physical or mental disability.

B. Documentation of how disabling conditions and other related factors are preventing preparing for, retaining or obtaining suitable employment.

C. Reasonable expectations that service will result in suitable employment.

For extended evaluation services

A. Above

B. Above

C. The need to determine whether services will benefit to the point of securing suitable employment.

G. Eligibility for services

You have applied for services from DORS. A determination of eligibility must be made prior to provision of services and you are entitled to that determination.

Diagnostic services required to determine eligibility.

Objective	Anticipated Achievement Date	Service or Activity	Estimated Cost and Funding Source	Dates of Services

I have read and discussed with the DORS representative the statements in the Part I portion of my individualized program and fully understand them. I have been given, for my reference, a copy of this program and a list of services, including those in Group _____ which are available, as necessary, in this program

Signature of client _____

(Date)

Signature of client's witness (if client signs with his mark)

parent   (If client is a minor)

or representative (if any) _____

(Date)

I have given this client a copy of Part I of his program and a list of services available, and have identified services under Group _____ that are a part of his program.

Signature of DORS representative _____

(Date)

APPENDIX

9F

Application for Rehabilitation Services and Release Authority

STATE OF ILLINOIS

DIVISION OF VOCATIONAL REHABILITATION

APPLICATION FOR REHABILITATION SERVICES
AND
RELEASE AUTHORITY

I, the undersigned, hereby apply for services from the Division of Vocational Rehabilitation in order to become (or remain) employed. I authorize the release of medical records or other personal information to other agencies or individuals only for the purpose of developing and completing my rehabilitation program.

I understand my right to appeal decisions of the Division of Vocational Rehabilitation and the appeal procedure, both of which have been explained to me by the Rehabilitation Counselor or the Rehabilitation Counselor's representative signing below.

Date	Applicant's Signature

Parent, Guardian or Agent's Signature

The NOTIFICATION OF COMPLIANCE has been read to the applicant and, if appropriate, to the co-signer of this Application. I have explained both the RELEASE AUTHORITY and the RIGHT OF APPEAL.

The Division of Vocational Rehabilitation and its lawful employees, representatives or agents understand that any information received on the above client shall be treated in accordance with the federal regulations on confidentiality. Further, the applicant/client has been informed that he is entitled to any remedies available to him at law in case of unauthorized disclosure of any confidential information.

Date	Signature of Rehabilitation Counselor or Rehabilitation Counselor's Representative

CLIENT'S RIGHT OF APPEAL

Any applicant for or recipient of vocational rehabilitation services from the Illinois Division of Vocational Rehabilitation who is dissatisfied with any action with regard to the furnishing or denial of such services, may file a request for an administrative review and redetermination of that action to be made by supervisory staff of the Agency. If dissatisfied with the finding of the administrative review, he can request and will receive a fair hearing before the Agency Director or a person or persons designated by the Director.

NOTIFICATION OF COMPLIANCE

Services, assistance and other benefits of the Division of Vocational Rehabilitation are provided on a non-discriminatory basis as required by the Civil Rights Act of 1964 and Section 504 of the Rehabilitation Act of 1973. Applicants, clients and participants who believe that discrimination on the grounds of handicap, sex, religion, race, color or national origin is being practiced by the Illinois Division of Vocational Rehabilitation may file a written complaint with the State agency, the Federal agency or both. Complaints shall be addressed to the State Director, Illinois Division of Vocational Rehabilitation, 623 East Adams Street, Springfield, Illinois 62706, and must bear the personal signature of the individual making the complaint.

APPENDIX

9G

Release Form

State of Illinois
DEPARTMENT OF REHABILITATION SERVICES

Date _____

To:

Attention:

The specific information requested by the Department is:

Please send the information to

Name

Address

Telephone

INFORMATION	Client's Initials	INFORMATION	Client's Initials	INFORMATION	Client's Initials
School Transcripts		Psychiatric Evaluations		Hospital Records	
Financial Information		Medical Records/Reports		Psychological Testing	
Psychosocial Evaluations		Past Employment History		Academic Performance Record/ Achievement Testing	
Individualized Educational Program		Social History		Other:	

AUTHORITY FOR RELEASE OF INFORMATION

I hereby request and authorize you to release to the Illinois Department of Rehabilitation Services the above types(s) of information which you have or may receive, pertaining to my application for or provision of services.

I understand that DORS has the right to inspect and copy any information which is covered by this release. The disclosure of information may be in verbal or written form and a photocopy of this authorization may be accepted with the same authority as the original. I understand that I have the right to withdraw my consent in writing at any time. Unless I withdraw my consent, this consent will automatically expire 12 months from the date of my signature.

I fully understand that I have the right to withhold my consent for the disclosure of the records and communications and that the receiving of services from DORS or related agencies is not conditioned upon my signing this consent, and that there are no other consequences from those agencies for such refusal.

Client signature	Date	Client's date of birth (month, day, and year)
Witness signature	Date	Client's full name (print)
*Parents or guardian signature	Date	Client's Social Security number
**Witness signature	Date	Record number
Client's maiden name (Or any other used)		*If client is a minor, signature of a parent or guardian is required.

**If unable to write his (or her) name, the client or applicant should enter an 'X' or other mark. Signature of a second witness is required when the 'X' signature is used.

The Department of Rehabilitation Services and its employees, representatives or agents understand that any information received on the above client shall be treated in accordance with the federal regulations on confidentiality. Further, the applicant/client has been informed of the legal remedies he is entitled to.

APPENDIX

9H

Otologic Report

DIVISION OF VOCATIONAL REHABILITATION

OTOLOGICAL REPORT

DVR CASE NUMBER

AREA OUTLINED TO BE COMPLETED BY COUNSELOR

TO:

DATE

M.D.

FROM:

REHABILITATION COUNSELOR

COUNSELOR'S ADDRESS

PHONE

PATIENT'S LAST NAME   FIRST   MIDDLE   PATIENT'S AGE   PATIENT'S PHONE

PATIENT'S ADDRESS

OCCUPATION OR OBJECTIVE (x)

The following information will be used in determining eligibility for Vocational Rehabilitation services and providing same if applicant is eligible. Audiogram must be completed, and appropriate reference level indicated.

Ave. decibel loss: speech range only (500, 1000, 2000 CPS)

Air: Right _____dbs.   Left_____dbs.

Bone: Right_____dbs.   Left_____dbs.

Type of
Hearing Loss: Nerve_____Conduction_____Mixed_____

Characteristics of
Hearing Condition: Slowly
(check those that apply)   Stable_____Progressive_____Acute_____

Diagnosis & Etiology

_____

_____

_____

_____

_____

_____

_____

SPEECH RANGE

HEARING THRESHOLD LEVEL IN DECIBELS

-10 0 10 20 30 40 50 60 70 80 90 100 110 120

125 250 500 1000 2000 4000 8000
                              3000 6000

CYCLES PER SECOND   CHECK ONE

UNMASKED MASKED UNMASKED MASKED

O AIR RIGHT △   ⋈ BONE RIGHT ☐   _____1951 ASA REFERENCE LEVEL

x AIR LEFT ▽   ⋈ BONE LEFT ☐   _____1964 ISO REFERENCE LEVEL

Is hearing loss congenital?	Age at Onset?	Should use of Hearing Aid be considered?	Has applicant used a hearing aid?	Successfully?	*(If not, comment below)*
Yes_____ No_____		Yes_____ No_____	Yes_____ No_____	Yes_____ No_____	

Is there any medical objection to fitting the ear mold to either ear?   Yes_____ No_____Right_____ Left_____

Why?

Is this a type of hearing that could be amenable to aural surgery?   Yes_____ No_____

Does client have stable balance?   Yes_____No_____

(x) DOCTOR: Recommendations and comments. Include advice on working conditions to be avoided. If the occupation or job objective has been entered by the Counselor, please indicate if it is medically and acoustically advisable.

Date patient was examined	Date of this report	Signature
		M.D.

91

Hearing Clinic Referral

DATE FORWARDED TO STATE OFFICE

STATE OF ILLINOIS

DIVISION OF VOCATIONAL REHABILITATION

HEARING CLINIC REFERRAL

DATE_____

NAME OF CLIENT_____AGE_____SEX_____

ADDRESS_____PHONE_____

CLIENT'S USED APPLIANCE	TYPE	MAKE	MODEL NO.	DATE RECEIVED

COMPLETE ITEMS A THROUGH E BELOW

A. VOCATIONAL OBJECTIVE:_____

    I. WORKING CONDITIONS:

        a. TO WHAT EXTENT IS ORAL COMMUNICATION NECESSARY?   GREAT ☐   SMALL ☐   NONE ☐

        b. IS POOR HEARING AN INDUSTRIAL HANDICAP?   YES ☐   NO ☐

        c. IS TEMPERATURE HIGH?   YES ☐   NO ☐

        d. IS HUMIDITY HIGH?   YES ☐   NO ☐

        e. IS ENVIRONMENT NOISY?   YES ☐   NO ☐

B. AVOCATIONS:

    I. MOVIES YES ☐ NO ☐   4. TV YES ☐ NO ☐

    2. CHURCH YES ☐ NO ☐   5. RADIO YES ☐ NO ☐

    3. CLUBS YES ☐ NO ☐   6. OTHER_____

C. NAMES OF AIDS READILY AVAILABLE TO CLIENT:_____

_____

_____

D. TIME AT WHICH CLIENT WILL BE AVAILABLE FOR TESTING:_____

_____

E. PROBLEMS SEEN BY THE COUNSELOR:_____

_____

F. FAMILY MEMBERS AT HOME:

NAME	RELATIONSHIP		NAME	RELATIONSHIP
I.		4.		
2.		5.		
3.		6.		

COUNSELOR_____ TELEPHONE_____

ADDRESS_____

APPENDIX

9J

Hearing Aid Evaluation Report

STATE OF ILLINOIS
DIVISION OF VOCATIONAL REHABILITATION
HEARING AID EVALUATION REPORT

To:_____Date_____197____

The information requested concerning this person is to be used to determine his NEED FOR A HEARING AID and to use as a guide in providing such services if the person is found to be eligible. All information will be held strictly confidential. (Audiometric examination must be included.)

Counselor_____Address_____

NAME OF PATIENT_____Phone_____Age_____

Address_____Employment Objective_____

FINDINGS

Graph: LOSS IN DECIBELS (-10, Normal 0, 10, 20, 30, 40, 50, 60, 70, 80, 90, 100) vs frequencies (125, 250, 500, 750, 1000, 2000, 4000, 8000)

AIR   BONE   SPEECH LOSS
Right Ear = O   Right Ear = ⌐
Left Ear = X   Left Ear = ⌐   _____DB

UNAIDED

		SPEECH RECEPTION THRESHOLD	DISCRIMINATION (% CORRECT)
MON-AURAL	RIGHT EAR	db	%
	LEFT EAR	db	%
BINAURAL		db	%

DID CLIENT HAVE HIS OWN AID WITH HIM?

YES ☐   NO ☐

MAKE_____

MODEL_____

HEARING AIDS TESTED	SPEECH RECEPTION THRESHOLD	DISCRIMINATION IN QUIET (% CORRECT)	IN NOISE (% CORRECT)	VOLUME SETTING	TOLERANCE SATISFACTORY	UNSATISFACTORY
1. Client's Own Aid	_____db					
2.	_____db					
3.	_____db					
4.	_____db					
5.	_____db					

RECOMMENDATIONS

HEARING AIDS RECOMMENDED:	NAME OR MAKE	MODEL NUMBER	RECEIVER	SETTING	VOLTAGE
(Most Acceptable)					
(Acceptable)					
(Acceptable)					
(Acceptable)					
(Acceptable)					

AUDITORY TRAINING IS   ☐ IMPERATIVE   ☐ RECOMMENDED   ☐ NOT RECOMMENDED

LIP READING TRAINING IS   ☐ IMPERATIVE   ☐ RECOMMENDED   ☐ NOT RECOMMENDED

COMMENTS:_____

_____

_____

_____

DATE_____197_____ SIGNATURE_____AUDIOLOGIST

APPENDIX

9K

Planned Goals, Objectives, and Service Activities

PLANNED GOALS, OBJECTIVES & SERVICE ACTIVITIES
Part II

Client _____ Date _____

Service Goals:

Program:

	IEP	IWRP	ICRP
	☐	☐	☐

Diagnostic Services	Extended Evaluation	Program Services	
☐	☐	☐	Amendment No. _____

Intermediate Objective	Anticipated Achievement Date	Service or Activity	Estimated Cost & Funding Source	Projected Dates	
				From	To

Page _____ of _____

Review Date _____

APPENDIX

9L

Evaluation Criteria and Client Views

EVALUATION CRITERIA & CLIENT VIEWS
Part III

Client _____   Date _____

IEP ☐   IWRP ☐   ICRP ☐   Extended Evaluation ☐   Program Services ☐   ☐ Amendment No. _____

Progress Evaluation Plan: (Review dates, methods and criteria)

CLIENT VIEWS
(For completion by client and/or his representative)

1. Do you fully understand the function and purpose of this Written Program?   Yes _____ No _____

2. Do you feel you had sufficient input in developing this plan?   Yes _____ No _____

3. Do you feel the services provided will help you reach your rehabilitation or educational goals?   Yes _____ No _____

4. Do you feel all necessary or desirable services have been included in your plan?   Yes _____ No _____
   If no, what services do you feel should be included?

5. Do you understand your rights of appeal?   Yes _____ No _____

If you wish to explain any answer to the questions above or make any other statement, use the space provided below. Use additional sheets if needed.

_____

_____

_____

_____

_____

_____

_____

_____

Client signature _____
                                                                    Date

Signature of client's witness (if client signs with his mark)
                    parent (if client is a minor)
                    or representative (if any) _____
                                                                    Date

DORS representative _____
                                                                    Date

Page ____ of _____   Review date _____

359

10

Community Aural Rehabilitation Programs

Jerome G. Alpiner, Ph.D.

Schow and Nerbonne (1980) summarize the settings in which aural rehabilitation for adults can take place.

(1) University and technical school settings
(2) Vocational rehabilitation
(3) Military-related facilities
(4) ENT clinic/private practice
(5) Community, hospital, and university hearing clinics
(6) Hearing aid dealers/dispensers

Although a variety of settings exist for services, there are few organized outreach mechanisms available to reach adults in the general mainstream of society for initial identification of hearing loss and follow up remediation.

Denson *et al.* (1977) conducted a survey of community colleges to determine (1) the extent and type of services in speech, hearing, or language screening remediation and improvement, (2) the extent and type of instruction in speech and language improvement, and (3) the extent and type of bilingual services in speech, hearing, or language presently offered to students and community members within the community college setting. In addition, the existence of plans to offer these services in the future was ascertained.

The community college was chosen because the authors state that it is the place where the last formal education for many people is received. Specific questions posed in the survey were as follows.

(1) What percentage of responding community colleges offer speech, hearing, or language services?
(2) What percentage of responding community colleges offer speech and/or hearing services in each of the following areas?
    (a) Screening
    (b) Evaluation
    (c) Remediation
(3) What percentage of responding community colleges offer instruction in speech and/or language improvement?
(4) What percentage of responding community colleges offer instruction to bilingual students?
(5) What percentage of responding community colleges indicate plans for implementing language, speech, or hearing services in the future?

A brief questionnaire was sent to the chief executive officer of 102 community colleges. Representatives of the colleges were asked to indicate on a checklist the availability of the following 9 services.

(1) Speech screening
(2) Hearing screening
(3) Speech evaluation
(4) Hearing evaluation
(5) Speech therapy
(6) Hearing therapy

(7) Speech improvement
(8) Language improvement
(9) Instruction for bilingual students

They were also asked to report the existence of plans to initiate any of the above services in the next 3 years.

66 of the 102 questionnaires were returned. 38% of the colleges offered no services. Of the 62% that did, almost all offered between 1 and 4 of the services listed while only 4 offered more. Little interest was shown in establishing future services. The results can be viewed both positively and negatively. On the positive side, some institutions were providing services in an area felt to be important to students and the community. This may be the only service available in the community. On the negative side, most schools provided minimal or no services. The most salient implication of the data presented is the necessity for community college personnel to consider the situation in their own institutions with respect to speech-language pathology and audiology services for their students and the community in which the college is located.

Stephens (1979) presents an aural rehabilitation program for the hearing-impaired adult in Denmark, which he refers to as the most comprehensive in the world. The present Danish system emerged from two Acts of Parliament in 1940 and 1951. The former established separate boards for pre-lingually deaf and for the hard-of-hearing, established hearing centers and vocational guidance bureaus, and provided remediation. The 1951 Act entitled every citizen to a free hearing aid and instruction in the use of residual hearing. When a person goes to one of the centers, he is given a basic audiologic examination. The physician decides whether the patient requires further testing, has a condition which may be treated medically or surgically, or needs a hearing aid. If no hearing aid is indicated, the person is sent to a hearing therapist for training to obtain maximal use of residual hearing. After selection of a hearing aid, the patient is given some basic instruction and then an impression for an ear mold is made. Once the ear mold is received, the patient is called back for an instruction course. The patient will have 1 or 2 lessons of 1/2 to 1 hour and then be given an appointment for a follow-up session 6 weeks later.

If at this point the patient is having difficulty, a social welfare assistant visits the home to give the patient more intensive training. If trouble still persists, he may be referred to the State Hearing Institute. The patient is then evaluated and assigned to any special classes which may be appropriate. These may include auditory training, hearing tactics, speechreading and the mouth-hand system. The patient, according to his needs, may spend a variable amount of time at the State Hearing Institute. When the staff is satisfied that the client has been adequately rehabilitated, he will be referred back to the local hearing center. Overall, it is indicated that the success of the Danish system is a result of its comprehensiveness rather than the use of highly sophisticated techniques.

Markides *et al.* (1979) outline the official policy of the British Society of Audiology on aural rehabilitation for hearing-impaired adults. Its major purpose is to present basic information from that policy pertaining to the aural rehabilitation needs of hearing-impaired adults. They emphasize that it is important for hearing impairment to be detected and diagnosed as early as possible. Early identification of hearing loss will also facilitate the aural rehabilitation process, especially for those patients suffering from progressive hearing loss. The most important matter is not only the availability of different types of hearing aids but the actual use of them by the patients. The hearing-impaired person also needs to be taught strategies in lipreading. Since the hard-of-hearing adult has normal speech, the aim in therapy is to teach the client to retain good sound production in order to conserve already acquired normal speech. Some of the psychosocial and vocational problems which face a hearing-impaired person also can be minimized by educating family members, friends, and employers.

Various concepts for aural rehabilitation programs appear to exist. In any program, it seems that initial identification of hearing loss is a major requisite. The establishment of a comprehensive community aural rehabilitation program can be a complex process if it is to be effective. Approaches to this situation are considered.

O'Neill and Oyer (1966) indicate that the primary objectives of hearing conservation programs are to locate the hearing-impaired and to help them obtain necessary medical and educational assistance. They state further that locating persons with hearing loss in the community is a significant undertaking. According to Smith and Porter (1958), there are various definitions of a community. To the average citizen it usually means a political subdivision, a geographical area within a political subdivision, or a group of individuals with a common interest.

When attempting to establish a community hearing conservation program, individuals with a common interest are the most important consideration. They may be found in education, social, and health agencies, civic organizations, universities, businesses, and industries. For any program to be implemented and sustained, persons within the community must be cognizant of the need for such a program. Typical members of a community may not know of existing needs until made aware of them. Smith and Porter (1958) state that communities are not psychologicly ready to assume the responsibility for a hearing conservation program unless they are absolutely convinced that the need exists.

Specific areas of concern have been outlined by Alpiner et al. (1973). Awareness of these concerns is a prerequisite for establishing a community hearing conservation program.

(1) Community programs need to be situated in strategic locations to serve all adults with hearing impairment. Not all hearing-impaired persons are found in large communities where services are generally available. Some hearing-impaired citizens live in smaller and rural communities where the population does not justify employing full time audiologists. Thousands of extended care facilities are located throughout the country and services are not generally available for their residents. In addition, most communities have no provisions for screening adults.

(2) All populations must be served. If screening programs are developed within communities, the need to provide follow-up remediation service also exists. Conservative estimates have indicated that there are at least 10 million persons with a significant degree of hearing impairment in the United States.

(3) Actual types of programs will vary among communities. Usually rural areas have no services available. Most metropolitan areas offer services in a variety of facilities: university centers, community centers, hospital clinics, otologists' offices, private practitioners' offices, and so forth, but there is no real mechanism to ensure that adults will utilize them. Some exceptions occur when referrals are made by otologists, other physicians, and certain community agencies. Holanov (1976) emphasizes that the majority of adults who need rehabilitative services generally do not receive them. This is due to either a lack of interest or uncertainty regarding where to go for help. Frequently, clients say that they found out about lipreading in the yellow pages of the telephone directory or through public service announcements in the newspapers or on the radio. The majority of clients do not come from direct otologic or hearing aid dealer referral sources. Individuals from rural areas frequently come to an urban center for evaluation on a one-visit basis, return to their home community, and find that no rehabilitation or follow-up services are available.

(4) Personnel serving the hearing-impaired should be qualified to perform the task for which they have been trained. For audiologic assessment, hearing aid evaluation, and rehabilitative services, personnel should be ASHA-certified (this certification is the criterion for provision of quality service and consumer protection). We cannot ignore the use of support personnel such as audiology assistants, who may be able to engage in some aspects of audiology under the supervision of an ASHA-certified audiologist. If assistants are used, their roles need to be clearly defined.

(5) Financing community programs may be difficult. University programs are usually self-supporting but, with decreased federal aid, difficulties may be encountered when attempting to use university personnel to provide the manpower for community programs. Community centers, too, are generally self-sustaining, but tend to avoid public service programs because of inadequate funds. The same situation faces hospital programs and private practitioners. Homes for senior citizens usually provide no hearing services because funds are not available.

(6) Apparently many hearing aid dealers and physicians have not referred their clients for rehabilitation because they are not convinced of the value of these services. Audiologists have been negligent in promoting the value of rehabilitation. There appears to be a real need for in-service training or workshops designed to educate allied health professionals, hearing aid dealers, and the media in order to disseminate information about audiology to the public.

(7) Identification of those with hearing impairment is essential for implementing hearing conservation programs. The problem is where these people may be located and whether there is a realistic way to reach persons living in rural areas.

(8) Both short and long term goals need to be established to implement hearing conservation programs. Audiologists must assume that lead in development of community goals. Efforts need to be directed toward programs of hearing loss identification and remediation.

THE NEED FOR A COMMUNITY AURAL REHABILITATION PROGRAM

Members of a community need to be convinced that hearing loss is a prevalent problem affecting significant numbers of individuals. A helpful approach may be to outline and discuss the types of hearing impairment which affect individuals. Some of the more common losses about which the community could be educated are those due to noise exposure, the aging process, ototoxic drugs, middle ear infections, and various illnesses. A convincing reason for establishing a hearing conservation program might be, for example, the problem of noise pollution. The approach used could emphasize the fact that excessive noise has become a threat to the hearing of millions of American men and women.

The proliferation of loud machinery in industry, as well as the effects of sounds from street noises and others in the home, are slowly wearing away the hearing of many persons (Employers Insurance of Wausau, 1967). The hearing of people of all ages is declining at a rate faster than can be explained by the aging process alone. Sataloff and Michael (1973) emphasize that high-level noise sources produced in the environment not only cause loss of hearing but also create a nuisance effect in the home, at work, in recreation areas, and in the community at large. Acceptable national standards for control of noise pollution do not yet exist. Sataloff and Michael (1973) list several variabilities to consider in the relationship between noise and annoyance. These include the attitude of the listener toward the noise source, the history of individual noise exposure, activities and stresses upon the listener during these exposures, the hearing sensitivity of the listener, and other factors related to individual variability which cause wide differences in reactions to noise.

Although hearing conservation programs now exist in many industries and in the military, community-wide programs are not prevalent. A variety of noises in community environments poses threats to citizens who are unaware of the damaging effects of noise pollution. Table 10.1 indicates levels of some common noises in the environment. Many of the examples cited are prevalent in everyday living situations and should be areas of community concern. In attempting to interest community groups we will need to stress the potentially damaging physical effects of noise as well as psychologic stresses which may occur.

Development of Community Interest

In today's complex society, many worthy projects compete for community participation. It can no longer be assumed that a community is able to support all of them. The community must decide which projects will be of greatest benefit (Porter and Smith, 1973) and address itself to problem areas only after their priority is determined. A community may be inspired to act if an audiologist can effectively create awareness of the problems of its hearing-impaired citizens.

Table 10.1
Common Noise Exposures [a]

dBA Scale	Stimulus
dB	
0	Approximate threshold of hearing for younger ears at 1000 Hz
30	Whisper at 5 feet
40	Broadcast studio
35–40	Country residence
60	Average conversation
70	Automobile
75	Average office or home
70–85	Average street noise or radio
80–85	Data processing equipment in modern office
85–95	Machine shop
95–100	Food blender
90–110	Loud street noise
90–110	Discotheque
95–105	Inside subway car
100–110	Motorcycle
105–115	Power lawn mower
120	Thunderclap
140–145	.45 magnum pistol
150–170	Jet engine
150	Pain threshold

[a] Reprinted by permission from J. Katz, *Handbook of Clinical Audiology.* Baltimore: Williams & Wilkins, copyright 1972.

Porter and Smith (1973) cite examples of how groups of individuals within a community become motivated. One may become interested in program development because he is personally involved with the particular problem. Civic pride may be the basis of motivation for encouraging programming for another individual who may be sincerely interested in making his community a better place in which to live. Very often, we find these civic-minded persons actively involved in service organizations within their communities. Other individuals may be motivated for economic reasons. They may prefer to see hearing-impaired persons rehabilitated, employed, and contributing purchasing power to the community rather than taxing the community through unemployment compensation. Finally, some individuals feel the moral and spiritual need to help persons with handicapping conditions. The audiologist willing to assume the responsibility for developing community programs needs to be aware of these different groups since he should contact those most likely to help.

It is easy to recommend an idealistic plan for comprehensive care of all hearing-impaired persons. The goals are immediately evident and a variety of exciting activities in pursuit of these goals is not difficult to draft. Such a proposal would include every aspect of total audiologic attention for even the most inaccessible person, but the plan would ultimately fail. Limitations must be realized and accepted. Programs should be individualized to meet specific needs and available resources of the state or region to be served. For example, one may extol the potential benefits of a roving audiologic mobile unit that is professionally staffed and multi-functional. In this instance, effective transportation for both client and clinician is the primary concern. It might not be a realistic proposal for a particular community, however, since the funds might not be available.

Lack of adequate funds is the most restrictive factor in the development and conduct of programs. Monetary problems seem to pervade every aspect of our society. It is extremely difficult to obtain sufficient funds to allow programs the opportunity for successful and effective survival while attempting to accomplish established goals. Another limitation appears to be the need for quali-

fied, willing, and dedicated professionals to initiate programs and see them to completion. This is also related to financial considerations. More professionals might be motivated if the salary were acceptable or, in some cases, even available. It is important to be realistic about financial problems, which will certainly be encountered.

Creating a Community Program

Newman (1970) indicates that there is no comprehensive approach to services for people with communicative disorders. The lack of organization (non-system) is characterized by separateness at the community level. There is no coordination among speech and hearing centers, vocational rehabilitation agencies, university centers, health programs, educational institutions, and hearing aid dealers. Newman (1970) states that fiscal coordination, by United Way for example, is not enough. The agencies, the service-givers themselves, must be integrated. Successful establishment of hearing conservation programs in the community will depend on involving professional groups. Put another way, we must know community resources before contacting those who may be in a position to help develop the program.

Two basic elements are involved in developing a program for the hearing-handicapped: a "core of interest" and the "person" (Porter and Smith, 1973). The "core" is either a private or public agency. It may be composed of audiologists, physicians, hearing-impaired persons, or some combination of these individuals working together. The "person" is one who is regarded as a community leader.

An appropriate starting point is an assessment of existing resources within the community. It is possible that development or expansion of a hearing conservation program may be accomplished through other established health service programs. For example, a community without hearing services may have a health screening program for heart disease, diabetes, and high blood pressure. The hearing conservation program could be implemented by including hearing screening as part of the health program. Obviously, hearing screening is not a total hearing rehabilitation program, but it can serve as the embryo for future development.

Porter and Smith (1973) present six steps

which may be followed in establishing a comprehensive program. The first step is to identify the "core of interest" group. The second step is to interest a community leader who can organize local groups to study the problem. Selection of a temporary steering committee, consisting of representatives from lay organizations and professional groups, appointed by the community leader, is step three in the process. Step four involves using the steering committee as a resource to study the geographical area, identify the number of persons with hearing loss, determine what facilities and services are needed, inventory the available facilities and services, and identify the gaps in current programs needing to be filled for provision of complete services. The fifth step suggests that the steering committee call a community meeting of citizen representatives of all interest groups. The purpose of this meeting would be to determine whether the group wishes to organize for the development of adequate community services. Data obtained from the sample study would be presented. The sixth and final step is to recommend the action required to develop the more formal organization required to establish a community program.

The process represents a challenge for those interested in program development. It is important to remember that the efforts expended may not always result in the desired objectives. On a positive note, however, it may be possible to accomplish the goal by proceeding in a persistent and organized way.

This author was involved in a process similar to that described above, in a small Michigan community of about 25,000 persons. Although a speech clinician was employed in the public school system, there were no financial allocations for a school psychologist or for special education resource instructors. The school superintendent, when questioned about the lack of such services, suggested that a study be undertaken to justify additional programs. He indicated that any study would have to be done on a voluntary basis and without funding. It took several months to organize a steering committee consisting of representatives from service clubs, the clergy, business leaders in the community, social service agencies, and concerned parents. All agreed to participate in a geographic study to determine need. Funding was provided by

service clubs and businesses. A speaker's bureau was established and 25 volunteers agreed to talk to social, service, business, religious, and other groups in the community. More than one-half of the community's residents were reached through the speaker's bureau. Cooperation of the local media was largely responsible for the group's ability to reach such a large segment of the population.

The process took about 1 year. The task was not easy and it could not have been accomplished by the school clinician alone. It was a successful community effort. New school personnel were hired. In addition, it should be noted that a community group agreed to support a program for pre-school children. Programs were implemented where none had existed before.

A graduate student addressed herself to the difficulty of establishing community programs. In a term paper, she stated that volunteers must be involved and cooperation must be sought from a variety of channels. Public awareness campaigns require the active efforts of volunteers representing all aspects of the community. Local involvement is a prerequisite for any successful program of intervention. Lay people must be educated regarding the benefits to be derived from interaction with those offering help. The communication barrier can be surmounted by aggressive action. Unless we can find the mechanism to locate individuals lacking necessary audiologic services, programs cannot emerge. This student stated that we should not wait for the hearing-impaired adult to come to us; we must reach out to him.

Use of Audiology Assistants

Audiology assistants can be trained by ASHA certified audiologists to engage in provision of specified services. Assistants in the United States are primarily involved with providing support services in the public schools and their performance appears to be acceptable (Alpiner, 1970)). Assistants can perform these tasks with adults as well, and can provide considerable manpower assistance in community aural rehabilitation programs if they are trained appropriately and supervised adequately. In no way do they conflict with the professional responsibilities of the audiologist.

The ASHA Committee on Supportive Personnel (American Speech-Language-Hearing Association, 1981) has developed guidelines which may be followed in the use of supportive personnel. Following is a definition prepared by the Committee.

The term audiology assistant shall designate any person who, following academic and/or on-the-job training, provides clinical services as prescribed and directed by a certified audiologist. The audiologist shall maintain responsibility for services provided. Individuals who are enrolled in a training program or who have obtained a professional degree (*e.g.* B.A., B.S., A.B. degree) in speech-language pathology or audiology could be included within the definition of the term audiology assistant.

The following minimum qualifications can be considered in selecting individuals for employment as audiology assistants.

(1) A high school diploma or the equivalent.
(2) Communication skills adequate for the tasks assigned.
(3) Ability to relate to the clinical population being served.

Additional qualifications may be established according to the needs of the program and the population being served.

The assistant should be assigned tasks only at the discretion of the professional audiologist and should not be assigned tasks for which he has not been trained. Following completion of training, the assistant may engage only in those duties that are planned, designed, and supervised by the professional.

In addition to assisting audiologists in urban area programs, assistants may be of invaluable assistance in rural areas. They may plan logistics and serve as a liasion for the audiologist and clients between formal visits. The audiology assistant may be a volunteer or he may be paid, depending on circumstances within individual communities.

Urban Area Programs

After appropriate planning regarding implementation of a community program has taken place, hearing screening will follow. A variety of screening procedures exist in the United States. It is suggested that guidelines established by ASHA (American Speech and Hearing Association, 1975) be used. These guidelines recommend that screening be conducted at 1000, 2000, and 4000 Hz. The

screening level should be 20 dB HL (re: ANSI, 1969) at 1000 and 2000 Hz, and 25 dB HL at 4000 Hz. Some audiologist will include 500 Hz if ambient noise levels are low enough to avoid interference with the testing of this frequency. An inability to respond to any of these frequencies in either ear constitutes a failure. It is wise to repeat the screening once if there is an initial failure. Wilson and Walton (1974) found that rescreening resulted in 52% reduction in failures with school children. Data are not available regarding rescreening of adults. Tympanometry also should be a part of the screening program.

Failure in the screening procedure necessitates pure-tone audiometry. Depending on the audiologist's criteria, referrals will be made to an otologist for medical examination. Based on input from the audiologist and the otologist, a decision may be made regarding the need for rehabilitation and if it should include hearing aid evaluation.

It may be feasible to utilize audiologic service sites already established for screening locations. There are many speech and hearing centers in universities and hospitals in the United States. In addition to these facilities, numerous community hearing and speech agencies are in operation. Whether these facilities charge for the screening service probably depends on their financial structure. Some programs may be financed by United Way agencies, foundations, or other groups which provide the screening for a nominal fee or free of charge as a community service.

In larger metropolitan areas it may be possible for an agency to conduct screening in various locations on a periodic basis, covering all geographic areas at least once each year. This procedure would help eliminate some of the transportation problems which exist in larger cities. Personnel who assume the responsibility for the program will have to make decisions regarding the logistics of the screening programs within existing financial manpower resources. In university communities students may conduct the screening under the appropriate supervision of a certified audiologist. In other situations audiology assistants may perform the screening, also supervised by a certified audiologist.

It is important to indicate that persons failing the screening and follow-up pure-tone tests should be referred to a physician. If they have no physician, the names of several otologists in the area should be provided. In addition, clients should be given a handout listing the location and types of services available for rehabilitation. Physicians should also have access to the information about the rehabilitative services offered.

When rehabilitation is recommended after completion of the screening process, other decisions need to be made. If a hearing aid evaluation is recommended, the individual should be referred to the nearest facility providing audiologic services. Since the hearing aid evaluation is usually completed in one or two sessions, the travel problem for clients is not as involved as the therapy conducted on a continuing basis. Hearing aid orientation can be incorporated into the therapy program.

If individual or group rehabilitation is recommended for the client, available community options should be considered. In larger metropolitan areas, therapy may be available at any number of university, hospital, or community agency speech and hearing centers. Private practitioners may also provide hearing rehabilitation services. Suburban areas may pose more difficulties in terms of available services. Depending on available funding, hearing rehabilitation may be provided at various locations several times a year. Once again, fees may or may not be charged depending on the support for the programs.

The manpower for evening therapy can come from university or school audiologists in the community who desire extra employment. Audiologists from community agencies may be able to provide daytime therapy. Community agencies in some cities have satellite centers for suburban areas. Individuals in private practice may also maintain satellite offices. In cities where no university or community agency is available, it is possible that a school audiologist or speech pathologist may be available and willing to offer evening rehabilitation programs. Usually evening therapy will be offered by the clinician who assumes the initiative for making it known that services can be provided. Community efforts must be coordinated to provide effective service for as many hearing-impaired adults as possible.

Rural Area Programs

The problem of providing hearing service to rural America represents a complex but not a totally hopeless situation. The number of persons with hearing loss residing in rural areas is far less than in larger cities. Since it is difficult to justify the need for full-time professional persons, audiologists rarely choose to live in rural communities. There will be hearing-impaired individuals, however, in need of therapy. In the total process it will be easier to implement hearing screening programs than to provide rehabilitation on a continuing basis. Some State departments of health already provide screening services on a periodic basis, but remediation services usually are not available.

DeVoe (1974) says that it is difficult for people to travel long distances to a centrally located audiologic facility to receive services. It is equally difficult for personnel from a central facility to travel extensively to provide direct services. This situation led to the development and coordination of hearing conservation programs by the Montana State Department of Health and Environmental Sciences (DeVoe, 1974). In 1973, six regional audiology centers were operating in Montana. Each was well equipped and staffed by qualified audiologists to serve a multi-county area.

Before 1973, adults, particularly the elderly, had only minimal services available to them. Local family physicians and otologists in Billings, Montana, constantly received requests for services. County health nurses and the few available school clinicians showed justification for hiring a qualified audiologic consultant to serve locally, which in eastern Montana means within 100 miles. Additional justification for this program came from the information that hearing conservation counselling and ear protection were needed, especially for high school students and adults. The people in this rural area were exposed to long hours of noise from farm and ranch machinery.

Use of a mobile audiology van was considered in the planning stages. Due to the problems associated with winter travel, this was not implemented. Instead, it was decided to plan in terms of permanent facilities. No one agency could fund a regional program, so the costs were categorized according to salary, sound suite and equipment, space, clerical help, mileage and per diem, summer salary, and supplies and materials (DeVoe, 1974).

The hearing conservation coordinator contacted a number of individuals and groups in the geographic area, the "core of interest" discussed earlier (Porter and Smith, 1973), for support. The State Departments of Vocational Rehabilitation, Public Instruction, Health and Environmental Sciences, the Glendive Public Schools, the Youth Development Bureau/Rural America Project, the Division of Services for the Aging, and Action for Eastern Montana all expressed interest in this program and provided funds. It was planned to operate on a "no fee" basis and to serve all age ranges. An audiologist was hired to implement the program. The job involved doing public relations work, serving as liaison with the cooperating funding groups, and 32,000 miles of travel during the first year. This program effectively demonstrates that assistance can be provided in rural areas. Further, it emphasizes that a number of agencies can work together to provide services for children and adults by cost-sharing.

This author believes that there is a unique quality to rural area program development when the audiologist is qualified and willing to serve infants, school children, adults, and senior citizens. In essence, the audiologist has a general practice rather than a specialization with one age group.

COMMUNITY OUTREACH PROGRAMS

Because little published information is available regarding community aural rehabilitation programs in the United States, letters were sent to agencies listed in the Guide to Clinical Services, published by ASHA. Information on community programs was requested. Only 25 responses were received. A greater response had been anticipated, the assumption being that these agencies would have prepared materials available regarding their programs. Several programs will be described to provide information regarding what can be accomplished within a community.

New York League for the Hard-of-Hearing Program

The New York League's Community Outreach Program (New York League for the Hard-of-Hearing, 1980) has been in operation since 1972. Senior citizens have been the primary focus in this program. Hearing

screenings, complete audiologic evaluations, otologic evaluations, and hearing aid evaluations have been provided in its mobile unit. The mobile unit is a self-contained, fully equipped audiologic diagnostic center with a soundproof booth, required by the New York State Department of Health for testing nursing home patients. The van is licensed by the New York State Department as an out-of-hospital health facility. The services are available to nursing home patients who are interested in obtaining audiologic services. A minimum of seven patients must be scheduled per day. Information regarding the patients' living situation, communication abilities, motor dexterity, and degree of senility, if any, are obtained from the nursing home staff prior to testing so that the audiologist can better understand the patients' needs. Prior to hearing aid evaluations, custom-fitted earmolds can be made for each patient by the League or a local hearing aid dealer. Arrangements for dispensing of the recommended hearing aid can be made with the dealer or at the League. To ensure that a complete rehabilitative program is planned for each patient, in-service training sessions can be arranged to teach the nursing home staff how to better care for hearing impaired patients' daily living needs and their hearing aids. Fees for these services are normally charged to the nursing home.

Mid-Maine Medical Center Program

The F. T. Hill Center for Communication Disorders, located in Waterville, ME, serves outpatients in an area which includes a population of approximately 120,000 people (Olsen, 1981).

There are five programs in this outreach service. The first is a lipreading program in effect since 1972. The course has 10 lessons and includes a great deal of counselling with regard to hearing, hearing aids, and communication problems of each individual participating. Close relatives and friends are encouraged to sit in on the classes. Partial and full tuition scholarships for this 10-week course are available to individuals who would otherwise be unable to afford this service.

Another program offered is the loaner hearing aid program which began in 1972. It is generally for senior citizens who are living on very small monthly incomes and could not afford hearing aids any other way. The program has loaned over 700 hearing aids to individuals in mental health institutions and nursing homes, to elderly living at home, and in at least one particular case allowing a retired individual to return to work as he had wished to do. The person may return the aid when it is in need of repair which is free to the individual. They only request is that the individual return the aid when they no longer have any need for the aid. Local service clubs provided great assistance in locating hearing aids for the program to use.

The individual is reponsible for the cost of the hearing testing, counselling, and earmold but these fees can be on a sliding scale depending on the individual's income.

The third program to be described is a lecture offered to groups who have interest in the hearing impaired. The concept of a service club being involved with the hearing-impaired in other ways than just donating money seems to have appeal to many service clubs.

The parents of hearing-impaired children have a group which meets 6 times a year to review topics of interest to them. The group exchanges ideas and general information. The program is coordinated and developed by one of the teachers of the hearing-impaired on the staff.

The last program described is one in which free hearing testing is offered for individuals of all ages in various communities in South Central Maine. These clinics are for adults who have no other way of receiving hearing testing and counselling regarding hearing loss. These clinics are sponsored by a variety of agencies. This is the most popular outreach program offered by the center.

University of California, San Francisco Program

Owens, *et al.* (1978) describe a program in which a dispenser of hearing aids visits an audiology facility on a regular basis as a supplier. In this procedure, a California-licensed hearing aid dispenser visits the facility 2 days each week to work with 4 audiologists. The audiologists provide hearing aid evaluations, recommendations, orientation, and assume responsibility for general management and follow-up. The dispenser assumes responsibility for the provision of recom-

mended instruments and arranges payment for them.

The person is given a choice of going to an outside dispenser or to the dispenser in the clinic. If the patient has chosen an outside dispenser, he is given a written recommendation for the instrument selected. He is still urged to come to the orientation sessions and is especially urged to return for a hearing aid check. The orientation sessions, which take about an hour each, deal with care and maintenance of the aid and mold, telephone use, manipulation of the controls, introduction to some communication skills, such as visual cues and awareness of the limitations of the aid especially in noisy and reverberant situations. If special difficulties occur during the first 3 weeks, the person is urged to attend extra orientation sessions.

One year after the start of the program, a questionnaire was sent to all patients who had been seen for a hearing aid evaluation. After the first year, 86% of the patients were still wearing their aids. 111 of the subjects were contacted by telephone after 2 years and 86% ofthem were still wearing their aids. Of these, 95 persons still wear their aids, only 9 had returned for a 1-year check, and 31 accounted for a total of 43 problem visits. Problems tended to be classified as major or minor with minor problems being handled over the phone. The major problem usually required mailing the aid to the factory and providing a loaner aid. The experiences of this program in general, during the first 2 years, have led this group to favor complete management by the audiologist, including responsibility for earmold impressions and all follow-up problems. One weakness, for example, is that they have tried to restrict follow-up visits to the 2 days during which the dispenser is in the office. It seems incumbent to provide follow-up services at all times, preferably on the same day that the patient calls. The sole responsibility of the supplier would be to deliver the aids to the clinic.

University of Texas, Dallas Program

The University of Texas (1980) at Dallas, Callier Center for Communication Disorders, Adult Aural Rehabilitation program is offered exclusively as an "in-house" service. They receive referrals from physicians and self-referrals. They are now in the process of publishing a pamphlet on their program. The program is offered either in groups or on an individual basis. Sessions are scheduled for 1 hour weekly. The groups are limited to 5 persons per group and family members are encouraged to attend. Therapy runs for as long as it is deemed necessary to accomplish predetermined goals. The focus of the aural rehabilitation program is to develop better overall communicative success, especially by incorporating the habitual use of "communication strategies" into everyday life. This is accomplished through intensive counselling and discussion. Speechreading and auditory training, though not neglected, are emphasized in favor of a more realistic approach. There have been marked attitude changes as clients learn to accept their impairment. The Denver Scale of Communication Function is presently being used to document these changes.

Southeastern Connecticut Hearing and Speech Center Program

The Southeastern Connecticut Hearing and Speech Center conducts "Hear Well" classes at the local Senior Citizen's Center. Classes meet 1 hour a week for 10 weeks. Classes are open to anyone over 60 and spouses or close family members are invited to attend. There is no charge for attending the classes.

Emphasis is primarily on improving communication through better understanding of hearing impairment and the use of communication strategies for new hearing aid users. These classes provide in-depth hearing aid orientation. For those reluctant to admit a hearing problem, the classes provide a rationale for evaluation. People are made aware of the classes through the Senior Citizen's Center, newspaper articles and as a result of being seen at the Speech and Hearing Center. The program is in its third year with a series of classes each fall and spring. Attendance varies but averages around 12–15 people.

Community Speech and Hearing Center, Ventura, California Program

The Community Speech and Hearing Center in Ventura, California (1980), is a centrally located non-profit center. The center is a forum for public information, a source for professional education, a supervised training facility, and a resource for other facilities and agencies to provide speech and hearing services to clients.

Three major activities are offered: evaluation, therapy, and counselling. Evaluation consists of tests and observations to determine present abilities and to estimate potential for improvement. Therapy consists of speech reading, auditory training, and other activities designed to meet the needs of the individual. There are many group counselling activities for individuals and their families which are scheduled periodically throughout the year. The center relies on individual donations which are tax-deductible.

Wilmington, Delaware Medical Center Program

The Wilmington, Delaware Medical Center Speech and Auditory Program (1980) provides basic audiology services. There are standard fees for services but no one is denied services if they cannot pay. EARS (Early Audiologic and Rehabilitation Services) is a program newly funded by the Division of Aging and Administered by the Division of Public Health, Office of Speech and Hearing Services.

EARS will provide help to elderly hearing-impaired Delaware residents who cannot afford the cost of hearing aids and related services. Most referrals to this center come from physicians but many come from community and state agencies, as well as self-referrals.

Washington, D. C. Hospital Center Program

The Washington, D. C. Hospital Center (1980) provides the basic services for the hearing-impaired. Once audiometric testing has been done, further testing is done to determine if hearing loss can be helped by a hearing aid. Once it is determined a hearing aid will be helpful, additional tests are conducted to determine which hearing aid will be best for the individual. As part of the Hearing Aid Program, an audiologist will fit the aid to the individual's earmold, make necessary modifications for wearing and listening comfort, and help clients become accustomed to it.

The Center charges a fee for all services, some of which may be taken care of by insurance. The person has a choice of where to buy the aid, through the Center or a hearing aid dealer. If purchased through the Center, the total amount of the hearing aid will be refunded if it is determined the hearing aid is not beneficial.

The Hearing Aid Program provides the individual with an opportunity to get used to wearing the aid in a variety of settings and to discuss with the audiologist any difficulty which may be experienced. The Center maintains contact long after the provision of the individual's aid. Questions about the aid can be asked at anytime. If there is need for repair, the Center will send it to an authorized dealer and provide the person with a loaner aid.

The Center also provides pamphlets which explain services as well as educate persons regarding the hearing aid.

The Boston Guild Program

The major emphasis of the program sponsored by the Boston Guild for the Hard of Hearing (Kennedy, 1981) is outreach programs which stress hearing conservation through early case finding. The Guild has two self-contained, completely equipped mobile units. Since 1970, the program has given hearing screening tests in 69 communities outside Boston. The mobile units are used to screen adults in local communities cooperating with boards of health and sponsoring service clubs. Other uses of the mobile units are the screening of preschool children in headstart programs and in private nursery schools. This program includes impedance tests as well as screening. A description of the Guild's cooperative plan follows.

(1) The Guild provides the mobile unit and a clinically certified audiologist for a chosen location.

(2) A master plan for publicity is prepared by the Guild and provided to the local health department for dissemination to the media. Names of as many locally participating people as possible (health officer, mayor, or head of board of selection, service club president, or head of service committee) appear in the releases.

(3) A receptionist provided by the sponsoring group assists the audiologist in seeing that everyone taking the test fills out a questionnaire, gives out free educational materials, and collects a 1-dollar fee.

(4) A list of test failures is given to the health department for follow-up. The department also 546receives questionnaires which have been comreceives questionnaires which have been completed by persons taking the test.

(5) Health department nurses follow up test failures by letter or telephone.

The sponsoring service clubs often request a speaker to explain the project, and will contribute $200.00 toward the cost of a maximum 2-day program in a community. If sponsoring groups such as the Council on Aging or Visiting Nurses pay the full cost of $160.00 a day, there is no charge for tests. Screening tests are occasionally administered free of charge at health fairs or multi-service centers in depressed areas. The mobile unit is also used for baseline testing in industries too small to set up their own hearing conservation programs.

An information and referral service handled 6400 requests in 1980. In addition, orientation lectures are held for nurses in training, schools of practical nursing, nursing home supervisors, personnel executives, social workers, rehabilitation counsellors, public welfare supervisors, and guidance counsellors.

The majority of clients using the Guild's hearing aid evaluation and counselling services are adults in the older age group but the outreach program includes many pre-school children. Six lipreading classes for adults are held yearly at the agency. A program of training volunteer lipreading teachers to work with the elderly in outlying communities has been in operation for 6 years. Forty-two volunteer teachers have been trained in a 40-hour course. Free lipreading classes for the elderly have been held in 40 communities.

A brochure describing the Guild's hearing aid evaluation service indicates the following.

"The Boston Guild provides a unique, highly personalized, non-commercial audiological testing and hearing aid evaluation service. It is by appointment only and takes one and one-half hours. If tests indicate that a hearing aid may help, you will be evaluated with different, appropriate hearing aids to determine the one most suitable for you. You will then be referred to a reputable hearing aid dealer who will fit you with the aid we recommend. In addition, free follow-up sessions are available every Thursday morning at the Guild without appointment. The fee for this complete service is $60.00. The comprehensive professional services are available at low cost thanks to a small endowment from hearing-impaired persons themselves and from partial support of the United Way of Massachusetts. To minimize billing costs, clients are asked to pay the fee at the reception area at the time of appointment. If there is financial need, fees can be adjusted by contacting the Guild's counselor by letter or phone before the appointment."

To this author, the most relevant aspect of the programs described is the fact that community programs can be implemented. Considerable energy must be expended if change is to be effected. We have a major role to play if we are sincerely interested in involvement and the challenge offered by helping people with hearing impairment.

Whether the community aural rehabilitation program is one which has been in existence for some time or relatively new, justification for its continued existence must be established. The community must be convinced that the program is an integral and important part of the total health care system. Goldstein (1971) states that we can evaluate program performance by asking the following questions.

(1) How important is the problem toward which the program has been directed?
(2) How much of the problem was solved?
(3) How effectively did the activities attain their objective?
(4) What was the cost in resources of attaining the objectives?

Goldstein (1971) indicates that there are no standards for determining or measuring appropriateness. The ability to measure program effectiveness, adequacy, and efficiency depends on whether measurable statements about the components of programs can be provided. We must agree in advance how health status should be measured.

References

ALPINER, J. G., *The Utilization of Supportive Personnel in Speech Correction in the Public Schools.* Denver: Colorado State Department of Education (1970).
ALPINER, J., MUSSEN, E., NORTHERN, J., REED, D., AND SODERBERG, M., Community aural rehabilitation programs. *J. Acad. Rehab. Audiol,* **6,** 31–34, (1973).
AMERICAN NATIONAL STANDARDS INSTITUTE, *Specifica-tions for Audiometers. ANSI S3.6—1969.* New York: American National Standards Institute, Inc. (1970).
AMERICAN SPEECH-LANGUAGE-HEARING ASSOCIATION, Guidelines for employment and utilization of supportive personnel. *ASHA,* **23,** 165–168 (1981).
AMERICAN SPEECH AND HEARING ASSOCIATION, Guidelines for identification audiometry. *ASHA,* **17,** 94–99 (1975).
COMMUNITY SPEECH AND HEARING CENTER, VENTURA, CALIFORNIA, personal communication (1980).
DENSON, T. A., LUBINSKI, R., BURKE, J. P., SCHIAVETTI, N., AND CHAPEY, R., The role of community colleges in providing language, speech, and hearing services. *Community/Junior College Research Quarterly,* **1,** 157–162 (1977).
DEVOE, M. F., Audiology in the big sky country. *Hear. Speech News,* **42,** 16–17,29 (1974).
EMPLOYERS INSURANCE OF WAUSAU, *Industrial Noise and Hearing Protection.* Wausau, WI: Employers Insurance Company (1967).
GOLDSTEIN, H., Principles of evaluation of public health services. In *Workshops on Speech Pathology and Audiology in Public Health.* Berkeley: University of California (1971).
HOLANOV, S., Public attitudes of adults regarding hearing. Paper presented at Annual Meeting of the Academy of Rehabilitative Audiology, Houston, Texas (1976).
KENNEDY, C. K. (BOSTON GUILD FOR THE HARD-OF-HEARING), personal communication (1981).
MARKIDES, A., BROOKS, D. N., HART, F. G., AND STEPHENS, S. D. G., Aural rehabilitation of hearing-impaired adults. *Br. J. Audiol.* **13,** 7–14 (1979).
NEWMAN, E., The future for rehabilitation. *Hear. Speech News,* **38,** 16–17,20 (1970).
NEW YORK LEAGUE FOR THE HARD-OF-HEARING, personal communication (1980).
OLSEN, B., Mid-Maine Medical Center, personal communication (1981).
OWENS, E., GERBER, C., AND UKEN, D., Two years of a program in hearing related services. *Arch. Otolaryngol.,* **104,** 495–500 (1978).
PORTER, E. B., AND SMITH, J. H., Hearing loss, a community loss. *Hear. Speech News,* **41,** 20–21,28 (1973).
SATALOFF, J., AND MICHAEL, P. L., *Hearing Conservation.* Springfield, IL: Charles C Thomas (1973).
SCHOW, R. L., AND NERBONNE, M. A., *Introduction to Aural Rehabilitation.* Baltimore: University Park Press (1980).
SMITH, J. H., AND PORTER, E. B., *Hearing Loss, A Community Loss.* Washington, D. C.: American Hearing Society (1958).
STEPHENS, S. D. G., Rehabilitation of the hearing impaired adult in Denmark. *Clin. Otolaryngol.,* **4,** 95–98 (1979).
UNIVERSITY OF TEXAS (DALLAS), personal communication (1980).
WASHINGTON, D. C. HOSPITAL CENTER, personal communication (1980).
WILMINGTON, DELAWARE MEDICAL CENTER, personal communication (1980).
WILSON, W., AND WALTON, W. K., Identification audiometry accuracy: evaluation of a recommended program for school-age children. *Language, Speech and Hearing Services in Schools,* **5,** 132–142 (1974).

11

Toward a Scientific Basis for Rehabilitative Audiology

Jerry V. Tobias

EMPIRICISM

Once upon a time, not so long ago, I lost the friendship of a particularly pleasant and attractive person who called to tell me that we could not meet as planned that afternoon because of an automobile problem: my friend had come within a hairsbreadth of being hit by a rather large car. "I knew there'd be a problem today. My horoscope said I'd have an accident." I should have clucked sympathetically. But my friend was unhurt, and I was trained to measure things, so instead I applied my interest in numbers.

"How many signs of the zodiac are there?" I asked.

"Twelve."

"And how many people in the United States?"

"I don't know—more than 200 million, I guess."

"Okay. How many of those 200 million have your sign?"

My friend didn't have a calculator handy, but I did, and the answer was something near 17 million. I said so. Then I made my mistake: I said that I could hardly wait for the evening newspaper to come out with its report of 17 million accidents that day.

My friend thought I wasn't taking the matter seriously enough.

Once upon another time, a longer time ago, during an oral examination, a teacher of mine asked for a conclusion about a particular kind of pathological problem and its effect on people who might suffer from it. We had seen only one case and read about a couple of others, so I said that I didn't know how to draw conclusions based on the clinical impression I had. The professor asked, "What do you have against clinical impressions?" and I had quite a bit of trouble answering. I talked about the imprecision of simple uncontrolled observations (but I recognized that often such observations are not only the total information available but that they are the source of ideas that lead to good, scientific experiments in the laboratory or in the clinic) and the commonly misleading generalizations that stem from studying or even measuring individuals or groups of individuals who have some specific characteristic in common (but I also recognized that sometimes those generalizations turn out to be true or at least based in truth). I finally came to the underlying concept that led me to my original answer: empirical measurement such as we had been doing is no substitute for scientific measurement when you want to develop usefully predictive theories.

My teacher was not awfully pleased.

The difference between empirical measurement and scientific measurement of people comes clear when you study the history of neurophysiology, particularly the part that deals with which parts of the brain receive information about and control which functions. The concept of cortical localization goes back to a time long before techniques existed to record brain potentials or to stimulate small segments of the nervous system.

Once upon a time, a long time ago, the original localization experiments were done by an anatomist named Franz Joseph Gall. He worked during the late eighteenth and early nineteenth centuries.

Empirical behavioral research, such as every research worker did in those days, is characterized by the study of cases or subjects who display the attributes you are interested in.

Scientific behavioral research, such as most research workers do today, is characterized by the comparison of cases or subjects who display the attributes you are interested in with others who do not display those attributes or by the comparison of cases or subjects who have received a particular treatment with others who have not.

Some other factors differentiate between the empirical and the scientific study, but for this discussion, the question of experimental controls (as the people who do not display the attribute or have not received the experimental treatment are called) is the critical one.

Gall, working with his colleague Johann Caspar Spurzheim, was an empiricist with a remarkable insight into the workings of the brain. He was convinced that the location of a burst of brain activity defined the nature of the visible response. Thus, Gall made the early steps that now permit the interpretation of electroencephalograms, the success of many kinds of brain surgery, and the measurement of evoked cortical and subcortical responses to externally applied signals. Gall and Spurzheim finished their books on the subject five years before Pierre Paul Broca's birth and fifty years before Korbinian Brodmann's (Broca and Brodmann are the names people most often think of in connection with the development of theories of the localization of cerebral function; they almost never think of Gall and Spurzheim).

When Gall and Spurzheim tried to figure out how to demonstrate the truth of their contention, they had to use the methods that were available in the 1810s or methods they could invent that were based on contempo-

rary methods. They knew that they couldn't successfully open living skulls and poke around inside, but they were anatomists and they had access to occasional cadavers for study. They ran a few tests and concluded that the skull fits like a cap over the brain and that its thickness is pretty constant. A scientific (rather than empirical) investigator would have made such measurements on a large number of skulls and would have studied variability; in the early nineteenth century, that wasn't considered important. The result is that their conclusions, although probably fairly accurate for the small sample they used, wouldn't hold up today.

Then, working from the skullcap assumption and the constant thickness assumption, they began collecting people with extreme behavior patterns in certain categories. They found a person who was a poet. They found one who was a fighter. Another was lazy. One was amorous. These people and dozens more were studied carefully and thoroughly, with Gall and Spurzheim recording overdeveloped areas for each person, and when they were through, they published an atlas of brain regions, much as Brodmann did about a hundred years later. Gall named the system "craniology." Spurzheim called it "phrenology."

They made two errors that we would now consider to be critical: the lesser of these is the one that a modern reader laughs about, and that is their assumption about the skull surface replicating the brain surface; the greater mistake was their dependence on empirical research. If their feisty subject had a lump on his skull, they were led by the skull assumption to assume, not that he'd been hit there (for instance), but that an underlying lump on his brain defined his bellicosity. The empirical method led them to believe that *everyone with a similar personality characteristic had a similar lump.*

Had the scientific method been available to them, they would have tested many fighters and they would have contrasted those people's lumps with the lumps of nonfighters. And they'd have rapidly found the impropriety of the skull-thickness assumption. As it was, they did the best empirical research that they knew how to do in those days. Yet instead of recognizing the work as a classic and important forerunner (which it is) of modern neurophysiology, neurosurgery, and neuroscience, we laugh at it.

My teacher who wanted to make a generalization based on a case observation and my friend who wanted to believe a horoscope were making Gall's mistake. They knew of a circumstance or two or ten in which the kinds of conclusion-jumping that they were interested in had seemed to fit the facts, and they didn't bother or had not yet been able to look at additional evidence or to study contradictory cases or to perform controlled scientific experiments.

The eagerness to believe, in both instances, takes on the form of a kind of superstition. The superstitious nature of decisions based on astrology is recognized by many—maybe most—people. The superstitious nature of decisions based on case reports is disguised, and, because case reports so often have led to ideas that have in turn led to good scientific research, most people overlook the errors, ignore (as Gall did) the cases that don't match the model, and forget the skepticism that they were taught to apply to research findings during the fraction of a semester when the scientific method was discussed.

RESEARCH IN THE CLINIC

Despite mankind's long, sometimes silly history of drawing questionable conclusions from nonscientific case observations, studies of clinical cases need not be based in superstition. In fact, if a clinical worker understands how to plan diagnostic and therapeutic activities appropriately, each client or patient can become a scientific-research resource.

Before I sketch some of the kinds of approaches one might take, let me list the areas in which a rehabilitative audiologist might want to conduct single-subject experiments.

To practice rehabilitative audiology, one simply helps hearing-impaired people to learn to understand what they hear and, sometimes, to learn to talk so that others can understand what they say. In order to create an atmosphere in which clients or patients will be receptive to help, one must also counsel them about potential difficulties and help them to accept the handicapping nature of hearing loss. Finally, one needs to develop

and maintain cordial relationships with members of other professions that are concerned with physical and mental health, with rehabilitation, and with society. All four of these primary functions—improving hearing, improving speech, improving self-acceptance, and improving professional interactions— can be subjects of research, and an audiologic practitioner might want to apply scientific principles to the study of any of them. By training and inclination, most audiologists will prefer to work on the first two, but the techniques I'll talk about are certainly applicable to all sorts of issues.

Laboratory research is the sort that we commonly think of when someone mentions *science*. That's the variety that our instructors usually tell us about in college, and that's the kind that the preponderance of journal articles discuss. Laboratory research is valuable, important, and, for some kinds of problems, necessary. Yet, immediately useful information is more likely to arise from single-subject (if you want to sound high class, say within-subject, and if you want to sound fancy, say intra-subject) clinical studies than from laboratory research.

The single subject of the within-subject clinical experiment is the same client or patient with whom you would be working anyway. An experiment can easily be incorporated into the normal testing, teaching, and counseling periods without interfering with the subject's progress. Indeed, some people may be led to more rapid improvement by experimental audiologists than by the ones who follow procedures that they have tried before and therefore believe to be true. Part of the reason is that new concepts may be developed experimentally, but a bigger part is that people aren't alike. Some kinds of experiments help to determine which of several procedures will work best on the particular person being studied.

Case reports are not scientific documents. Generally, such reports are just descriptions, sometimes lengthy ones (maybe because the writer doesn't know how to separate what's important from what's unimportant), based on uncontrolled observation. They are easy to write, and once in a while a reader may garner an insight into a client's problems, but those small virtues are outweighed by the purely subjective nature of the writing and reading. Most of the material is in the form of statements of opinion, and when quantitative matter *is* included, it often suffers from the same kinds of flaws that misled Gall and Spurzheim.

Case studies, on the other hand, can frequently be important additions to knowledge. (Remember, please, that the term *report* or *study* used by an author does not differentiate between reports and studies; only the content will tell a reader which is which.) They follow comparatively modern research designs that use the subject not only as the experimental case, but as the control case too. An especially easy method calls for comparisons between the results one gets using one procedure with the client and the results one gets using another, alternative procedure; then, in order to minimize the drawing of mistaken conclusions, one goes back to the beginning to repeat both the first and second treatments (or tests or teaching methods or whatever is being investigated) to see whether the results are a consequence of the procedure or of something else (Hersen and Barlow, 1976; Barlow and Hayes, 1979). Repetitions of the cycle may continue several more times, depending on the nature of the question and the importance of correctly interpreting the outcome.

In a study of teaching methods, for example, these alternations of procedures will not be made in rapid succession. Instead, the first method will be used for a predetermined number of sessions (maybe only one, but maybe several), during and immediately following which measurements of improvement or change are made. Then the other method will be used for a similar number of sessions, during and following which measurements are made. And so on. Each procedure must be given a long enough time to produce some effect—if in fact that procedure can produce any effect.

The reason for using the method-comparing process and the cycling of one technique (call it A) with another (call it B), then with one again and another again (call the whole series ABAB) is that you haven't shown the efficacy of what you did unless you can show that what you tried led to the observed effect on the client or patient. Suppose that the passage of time is all that's required to make a change in your client. If you only used technique A, you might be fooled into believing that the change was a function of A. If you only tested A-followed-by-B, you might be fooled into believing that A helped some but that B helped more. But if you tried ABAB, the data (in a situation in which time is the effective factor) would show a continuous improvement. That wouldn't necessarily mean that neither A nor B helped. But it would mean either that they were about equally useful or that some external element—such as time—was more important than either of them. Additional experimentation, carefully planned, could tell you which.

In general, though, what you learn is that either A or B is consistently more effective. For example, if A creates an increase in the desired performance, then B shows an increase too, but smaller than A's, you are on the track of learning which technique will work better with your client. If, when you return to A for the second (or third or fourth) time, the increase grows large again, and when you return to B it grows small again, you know to concentrate the rest of your work on that problem on technique A. Once you have successfully replicated your experiment, you can discard the poorer procedure and work with your client in the manner that is best for that particular person.

Logic dictates that sometimes the best comparison is between using a treatment and using no treatment; the data from such an experiment can tell you whether the treatment was worth using at all. However, for some kinds of case studies, ethical considerations should prevent you from performing this "best" experiment. As rehabilitative-audiologist experimenters, we have to exercise our best judgment about withholding treatment from someone who has come to us for help. Refusing to do anything at all for a while may lead to critically important information about what to do for that person, but it also has the potential of creating psychological or developmental problems. The difficulty is less troublesome when you work with adults than when you work with children, but it is real, nevertheless, for some members of any age group. (Withholding treatment from some young children during a developmentally critical period may have far-reaching negative effects.) One must be careful to make these decisions on the basis of what is best for the client, because it's tempting to make them in ways that will "make the experiment come out right."

Unlike laboratory studies, single-subject experimental studies can be individualized to meet the specific and special needs of a given client or patient. For example, if you find yourself having to work with a person who has had a blow to the head, you won't be able to figure out how to approach that problem by generalizing from what you've seen of other people suffering from head injuries; those cases are just too different from each other. As Costello (1979) put it, "Whoever found . . . a homogeneous group of aphasic patients?"

Further, it's easy to forget that laboratory research findings, no matter how significant, may be totally useless in the clinic. Statistical significance—the kind that's reported in the usual journal article—tells whether the average scores in two populations (of people, of test scores, of whatever the research was designed to measure) are far enough apart to be truly different.[1] In a study in which a large number of people or a large number of test scores (or whatever) make up the populations that are under comparison, significant differences can sometimes be found for averages that are very close together. But an individual measurement that went into the calculation of the average for Population 1 might itself be far away from that average. And an individual measurement that went into the calculation of the average for Population 2 might be far away from its population average too. Looking at those individual measurements one at a time, you might be completely unable to judge which population either one came from. That is, the masses of data from all the subjects form distribution curves that are, statistically and graphically, clearly separate from each other. Yet when someone asks you to look at a single test score and pick which

distribution it came from, most of the time you cannot do it—the curves overlap too much.

Figuring out how to treat a client or patient who comes to you for help is the same as being asked to look at a single score. For some kinds of tests, the populations are far enough apart that you can tell right away which distribution the score came from: pure-tone air- and bone-conduction audiometry separate the populations of conductive and nonconductive hearing losses by enough to make those tests clinically valuable for that differentiation. For more kinds of tests, the job is awfully hard: tympanography separates the populations of otosclerotic and nonotosclerotic pathologies, but only in a few percent of the cases will an individual result be extreme enough to tell you which population it came from. (That isn't to say that tympanography is clinically useless, but only that it is not much help in finding otosclerosis.)

Single-subject research designs of the sort outlined above, and of a number of other sorts too, are detailed in the book *Single Case Experimental Designs* by Hersen and Barlow (1976). To follow their recommendations, you must apply a little more rigor than some clinicians normally take into their work, but that in itself is valuable. More than that, the resulting case studies increase your potential for helping the clients you see today, increase your insight into how to help future clients, and help the profession when you publish reports of your studies.

SAMPLES OF USEFUL RESEARCH

Much of the writing on rehabilitative audiology has been anecdotal or descriptive. People say what they like to do with their patients or clients, and they tell stories about their special successes. They believe in what they do and want others to follow along. But most are only empiricists who collect evidence to support a viewpoint. Hardly any are scientists who develop their viewpoints *after* collecting and weighing the evidence.

We have comparatively few controlled, scientific experiments to draw upon. Some of those few have been laboratory studies, and some have been single-subject studies. Some have managed to combine the advantages of laboratory work with the advantages of sin-

---

[1] Actually, "truly different" isn't quite an accurate description, although, for this discussion, it's close enough. But for the sake of accuracy, *significantly different* populations have averages—means, most of the time—that are far enough apart that we can say that there is only a small chance that the separation could have occurred by accident.

gle-subject work; some have managed to combine the disadvantages.

Only a few topics have been looked at experimentally,[2] and a majority of them have been directed toward problems of children rather than adults. However, despite this book's emphasis on adults' problems, I am going to include some of the research on children in the following sketch of a few of the kinds of studies that have been done. The reason is that those experiments have applications to the whole population of hearing-impaired people, without regard for their ages.

In the section on "Research in the Clinic," I listed major components of a rehabilitative audiology program: counseling, helping the hearing-impaired person to understand what is said, teaching that person how to be understood by a listener, and developing and maintaining good professional relationships. The topics are all amenable to scientific study, but research on counseling and research on professional interactions belong, for the most part, in other disciplines. What follows, then, is limited to speech recognition and speech production. Hearing aids are touched on only lightly because they are covered in Chapter 3. Speech production is touched on only lightly because not much research has been published on speech production by the hearing impaired.

For at least 50 years, we have recognized that a listener's ability to understand speech that is being transmitted under difficult conditions (in high noise, at a low intensity, through a deaf ear) depends not only on the sound that reaches that listener's ear, but also on cues that arrive via other sense organs. For instance, a speech signal can be made less intelligible by adding masking noise to it. Suppose you keep adding noise until a normal-hearing listener can understand only 10 or 15% of the words. This test subject has never had any need to lipread and cannot be expected to have learned the techniques of

recognizing speech sounds visually by analyzing the positions of the talker's lips, jaw, and tongue. Despite that fact, letting the listener look at the talker produces dramatic improvements in intelligibility (Sumby and Pollack, 1954). For words from a restrictively small vocabulary (where one might expect that only a little information is necessary in order for a listener to figure out which word was being spoken), scores rise to 90% or more. For words from a larger vocabulary (which are less predictable), scores rise to only 40 or 50%, but even that is a significant improvement. Had the tests been done with connected discourse—speech in which one part of the message depends on other parts, creating a higher level of redundancy in the speech signals than one finds in lists of unrelated signal words—the scores might have risen considerably higher than 50% when visual information was added to auditory. (Although the Sumby and Pollack experiments found a limiting value of about 40% intelligibility for large vocabularies, other research indicates that continued increase in vocabulary size—that is, word-list size—leads to continued decrease in intelligibility. Nevertheless, the added redundancy of connected discourse suggests that real speech might behave more like single words from a small vocabulary and be considerably more intelligible than 40 or 50%.)

As C. V. Hudgins (1954) suggested, "the goal of our auditory training program for the profoundly deaf will be something less than that of establishing a hearing vocabulary or developing verbal discrimination by ear alone. . . . We can measure progress, however, in terms of the degree to which auditory perception supplements visual perception when both are applied simultaneously. . . ." He went a bit further than that, in fact, by saying that teaching speech perception and production to the deaf requires a multisensory approach (including touch as well as vision and hearing), even for the profoundly deaf for whom one might expect acoustic signals to be completely ineffective. He did some single-subject studies of hearing-impaired children that are comparable to the work on normal-hearing young adults reported by Sumby and Pollack (1954). He compared the speech intelligibility that results from hearing alone and from vision

---

[2] I exclude areas that are important to the practice of rehabilitative audiology but that do not stem from it. For example, learning theory, psychoacoustics, linguistics in its various forms, sociology, psycho- and neuropathology, and some additional fields all are necessary for a practitioner to have studied and to understand. But, although they are pertinent, they are not the specific preserve of this profession.

alone with the intelligibility from both together. For those children whom he classified as "partially deaf," the combination of hearing and vision gave scores of 79 to 98%, an improvement ranging from 12 to 44% over hearing alone and from 19 to 23% over lipreading alone. For those children whom he classified as "profoundly deaf," the combination of hearing and vision gave scores of 42 to 91%, an improvement ranging from 27 to 72% over hearing alone (a potentially misleading set of numbers because, for most of these children, hearing alone produced zero or near-zero intelligibility) and from a decrement of 7% (for one highly variable child) through an insignificant 0 or 1% (for several) to a high of 35% over lipreading alone. The average improvement over lipreading alone for the 13 children he tested was about 7%.

Three points need commentary. First, these scores come at the end of 3, 4, 5, or 6 years of training in special classrooms; when they were tested prior to training, these same children had far poorer scores. However, the trends were similar. Second, some authorities suggest that improvements that average only 7% or so are scarcely worth the trouble of fitting hearing aids to the profoundly deaf, but one can argue in rebuttal that, for a person who can lipread only half or two-thirds of the words that are spoken in these tests, an increase of 7 or 10% is a major addition to the information available. When the messages being received have context, as in everyday speech, the numbers will be even higher. Surely for these people, every little bit not only helps but is necessary for adequate functioning. Third, I need to say that the averages result from my own arithmetic, not Hudgins's. He, quite rightly, recognized the highly individual nature of each child's performance and reported their performances separately. Only single-subject studies are appropriate here, and the selection of treatment and of training procedures for each child needs to be made on the basis of that child's status. Averages are valuable if one is trying to decide, for example, whether a new, untrained person ought to be given a hearing aid; in that situation, a guess based on population statistics will help. But once one begins to gather data on a person's progress, that person has to be considered separately from anyone else with regard to many kinds

of information. That individuality is maintained both in the clinical setting and in the research setting.

The preponderance of the research that has been done since the Hudgins (1954) report is on related topics, expanding, extending, and refining his findings. This sort of replication, repetition, modification, confirmation, and reconfirmation is a critical part of scientific research. Only when an experimental result proves to be consistently repeatable is its truth satisfactorily demonstrated. A primary reason that journal editors so strongly insist that the method, the procedure, and the equipment used be spelled out in close detail is to insure that a person who wants to try to replicate the study can do so. Often, slight changes in method lead to large changes in results, so the accuracy of the description is essential. (The other major reason for including those details is so that a reviewer or a reader can judge the appropriateness of the experiment to the question whose answer is being sought.) Remember that the key to progress in science is skepticism and doubt, not only about reports and studies done by other people, but about your own as well. Faith in the written word and acceptance of authority have no place in the reading and writing of reports of laboratory experiments, of single-subject clinical experiments, or even of clinical progress.

I won't review the dozens of articles that follow in Hudgins's path, but I will mention a few of them.

In 1972, Erber compared normal-hearing children and adults with profoundly deaf children in their ability to lipread with and without accompanying sound. Unlike Hudgins, he used two sorts of sounds: one was the speech that was being watched (used only with the deaf children); the other was a noise whose intensity and time patterns matched those of the speech, but whose waveform did not. The six deaf children he tested averaged about 11% higher when the sound of the speech was added to the lipreading-alone condition. Everyone averaged 6 to 8% higher when the shaped noise was added. Erber suggested that these improvements that range from 6 to 11% are essentially equivalent to each other, although the paper doesn't include either the individual scores for us to check or a statistical analysis to confirm that conclusion. Nevertheless, whether the numbers are statistically different or not, certainly the fact that a modulated noise creates an increase in performance level that is about the same size as the Hudgins (1954) 7% has to be meaningful. It says that unrecognizable sounds that convey information about rhythm may be as useful as amplified speech in improving the understandability of word lists for the profoundly deaf listener. And that suggests some other kinds of experiments— experiments with sense organs besides ears as the conductors of rhythm information.

During World War II and for 20 years or so afterwards, a number of scientists tried to find ways to transmit speech signals to workers in noisy environments by attaching sets of electrodes or of vibrators to the arm, the chest, the back, or another part of the body. The effectiveness of such transmissions was poor. Further, electrical stimulation proved to be hard to control adequately: once the intensity of the shock rose above the threshold, an extra 10 or 20 dB would be enough to cause pain, and a worker's external and internal environments constantly change the threshold. Neither electrodes nor vibrators seemed capable of transmitting enough information to produce anything even close to the equivalent of an ear's response to the simplest spoken message, so, for a long time, research on and interest in "skin speech" ceased.

But research on using such devices as adjuncts to lipreading was only beginning.[3] Single-channel, dual-channel, and multi-channel devices have been tried. Let me tell you about a study done at the complex end of that dimension. Sparks et al. (1979) tested a system that split speech signals into 36 adjacent frequency bands of varying widths, then split each band into 8 intensity-range segments, making a total of 288 information-carrying channels. Each channel sent its message to one electrode, and the rectangular array of 288 electrodes was fitted into a cushioned elastic belt that was "applied to the abdomen of the wearer," one of three normal-hearing

young women. One may question some of the details of how tests were performed, and that sort of questioning is necessary in order to interpret the value of the results. For example, in this study, one may ask whether the sensory receptors of the abdomen are as capable of discriminating 288 closely spaced stimulation positions as the hand or arm or tongue might be (although those parts of the body offer less surface for the attachment of electrodes); the question is important because better results might have been obtained had a different part of the body been used. Also, one may wonder whether acoustic cues to speech were adequately removed by the earplugs and masking noise that were used. Earplugs make insignificant changes in the signal-to-noise ratio, and the masking noise was presented at only 80 dB SPL; we already know from the Sumby and Pollack (1954) study that the availability of lipreading to normal-hearing listeners makes speech intelligible even when it's masked at an extremely detrimental signal-to-noise ratio.

Despite our not knowing as much about the test conditions as we'd like, the results are instructive. For at least the first 12 or 15 hours of testing (at 1 hour per day), the scores with the belt were a consistent 10 or 15% better than the scores by lipreading alone. After 12 hours (by which time her scores had risen to 50%), one subject's results for the belt and the nonbelt conditions became quite similar to each other—you can't tell by looking at the scores whether she was using the electrode array or not.

The authors noted that this multi-channel device produced improvements that are inferior to those found elsewhere for a two-channel device. Inferior may be too strong a word, but certainly the results of this study show the multi-channel system to be no better than the two-channel, another hint that the effective information may be in the rhythm or the prosody of the speech.

Lipreading efficiency can be predicted, on the basis of external evidence, to be limited to 30 or 40%; no more than that proportion of speech sounds can be seen—the rest are hidden inside the mouth. (No one has done the study that will tell us whether the visible sounds are used in normal conversation more frequently, less frequently, or the same as the invisible sounds. That information might

---

[3] That's not quite true: R. H. Gault (1928) was using a hollow tube to carry vibrations from a talker's mouth to a listener's hand starting around 1924, and those vibrations improved lipreading scores by about 10%. Following that work, though, nothing much happened until the 1970s.

change the numbers a little.) When an extra set of cues is provided by a skin stimulator or by near-threshold, distorted, or masked sound, a 10 or 15% improvement occurs. On that foundation of reasoning, together with the actual data we've looked at, we can say that, for a speech signal that is transmitted well optically but poorly acoustically, scores higher than 60% are rare. Still, Hudgins (1954) reported that about a quarter of the profoundly deaf children he studied did better than that. A few of them did a lot better. Some mysteries remain. If you wonder how lipreading alone is postulated to be capable of producing intelligibility scores of 40%, but manages to make 50% improvements when it is added to poor hearing and leads to scores of 60% and sometimes more when it is used by the profoundly deaf, I wonder too. Something special is going on somehow. The answers are simply not known. Yet.

Let me sample a few other studies of speech understanding before going on to the less extensive categories of education and speaking.

A vibrator or electrode—and maybe a distorted voice—carries timing information to the lipreader. If that timing information happens to be related to voicing, as it likely is in most of the conditions that have been tested, then it may provide information about something more than rhythm: it may help with consonant discrimination by letting the listener discriminate among sounds that look alike (homophenous sounds). Voicing and voice-onset-time data can help a listener to tell the difference between members of a homophenous group such as /p/, /b/, and /m/. Walden et al. (1974) wondered whether they could predict the amount of improvement in test scores on the basis of how much confusion about homophenous sounds the combination of vision and hearing could clear up. After testing 100 men who had a wide range of audiometric configurations, they calculated the value of their prediction formula and determined that it could account for about half of the improvement, a statistically good result that isn't very valuable in the clinic.

When an experimental investigation looks at an old problem in a novel way and comes up with results that are similar to those that were found previously, that study strengthens

the acceptability of the earlier work. Steele et al. (1978) used a modern technique to measure the relative contributions of vision and hearing to the understanding of speech. Instead of measuring the proportion of correct responses for a particular amount of distortion (or noise or hearing loss or whatever), they used an adaptive procedure in which they adjusted the signal-to-noise ratio until they got a preselected percentage of correct answers. They chose two performance levels for their measurements: one near the high end and one near the low end of the linear segment of the curve that describes the effect of noise on intelligibility. For the normal-hearing young adults they tested, the addition of vision to a hearing-only situation was worth 13 or 14 dB. In addition, the changes in signal-to-noise ratio that were necessary for them to shift from one performance level to the other are comparable to what Sumby and Pollack (1954) reported, helping to confirm the accuracy of both studies.

This 13- or 14-dB improvement is equivalent to a 50% increase in the understandability of the speech.[4] Once again, the data indicate that visual information may be more valuable in the interpretation of difficult speech transmissions than is auditory information. Certainly, the studies that have been done so far point to that interpretation in the situation in which clear vision and fuzzy hearing are involved. An auditory signal added to a visual signal for a person who can lipread may be worth an extra 15% in intelligibility. A visual signal added to an auditory one may be worth an extra 50%.

A recommendation can be drawn from that set of numbers. Like all recommendations for clinical practice, whether drawn from research or nonresearch information, it needs to be looked at skeptically and to be reevaluated from time to time. For the moment, though, it makes sense to recognize that lipreading is a major factor in the understanding of speech and that, despite arguments to the contrary by a number of authorities (see Best,

---

[4] A 50% increase in a score can only be measured when the original score is small. If your hearing-only scores were 70, 80, or 90%, then, no matter how carefully you ran your experiment, you would never get a score higher than 100%. This silly-sounding principle has occasionally tripped up highly experienced research workers.

1978) who question the usefulness of lipreading training, such training is fundamental to successful rehabilitation. When the teaching of lipreading doesn't lead to results that meet our expectations, we need to develop new methods, and certainly current methods of training and methods for testing progress need an awful lot of work. They will continue to need it for a long time to come.

Lipreading alone isn't enough, though. When a person is limited to understanding only a minor fraction of what's being said, an extra 7 to 15% is precious. That little bit more can make the difference between success and failure, so it has to be cultivated. It is the amount of improvement that acoustic, vibratory, or electrical stimulation can provide, and since hearing aids are technologically further advanced than vibrators or shockers, auditory training is the recommended approach even for the profoundly deaf client or patient. Of course, the clinician ought to conduct single-subject experiments as a part of the rehabilitation program, and one set of those experiments needs to be devoted to a demonstration of whether auditory training is worthwhile for that particular person. Because each person is different, or because we don't know enough yet to be able to discover which ones are alike, a demonstration of the merit of auditory training (and lipreading and anything else that is done) has to be made anew for each person.

Is age a factor in a person's ability to succeed in a rehabilitation program? Or, to be more precise, does something that happens to us as we grow older affect our ability to succeed? The something might be a greater susceptibility to mental or physical fatigue, for example; it might be experience; it might be something that no one has thought of yet. Shoop and Binnie (1979) considered whether some age-influenced process changes the visual perception of speech. Their subjects were people in a broad range of age groups, all of whom had normal hearing and normal or corrected-to-normal vision. They found a decrement in performance as their subjects' ages increased. Age is indeed a factor, and that may mean that different training procedures have to be worked out, that different schedules of work with older people need to be arranged, that more work is necessary in order to reach a given level of performance,

or that older people have lower plateaus that mark the maximum progress they can make. Or it may mean none of those things; the tests were run only on normal subjects, and not one of the interpretations I just made has been tested scientifically.

We've talked at length about distortions of the acoustic signal. Erber (1979) distorted the optical signal. By moving a rough-surfaced Plexiglas screen to points at various distances in front of the talker, he created a continuum of visual fuzziness. Not unexpectedly, he found that optical degradation is an effective way to interfere with communication, just as acoustic degradation is. That the finding seems obvious does *not* mean that the work shouldn't have been attempted and reported. Obvious conclusions sometimes turn out to be false, and even when one proves to be true, valuable information can be garnered from the quantification of the phenomenon.

In his discussion of the work, Erber suggested several clinical applications for the screen. A couple of the more interesting ones are its use (1) to show severely hearing-impaired clients the value of amplification as a lipreading aid under poor optical conditions and (2) "to guide a child's use of acoustic cues as an aid to lipreading." In other words, by making experimental reductions in the amount of information available to the eye, one may force the person's auditory system to work harder and thereby to accept a larger role in the speech-understanding process. The idea is intuitively appealing, but, so far as I know, no studies have been done to tell us whether that weaning-away-from-vision is desirable.

An exceptionally complete, exceptionally thoughtful, and exceptionally readable review of what we know about hearing aids and their value for wearers was recently published by a group of research workers from the Massachusetts Institute of Technology (Braida *et al.* 1979). After critical readings of hundreds of reports of experiments on amplification, signal compression, and signal coding, the authors of that review concluded that "the research ... is far from inspiring." The data from studies of frequency/gain characteristics of hearing aids are inadequate. The impairments of the subjects in the experiments have been poorly characterized. Test materials are not suited to the tasks they're used for. Recent technical advances haven't yet been incorporated into hearing aids, so laboratory studies and clinical studies contradict each other. In fact, discrepancies among laboratory studies suggest that considerably more research will have to be done before we can make any sense out of such problems as how to select optimum types and levels of signal compression. Training methods are inadequate and are not long enough, intense enough, or consistent enough. And so on and so on.

Our lack of knowledge about amplification, which may be the portion of rehabilitative audiology upon which the largest quantity of controlled scientific research has been done, is nearly as great as our lack of knowledge about the rest of the field.

And when we look at the newest kind of hearing aid, the cochlear implant, not surprisingly, we discover that most of our knowledge of effectiveness or ineffectiveness is based in descriptions—instead of tests—of auditory behavior. At best, information is only derived from empirical studies; science is not much a part of cochlear implantation so far. In 1961, Békésy, discussing fads and procedures for which the scientific basis was limited, poor, or unknown, said that "more preliminary experiments could and should be done on animals before surgical experiment is undertaken on human patients." Surgical invasion of the inner ear for the purpose of implanting wires is certainly experimental today. Basic physiological, psychoacoustic, neurological, and immunological background data are almost completely lacking. Even if those problems were solved, we still don't know how to encode the signals that the wires carry, and when we learn to do that, we still won't know how to train the patient to use the information in a way that would improve on the use that we know can be made of an externally applied vibrator.

In fact, training methods, training aids, and training patterns underlie a lot of rehabilitative activity. We are terribly ignorant. Research is sparse.

At the National Technical Institute for the Deaf in Rochester, New York, a computer-assisted procedure for teaching lipreading is being studied (Cronin, 1979; Sims *et al.* 1979). It uses a "data analysis video interactive device" called DAVID, which permits rapid access to any of 100 or more segments of videotape. DAVID can ask a question and, in response to a typewritten answer, repeat the question, rephrase it, go on to another statement based on the answer, change to a new question, or do whatever it is instructed—programmed—to do. In the first experiments run with DAVID, it seems to have been as good a teacher as the person who taught a group of control students in a conventional classroom situation.

An obvious advantage of using DAVID, particularly if it continues to do as well as the classroom teacher, is that it can be used without the presence of the human instructor, who can be working on other kinds of problems with other people. A less obvious advantage, but one that may turn out to be even more valuable, is that, because it analyzes the student's difficulties and selects lipreading material accordingly, it can rapidly move through the easy parts and extend practice on the material that is particularly hard for that student to master.

Gulian (1981) reported on another sort of training system—one that was designed to help teach hearing-impaired children to produce acceptable vowel sounds when they speak. The Computer Vowel Trainer (CVT) that she used is one of a number of such visual-aids-for-speech-training that have been talked about and built over the past 100 years or so. The CVT presents a pattern on a computer's display screen. The talker tries to reproduce the pattern by saying a vowel into a microphone, which in turn is fed into the computer and results in a pattern on the screen. The talker can see whether the vowel is close to or distant from the model, and the system is adjustable as to how precise or how sloppy a match it will accept. The CVT then provides the talker with a report of whether the attempt is acceptable or not.

Gulian recognized that "However impressive the technology of an aid, however interesting the theoretical rationale underlying its use, and however suggestive the successes achieved in single cases, its usefulness can be demonstrated only by objective assessments." And so she proceeded to compare an experimental group of profoundly deaf children with a matched control group who were trained according to the same schedule, but by a human teacher. Over an 18-month period, a faster-than-linear kind of learning was found, apparently accelerated by long pauses in the training: during a training cycle of, say, ten sessions, little progress was seen; when the work was resumed two or more months later, scores were higher than they had ever been before. Repeated cycles of vowel work and no vowel work led to successive leaps in performance.

At the end of the 18-month program, according to judges who listened to the children's speech, the CVT group and the traditionally trained group did about equally well (they were approximately 40% intelligible), with the CVT group a few percentage points better. But when training halted for both groups, an interesting and instructive change took place. After a month or so, both groups improved to about 50% understandable. Then, the CVT group continued to improve, but the control group began to decline. Nine months following the cessation of training, the control group had fallen back to 30%; the CVT group had climbed to and maintained about 60%. The people who had been given traditional training showed the often-reported decline in performance once they were out of the clinical situation. The machine-trained people did not.

Only one obvious difference between a human teacher and a computer teacher appears in this study. As Gulian said, the human teacher's evaluation criteria "cannot be constant and are influenced by a great number of variables (familiarity with the characteristics of the deaf speech and/or with the specific speaker, previously formed opinions of his or her proficiency, extent of teaching, etc.). The built-in criteria of the CVT ensure that an utterance has to meet the same precision whenever it is produced. . . ." The strong indication is that applying perfectly consistent criteria during training helps to prevent the extinguishing of the learned behavior.

Another kind of training problem was looked at by Walden et al. (1981), who wondered if concentrating training efforts on one portion of the speech-understanding problem—consonant recognition—might lead to better overall performance. They worked with three groups of men who had predominantly high-frequency, sensorineural hearing losses. All three were enrolled in a short aural rehabilitation program. One experimental group received, in addition, individual training on lipreading consonants. Another experimental group received, in addition to the aural rehabilitation program, individual training on auditory recognition of consonants. The third group received neither of the experimental treatments and served as a control.

The authors recognized that their experimental technique created a number of problems that confound the interpretation of the results, which were that, although all three groups improved in their ability to recognize consonants, the two experimental groups improved significantly more than the control group did. Of course, the extra, individualized training that the experimental groups received may account for that result, but it may not. Another experiment with a different kind of treatment of the control group will have to be done to tell us. But the study hints at a teaching technique that may some day be shown to be useful: concentrating on a portion of a problem in disordered communication might lead to a greater improvement than working on everything at once does. (Some studies in behavior shaping, in pedagogy, and in learning hint at the same thing.) However, until the completion of new, well designed, carefully controlled, scientific experiments on this kind of person—experiments developed to help tell us if that statement is true—we will not be able to make a rational judgment.

A set of experiments on quite a different topic (Tobias and Irons, 1973) led to another idea that might be applicable to the training of hearing-impaired people. The subjects in this study, normal-hearing young adults, were taught to "shadow" speech. That is, they repeated what they heard as they heard it. Then they listened to badly masked or badly distorted continuous-speech signals (paragraphs from the *Reader's Digest*) and were tested to measure changes in their ability to understand what was being said. As time passed, their experience increased, and they were able to change their beginning scores of 15 or 20% up to final scores of 70 or 80%.

Most of the subjects were asked to shadow continuously so that progress could be monitored at every moment. Just like Gulian's (1981) children, they improved for a while, came to rest at a plateau value, then showed a major improvement after a long time away from the test situation. (In Gulian's work, though, the students worked for a month or so and then took 2 months off before returning to the task; in this investigation, the listeners worked for an hour—reaching the plateau in about half an hour—and then took a week or two off.) One group of subjects was treated differently: they did not have to shadow continuously. They'd be tested for a minute or two every once in a while, but outside of that, they just listened to the distorted speech without repeating what they were hearing. That group improved all the way up to the maximum in just one session. Tobias and Irons took precautions to insure that the result was not an effect of shadowing ability. They suggested that a higher level of motivation might be creating that level of performance. Whatever the reason, though, the subjects who were not asked to respond while they were listening learned faster and more thoroughly than the others, they remembered the details of what they had heard (the others didn't), and they reached their maximum capacity much sooner, which suggests that perhaps we err when we require immediate responses from the people we work with on speech production, auditory training, and lipreading.

Experiments have not been done to confirm that this guess about the usefulness of a novel teaching method is anywhere near correct. We've looked at other interpretations of other research results, and as with them, this one offers no more than a suspicion of an inkling that an idea might have some value. The required research hasn't been done yet.

One other finding from the Tobias and Irons (1973) experiments may turn out to have some interest for rehabilitative audiologists. In part of their study, they increased the listening difficulty so that beginning scores fell to 5 or 10% instead of 15% and above. People who listened under those conditions never reached intelligibility scores beyond about 50%, no matter how long they practiced. Could that outcome mean that people who lose their hearing suddenly might never learn to use amplification adequately unless they get a good hearing aid immediately? Or (to extend the speculation further) could it mean that children who are born with high-moderate to severe hearing losses might never learn to make adequate use of their residual hearing—or maybe that they

might never learn to talk—unless they get to hear at least 15% of the speech around them at a very early age? I don't know, of course, because the experiments to test those questions have not been designed or run. But they could be if someone with access to an appropriate clinical population were interested enough.

Every good scientific study (and many of the not-so-good ones) has implicit in it the seeds of other studies. Usually, only the idea is there, but sometimes so is the method and the instrumentation. Twenty- and thirty-year-old publications can be as inspiring as the newest, and from time to time, forgotten concepts are rediscovered in older articles and found to be productive.

The number of existing laboratory and single-subject studies that could help a rehabilitative audiologist far exceeds the ones reported in this chapter. Some of them are cited in other parts of this book. Lots more are in any of a dozen journals (old and recent issues alike), in published proceedings of conferences, in the manuscripts of papers presented at the conventions of professional and technical societies, and in the conversations of colleagues. Just remember to read and listen critically and skeptically.

I could conclude this "Samples of Useful Research" section by saying that every aspect of rehabilitative audiology needs extensive research—and that's a fact—but a more useful approach to discussing our new directions is available.

NEW DIRECTIONS

Recently (National Institute of Neurological and Communicative Disorders and Stroke, 1979), hundreds of experts in speech-language pathology and audiology, in clinical medicine, in medical science, in psychological and physiological acoustics, in engineering, and in a number of other related specialties collaborated in the preparation of a report on the current status and future research needs of the field of communicative disorders. Most of this "New Directions" section is quoted directly from that report.

The selected quotations[5] are only a small

---

[5] The number following each quotation specifies the page(s) of the report (National Institute of Neurological and Communicative Disorders and Stroke, 1979) from which it was taken.

proportion of the suggestions and recommendations that the group made with regard to hearing. I have chosen material that has the potential to affect the practice of rehabilitative audiology directly, which means that I've left out a lot that was written about needs in diagnostic testing, in medicine and surgery, in neurophysiology, in pharmacology, in prevention of hearing pathology, and so on. I have discriminated (a little) against recommendations that are primarily aimed at the treatment of children since this book is concerned with the rehabilitation of adults.

Most of the problems of the near future are likely to be solved by laboratory research, but all of them are sure to benefit from the contributions of rehabilitative audiologists. Among the quoted comments and suggestions, you may find some that can be approached, at least in part, through single-subject studies or through evaluations of groups of clients or patients in an audiologic practice.

The Research-Needs List

"Can the new high-frequency emphasis hearing aids be used for patients with noise-induced and related high-frequency neural hearing losses?" (52)

"Since the risk for hearing loss and other communicative disorders (e.g., aphasia following stroke) increases with age, it is important to study the interactions between language and the relearning of spoken communication . . . Among the more broadly sketched questions, we include studies of [social and emotional effects of] hearing loss on the aged populations. Does auditory habilitation really help older patients communicate more effectively? . . . Studies comparing the communicative abilities of institutionalized and noninstitutionalized aged patients might provide useful data. Practical suggestions might emerge, such as enlarging hearing-aid controls so that the elderly will have less trouble manipulating switching devices. Because brain stem dystrophies have been reported in the aged, the study of binaural hearing-aid amplification may be an especially provocative issue for research." (56)

"Support should be given to studies of . . . the efficacy of habilitation programs." (60)

"What are the critical periods during which

hearing loss leads to central dystrophies? Are the effects of auditory deprivation reversible?" (79)

"Important findings have . . . been obtained regarding recognition and memory in tonal sequences. These findings are of importance in the study of central processing mechanisms as well as in providing a basis for studies of auditory perceptual learning, an area relevant to the development of practical auditory rehabilitation strategies.

"Of particular importance for the development of effective diagnostic, intervention, and rehabilitation strategies is the study of auditory perception in the hearing-impaired. For some time, research on the psychoacoustics of the hearing-impaired has paralleled that of normal psychoacoustics, but on a much smaller scale and usually several, if not many, years after the normal studies." (93)

"A pervasive problem in the psychoacoustics of the hearing impaired is that of individual differences. Not only are differences between subjects large, but there are often major interactions between subjects and the quantities being measured, some subjects showing effects that are opposite to those shown by other subjects. It is also both more difficult and more time-consuming to obtain data on the hearing-impaired as compared to subjects with normal hearing. The cumulative effect of these difficulties is that there is a paucity of psychoacoustic data on the hearing-impaired, and there have been only a few scattered attempts at developing psychoacoustic models of the impaired auditory system." (93)

"In order to understand auditory communication and disorders of communication it is essential that the processing of complex stimuli by the auditory system be understood. An understanding of the auditory processing of speech and speech-like stimuli is of particular importance. An abiding question is whether the nature of speech perception by the hearing-impaired is a simple consequence of the damage to the auditory system or the symbiotic effect of the damage and the lack of n'rmal experience with speech. Careful comparisons between prelingually and postlingually deafened persons' perception of speech would help answer these questions." (97)

"The psychophysics of direct electrical stimulation is a controversial area. At present, a few hearing-impaired persons have electrodes implanted in their cochlea, and detailed information on the electrical correlates of auditory sensation should be obtained from this population. Further implantation of electrodes in the human cochlea should be limited until such information is available. If in the future there is sufficient justification for additional implantation of electrodes in the human cochlea, then it is essential that these studies be rigorously controlled and that comprehensive pre- and postoperative audiological information be obtained on each subject. An important consideration in the study of electrical stimulation in the existing population of persons with cochlear implants is to separate out the electrical signal-transmission characteristics of the stimulating device from the auditory coding of electrical stimuli. In order to do this, the electrical input to the auditory system should be monitored directly." (99)

"Research on the psychoacoustics of the impaired auditory system should be increased substantially with due weight given to the development of quantitative theories of impaired auditory perception and the development of more effective diagnostic tests and rehabilitation procedures." (103)

"The psychophysics of direct electrical stimulation of the auditory system should be studied." (103)

"Since methodological problems occur throughout psychoacoustics, especially in the study of important new areas, methodological issues should be studied in their own right rather than as appendages to ongoing studies." (103)

"In order to derive more effective ways of prescribing hearing aids and for assessing their performance in speech communication, it is necessary to know more about how speech is perceived by the hearing-impaired. Studies should be designed to determine which features of speech are perceived by the hearing-impaired and how they relate to audiological measures of the subject's residual hearing." (110)

"A common problem reported by almost all hearing-aid users is the severely disruptive effects of unwanted sound on the desired speech message. Methods for reducing the effects of background noise in hearing-aid use need to be thoroughly explored. These may include the use of sophisticated signal processing techniques . . . as well as other, simpler expedients such as improved microphone placement." (110)

"The simplest monaural hearing aid consists essentially of an amplifier with frequency-selective gain and a simple form of amplitude limiting such as peak-clipping. At present, it is not known how to determine the optimum frequency-gain characteristic and clipping level. The results of recent research from several independent laboratories indicate that there are ways of shaping the frequency-gain characteristic for individual hearing-aid users so as to obtain significantly improved performance. Once the optimum frequency-gain characteristic and method of amplitude limiting for a given individual have been determined, the performance obtained under those conditions could serve as a touchstone for evaluating other sensory aids. Determining the optimum monaural system in each ear would also appear as a useful first step toward finding the optimum binaural hearing aid. A contingent problem is the development of an effective clinical procedure for obtaining, within the practical constraints imposed by clinical testing, a good approximation to this optimum set of characteristics.

"A problem of long standing is that of determining whether a binaural hearing aid is superior to a monaural hearing aid. Unfortunately, early attempts to resolve this problem led to inconclusive results. The problem is considerably more complicated than originally believed. Since binaural processes in the hearing-impaired are not fully understood, it is not known how binaural interactions should be taken into account in the prescriptive fitting of binaural hearing aids. Binaural interactions may even play a part in the prescriptive fitting of monaural hearing aids, if there is significant residual hearing in the unaided ear. A further complicating factor is that there are several different ways of routing signals from one or more microphones to either or both ears (the so-called CROS hearing aid, and variations of it).

"A fundamental weakness of previous attempts to solve the monaural-binaural controversy was that there was no well-established way of determining the optimum monaural or binaural amplification system for purposes of comparison. For example, in those studies in which no significant advantage was reported for the binaural hearing aid, the finding could have been a result of using a less-than-optimum binaural aid rather than the implied conclusion that binaural amplification is of little practical benefit." (110–111)

"Among the most pressing problems is that of determining why the prognosis for hearing aids among the elderly is so poor. Considering that the incidence of hearing impairment increases dramatically with the elderly, this is a problem of particular importance." (113)

"The possibility of radically recoding the speech signal so that it is entirely within the residual hearing of the hearing-impaired listener offers some hope for the long term. In order to do so, basic research is needed to establish general principles of transposition. Information is needed on what general cues can be transmitted in this way, rather than pursuing idiosyncratic studies on individual devices.

"For the short term, it is likely that small gains could be obtained by nonradical processing of the speech signal (e.g., adaptive frequency shaping, moderate frequency lowering). Optimum parameters of such systems should be developed, and practical procedures for prescribing the devices, for assessing their performance, and for providing training in their use should be pursued." (115)

"The development of wearable tactual or visual aids is of particular importance. A criticism of early research on tactual and/or visual aids is that the subject was only exposed to the display for limited periods of time. With a wearable display, the exposure to the display can be extended considerably. Length of exposure may well be one of the critical variables in developmental studies. The effect of prolonged exposure on ability to discriminate and to learn various tactual (or visual) patterns needs to be studied. . . . From the clinical standpoint, it is important to develop general principles whereby supplemental visual and/or tactual sensory aids would be prescribed. In broad terms, many of the issues are similar to those encountered with hearing aids: To what extent is individualized fitting . . . necessary for the optimal or near-optimal use of such an aid? What are the training needs for the effective use of such

an aid? In what practical ways can the effectiveness of the fitted aid be assessed reliably?" (118)

". . . the range of [speech] errors produced by all the deaf is extensive, and it is important to determine which errors are most damaging to intelligibility.

"Basic research is needed in order to develop quantitative models of speech production in the deaf." (126)

"Speech-training aids of various kinds should fit in the overall strategy for speech training. As a general principle, it is important to train the deaf speaker to make maximal use of his or her residual hearing. Effective acoustic amplification should be viewed as an essential requirement of any speech-training strategy.

"The potential value of many of the speech-training aids that have already been developed is being wasted because teachers do not know how to use them. The emphasis in developing these speech-training strategies should be on principles of usage rather than on device-specific procedures. . . . If a supplemental display of some kind is used and the required speech skill is learned, efficient methods of weaning the student from the display need to be developed.

At present, there is little quantitative information on the relative advantages (in terms of either increased proficiency or reduced learning time) in using the various speech-training aids that are available." (127)

"Although there have been important advances in the development of laboratory instruments for analyzing the speech of the deaf, there is an urgent need for the development of practical tests or measuring instruments that can be used in a classroom setting." (127)

"The thrust of most research on speech training of the deaf has been with respect to the needs of hearing-impaired children. The special problems of the deaf adult need to be identified, and appropriate training procedures developed. The range of problems encountered is likely to be much larger than for deaf children because of the diverse nature of the adult population. The proportion of post-lingually deafened persons necessarily increases with age, and it is likely that they will need different speech-training procedures. For example, maintenance of previously acquired speech skills may be a special problem for this group." (128)

"A ubiquitous problem in speech training, as in habilitation in general, relates to the skills of the trainer. There are wide variations in skills of teachers and clinicians working with the hearing-impaired. . . . Research in this area could help specify the skills required of the professionals and methods to train them." (128)

"Innovative uses of the telephone and broadcast media for enhancing the quality of life of the communicatively impaired, particularly those who are home-bound, need to be investigated." (130)

"Alerting and warning systems for the hearing-impaired have been found very useful. However, they lack uniformity and are not always designed for maximum effectiveness. Studies should be conducted to determine the most effective form of alerting and warning signals, and standards should be developed for their widespread use." (130–131)

"Emphasis should be placed on methods for improving the efficacy of hearing aids. This includes improved methods for evaluation, prescription, and habilitation . . . ." (131)

"[We should] examine the long-term effects of various modes of communication (Oral, Manual, and Total) and the use of appropriate sensory aids." (132)

"[We need] both basic and clinical studies of auditory deprivation. . . . This area is one of the most important developing scientific frontiers in the field of hearing." (136)

"Of particular importance is the psychoacoustics of the hearing-impaired. Although good work has been done in this area, the rate of progress has been insufficient considering the enormity of the problem and its implications for effective prevention, intervention and management of auditory disorders." (136–137)

"Although needs differ across different types of sensory aids, there are common research principles that pertain to all aids. Research on general methods of evaluating sensory aids is sorely needed. Within this framework there is a pressing need for realistic tests of communication ability (with and without a sensory aid). An equally pressing problem is that of developing effective habilitation strategies. One of the shortcomings of earlier

research on sensory aids is that evaluation and training have often been device-specific, with little scope for generalization to other sensory aids. If general principles subject to experimental evaluation can be developed, it is likely that coordinated comprehensive habilitation strategies of proven effectiveness could be developed. A problem of particular importance in the management of the severely hearing-impaired is the role of mode of communication. There are substantial differences between Oral and Total education philosophies, and an unbiased study is needed that would demonstrate unambiguously the relative merits of those approaches." (138–139)

"Whatever the specific form of the sensory aid, the aspect of wearability brings a new factor into play—that of prolonged stimulation. Very little is known about the effects of prolonged exposure to supplemental stimulation (visual or tactual), particularly during the early years of life. Basic research is needed in order to learn how best to take advantage of available technology." (139)

"There are a number of special considerations that need to be taken into account when working with the elderly. Individual differences in life history are typically much larger in the elderly population. There may also be important ancillary problems involving other modalities or the central processing system. The incidence of hearing impairment is substantially greater among the elderly than for any other age group. All of these factors need to be taken into account in developing sensory aids and realistic evaluation and rehabilitation strategies to be used with this age group." (140)

Comment about the List

All the problems that research workers have been tackling seem to need still more work. All the procedures, techniques, tools, methods of teaching, and tests that we use in the clinic seem either to have been inadequately validated or never to have been validated at all. Nearly everything that goes on in a rehabilitation program is, according to the NINCDS-selected panel of experts, subject to doubt as to its effectiveness and, therefore, is in need of investigation. Anyone who is willing to question, to doubt, to take the care that is required of a researcher, and to follow the rules of good scientific experimentation can participate—and should. We just don't know enough yet.

SKEPTICISM

It's easier to talk about what you already know than about how you can learn something new. As a result, people in all walks of life prefer to take a philosophical rather than a scientific approach to problem solving. So instead of talking to each other about facts, we mostly share guesses and feelings. Even when we have to decide the most important matters, we end up not by gathering data, but by gathering opinions.

We share ignorances in preference to figuring out how to measure the breadth of a problem or how to search for a rational solution to it. As one of my professors put it, a discussion is a lot less work when you're unencumbered by facts.

Many of our best known, most successful authority figures are as unencumbered as anybody. Every field has the same trouble. Diet books consistently climb to the top of the best-seller lists despite their lack of basis in sound nutritional research. Some of those books can hurt you, but their authors claim to be authorities, and so thousands of people buy what they write. Exercise books do nearly as well and can do nearly as much harm. Self-help psychology is often in the same category. We approach all these writings with our good sense overwhelmed by our eagerness to accept authority.

Let me recommend an alternative approach. Don't accept an authority's title or institutional affiliation or publication list as a sign of universal wisdom. Always doubt what an engineer tells you about the difference between mushrooms and toadstools or what a biologist tells you about auto repairs. Never mind that they teach at Oxford and are highly respected for the books and articles that they've written in their own specialty areas.

What's more, don't be very accepting of what authorities—or nonauthorities—say about their own fields. Be critical. Probe for facts.

Don't accept what's been printed as if publication were adequate proof of merit. The editor may have been ignorant or badly advised or may have thought that the article or book was worth publishing because it was controversial or harmless or attractive or supportive of her or his prejudices. Or maybe some space had to be filled and nothing else was available.

Don't fall victim to the disease of believing that a problem has been solved when it has only been named. An easy example comes from the family of authors, popular both with the public and with members of their profession, who instruct people on how to describe behavior patterns—not how to diagnose them or treat them—just how to describe them. One may tell you, for instance, how to recognize your "child," your "adult," and your "parent," all of which are supposed to name segments of your diverse and variable personality. Then you know enough to say such things as, "That was an argument between your child and my parent," as if the naming were equivalent to or better than clarifying the reasons for the argument, for the direction it took, and for the way it ended. Nonsense.

We are no better. We haggle over whether to name an entity *lipreading* or *speechreading*, whether to identify a process as *habilitation* or *rehabilitation*, whether we offer *treatment* or *remediation* (an especially ugly coinage), whether the adjective should be *audiological* or *audiologic*. When we reach a temporary conclusion to one of those discussions, we believe we have solved an important problem!

Although a description is longer, in this context it is not much better than a name. A description should not be accepted as a substitute for a diagnosis or a therapy, and it cannot replace data from a controlled scientific experiment.

Instead of all that describing and name calling, instead of fussing about the superficial aspects of our work, we ought to try to get on with performing it.

Look for ways to advance what we do. Remember what is critical to the growth of the profession. Question attempts to preserve the way things are done today. Preserve your skepticism. Preserve your doubting state of mind. And above all, look for the underlying causes of the phenomena you read and hear about, observe, and participate in. Then, when you can, test to see if the causes you found are real. And then test again and again.

INTEGRATION

Once upon a time,[6] 3,000 years ago in fact, the Chinese wore eyeglasses. Within a few hundred years, the Assyrians and Greeks (and later, the Romans) began using carved crystal lenses and curved bottles of water to start fires and to magnify things.

It took until the thirteenth century A.D. before anyone wrote about magnifying glasses. Two more centuries slipped by before scholars began to want telescopes and started doing serious research. Then, near the end of the sixteenth century, Zacharias Janssen misaligned a lens he'd been messing around with, and instead of the telescope that he'd been expecting, he got the first microscope. It was 6 feet long. This breakthrough intrigued other messers around (Galileo and Kepler, for example), who added attachments and variations such as focusing knobs and clearer glass.

In the early eighteenth century, Anton van Leeuwenhoek ran some systematic studies of microscope lenses. He did it because he wanted to see the little animals that live in water and in blood, and he was *able* to do it because lens grinding had just been invented. He could grind predetermined changes into the curvature of his lenses and create variations that were unavailable to the users of the older, molded lenses. So he varied the size and shape of the glass and measured how much bigger or smaller and how much better or worse the image got. Before he was through, he'd built himself at least a hundred microscopes.

For another 150 years, until 1873 and a little beyond, various research workers and instrument makers fiddled around with the components of the microscope and improved its power and clarity somewhat.

But in 1873, Ernst Abbe published his theoretical treatise on how lenses in microscopes modify images. From then on, an instrument maker could decide ahead of time what result was wanted and then select the glass and grind the lenses to create a microscope that would produce that result—quite the opposite of what had been the necessary approach previously.

The "what if" experiments of the first 2900 years of research on magnifiers led to vast improvements in microscopy and, as a result, to immeasurable increases in our knowledge of the world in which we live and in our ability to cope with that world. Yet, as Burgh (1974) put it, "If the theories discussed in Abbe's book had not been followed, today's microscopes would form very poor, inferior images." Abbe's attempt to find basic principles to describe the relations that had been charted and graphed for hundreds of years led him to a simple set of formulas that not only supplanted the trial-and-error results of van Leeuwenhoek and Galileo, but instantaneously made possible the manufacture of superior glass and the construction of superior optical systems that were capable of performing the old tasks with previously unimagined precision and ease and even of performing previously unimagined tasks.

When Abbe put aside the let-me-try-something-new-and-see-what-it-does method that had led all his predecessors to rapid but small advances in microscope design, he must have known that failure would be expensive. By spending his time in planning and in searching through the data for keys to the relations among observations, he gave up the chance to keep his potential failures small. A failure for van Leeuwenhoek meant only that he needed to grind another lens; failure for Abbe would have meant the loss of years spent in study.

But he didn't lose. In fact, he succeeded so well that people stopped working in that branch of optics until quite recently.

In rehabilitative audiology, we are not yet ready for an Abbe to come along. No one can devise a theory or write out predictive formulas or systematize the charts, tables, and graphs filled with data when the charts, tables, and graphs are nearly nonexistent. Most of us are beyond the thirteenth century (when Roger Bacon, the first writer on magnification, said everything that seemed to be important at the time: glasses were helpful for old folks who wanted to read). We know a bit about the physics of hearing aids and a modicum about pedagogy and a snippet about how to apply learning theory. But in general, we are still in the 1730s, starting to do the trial-and-error experiments, making

---

[6] The pertinence of the microscope metaphor was first noted by Békésy (1961). The history is based on Burgh (1974).

painfully small advances in teaching the hearing impaired to talk and to listen.

Workers in the field are, for one reason or another, seldom trying to add to the store of knowledge about what is effective and what isn't. Anecdotes are common; data are not.

Part of the problem stems from devotion to untested concepts. Manualists know people who have succeeded without oral training, and so, like Gall and Spurzheim with their reports of bumps on skulls, manualists conclude that manualism is the ideal solution for everyone. Oralists know people who have succeeded without manual training, and so they conclude that oralism is the ideal solution for everyone. Proponents of each of those extreme views, together with proponents of total communication, seem to prefer to accept on faith the reasonableness of writers and speakers who tell about cases that meet their expectations and to slough off equally sketchy reports from writers and speakers whose cases seem to support a different bias.

Similar sorts of fervor seize people who recommend only one sort of hearing-aid fitting (monaural, binaural, CROS, or whatever) or who follow one or another method for teaching lipreading. In nearly every instance, their choices result from reliance on unquantified and usually unquantifiable observations of selected cases or from acceptance of the recommendations of an authority who in turn relies on unquantified and unquantifiable observations of selected cases.

Please don't get me wrong: these people are usually not charlatans or frauds. They believe in the truth and the efficacy of what they say and do. Often, they help their clients and patients toward an improved state of mind and being. But think how much better they would do if, instead of depending on faith, tradition, authority, and orthodoxy, instead of recycling their current beliefs each time a new client arrived, they began to perform some controlled, single-subject experiments and then reported the results for others to see, to review, to criticize, and to try to replicate. Such research can advance knowledge while it helps today's patient, and it is certain to teach us how to help tomorrow's patient faster and more effectively.

The most valuable solutions to clinical problems in other disciplines have come about through integrated attacks: laboratory research, clinical research, and case observation have all played roles. Rarely, the same person (or the same team) has undertaken the whole spectrum of work. But differences in temperaments and talents often keep the laboratory worker out of the clinic and the clinical worker out of the laboratory.

In our field, finally, the two kinds of worker are beginning again to read each other's journals, to talk together about each other's problems, and generally to recognize that neither can advance very far without drawing on the knowledge, the work, and the talent of the other. In order to move out of the eighteenth century, we have to start producing first-rate clinical research, and that means an integration of laboratory techniques and approaches with clinical techniques and approaches so that, ultimately, we can put together a theoretical structure that can do for rehabilitative audiology what Abbe's theoretical structure did for microscopy.

References

BARLOW, D. H., and HAYES, S. C., Alternating treatments design: one strategy for comparing the effects of two treatments in a single subject. *J. Appl. Behav. Anal.*, **12**, 199–210 (1979).

BÉKÉSY, G. V., Are surgical experiments on human subjects necessary? *The Laryngoscope*, **71**, 367–376 (1961).

BEST, L. G., Research aspects of rehabilitative audiology. In J. G. Alpiner (Ed.), *Handbook of Adult Rehabilitative Audiology*. Baltimore: Williams & Wilkins (1978).

BRAIDA, L. D., DURLACH, N. I., LIPPMANN, R. P., HICKS, B. L., RABINOWITZ, W. M., and REED, C. M., Hearing aids—a review of past research on linear amplification, amplitude compression, and frequency lowering. In *ASHA Monographs*. Vol. 19. Rockville, MD: American Speech-Language-Hearing Association (1979).

BURGH, D. A., Microscope. In R. M. Besançon (Ed.), *The Encyclopedia of Physics*. 2nd Ed. New York: Van Nostrand Reinhold Company (1974).

COSTELLO, J. M., Clinicians and researchers: a necessary dichotomy? *J. Nat. Student Speech Hear. Assoc.*, **7**, 6–26 (1979).

CRONIN, B., The DAVID system: the development of an interactive video system at the National Technical Institute for the Deaf. *Am. Ann. Deaf*, **124**, 616–618 (1979).

ERBER, N. P., Auditory-visual perception of speech with reduced optical clarity. *J. Speech Hear. Res.*, **22**, 212–223 (1979).

ERBER, N. P., Speech-envelope cues as an acoustic aid to lipreading for profoundly deaf children. *J. Acoust. Soc. Am.*, **51**, 1224–1227 (1972).

GAULT, R. H., Interpretation of spoken language when the feel of speech supplements vision of the speaking face. *Volta Rev.*, **30**, 379–386 (1928).

GULIAN, E., Computer-based aids, motor control, and speech acquisition by the deaf. In J. V. Tobias and E.

D. Schubert (Eds.), *Hearing Research and Theory, Volume 1.* New York: Academic Press (1981).

HERSEN, M., and BARLOW, D. H., *Single Case Experimental Designs: Strategies for Studying Behavior Change.* New York: Pergamon Press (1976).

HUDGINS, C. V., Auditory training: its possibilities and limitations. *Volta Rev.,* **56,** 339–349 (1954).

NATIONAL INSTITUTE OF NEUROLOGICAL AND COMMUNICATIVE DISORDERS AND STROKE, *Report of the Panel on Communicative Disorders to the National Advisory Neurological and Communicative Disorders and Stroke Council, NIH Publication No. 81-1914.* Washington, D. C.: National Institutes of Health (1979).

SHOOP, C., and BINNIE, C. A., The effects of age upon the visual perception of speech. *Scand. Audiol.,* **8,** 3–8 (1979).

SIMS, D., VONFELDT, J., DOWALIBY, F., HUTCHINSON, K., and MYERS, T., A pilot experiment in computer assisted speechreading instruction utilizing the data analysis video interactive device (DAVID). *Am. Ann. Deaf,* **124,** 618–623 (1979).

SPARKS, D. W., ARDELL, L. A., BOURGEOIS, M., WIEDMER, B., and KUHL, P. K., Investigating the MESA (Multipoint Electrotactile Speech Aid): the transmission of connected discourse. *J. Acoust. Soc. Am.,* **65,** 810–815 (1979).

STEELE, J. A., BINNIE, C. A., and COOPER, W. A., Combining auditory and visual stimuli in the adaptive testing of speech discrimination. *J. Speech Hear. Disord.,* **43,** 115–122 (1978).

SUMBY, W. H., and POLLACK, I., Visual contribution to speech intelligibility in noise. *J. Acoust. Soc. Am.,* **26,** 212–215 (1954).

TOBIAS, J. V., and IRONS, F. M., Reception of distorted speech. In W. D. Ward (Ed.), *Proceedings of the International Congress on Noise as a Public Health Problem.* Washington: Environmental Protection Agency (1973).

WALDEN, B. E., ERDMAN, S. A., MONTGOMERY, A. A., SCHWARTZ, D. M., and PROSEK, R. A., Some effects of training on speech recognition by hearing impaired adults. *J. Speech Hear. Res.,* **24,** 207–216 (1981).

WALDEN, B. E., PROSEK, R. A., and WORTHINGTON, D. W., Predicting audiovisual consonant recognition performance of hearing-impaired adults. *J. Speech Hear. Res.,* **17,** 270–278 (1974).

Author Index

Subject Index